Nursing

Informatics
and the Foundation of Knowledge

The Pedagogy

Nursing Informatics and the Foundation of Knowledge, Second Edition drives comprehension through various strategies that meet the learning needs of students while generating enthusiasm about the topic. This interactive approach addresses different learning styles, making this the ideal text to ensure mastery of key concepts. The pedagogical aids that appear in most chapters include the following:

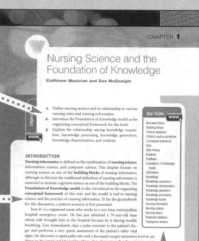

CHAPTER OBJECTIVES

These objectives provide instructors and students with a snapshot of the key information they will encounter in each chapter. They serve as a checklist to help guide and focus study.

CHAPTER INTRODUCTIONS

Found at the beginning of each chapter, chapter introductions provide an overview of the importance of the chapter's topic. They also help keep students focused as they read.

KEY TERMS

Found in a list at the beginning of each chapter and in bold within the chapter, these terms will create an expanded vocabulary in evidence-based practice. The 'www' icon directs you to the companion website **http://go.jblearning.com/mcgonigle** to see these terms in an interactive glossary and use flashcards and word puzzles to nail the definitions.

RESEARCH BRIEFS

Many chapters have research briefs presented in text boxes to encourage the reader to access current research. These briefs include important findings related to the topics in the book.

creasing safety concerns. Schools of nursing will embrace nursing science as they strive to meet the needs of changing student populations and the increasing complexity of healthcare environments.

SUMMARY

This chapter provides an overview of nursing science and how nursing science relates to typical nursing practice roles, nursing education, and nursing research. The Foundation of Knowledge model was introduced as the organizing conceptual framework for this book. Finally, the relationship of nursing science to nursing informatics was discussed. In subsequent chapters the reader will learn more about how nursing informatics supports nurses in their many and varied roles. In an ideal world nurses would embrace nursing science as knowledge users, knowledge managers, knowledge developers, knowledge engineers, and knowledge workers.

THOUGHT-PROVOKING Questions [www.]

1. Imagine you are in a social situation and someone asks you, "What does a nurse do?" Think about how you will capture and convey the richness that is nursing science in your answer.
2. Choose a clinical scenario from your recent experience and analyze it using the Foundation of Knowledge model. How did you acquire knowledge? How did you process knowledge? How did you generate knowledge? How did you disseminate knowledge? How did you use feedback, and what was the effect of the feedback on the foundation of your knowledge?

For a full suite of assignments and additional learning activities, use the access code located in the front of your book to visit this exclusive website: http://go.jblearning.com/mcgonigle. If you do not have an access code, you can obtain one at the site. [www.]

References

American Association of Colleges of Nursing. (2008, October 20). The Essentials of Baccalaureate Education for Professional Nursing Practice. Retrieved from American Association of Colleges of Nursing Web site: http://www.aacn.nche.edu/Education/pdf/ BaccEssentials08.pdf
American Nurses Association. (2003). Nursing's social policy statement (2nd ed.). Silver Spring, MD: Author.

CHAPTER SUMMARIES

Summaries are included at the end of each chapter to provide a concise review of material covered in each chapter. These summaries highlight the most important points in the chapter and describe what the future holds for each topic.

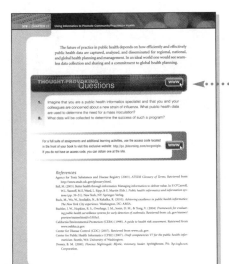

Case Study:
Early Detection of a Change in Condition [www.]

Mrs. C., an independent, 96-year-old woman, has a history of rehospitalization because of atrial fibrillation resulting from congestive heart failure (CHF) and hypertension.

After her most recent hospitalization, Mrs. C. was treated and released into home care at an agency in Washington. A home telemonitoring system that tracks and transmits patients' vital signs was placed in her home. The primary goal of placing this patient on the telemonitor was to provide daily monitoring of the patient's condition, thereby avoiding unnecessary rehospitalizations.

One morning, Mrs. C's telenurse detected an alarmingly low oxygen saturation level in the patient's transmitted data. As a result, the nurse telephoned Mrs. C. and asked her to retake her oxygen reading. The reading was confirmed and the telenurse contacted the patient's physician, who requested immediate transportation of the patient to the hospital emergency room. Medics were called and the patient was taken to the hospital, where she was diagnosed with a pulmonary embolism.

The prompt response resulted from early detection and timely intervention enabled by the home telehealth equipment and a home health nurse's oversight. One notable fact in this case is that although the primary goal of monitoring patients is to avoid unnecessary hospitalization, in this case the hospitalization was necessary for the patient as a result of her elevated blood pressure and compromised oxygen saturation levels. The patient was still asymptomatic at the time of detection. However, the telehealth intervention and subsequent hospitalization allowed for the embolism to be treated before any serious damage occurred.

Under the traditional home care model, this patient may only have been seen by a nurse two to three times a week. The clinician does not have knowledge of the patient's condition is between visits; however, having vital patient data tracked and transmitted daily allowed for rapid response that resulted in a positive outcome, perhaps a life-saving intervention for this patient.

DRIVING FORCES FOR TELEHEALTH

A significant increase is expected in the use of information technology tools in nursing venues in the coming decades. This use is affected by a number of factors in all of western society. The following factors are drivers of the growing trend toward telehealth and technology use and will influence nursing practice significantly in the next decades: demographic nursing and healthcare worker shortages; chronic diseases and conditions; the new, educated consumers; and excessive costs of healthcare services that are increasing in need and kind.

CASE STUDIES

Case studies encourage active learning and promote critical thinking skills in learners. Students can ask questions, analyze the situation they are presented with, and solve problems so they can learn how the information in the text applies to everyday practice online at **http://go.jblearning.com/mcgonigle**.

The future of practice in public health depends on how efficiently and effectively public health data are captured, analyzed, and disseminated for regional, national, and global health planning and management. In an ideal world one would see seamless data collection and sharing and a commitment to global health planning.

THOUGHT-PROVOKING Questions [www.]

1. Imagine that you are a public health informatics specialist and that you and your colleagues are concerned about a new strain of influenza. What public health data are used to determine the need for a mass inoculation?
2. What data will be collected to determine the success of such a program?

For a full suite of assignments and additional learning activities, use the access code located in the front of your book to visit this exclusive website: http://go.jblearning.com/mcgonigle. If you do not have an access code, you can obtain one at the site. [www.]

References

Agency for Toxic Substances and Disease Registry (2003). ATSDR Glossary of Terms. Retrieved from http://www.atsdr.cdc.gov/glossary.html.
Ball, M. (2003). Better health through informatics: Managing information to deliver value. In P. O'Carroll, W.J., Yasnoff, M.E. Ward, L. Ripp, & F. Martin (Eds.), Public health informatics and information systems (pp. 39–51). New York, NY: Springer-Verlag.
Buck, M., Wu, W., Soulakis, N., & Kukafka, R. (2010). Achieving excellence in public health informatics: The New York City experience. Washington, DC: AMIA.
Buehler, J. W., Hopkins, R. S., Overhage, J. M., Sosin, D. M., & Tong, V. (2004) Framework for evaluating public health surveillance systems for early detection of outbreaks. Retrieved from cdc. gov/mmwr/preview/mmwrhtml/rr5305a1.
California Environmental Protection (CEPA) (1998). A guide to health risk assessment. Retrieved from www.oehha.ca.gov.
Center for Disease Control (CDC) (2007). Retrieved from www.cdc.gov.
Center for Public Health Informatics (CPHI) (2007). Draft competencies V7 for the public health informatician. Seattle, WA: University of Washington.
Dossey, B. M. (2000). Florence Nightingale: Mystic, visionary, healer. Springhouse, PA: Springhouse Corporation.

THOUGHT-PROVOKING QUESTIONS

Each chapter includes specific questions students should be able to answer after reading through the chapter. The objectives are conveniently listed in a question format so that students can respond and email answers directly to their instructor. The 'www' icon directs you to the companion website **http://go.jblearning.com/mcgonigle** to answer each question and email your response to your instructor.

Nursing Informatics

SECOND EDITION

and the Foundation of Knowledge

Dee McGonigle, PhD, RN, FACCE, FAAN

Professor, Online-MSN Program
Chamberlain College of Nursing
Editor-in-Chief, *Online Journal of Nursing Informatics*
Member, Informatics and Technology Expert Panel (ITEP)
American Academy of Nursing

Kathleen Mastrian, PhD, RN

Associate Professor and Program Coordinator for Nursing
Pennsylvania State University, Shenango
Sr. Managing Editor, *Online Journal of Nursing Informatics*

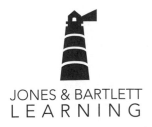

JONES & BARTLETT
LEARNING

World Headquarters
Jones & Bartlett Learning
5 Wall Street
Burlington, MA 01803
978-443-5000
info@jblearning.com
www.jblearning.com

Jones & Bartlett Learning books and products are available through most bookstores and online booksellers. To contact Jones & Bartlett Learning directly, call 800-832-0034, fax 978-443-8000, or visit our website, www.jblearning.com.

Substantial discounts on bulk quantities of Jones & Bartlett Learning publications are available to corporations, professional associations, and other qualified organizations. For details and specific discount information, contact the special sales department at Jones & Bartlett Learning via the above contact information or send an email to specialsales@jblearning.com.

Production Credits
Publisher: Kevin Sullivan
Acquisitions Editor: Amanda Harvey
Editorial Assistant: Rachel Shuster
Editorial Assistant: Sara Bempkins
Associate Production Editor: Cindie Bryan
Marketing Manager: Elena McAnespie
Associate Marketing Manager: Katie Hennessy
V.P., Manufacturing and Inventory Control: Therese Connell
Composition: Auburn Associates, Inc.
Cover Design: Scott Moden
Cover Image: © Leigh Prather/ShutterStock, Inc.
Printing and Binding: Malloy, Inc.
Cover Printing: Malloy, Inc.

To order this product, use ISBN: 978-1-4496-3174-1

Library of Congress Cataloging-in-Publication Data
Nursing informatics and the foundation of knowledge / [edited by] Dee McGonigle, Kathleen Mastrian.—2nd ed.
    p. ; cm.
  Includes bibliographical references and index.
  ISBN-13: 978-0-7637-9236-7 (pbk.)
  ISBN-10: 0-7637-9236-5 (pbk.)
  1. Nursing informatics. I. McGonigle, Dee. II. Mastrian, Kathleen Garver.
  [DNLM: 1. Nursing Informatics. 2. Knowledge. WY 26.5]
  RT50.5.N8693 2012
  651.5′04261—dc22

                                                                        2011000687
6048
Printed in the United States of America
16 15 14 13   10 9 8 7

Contents

Preface

The idea for this book originated with the development of nursing informatics (NI) classes, the publication of articles related to technology-based education, and the creation of the *Online Journal of Nursing Informatics (OJNI)*, which Dee McGonigle co-founded. Like most nurse informaticists, we fell into the specialty; our love affair with technology and gadgets and our willingness to be the first to try new things helped to hook us into the specialty of informatics. The rapid evolution of technology and its transformation of the ways of nursing prompted us to try to capture the essence of NI in a text.

We realized as we were developing the first edition, that we could not possibly know all there is to know about informatics and how it supports nursing practice, education, administration, and research. We also knew that our faculty roles constrained the opportunities for exposure to changes in this rapidly evolving field. Therefore, we developed a tentative outline and a working model of the theoretical framework for the book and invited participation from informatics experts and specialists around the world. We were pleased with the enthusiastic responses we received from some of those invited contributors and a few volunteers who heard about the book and asked to participate in their particular area of expertise. In this second edition, we invited the original contributors to revise and update their chapters. Not everyone chose to participate in the second edition, so we revised several of the chapters using the original work as a springboard. The revisions to the text were guided by the contributors' growing informatics expertise and the reviews provided by text-book adopters. In the revisions, we sought to do the following:

- Expand the audience focus to include nursing students from BS through DNP and nurses thrust into informatics roles in clinical agencies.
- Include, whenever possible, an attention-grabbing case scenario as an introduction or an illustrative case scenario demonstrating why the topic is important.
- Include important research findings related to the topic. Many chapters have *research briefs* presented in text boxes to encourage the reader to access current research.
- Focus on cutting edge innovations, meaningful use, and patient safety as appropriate to each topic.
- Include a paragraph describing what the future holds for each topic.

New chapters that were added to the book include technology and patient safety, system development life cycle, workflow analysis, gaming, simulation, and bioinformatics.

We believe that this book provides a comprehensive elucidation of this exciting field. The reader may notice that occasionally the contributing authors present similar information about a topic. We did not edit those similarities in every case, because we believe that it is important to preserve the perspectives of our expert contributors, and similar presentations of materials help to emphasize the importance of a particular topic.

The theoretical underpinning of the book is the Foundation of Knowledge model. The model is introduced in its entirety in Chapter 1, which discusses nursing science and its relationship to NI. We believe that humans are organic information systems constantly acquiring, processing, and generating information or knowledge both in professional and personal lives. It is a high degree of knowledge that characterizes humans as extremely intelligent, organic machines. Individuals have the ability to manage knowledge. This ability is learned and honed from birth. We make our way through life interacting with our environment and being inundated with information and knowledge. We experience our environment and learn by acquiring, processing, generating, and disseminating knowledge. As we interact in our environment, we acquire knowledge that we must process. This processing effort causes us to redefine and restructure our knowledge base and generate new knowledge. We then share (disseminate) this new knowledge and receive feedback from others. The dissemination and feedback initiates this cycle of knowledge over again because we acquire, process, generate, and disseminate the knowledge gained from sharing and reexploring our own knowledge base. As others respond to our knowledge dissemination and we acquire new knowledge, we engage in rethinking and reflecting on our knowledge, processing, generating, and then disseminating anew.

The purpose of this book is to provide a set of practical and powerful tools to ensure that the reader gains an understanding of NI and moves from information through knowledge to wisdom. Defining the demands of nurses and providing tools to help them survive and succeed in the Knowledge Era remains a major challenge. Exposing nursing students and nurses to the principles and tools used in NI helps to prepare them to meet the challenge of practicing nursing in the Knowledge Era while striving to improve patient care at all levels.

The text provides a comprehensive framework that embraces knowledge so that readers can develop their knowledge repositories and the wisdom necessary to act on and apply that knowledge. The book is divided into six sections. Section I covers the building blocks of NI: nursing science, information science, computer science, cognitive science, and the ethical management of information. Section II provides readers with a look at various perspectives on NI and NI practice as described by experts in the field. Section III covers the precare and care support functions of administrative applications of NI. Healthcare delivery applications including electronic health records (EHRs), clinical information systems, telehealth, patient safety, patient and community education, and care management are covered in Section IV. Section V presents subject matter on how informatics supports nursing education and nursing research. An introduction to bioinformatics, the future of NI, and a summary of the relationship of informatics to the Foundation of Knowledge model are presented in Section VI. The introduction to each section explains the relationship between the content of that section and the Foundation of Knowledge model. This book places the material within the context of knowledge acquisition, processing, generation, and dissemination. It serves both nursing students (BS to DNP/PhD) and professionals who need to understand, use, and evaluate NI knowledge. As nursing professors, our major responsibility is to prepare the practitioners and leaders in the field. Because NI permeates the entire scope of nursing (practice, administration, education, and research), nursing education curricula must include NI. Our primary objective is to develop the most comprehensive and user-friendly NI text on the market to prepare nurses for current and future practice challenges. In particular, this book provides a solid groundwork from which to integrate NI into practice, education, administration, and research.

Goals of this book are to

1. Impart core NI principles that should be familiar to every nurse and nursing student
2. Help the reader understand knowledge and how it is acquired, processed, generated, and disseminated
3. Explore the changing role of NI professionals
4. Demonstrate the value of the NI discipline as an attractive field of specialization

These goals help nurses and nursing students understand and use fundamental NI principles so that they efficiently and effectively function as current and future nursing professionals. The overall vision, framework, and pedagogy of this book offer benefits to readers by highlighting established principles while drawing out new ones that continue to emerge as nursing and technology evolve.

Acknowledgments

We are deeply grateful to the contributors who provided this text with a richness and diversity of content that we could not alone have captured. We especially wish to acknowledge the superior work of Alicia Mastrian, graphic designer of the Foundation of Knowledge model, which serves as the theoretical framework on which this text is anchored. We could never have completed this project without the dedicated and patient efforts of the Jones & Bartlett Learning staff, especially Kevin Sullivan and Cindie Bryan. Both fielded our questions and concerns in a very professional and respectful manner.

Dee acknowledges the undying love, support, patience, and continued encouragement of her best friend and husband, Craig, and her son, Craig, who has also made her so very proud. She sincerely thanks her cousins Judi, Camille, Glenn, Mary Jane, and Sonny, and her dear friends for their support and encouragement, especially Renee.

Kathy acknowledges the loving support of her family: husband Chip; children Ben and Alicia; sisters Carol and Sue; and parents Bob and Rosalie Garver. Kathy also acknowledges those friends who understand the importance of validation, especially Katie, Bobbie, Kathy, Anne, and Catherine.

Authors' Note

This text provides an overview of nursing informatics from the perspective of diverse experts in the field, with a focus on nursing informatics and the Foundation of Knowledge model. We want our readers and students to focus on the relationship of knowledge to informatics, a message all too often lost in the romance with technology. We hope you enjoy the text!

Contributors

Ida Androwich, PhD, RN, BC, FAAN
Loyola University Chicago
School of Nursing
Maywood, IL

Emily Barey, MSN, RN
Director of Nursing Informatics
Epic Systems Corporation
Madison, WI

Lisa Reeves Bertin, BS, EMBA
Pennsylvania State University
Sharon, PA

Brett Bixler, PhD
Pennsylvania State University
University Park, PA

Jennifer Bredemeyer, RN
Loyola University Chicago
School of Nursing
Skokie, IL

Sylvia M. DeSantis, MA
Pennsylvania State University
University Park, PA

Eric R. Doerfler, PhD, NP
Pennsylvania State University
School of Nursing
Middletown, PA

Judith Effken, PhD, RN, FACMI
University of Arizona
College of Nursing
Tucson, AZ

William Scott Erdley, DNS, RN
Niagara University
Niagara University, NY

Nedra Farcus, MSN, RN
Pennsylvania State University–Altoona
Altoona, PA

Kathleen M. Gialanella, JD, RN, LLM
Law Offices
Westfield, NJ
Associate Adjunct Professor
Teachers College, Columbia University
New York, NY
Adjunct Professor
Seton Hall University, College of Nursing & School of Law
South Orange & Newark, NJ

Denise Hammel-Jones, MSN, RN-BC, CLSSBB
Greencastle Associates Consulting
Malvern, PA

Nicholas Hardiker, PhD, RN
Senior Research Fellow
University of Salford
School of Nursing & Midwifery
Salford, UK

Glenn Johnson, MLS
Pennsylvania State University
University Park, PA

June Kaminski, MSN, RN
Kwantlen University College
Surrey, British Columbia, Canada

Julie Kenney, MSN, RNC-OB
Clinical Analyst Advocate Health Care
Oak Brook, IL

Margaret Ross Kraft, PhD, RN
Loyola University Chicago
School of Nursing
Maywood, IL

Wendy L. Mahan, PhD, CRC, LPC
Pennsylvania State University
University Park, PA

Heather McKinney, PhD
Pennsylvania State University
University Park, PA

Nickolaus Miehl, MSN, RN
Pennsylvania State University
Erie, PA

Peter J. Murray, PhD, RN, FBCS
Coachman's Cottage
Nocton, Lincoln, UK

Lynn M. Nagle, PhD, RN
Assistant Professor
University of Toronto
Toronto, Ontario, Canada

Ramona Nelson, PhD, RN-BC, FAAN, ANEF
Professor Emerita, Slippery Rock University
President, Ramona Nelson Consulting
Pittsburgh, PA

Nancy Staggers, PhD, RN, FAAN
Professor, Informatics
University of Maryland
Baltimore, MD

Jeff Swain
Instructional Designer
Pennsylvania State University
University Park, PA

Denise D. Tyler, MSN/MBA, RN-BC
Implementation Specialist
Healthcare Provider, Consulting
ACS, a Xerox Company
Dearborn, MI

The Editors also acknowledge the work of the following first edition contributors
(original contributions edited by McGonigle and Mastrian for second edition):

Kathleen Albright, BA, RN
Strategic Account Manager at GE Healthcare
Philadelphia, PA

Schuyler F. Hoss, BA
Northwest Healthcare Management
Vancouver, WA

Audrey Kinsella, MA, MS
Information for Tomorrow
Telehealth Planning Services
Asheville, NC

Susan M. Paschke, MSN, RN
The Cleveland Clinic
Cleveland, OH

Sheldon Prial, RPH, BS Pharmacy
Sheldon Prial Consultance
Melbourne, FL

Jackie Ritzko
Pennsylvania State University
Hazelton, PA

Marianela Zytkowsi, MSN, RN
The Cleveland Clinic
Cleveland, OH

Building Blocks of Nursing Informatics

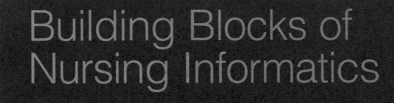

Nursing professionals are information-dependent knowledge workers. As health care continues to evolve in an increasingly competitive information marketplace, professionals, the knowledge workers, must be well prepared to make significant contributions by harnessing appropriate and timely information. Nursing informatics (NI), a product of the scientific synthesis of information in nursing, uses concepts from computer science, cognitive science, information science, and nursing science. NI continues to evolve as more and more professionals access, use, and develop the information, computer, and cognitive sciences necessary to advance nursing science for the betterment of patients and the profession. Regardless of future roles, it is clear that nurses need to understand the ethical application of computer, information, and cognitive sciences to advance nursing science.

To implement NI one must view it from the perspective of the current healthcare delivery system and specific, individual organizational needs, while anticipating and creating future applications in both the healthcare system and the nursing profession. Nursing professionals should be expected to discover opportunities to use NI; participate in the design of solutions; and be challenged to identify, develop, evaluate, modify, and enhance applications to improve patient care. This book is designed to provide the reader with the information and knowledge needed to meet this expectation.

Section I presents an overview of the building blocks of NI: nursing, information, computer, and cognitive sciences. Also included in this section is a chapter on ethical applications of healthcare informatics. This section lays the foundation for the remainder of the book.

Chapter 1 describes nursing science and introduces the Foundation of Knowledge model as the conceptual framework for the book. In this chapter, a clinical case scenario is used to illustrate the concepts central to nursing science. A definition of nursing science is also derived from the American Nurses Association definition of nursing. Nursing science is the ethical application of knowledge acquired through education, research, and practice to provide services and interventions to patients to maintain, enhance, or restore their health, and to acquire, process, generate, and disseminate nursing knowledge to advance the nursing profession. Information is a central concept and health care's most valuable resource. Information science and systems, together with computers, are constantly changing the way healthcare organizations conduct their business. This will continue to evolve.

To prepare for these innovations, the reader must understand fundamental information and computer concepts, covered in Chapters 2 and 3, respectively. Information science deals with the interchange (or flow) and scaffolding (or structure) of information and involves the application of information tools for solutions to patient care and business problems in health care. To be able to use and synthesize information effectively, one must be able to obtain, perceive, process, synthesize, comprehend, convey, and manage the information. Computer science deals with understanding the development, design, structure, and relationship of computer hardware and software. This science offers extremely valuable tools that, if used skillfully, can facilitate the acquisition and manipulation of data and information by nurses, who can then synthesize these into an ever-evolving knowledge and wisdom base. This not only facilitates professional development and the ability to apply evidence-based practice decisions within nursing care, but if disseminated and shared, can advance the profession's knowledge base. The development of knowledge tools, such as the automation of decision making and strides in artificial intelligence, has altered the understanding of knowledge and its representation. The ability to structure knowledge electronically facilitates the ability to share knowledge structures and enhance collective knowledge.

As discussed in Chapter 4, cognitive science deals with how the human mind functions. This science encompasses how people think, understand, remember, synthesize, and access stored information and knowledge. The nature of knowledge, how it is developed, used, modified, and shared, provides the basis for continued learning and intellectual growth.

Chapter 5 focuses on ethical issues associated with managing private information with technology and provides a framework for analyzing ethical issues and supporting ethical decision making.

The material within this book is placed within the context of the Foundation of Knowledge model (shown in Figure I-1 and periodically throughout the book, but more fully introduced and explained in Chapter 1). The Foundation of Knowledge model is used throughout the text to illustrate how knowledge is used to meet the needs of healthcare delivery systems, organizations, patients, and nurses. It is through interaction with these building blocks—the theories, architecture, and tools—that one acquires the bits and pieces of data necessary, processes these into information, and generates and disseminates the resulting knowledge. Through this dynamic exchange that includes feedback, one continues the interaction and use of these sciences to input or acquire, process, and output or disseminate generated knowledge. Humans experience their environment and learn by acquiring, processing, generating, and disseminating knowledge. When one then shares (disseminates) this new knowledge and receives feedback on the knowledge they have shared, the feedback initiates the cycle of knowledge all over again. As one acquires, processes, generates, and disseminates the knowledge, they are motivated to share, rethink, and explore their own knowledge base.

FIGURE

I-1   Foundation of Knowledge model.

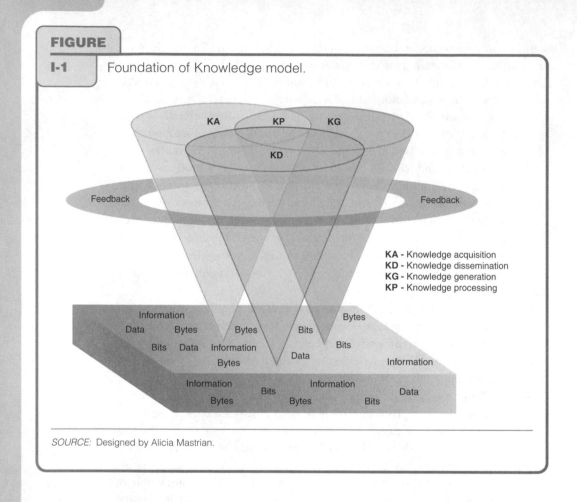

KA   KP   KG

KD

Feedback   Feedback

KA - Knowledge acquisition
KD - Knowledge dissemination
KG - Knowledge generation
KP - Knowledge processing

Information   Bytes
Data   Bytes   Bytes   Bits
Bits   Data   Information   Bits
Bytes   Data   Information
Information   Information   Data
Bytes   Bits   Bytes   Bits

SOURCE: Designed by Alicia Mastrian.

This complex process is captured in the Foundation of Knowledge model. Reading the chapters in Section I, the reader is challenged to think about how the model can help them to understand the ways in which one acquires, processes, generates, disseminates, and then receives feedback on their new knowledge of the building blocks of NI.

CHAPTER 1

Nursing Science and the Foundation of Knowledge

Kathleen Mastrian and Dee McGonigle

1. Define nursing science and its relationship to various nursing roles and nursing informatics.
2. Introduce the Foundation of Knowledge model as the organizing conceptual framework for the book.
3. Explain the relationship among knowledge acquisition, knowledge processing, knowledge generation, knowledge dissemination, and wisdom.

WWW

Key Terms **WWW**

Borrowed theory
Building blocks
Clinical databases
Clinical practice guidelines
Conceptual framework
Data
Data mining
Evidence
Feedback
Foundation of Knowledge
  model
Information
Knowledge
Knowledge acquisition
Knowledge dissemination
Knowledge generation
Knowledge processing
Knowledge worker
Nursing informatics
Nursing science
Nursing theory
Relational database
Transparent wisdom

INTRODUCTION

Nursing informatics is defined as the combination of **nursing science**, information science, and computer science. This chapter focuses on nursing science as one of the **building blocks** of nursing informatics, although in this text the traditional definition of nursing informatics is extended to include cognitive science as one of the building blocks. The **Foundation of Knowledge model** is also introduced as the organizing **conceptual framework** of this text, and the model is tied to nursing science and the practice of nursing informatics. To lay the groundwork for this discussion, a patient scenario is first presented.

Tom H. is a registered nurse who works in a very busy metropolitan hospital emergency room. He has just admitted a 79-year-old man whose wife brought him to the hospital because he is having trouble breathing. Tom immediately clips a pulse oximeter to the patient's finger and performs a very quick assessment of the patient's other vital signs. He discovers a rapid pulse rate and a decreased oxygen saturation level in addition to the rapid and labored breathing. Tom determines that the patient is not in immediate danger and that he does not require intubation. Tom focuses his initial attention on easing the patient's labored breathing by elevating the head of the bed and initiating oxygen treatment; he then hooks the patient up to a heart monitor.

Tom continues to assess the breathing status as he performs a head-to-toe assessment of the patient that leads to the nursing diagnoses and additional interventions necessary to provide comprehensive care to this patient.

Consider Tom's actions and how and why he intervened as he did. Tom relied on the immediate **data** and information that he acquired during his initial rapid assessment to deliver appropriate care to his patient. Tom also used technology (pulse oximeter and heart monitor) to assist with and support the delivery of care. What is not immediately apparent, and some would argue is transparent (done without conscious thought), is the fact that during the rapid assessment, Tom reached into his **knowledge** base of previous learning and experiences to direct his care, so that he could act with **transparent wisdom**. He used both **nursing theory** and **borrowed theory** to inform his practice. Tom certainly used nursing process theory, and he may have also used one of several other nursing theories, such as Rogers's science of unitary human beings, Orem's theory of self-care deficit, or Roy's adaptation theory. In addition, Tom may also have applied his knowledge from some of the basic sciences, such as anatomy, physiology, psychology, and chemistry, as he determined the patient's immediate needs. Information from Maslow's hierarchy of needs, Lazarus's transaction model of stress and coping, and the health belief model may also have helped Tom practice professional nursing. He gathered data, then analyzed and interpreted that data to form a conclusion—the essence of science. Tom has illustrated the practical aspects of nursing science.

The American Nurses Association (2003) defines nursing in this way: "Nursing is the protection, promotion, and optimization of health and abilities, prevention of illness and injury, alleviation of suffering through the diagnosis and treatment of human response, and advocacy in the care of individuals, families, communities, and populations" (p. 6). Thus, the focus of nursing is on human responses to actual or potential health problems and advocacy for various clients. These human responses are varied and may change over time in a single case. Nurses must possess the technical skills to manage equipment and perform procedures; the interpersonal skills to interact appropriately with people; and the cognitive skills to observe, recognize, and collect data, analyze and interpret data, and reach a reasonable conclusion that forms the basis of a decision. At the heart of all of these skills lies the management of data and information. This is a definition of nursing science as the ethical application of knowledge acquired through education, research, and practice to provide services and interventions to patients to maintain, enhance, or restore their health and to acquire, process, generate, and disseminate nursing knowledge to advance the nursing profession.

Nursing is an information-intensive profession. The steps of using information, applying knowledge to a problem, and acting with wisdom form the basis of nursing practice science. **Information** is data that are processed using knowledge.

For information to be valuable, it must be accessible, accurate, timely, complete, cost effective, flexible, reliable, relevant, simple, verifiable, and secure. Knowledge is the awareness and understanding of a set of information and ways that information can be made useful to support a specific task or arrive at a decision. In the case example, Tom used accessible, accurate, timely, relevant, and verifiable data and information. He compared that data and information to his knowledge base and previous experiences to determine which data and information were relevant to the current case. By applying previous knowledge to data, he converted data into information and information into new knowledge, an understanding of what nursing interventions were appropriate in this case. Thus, information is data made functional through the application of knowledge.

Humans acquire data and information in bits and pieces and then transform the information into knowledge. The information-processing functions of the brain are frequently compared to those of a computer and vice versa (discussed further in Chapter 4). Humans can be thought of as organic information systems constantly acquiring, processing, and generating information or knowledge in their professional and personal lives. Individuals have an amazing ability to manage knowledge. This ability is learned and honed from birth as one makes their way through life interacting with the environment and being inundated with data and information. One experiences the environment and learns by acquiring, processing, generating, and disseminating knowledge. Tom acquired knowledge in his basic nursing education program and continues to build his foundation of knowledge by such activities as reading nursing research and theory articles, attending continuing education programs, consulting with expert colleagues, and using **clinical databases** and **clinical practice guidelines**. As he interacts in the environment, he acquires knowledge that must be processed. This processing effort causes him to redefine and restructure his knowledge base and generate new knowledge. He can then share (disseminate) this new knowledge with other colleagues, and he may receive **feedback** on the knowledge that he shares. This dissemination and feedback builds the knowledge foundation anew as he acquires, processes, generates, and disseminates new knowledge as a result of his interactions. As others respond to his **knowledge dissemination** and he acquires yet more knowledge, he is engaged to rethink, reflect on, and re-explore his **knowledge acquisition**, thus processing, generating, and then disseminating anew. This process is captured in the Foundation of Knowledge model, used as an organizing framework for this text.

At its base, the model has bits, bytes (computer terms for chunks of information), data, and information in a random representation. Growing out of the base are separate cones of light that expand as they reflect upward and represent knowledge acquisition, **knowledge generation**, and knowledge dissemination. At the intersection of the cones and forming a new cone is **knowledge processing**. Encircling and cutting through the knowledge cones is feedback that acts on and may transform any or all aspects of knowledge represented by the cones. One should imagine the model as a dynamic figure with the cones of light and the feedback rotating and interacting rather than remaining static. Knowledge acquisition, knowledge generation, knowledge dissemination, knowledge processing, and feedback are constantly evolving for nurse scientists. The transparent effect of the cones is deliberate and is intended to suggest that as knowledge grows and expands its use becomes more transparent—one uses it during practice without even being consciously aware of what aspect of knowledge is being used at any given moment.

FIGURE 1-1   Foundation of Knowledge model.

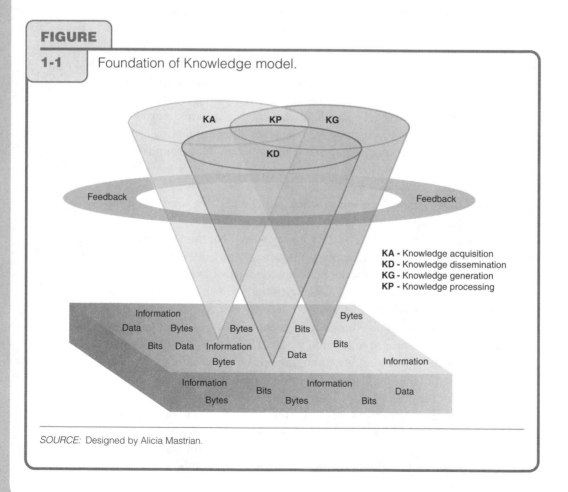

SOURCE: Designed by Alicia Mastrian.

An experienced nurse, thinking back to the novice years, may recall feeling like their head was filled with bits of data and information that did not form any type of cohesive whole. As the model depicts, the processing of knowledge begins a bit later (imagine a time line applied vertically) with early experiences on the bottom and expertise growing as the processing of knowledge ensues. Early on in a nurse's education conscious attention is focused mainly on knowledge acquisition, and they depend on their instructors and others to process, generate, and disseminate knowledge. As the nurse becomes more comfortable with the science of nursing, they begin to take over some of the other Foundation of Knowledge functions. However, to keep up with the explosion of information in nursing and health care, one must continue to rely on the knowledge generation of nursing theorists and researchers and the dissemination of their work. In this sense, nurses are committed to lifelong learning and the use of knowledge in the practice of nursing science.

This book uses the Foundation of Knowledge model, reflecting that knowledge is a powerful tool and that nurses focus on information as a key building block of knowledge. The application of the model is described in each section of the book to help the reader understand and appreciate the foundation of knowledge in nursing science and how it applies to nursing informatics. All of the various nursing roles (practice, administration, education, research, and informatics) involve the science of nursing. Nurses are **knowledge workers**, working with information and generating information and knowledge as a product. They are knowledge acquirers, providing convenient and efficient means of capturing and storing knowledge. They are knowledge users, individuals or groups who benefit from valuable, viable knowledge. Nurses are knowledge engineers, designing, developing, implementing, and maintaining knowledge. They are knowledge managers, capturing and processing collective expertise and distributing it where it can create the largest benefit. They are knowledge developers or generators, changing and evolving knowledge based on the tasks at hand and information available.

In the case scenario, at first glance one might label Tom as a knowledge worker, a knowledge acquirer, and a knowledge user. However, stopping here might sell Tom short in his practice of nursing science. Although he acquired and used knowledge to help him achieve his work, he also processed the data and information he collected to develop a nursing diagnosis and a plan of care. The knowledge stores Tom used to develop and glean knowledge from valuable information are generative (having the ability to originate and produce or generate) in nature. For example, Tom may have learned something new about his patient's culture from the patient or his wife that he will file away in the knowledge repository of his mind to be used in another similar situation. As he compares this new cultural information to what he already knows, he may gain insight into the effect of culture on a patient's response to illness. Thus, Tom is a knowledge generator. If he shares this newly acquired knowledge with another practitioner, and as he records his observations and his conclusions, he is then disseminating knowledge. Tom is also using feedback from the various technologies he has used to monitor his patient's status. He may also use feedback from laboratory reports or even other practitioners to help him rethink, revise, and apply the knowledge about this patient that he is generating.

Knowledge must also be viable. Knowledge viability refers to applications (most technology based) that offer easily accessible, accurate, and timely information obtained from a variety of resources and methods and presented in a manner so as to provide the necessary elements to generate new knowledge. In the case scenario, Tom may have felt the need to consult an electronic database or a clinical guidelines repository that he has downloaded on his PDA or that reside in the emergency room's networked computer system to assist him in the development of a comprehensive care plan for his patient. In this way, Tom is also using technology and **evidence** to support and inform his practice. It is also possible in this scenario that an alert may appear in the electronic health record or the clinical information system (CIS) reminding Tom to ask about influenza and pneumonia vaccines. Clinical information technologies that support and inform nursing practice and nursing administration are an important part of nursing informatics and are covered in detail in Sections III and IV of this text. Technologies that support and inform nursing education and nursing research are covered in Section V.

This book provides a framework that embraces knowledge so that the reader can develop the wisdom necessary to apply what they have learned. Wisdom is the application of knowledge to an appropriate situation. In the practice of nursing science, one expects actions directed by wisdom. Wisdom uses knowledge and experience to heighten common sense and insight to exercise sound judgment in practical matters. It is developed through knowledge, experience, insight, and reflection. Wisdom is sometimes thought of as the highest form of common sense resulting from accumulated knowledge or erudition (deep, thorough learning) or enlightenment (education that results in understanding and the dissemination of knowledge). Wisdom is the ability to apply valuable and viable knowledge, experience, understanding, and insight while being prudent and sensible. Knowledge and wisdom are not synonymous because knowledge abounds with others' thoughts and information, whereas wisdom is focused on one's own mind and the synthesis of experience, insight, understanding, and knowledge. Wisdom has been called the foundation of the art of nursing.

Some nursing roles might be viewed as more focused on some rather than other aspects of the foundation of knowledge. One might argue that nurse educators are primarily knowledge disseminators and nurse researchers are knowledge generators. Although the more frequent output of their efforts can certainly be viewed in this way, it is important to realize that nurses use all of the aspects of the Foundation of Knowledge model regardless of their area of practice. For nurse educators to be effective, they must be in the habit of constantly building and rebuilding their foundation of knowledge about nursing science. In addition, as they develop and implement curricular innovations, they must also evaluate the effectiveness of those changes. In some cases, they use formal research techniques to achieve this and are therefore generating knowledge about the best and most effective teaching strategies. Similarly, nurse researchers must acquire and process new knowledge as they design and conduct their research studies. All nurses have the opportunity to be involved in the formal dissemination of knowledge via their participation in professional conferences, either as presenters or attendees. In addition, some nurses disseminate knowledge by formal publication of their ideas. In the cases of conference presentation and publication, nurses may receive feedback that stimulates rethinking about the knowledge they have generated and disseminated, thus prompting them to acquire and process anew.

All nurses, regardless of the practice arena, must use informatics and technology to inform and support that practice. The case scenario discussed Tom's use of various monitoring devices that provide feedback on the physiologic status of the patient. It was also suggested that Tom might consult a clinical database or nursing practice guidelines residing on a PDA or a clinical agency network as he develops an appropriate plan of action for his nursing interventions. Perhaps the CIS in the agency supports the collection of data about patients in a **relational database**, providing an opportunity for **data mining** by nursing administrators or nurse researchers. Thus, administrators and researchers can glean information about best practices and what improvements are necessary to deliver the best and most effective nursing care (Swan, Lang, & McGinley, 2004).

The future of nursing science and nursing informatics is closely associated with nursing education and nursing research. Skiba (2007) suggests that techno-savvy and well-informed faculty are needed who can demonstrate the appropriate use of technologies to enhance the delivery of nursing care. Along those lines, Greenfield (2007) conducted research among nursing students to determine the effectiveness of PDA technology applied to medication administration. Her study makes a good case for incorporating PDA technology into nursing curricula. Girard (2007) discussed cutting-edge operating room technologies, such as nanosurgery using nanorobots, smart fabrics that aid in patient assessment during surgery, biopharmacy techniques for the safe and effective delivery of anesthesia, and virtual reality training. She makes an extremely provocative point about nursing education: "Educators will need to expand their knowledge and teach for the future and not the past. They must take heed that the old tried-and true nursing education methods and curriculum that has lasted 100 years will have to change, and that change will be mandated for all areas of nursing ..." (p. 353).

Bassendowski (2007) specifically addresses the potential for the generation of knowledge in educational endeavors as faculty apply new technologies to teaching and the focus shifts away from individual to group instruction that promotes sharing and processing of knowledge.

Several key national groups are promoting the inclusion of informatics content in nursing education programs. These initiatives include the National League for Nursing (NLN, 2008), the Quality and Safety Education for Nurses (Cronenwett et al., 2007) report, the Technology Informatics Guiding Education Reform (TIGER) Initiative (2007), and the American Association of Colleges of Nursing (AACN, 2008).

The NLN (2008) Position Statement, Preparing the Next Generation of Nurses to Practice in a Technology-Rich Environment: An Informatics Agenda, challenges nurse educators to prepare informatics-competent nurses who can practice safely in a technology-rich healthcare environment. In the Quality and Safety Education for Nurses (2007) report, Cronenwett and colleagues identified several core competencies for nursing education. One competency specifically addressed nursing informatics: "Use information and technology to communicate, manage knowledge, mitigate error, and support decision-making" (p. 129). Another addressed the appropriate use of data and information in nursing practice to promote quality improvement: "Use data to monitor the outcomes and processes and use improvement methods to design and test changes to continuously improve the quality and safety of health care systems" (p. 127).

The TIGER (2007) initiative identifies a key purpose, "to create a vision for the future of nursing that bridges the quality chasm with information technology, enabling nurses to use informatics in practice and education to provide safer, higher-quality patient care" (p. 4). The pillars of the TIGER vision include the following:

- Management and Leadership: Revolutionary leadership that drives, empowers, and executes the transformation of health care.
- Education: Collaborative learning communities that maximize the possibilities of technology toward knowledge development and dissemination, driving rapid deployment and implementation of best practices.
- Communication and Collaboration: Standardized, person-centered, technology-enabled processes to facilitate teamwork and relationships across the continuum of care.

- Informatics Design: Evidence-based, interoperable intelligence systems that support education and practice to foster quality care and safety.
- Information Technology: Smart, people-centered, affordable technologies that are universal, useable, useful, and standards-based.
- Policy: Consistent, incentives-based initiatives (organizational and governmental) that support advocacy and coalition-building, achieving and resourcing an ethical culture of safety.
- Culture: A respectful, open system that leverages technology and informatics across multiple disciplines in an environment where all stakeholders trust each other to work together towards the goal of high quality and safety (p. 4).

The Essentials of Baccalaureate Education for Professional Nursing Practice (AACN, 2008, pp. 18-19) includes the following technology-related outcomes for baccalaureate nursing graduates:

1. Demonstrate skills in using patient care technologies, information systems, and communication devices that support safe nursing practice.
2. Use telecommunication technologies to assist in effective communication in a variety of healthcare settings.
3. Apply safeguards and decision-making support tools embedded in patient care technologies and information systems to support a safe practice environment for both patients and healthcare workers.
4. Understand the use of CIS systems to document interventions related to achieving nurse-sensitive outcomes.
5. Use standardized terminology in a care environment that reflects nursing's unique contribution to patient outcomes.
6. Evaluate data from all relevant sources, including technology, to inform the delivery of care.
7. Recognize the role of information technology in improving patient care outcomes and creating a safe care environment.
8. Uphold ethical standards related to data security, regulatory requirements, confidentiality, and clients' right to privacy.
9. Apply patient care technologies as appropriate to address the needs of a diverse patient population.
10. Advocate for the use of new patient care technologies for safe, quality care.
11. Recognize that redesign of workflow and care processes should precede implementation of care technology to facilitate nursing practice.
12. Participate in the evaluation of information systems in practice settings through policy and procedure development.

The report suggests the following sample content for achieving these student outcomes (AACN, 2008, pp. 19-20):

- Use of patient care technologies (e.g., monitors, pumps, computer-assisted devices)
- Use of technology and information systems for clinical decision making
- Computer skills that may include basic software, spreadsheet, and healthcare databases
- Information management for patient safety
- Regulatory requirements through electronic data-monitoring systems
- Ethical and legal issues related to the use of information technology, including copyright, privacy, and confidentiality issues
- Retrieval information systems, including access, evaluation of data, and application of relevant data to patient care
- Online literature searches
- Technologic resources for evidence based practice
- Web-based learning and online literature searches for self and patient use
- Technology and information systems safeguards (e.g., patient monitoring, equipment, patient identification systems, drug alerts and IV systems, and barcoding)
- Interstate practice regulations (e.g., licensure, telehealth)
- Technology for virtual care delivery and monitoring
- Principles related to nursing workload measurement and resources and information systems
- Information literacy
- Electronic health record and physician order entry
- Decision support tools
- Role of the nurse informaticist in the context of health informatics and information systems

This text is designed to include the necessary content to prepare nurses for practice in the ever changing and technology-laden healthcare environments.

Goossen (2000) believes that the focus of nursing informatics research should be on the structuring and processing of patient information and how these inform nursing decision making in clinical practice. The increased use of technology to enhance nursing practice, nursing education, and nursing research will open new avenues for acquiring, processing, generating, and disseminating knowledge.

In the future, nursing research will contribute significantly to the development of nursing science. Technologies and translational research will abound and clinical practices will be evidence based, thus improving patient outcomes and decreasing safety concerns. Schools of nursing will embrace nursing science as they strive to meet the needs of changing student populations and the increasing complexity of healthcare environments.

SUMMARY

This chapter provides an overview of nursing science and how nursing science relates to typical nursing practice roles, nursing education, and nursing research. The Foundation of Knowledge model was introduced as the organizing conceptual framework for this book. Finally, the relationship of nursing science to nursing informatics was discussed. In subsequent chapters the reader will learn more about how nursing informatics supports nurses in their many and varied roles. In an ideal world nurses would embrace nursing science as knowledge users, knowledge managers, knowledge developers, knowledge engineers, and knowledge workers.

THOUGHT-PROVOKING Questions

WWW

1. Imagine you are in a social situation and someone asks you, "What does a nurse do?" Think about how you will capture and convey the richness that is nursing science in your answer.

2. Choose a clinical scenario from your recent experience and analyze it using the Foundation of Knowledge model. How did you acquire knowledge? How did you process knowledge? How did you generate knowledge? How did you disseminate knowledge? How did you use feedback, and what was the effect of the feedback on the foundation of your knowledge?

For a full suite of assignments and additional learning activities, use the access code located in the front of your book to visit this exclusive website: http://go.jblearning.com/mcgonigle. If you do not have an access code, you can obtain one at the site.

WWW

References

American Association of Colleges of Nursing. (2008, October 20). The Essentials of Baccalaureate Education for Professional Nursing Practice. Retrieved from American Association of Colleges of Nursing Web site: http://www.aacn.nche.edu/Education/pdf/ BaccEssentials08.pdf

American Nurses Association. (2003). *Nursing's social policy statement* (2nd ed.). Silver Spring, MD: Author.

Bassendowski, S. (2007). NursingQuest: Supporting an analysis of nursing issues. *Journal of Nursing Education, 46*(2), 92–95. Retrieved from Education Module database [document ID: 1210832211].

Cronenwett, L., Sherwood, G., Barnsteiner J., Disch, J., Johnson, J., Mitchell, P., …Warren, J. (2007). Quality and safety education for nurses. *Nursing Outlook, 55*(3), 122–131.

Girard, N. (2007). Science fiction comes to the OR. *Association of Operating Room Nurses. AORN Journal, 86*(3), 351–353. Retrieved from Health Module database [document ID: 1333149261].

Goossen, W. (2000). Nursing informatics research. *Nurse Researcher, 8*(2), 42. Retrieved from ProQuest Nursing & Allied Health Source database [document ID: 67258628].

Greenfield, S. (2007). Medication error reduction and the use of PDA technology. *Journal of Nursing Education, 46*(3), 127–131. Retrieved from Education Module database [document ID: 1227347171].

National League for Nursing. (2008). Preparing the next generation of nurses to practice in a technology rich environment: An informatics agenda. (Position Statement). Retrieved from: http://www.nln.org/aboutnln/PositionStatements/informatics_052808.pdf

Skiba, D. (2007). Faculty 2.0: Flipping the novice to expert continuum. Nursing Education Perspectives, 28(6), 342–344. Retrieved from ProQuest Nursing & Allied Health Source database [document ID: 1401240241].

Swan, B., Lang, N., & McGinley, A. (2004). Access to quality health care: Links between evidence, nursing language, and informatics. *Nursing Economics, 22*(6), 325–332. Retrieved from Health Module database [document ID: 768191851].

Technology Informatics Guiding Education Reform. (2007). Evidence and Informatics Transforming Nursing: 3-Year Action Steps Toward a 10-year Vision. Retrieved from The Tiger Initiative website: http://www.aacn.nche.edu/Education/pdf/TIGER.pdf

CHAPTER 2

Introduction to Information, Information Science, and Information Systems

Dee McGonigle and Kathleen Mastrian

Objectives

1. Reflect on the progression from data to information to knowledge.
2. Describe the term *information*.
3. Assess how information is acquired.
4. Explore the characteristics of quality information.
5. Describe an information system.
6. Explore data acquisition or input and processing or retrieval, analysis, and synthesis of data.
7. Assess output or reports, documents, summaries alerts, and outcomes.
8. Describe information dissemination and feedback.
9. Define information science.
10. Assess how information is processed.
11. Explore how knowledge is generated in information science.

Key Terms www

Acquisition
Alerts
Analysis
Chief information officer
Chief technical officer
Chief technology officer
Cloud computing
Cognitive science
Communication science
Computer-based
   information system
Computer science
Consolidated health
   informatics
Data
Dissemination
Document
Electronic health record
Federal Health
   Information Exchange
Feedback
Health information
   exchange
Health Level Seven
Indiana Health Information
   Exchange
Information
Information science

Continues

INTRODUCTION

This chapter explores information, **information systems** (IS), and information science. The key word is information. Healthcare professionals are **knowledge workers**, and deal with information on a daily basis. There are many concerns and issues that arise with healthcare information, such as ownership, access, disclosure, exchange, security, privacy, disposal, and dissemination. With the gauntlet of an **electronic health record** being set, public and private sector stakeholders have been collaborating on a wide-ranging variety of healthcare information solutions. These initiatives include **Health Level Seven** (HL7), **Consolidated Health Informatics's** (CHI's) eGov initiative, the **National Health Information Infrastructure** (NHII), the **National Health Information**

Network (NHIN), **Next-Generation Internet** (NGI), **Internet2**, and iHealth record. There are also **health information exchange** (HIE) systems, such as Connecting for Health, the eHealth initiative, the **Federal Health Information Exchange** (FHIE), the **Indiana Health Information Exchange** (IHIE), the **Massachusetts Health Data Consortium** (MHDC), the **New England Health EDI Network** (NEHEN), the State of New Mexico **Rapid Syndromic Validation Project** (RSVP), the Southeast Michigan e-Prescribing Initiative, and the Tennessee Volunteer eHealth Initiative (Goldstein, Groen, Ponkshe, & Wine, 2007). The most recent initiative, the HITECH Act, has set 2014 as the deadline for electronic health records (see Chapter 10). It is quite evident from the previous brief listing that there is a need to remedy healthcare **information technology** concerns, challenges, and issues faced today. One of the main issues deals with how healthcare information is managed to make it meaningful. It is important to understand how people obtain, manipulate, use, share, and dispose of information. This chapter deals with the information piece of this complex puzzle.

INFORMATION

Suppose someone states the number 99.5. What does that mean? It could be a radio station or a score on a test. Now, if someone says that Ms. Howsunny's temperature is 99.5°F, what does that convey? It is then known that 99.5 is a person's temperature. The data (99.5) were processed to the information that 99.5° is a specific person's temperature. **Data** are raw facts. Information is processed data that has meaning. Healthcare professionals constantly process data and information to provide the best care possible for their patients.

There are many types of data, such as alpha, numeric, audio, image, and video data. Alpha data refers to letters and numeric refers to numbers, and alphanumeric data includes both letters and numbers. This includes all text and the numeric outputs of digital monitors. Some of the alphanumeric data encountered by healthcare professionals are in the form of patients' names, identification numbers, or medical record numbers. Audio data refer to sounds, noises, or tones. There are monitor alerts or alarms, taped or recorded messages, and other sounds. Image data include graphics and pictures, such as graphic monitor displays or recorded electrocardiograms, radiographs, MRIs, and CT scans. Video data refer to animations, moving pictures, or moving graphics. One may review the ultrasound of a pregnant patient; examine a patient's echocardiogram; watch an animated video for professional development; or learn how to operate a new technology tool, such as a pump or monitoring system.

The integrity and quality of the data, rather than the form, are what matter. Integrity refers to whole, complete, correct, and consistent data. Data integrity can be compromised through human error; viruses, worms, other bugs; hardware failures or crashes; transmission errors; or hackers entering the system. Information technologies help to decrease these errors by putting into place safeguards, such as backing up files on a routine basis, error detection for transmissions, and developing user **interfaces** that help people enter the data correctly. High-quality data are relevant and accurately represent their corresponding concepts. Data are dirty when there are errors in the database, such as duplicate, incomplete, or outdated records. One author (D.M.) found 50 cases of tongue cancer in a database she examined for data quality. When the records were tracked down and analyzed, and the dirty data were removed, there was only one case of tongue cancer. The same person had been entered erroneously 49 times. The major problem was with the patient's identification number and name. The numbers were changed or his name was misspelled repeatedly. If researchers had just taken the number of cases in that defined population as 50, they would have concluded it was an epidemic, resulting in flawed information that is not meaningful. Therefore, it is imperative that data be clean if the goal is quality information. The data that are processed into information must be of high quality and integrity to create meaning to inform assessments and decision making.

To be valuable and meaningful, information must be of good quality. Characteristics of valuable, quality information include accessibility, security, timeliness, accuracy, relevancy, completeness, flexibility, reliability, objectivity, utility, transparency, verifiability, and reproducibility. Accessibility is a must; the right user must be able to have the right information at the right time and in the right format to meet his or her needs. Getting meaningful information to the right user at the right time is as vital as generating the information in the first place. The *right user* refers to an authorized user who has the right to obtain the data and information he or she is seeking. Security is a major challenge because unauthorized users must be blocked while the right user is provided with open, easy access (see Chapter 15). Timely information means that it is available when it is needed for the right purpose and at the right time. Knowing who won the lottery last week does not help one to know if he or she won it today. Accurate information means that there are no errors in the data and information. Relevant information is subjective in the fact that the user must have information that is relevant or applicable to his or her needs. If one is trying to decide whether or not a patient needs insulin and only the patient's CT scan information is available, this information is not relevant for that current need. However, if one needed information about the CT scan, then the information is relevant. Complete information contains all of the necessary essential data. If one needs to contact the only relative listed for the patient and his or her contact information is listed but the approval for them to be a contact is missing, this information is considered incomplete. Flexible information means that it can be used for a variety of purposes. Information concerning the inventory of supplies on a nursing unit can be used by nurses who need to know if an item is available for use for a patient. The nurse manager accesses this information to help decide what supplies need to be ordered and to determine what items are used often and to do an economic assessment of any waste. Reliable information comes from reliable or clean data and authoritative and credible sources. Objective information is as close to the truth as one can get. It is not subjective or biased but rather is factual and impartial. If someone states something, it must be determined if that person is reliable and if what he or she is stating is objective or tainted by his or her own perspective. Utility refers to the ability to provide the right information at the right time to the right person for the right purpose. Transparency allows users to apply their intellect to accomplish their tasks while the tools housing the information disappear. Verifiable information means that one can check to verify or prove that it is correct. Reproducibility refers to the ability to produce the same information again. The value relates directly to how the information informs decision making.

Information is acquired either by actively looking for it or by having it conveyed by the environment. All of the senses (vision, hearing, touch, smell, and taste) are used to gather input from the surrounding world, and as technologies mature, there will be more and more **input** through the senses. Currently, people receive information from computers (output), through vision, hearing, or touch (input), and the response (output) to the computer (input) is the interface with technology. Gesture recognition is increasing and interfaces that incorporate it will change the way people become informed (see Box 2-1). Many people access the Internet on a daily basis seeking information or imparting information. One is constantly becoming informed, discovering, or learning; becoming reinforced, rediscovering, or relearning; and purging what has been acquired. The information acquired is added to the knowledge base. **Knowledge** is the awareness and understanding of a set of information and ways that information can be made useful to support a specific task or arrive at a decision. This knowledge building is an ongoing process engaged in while one is conscious and going about his or her normal daily activities.

INFORMATION SCIENCE

Information science has evolved over the last 50 some years as a field of scientific inquiry and professional practice. Information science can be thought of as the science of information, studying the application and usage of information and

BOX

2-1

Gesture Recognition in Surface and iTable Computing

These surfaces are multitouch, gesture recognition interfaces that interpret human gestures by means of mathematical algorithms to manipulate digital content for one or multiple users.

According to McGonigle (2009), one should not get too attached to the mouse and keyboard, because they are going to be outdated soon if Microsoft and PQ Labs have their way. Microsoft has introduced the Surface and PQ Labs is building custom iTables (Kumparak, 2009). Have you ever thought of digital information you can touch and grab? Microsoft and PQ Labs are leading us into the next generation of computing, surface or table computing.

Surface or table computing consists of a multitouch, multiuser interface that allows one to "grab" digital information, collaborate, share, and store without using a mouse or keyboard, just the hands and fingers and such devices as a digital camera and PDA. This interface generally rests on top of a table and is so advanced that it can actually sense objects, touch, and gestures from many users (Microsoft, 2008).

Imagine entering a restaurant and interacting with the menu through the surface. Once you have completed your order you can begin computing by using the capabilities built into the surface or using your own device, such as a PDA. For example, one could set the PDA on the surface and download images, graphics, and text to the surface. You could even communicate using full audio and video with others while waiting for the order. When finished eating, set your credit card on the surface where it is automatically charged, and pick up your credit card and leave. That is a different kind of eating experience, but one that will become commonplace for the next generation of users.

This new age of computing is currently available in Las Vegas and in select casinos, banks, restaurants, and hotels throughout the United States and Canada.

Explore this new interface, which will forever change how people interact and compute. Think of the ramifications for health care....

References

Kumparak, G. (2009). Look out, Microsoft Surface—The iTable might just trump you in every way. Retrieved from http://www.crunchgear.com/2009/01/10/look-out-microsoft-surface-the-itable-might-just-trump-you-in-every-way/

McGonigle, D. (2009). Editorial: Microsoft surface tension? iTable. *Online Journal of Nursing Informatics (OJNI), 13*(2). Available at http://ojni.org/13_2/dee.htm

Microsoft Surface. (2008). Microsoft Surface: General Questions. Retrieved from http://www.microsoft.com/SURFACE/about_faqs/faqs.aspx

knowledge in organizations and the interface or interaction between people, organizations, and IS. It is an extensive, interdisciplinary science that integrates features from **cognitive science**, **communication science**, **computer science**, **library science**, and **social sciences**. Information science is primarily concerned with the input, processing, output, and feedback of data and information through technology integration with a focus on comprehending the perspective of the **stakeholders** involved and then applying information technology as needed. It is systemically based, dealing with the big picture rather than individual pieces of technology. Information science can be related to determinism. It is a response to technologic determinism, the belief that technology develops by its own laws, that it realizes its own potential, limited only by the material resources available, and must therefore be regarded as an autonomous system controlling and ultimately permeating all other subsystems of society (Web Dictionary of Cybernetics and Systems, 2007, para. 1).

This approach sets the tone for the study of information as it applies to itself, the people, the technology, and the varied sciences that are contextually related depending on the needs of the setting or organization; what is important is the interface between the stakeholders and their systems and how they generate, use, and locate information. According to Cornell University (2010), "Information Science brings together faculty, students and researchers who share an interest in combining computer science with the social sciences of how people and society interact with information" (para. 1). Information science is an interdisciplinary, people-oriented field that explores and enhances the interchange of information to transform society, communication science, computer science, cognitive science, library science, and the social sciences. Society is dominated by the need for information, and knowledge and information science focuses on systems and individual users fostering user-centered approaches that enhance society's information capabilities, effectively and efficiently linking people, information, and technology. This impacts the configuration and mix of organizations and influences the nature of work or how knowledge workers interact with and produce meaningful information and knowledge.

INFORMATION PROCESSING

Claude E. Shannon is considered the father of information theory (Horgan, 1990) and thought of information processing as the conversion of latent information into manifest information. Latent information is that which is not yet realized or apparent, whereas manifest information is obvious or clearly apparent. According to O'Connor and Robertson (2005), "Shannon believed that information was no different than any other quantity and therefore could be manipulated by a machine" (para. 13).

Information science enables the processing of information. This processing links people and technology. Humans are organic ISs, constantly acquiring, processing, and generating information or knowledge in their professional and personal lives. It is a high degree of knowledge that characterizes humans as extremely intelligent organic machines. The premise of this book revolves around this concept and is organized on the basis of the Foundation of Knowledge model: knowledge **acquisition**, knowledge processing, knowledge generation, and knowledge dissemination.

Information is data that are processed using knowledge. For information to be valuable or meaningful, it must be accessible, accurate, timely, complete, cost effective, flexible, reliable, relevant, simple, verifiable, and secure. Knowledge is the awareness and understanding of an information set and ways that information can be made useful to support a specific task or arrive at a decision. As an example, if one were going to design a building, part of the knowledge necessary for developing a new building is understanding how the building will be used, how large of a building is needed compared to the available building space, and how many people will have or need access to this building. Therefore, the work of choosing or rejecting facts based on their significance or relevance to a particular task, such as designing a building, is also based on a type of knowledge used in the process of converting data into information. Information can then be considered data made functional through the application of knowledge. The knowledge used to develop and glean knowledge from valuable information is generative (having the ability to originate and produce or generate) in nature. Knowledge must be viable. Knowledge viability refers to applications that offer easily accessible, accurate, and timely information obtained from a variety of resources and methods and presented in a manner so as to provide the necessary elements to generate knowledge.

Information science and computational tools are extremely important in enabling the processing of data, information, and knowledge in health care. The hardware, software, networking, algorithms, and human organic ISs work together to create meaningful information and generate knowledge. The links between information processing and scientific discovery are paramount. However, without the ability to generate practical results that can be disseminated, the processing of data, information, and knowledge is for naught. It is the ability of machines (inorganic ISs) to support and facilitate the functioning of people (human organic ISs) that refines, enhances, and evolves nursing practice by generating knowledge. This knowledge represents five rights: the right information, accessible by the right people in the right settings, applied the right way at the right time. It is also the struggle to integrate new knowledge and old knowledge to enhance wisdom. Wisdom is the ability to act; it assumes actions directed by one's own wisdom. Wisdom uses knowledge and experience to heighten common sense, and insight to exercise sound judgment in practical matters. It is developed through knowledge, experience, insight, and reflection. Wisdom is sometimes thought of as the highest form of common sense resulting from accumulated knowledge or erudition (deep, thorough learning) or enlightenment (education that results in understanding and the dissemination of knowledge). It is the ability to apply valuable and viable knowledge, experience, understanding, and insight while being prudent and sensible. Knowledge and wisdom are not synonymous because knowledge abounds with others' thoughts and information, whereas wisdom is focused on one's own mind and the synthesis of one's own experience, insight, understanding, and knowledge. If clinicians are inundated with data without the ability to process it, the situation results in too much data and too little wisdom. That is why it is crucial that clinicians have viable ISs at their fingertips to facilitate the acquisition, sharing, and use of knowledge while maturing wisdom; it is a process of empowerment.

INFORMATION SCIENCE AND THE FOUNDATION OF KNOWLEDGE

Information science is a multidisciplinary science that involves aspects from computer science, cognitive science, social science, communication science, and library science to deal with obtaining, gathering, organizing, manipulating, managing, storing, retrieving, recapturing, disposing of, distributing, or broadcasting information. Information science studies everything that deals with information and can be defined as the study of ISs. This science originated as a subdiscipline of computer science, to understand and rationalize the management of technology within organizations. It has matured into a major field of management; is an important area of research in management studies; and has expanded to examine the human–computer interaction, interfacing, and interaction of people, ISs, and corporations. It is taught at all major universities and business schools worldwide. Organizations have become intensely aware of the fact that information and knowledge are potent resources that must be cultivated and honed to meet their needs. Thus, information science or the study of ISs, the application and usage of knowledge, focuses on why and how technology can be put to best use to serve the information flow within an organization.

Information science impacts information interfacing, influencing how people interact with information and subsequently develop and use knowledge. The information one acquires is added to one's knowledge base. Knowledge is the awareness and understanding of an information set and ways that information can be made useful to support a specific task or arrive at a decision.

Healthcare organizations are affected by and rely on the evolution of information science to enhance the recording and processing of routine and intimate information while facilitating human-to-human and human-to-systems communications, delivery of healthcare products, dissemination of information, and enhancement of the organization's business transactions. The benefits and enhancements of information science technologies have also brought risks, such as glitches and loss of information and hackers who can steal identities and information. Solid leadership, guidance, and vision are vital to the maintenance of cost-effective business performance and cutting-edge, safe information technologies for the organization. This field studies all facets of the building and use of information. The emergence of information science and its impact on information has also influenced how people acquire and use knowledge.

Information science has had a tremendous impact on society and will expand its sphere of influence as it continues to evolve and innovate human activities at all levels. What visionaries only dreamed of is now possible and part of reality. The future has yet to unfold in this important arena.

INTRODUCTION TO INFORMATION SYSTEMS

Consider the following scenario. You have just been hired by a large healthcare facility. You enter the personnel office and are told that you will have to learn a new language to work on the unit where you have been assigned. This language is just used on this unit. If you had been assigned to a different unit, you would have to learn another language that is specific to that unit, and so on. Therefore, interdepartmental sharing and information exchange (known as interoperability) is severely hindered. This is how workers used to operate in health care—in silos. There was a system for the laboratory, one for finance, one for clinical departments, and so on. Learning the importance of communication, tracking, and research, there are now integrated ISs that handle the needs of the entire organization.

Information and information technology have become major resources for organizations, and health care is no exception (see Box 2-2). Information technologies help to shape a healthcare organization, in conjunction with personnel, money, materials, and equipment. Many healthcare facilities have hired **chief information officers** (CIOs) or **chief technical officers** (CTOs), also known as **chief technology officers**. The CIO is involved with the information technology **infrastructure** and this role is sometimes expanded to chief knowledge officer. The CTO is focused on organizationally based scientific and technical issues and is responsible for technologic research and development as part of the organization's products and services. The CTO and CIO must be visionary leaders for the organization, because so much of the business of health care relies on solid infrastructures that generate potent and timely information and knowledge. The CTO and CIO are sometimes interchangeable positions, but in some organizations the CTO reports to the CIO. These positions will become paramount as companies

BOX

2-2

Examples of Information Systems

Information System	How It Is Used
Clinical Information System (CIS)	Comprehensive and integrative systems that manage the administrative, financial, and clinical aspects of a clinical facility; it should help to link financial and clinical outcomes. One example is the electronic health record (EHR).
Decision Support System (DSS)	Organizes and analyzes information to help decision makers formulate decisions when they are unsure of their decision's possible outcomes. After gathering relevant and useful information, develops "What-If" models to analyze the options or choices and alternatives.
Executive Support System	Collects, organizes, analyzes, and summarizes vital information to help executives or senior management with strategic decision making. Provides a quick view of all strategic business activities.
Geographic Information System (GIS)	Collects, manipulates, analyzes, and generates information related to geographic locations or the surface of the earth; provides output in the form of virtual models, maps, or lists.
Management Information Systems (MIS)	Provides summaries of internal sources of information, such as information from the transaction processing system and develops a series of routine reports for decision making.
Office Systems	Facilitates communication and enhances the productivity of users needing to process data and information.
Transaction Processing System (TPS)	Processes and records routine business transactions, such as billing systems that create and send invoices to customers, and payroll that generates employee's pay stubs and wage checks and calculates tax payments.
Hospital Information System (HIS)	Manages the administrative, financial, and clinical aspects of a hospital enterprise. It should help to link financial and clinical outcomes.

continue to shift from being product oriented to knowledge oriented and as they begin emphasizing the production process itself rather than the product. In health care, ISs must be able to handle the volume of data and information necessary to generate the needed information and knowledge for best practices, because the goal is to provide the highest quality of patient care.

INFORMATION SYSTEMS

ISs can be manually based, but for the purposes of this text, the term refers to **computer-based information systems** (CBISs). According to Jessup and Valacich (2008), computer-based ISs "are combinations of hardware, software and telecommunications networks that people build and use to collect, create, and distribute useful data, typically in organizational settings" (p. 10). Along those lines, ISs are also defined as "a set of interrelated components that collect, manipulate, store and disseminate data and information and provide a feedback mechanism to meet an objective" (Stair & Reynolds, 2008, p. 4). ISs are designed for specific purposes within organizations. They are only as functional as the decision-making, problem-solving skills, and programming potency built in and the quality of data and information inputted (see Chapter 12). The capability of the IS to disseminate, provide feedback, and adjust the data and information based on these dynamic processes is what sets them apart. The IS should be a user-friendly entity that provides the right information at the right time and in the right place.

An IS acquires data or inputs; processes data that consists of the retrieval, **analysis**, or **synthesis** of data; disseminates or outputs in the form of reports, documents, summaries, alerts, prompts, or outcomes; and provides for responses or feedback. Input or data acquisition is the activity of collecting and acquiring raw data. Input devices are combinations of hardware, software, and **telecommunications** and include keyboards, light pens, touch screens, mice or other pointing devices, automatic scanners, and machines that can read magnetic ink characters or lettering. In receiving a pay-per-view movie, the viewer must input the chosen movie, verify the purchase, and have a payment method approved by the vendor. The IS must acquire this information before one can receive the movie.

Processing, the retrieval, analysis, or synthesis of data refers to the alteration and transformation of the data into helpful or useful information and outputs. The processing of data can range from storing it for future use to comparing the data, making calculations, or applying formulas, to taking selective actions. Processing devices are combinations of hardware, software, and telecommunications and include processing chips where the central processing unit (CPU) and main memory are housed. According to Schupak (2005), the bunny chip could save the pharmaceutical industry money while sparing "millions of furry creatures, with a chip that mimics a living organism" (para. 1). The HµREL Corporation has developed environments or biologic ISs that reside on chips and actually mimic the functioning of the human body. Therefore, researchers can test for both the harmful and beneficial effects of drugs, including those that are considered experimental and that could be harmful if used in human and animal testing. These chips also allow researchers to monitor the drug's toxicity to the liver and other organs.

A patented HμREL microfluidic "biochip" comprises an arrangement of separate but fluidically interconnected "organ" or "tissue" compartments. Each compartment contains a culture of living cells drawn from, or engineered to mimic primary functions of the respective organ or tissue of a living animal. Microfluidic channels permit a culture medium that serves as a "blood surrogate" to recirculate as in a living system, driven by a microfluidic pump. The geometry and fluidics of the device are fashioned to simulate the values of certain related physiologic parameters found in the living creature. Drug candidates or other substrates of interest are added to the culture medium and allowed to recirculate through the device. The effects of drug compounds and their metabolites on the cells within each respective organ compartment are detected by measuring or monitoring key physiologic events. The cell types used may be derived from either standard cell culture lines or primary tissues (HμREL Corporation, 2010, para. 2-3). As these new technologies continue to evolve, more and more robust ISs that can handle a variety of biological and clinical applications will be seen.

In the movie rental example, the IS must verify the data entered and then process the request by following the steps necessary to provide access to the movie that was ordered. This processing must be instantaneous in today's world where everyone wants it now. After the data is processed, it is stored. In this case, the rental must also be processed so the vendor receives payment for the movie, whether electronically, via a credit card or checking account withdrawal, or by generating a bill for payment.

Output or **dissemination** produces helpful or useful information that can be in the form of reports, documents, summaries, alerts, or outcomes. **Reports** are designed to inform and are generally tailored to the context of a given situation or user or user group. Reports may include charts, figures, tables, graphics, pictures, hyperlinks, references, or other documentation necessary to meet the needs of the user. **Documents** represent information that can be printed, saved, e-mailed or shared, or displayed. **Summaries** are condensed versions of the original designed to highlight the major points. **Alerts** are warnings, feedback, or additional information necessary to assist the user in interacting with the system. **Outcomes** are the expected results of input and processing. **Output** devices are combinations of hardware, software, and telecommunications and include sound and speech synthesis outputs, printers, and monitors. Continuing with the movie rental example, the IS must be able to provide the consumer with the movie ordered when it is wanted and somehow notify the purchaser that he or she has indeed purchased the movie and is granted access. The IS must also be able to generate payment either electronically or by generating a bill, and storing the transactional record for future use.

Feedback or responses are reactions to the inputting, processing, and outputs. In ISs, feedback refers to information from the system that is used to make modifications in the input, processing actions, or outputs. In the movie rental example, what if the consumer accidentally entered the same movie order three times and only wanted to order the movie once? The IS would determine that more than one movie order is out of range for the same movie order at the same time and provide feedback. The feedback is used to verify and correct the input. If undetected, this error would result in an erroneous bill and decreased customer satisfaction while creating more work for the vendor, who would have to deal with the customer to resolve this problem. Section IV of this book provides detailed descriptions of clinical ISs that operate on these same principles to support healthcare delivery.

SUMMARY

ISs deal with the development, use, and management of an organization's information technology (IT) infrastructure. An IS acquires data or inputs; processes data that consist of the retrieval, analysis, or synthesis of data; disseminates or outputs in the form of reports, documents, summaries, alerts, or outcomes; and provides for responses or feedback. Quality decision-making and problem-solving skills are vital to the development of effective, valuable ISs. Organizations are recognizing that their most precious asset is their information, represented by their employees, experience, competence or know-how, and innovative or novel approaches, all of which are dependent on a robust information network that encompasses the information technology infrastructure.

In an ideal world, one would see ISs that are fluid in their ability to adapt to any and all users' needs. They would be Internet oriented and global, where resources are available to everyone. Think of **cloud computing**; this is just a beginning point from which ISs will expand and grow in their ability to provide meaningful information to their users. As technologies advance, so will the skills and capabilities to comprehend and realize what ISs can become.

It is important to continue to develop and refine functional, robust, visionary ISs that meet the current meaningful information needs while evolving to handle future information and knowledge needs of the healthcare industry.

THOUGHT-PROVOKING Questions

1. How do you acquire information? Choose 2 hours out of your busy day and try to take note of all of the information that you receive from your environment. Keep diaries denoting where the information came from and how you knew it was information and not data.

2. Reflect on an IS that you are familiar with, such as the automatic banking machine. How does this IS function? What are the advantages of using this system (i.e., why not use a bank teller instead)? What are the disadvantages? Are there enhancements that you would add to this system?

3. In health care, think about a typical day of practice and describe the setting. How many times does the nurse interact with ISs? What are the ISs that we interact with, and how do we access them? Are they at the bedside, handheld, or station based? How does their location and ease of access impact nursing care?

4. Briefly describe an organization and discuss how our need for information and knowledge impacts the configuration and mix of that organization with other organizations. Also discuss how the need for information and knowledge influences the nature of work or how knowledge workers interact with and produce information and knowledge in this organization.

5. If you could only meet four of the rights discussed in this chapter, which one would you omit and why? Also, provide your rationale for each right you chose to meet.

For a full suite of assignments and additional learning activities, use the access code located in the front of your book to visit this exclusive website: http://go.jblearning.com/mcgonigle. If you do not have an access code, you can obtain one at the site.

References

Cornell University. (2010). Information science. Retrieved from http://www.infosci.cornell. edu/

Goldstein, D., Groen, P., Ponkshe, S., & Wine, M. (2007). *Medical informatics 20/20*. Sudbury, MA: Jones and Bartlett.

Horgan, J. (1990). Claude E. Shannon: Unicyclist, juggler and father of information theory. Retrieved from http://www.ecs.umass.edu/ece/hill/ ece221.dir/shannon.html

HμREL Corporation. (2010). Human-Relevant. HμREL. Technology Overview. Retrieved from http://www.hurelcorp.com/overview.php

Jessup, L., & Valacich, J. (2008). *Information systems today* (3rd ed.). Upper Saddle River, NJ: Pearson Prentice Hall.

O'Connor, J., & Robertson, E. (2005). Claude Elwood Shannon. Retrieved from http://www.thocp .net/biographies/shannon_claude.htm

Schupak, A. (2005). Technology: The bunny chip. Retrieved from http://members.forbes.com/ forbes/2005/0815/053.html

Stair, R., & Reynolds, G. (2008). *Principles of information systems* (8th ed.). Boston, MA: Thompson Course Technology.

Web Dictionary of Cybernetics and Systems. (2007). Technological determinism. Retrieved from http://pespmc1.vub.ac.be/asc/TECHNO_ DETER.html

CHAPTER 3

Computer Science and the Foundation of Knowledge Model

June Kaminski

WWW

Objectives

1. Describe the essential components of computer systems including hardware and software.
2. Recognize the rapid evolution of computer systems and the benefit of keeping up to date with current trends and developments.
3. Analyze how computer systems function as tools for managing information and generating knowledge.
4. Define the concept of human–technology interfaces.
5. Articulate how computers can support collaboration, networking, and information exchange.

Key Terms

WWW

Acquisition
Applications
Arithmetic logic unit (ALU)
Binary system
Basic input/output system (BIOS)
Bit
Bus
Byte
Cache memory
Central processing unit (CPU)
Communication software
Compact disc read-only memory (CD-ROM)
Compact disc-recordable (CD-R)
Compact disc-rewritable (CD-RW)
Compatibility
Computer
Computer science
Conferencing software
Creativity software
Databases
Degradation
Desktop
Digital video disc (DVD)
Digital video disc-recordable (DVD-R)

Continues

INTRODUCTION

In this chapter, the discipline of **computer science** is introduced through a focus on computers and the **hardware** and software that make up these evolving systems. Computer science offers extremely valuable tools that, if used skillfully, can facilitate the acquisition and manipulation of data and **information** by nurses, who can then synthesize these into an evolving **knowledge** and **wisdom** base. This can facilitate **professional development** and the ability to apply evidence-based practice decisions within nursing care, and if disseminated and shared, can also advance the professional knowledge base. This chapter begins with a look at common computer hardware, followed by a brief overview of operating, productivity, creativity, and communication software. The chapter concludes with a glimpse at how computer systems help to shape knowledge and collaboration, and an introduction to human–technology interface dynamics.

THE COMPUTER AS A TOOL FOR MANAGING INFORMATION AND GENERATING KNOWLEDGE

Throughout history, various milestones have signaled discoveries, inventions, or philosophic shifts that spurred a surge in knowledge and understanding within the human race. The advent of the **computer** is one such milestone, one that has sparked an intellectual metamorphosis whose boundaries have yet to be fully understood. Computer **technology** has ushered in what has been called the "**information age**," an age when data, information, and knowledge are both accessible and able to be manipulated by more people than ever before in history. How can a mere machine provide such a revolutionary state of knowledge potential? To begin to answer this question, it is best to examine the basic structure and components of computer systems.

Essentially, a computer is an electronic information-processing machine that serves as a tool to manipulate data and information. The easiest way to begin to understand computers is to realize they are input–output systems. These unique machines accept data inputted via a variety of devices, process data through logical and arithmetic rendering, store the data in **memory** components, and output data and information to the user.

Since the advent of the first electronic computer in the mid 1940s, computers have evolved to become essential tools in every walk of life, including the profession of nursing. The complexity of today's computers has skyrocketed and will continue to do so. "Computing has changed the world more than any other invention of the past hundred years, and has come to pervade nearly all human endeavors. Yet, we are just at the beginning of the computing revolution; today's computing offers just a glimpse of the potential impact of computers" (Evans, 2010, p. 3). Major computer manufacturers and researchers, such as Intel, have identified the need to design computers to mask this growing complexity. The sophistication of computers is evolving at amazing speed, yet ease of use or user-friendly aspects are also increasing accordingly. This is achieved by honing hardware and software capabilities until they work seamlessly together to ensure **user-friendly**, intuitive tools for users of all levels of expertise. Box 3-1 provides information about computing surfaces.

According to Intel Corporation's Technology Research team, the goal is "technology that just works." "To conceal complexity, Intel Research is looking at a number of solutions by:

- Relating user mental models with complex systems and technology to improve the use and adaptation of systems across devices and contexts.

BOX
3-1

Microsoft Surface Tension? iTable.

Dee McGonigle

Do not get too attached to your mouse and keyboard because they are going to be outdated soon if Microsoft and PQ Labs have their way. Microsoft has introduced the **Surface** and PQ Labs is building custom iTables according to Kumparak (2009). Have you ever thought of digital information one can touch and grab? Microsoft and PQ Labs are leading us into the next generation of computing: Surface or Table computing.

Surface or Table computing consists of a multitouch, multiuser interface that allows one to "grab" digital information, collaborate, share, and store without using a mouse or keyboard, just the hands and fingers, and such devices as a digital camera and personal digital assistant (PDA). This interface generally rests on top of a table and is so advanced that it can actually sense objects, touch, and gestures from many users (Microsoft, 2008).

Imagine entering a restaurant and interacting with the menu through the surface. Once you have completed your order you can begin computing by using the capabilities built into the surface or using your own device, such as a PDA. You can set the PDA on the surface and download images, graphics, and text to the surface. You can even communicate with others using full audio and video while waiting for your order. When you are done eating, all you have to do is set your credit card on the surface and it is automatically charged. You pick up your credit card and leave. Now, that is a different kind of eating experience and will become commonplace for the next generation of users.

You might be asking when this new age of computing will be touched by typical users: right now in Las Vegas, but also in select casinos, banks, restaurants, and hotels throughout the United States and Canada.

I urge you to explore this new interface, which will forever change how we interact and compute. Think of the ramifications for health care...

Continues

Continues

Key Terms Continued

Monitor
Motherboard
Mouse
MPEG-1 Audio Layer-3 (MP3)
Networks
Nonsynchronous
Office suite
Open source
Operating system (OS)
Palm computers
Parallel port
Peripheral component interconnection (PCI)
Personal computer (PC)
Personal digital assistants (PDAs)
Plug and play
Port
Portability
Portable operating system interface for UNIX (POSIX)
Power supply
Presentation
Processing
Productivity software
Professional development
Programmable read-only memory (PROM)
Publishing
QWERTY
Random access memory (RAM)
Read-only memory (ROM)
Security
Serial port
Small computer system interface (SCSI)
Software
Sound card
Spreadsheet
Supercomputers
Synchronous

Continues

BOX *(Continued)*

3-1

References

Kumparak, G. (2009). Look out, Microsoft Surface—the
   iTable might just trump you in every way. Retrieved
   from http://www.crunchgear.com/2009/01/10/look-out-
   microsoft-surface-the-itable-might-just-trump-you-in-
   every-way/
Microsoft Surface. (2008). Microsoft Surface: General
   questions. Retrieved from
   http://www.microsoft.com/SURFACE/about_faqs/faqs.
   aspx

- Enabling devices to explore their environment to discover other devices and capabilities, and then form integrated "teams" that self organize for higher functionality and performance.
- Better control of failure modes, graceful **degradation** and self-healing across ensembles of devices.
- Zero-knowledge applications and interoperation." (Intel, 2008, para. 2).

A common example of complexity masked in simplicity is the evolution to "**plug and play**" computer add-ons, where a peripheral, such as an iPod or game console, can be simply plugged into a serial or other **port** and instantly used.

Computers are universal machines, because they are general-purpose, symbol-manipulating devices that can perform any task represented in specific programs. For instance, they can be used to draw an image, calculate statistics, write an essay, or record nursing care data. In a nutshell, computers can be used for data and information storage, retrieval, analyzation, generation, and transformation.

Most computers are based on scientist John Von Neumann's model of a processor-memory-input-output architecture. The logic unit and control unit are parts of the processor; the memory is the storage region; and the input and output segments are provided by the various computer devices, such as the keyboard, mouse, monitor, and printer. Recent developments have modified alternative configurations to the Von Neumann model, particularly the parallel computing model where multiple processors are set up to work together. Still, today's computer systems share the same basic configurations and components inherent in the earliest computers.

Components

Hardware

Computer hardware refers to the actual physical "body" of the computer and its components. There are several key components in the average computer that work together to shape a complex yet highly usable machine that serves as a tool for knowledge management, communication, and creativity.

Protection: The Casing The most noticeable component of any computer is the outer case. Desktop **personal computers** have either a **desktop** case, which lies flat, horizontally on a desk, often with the computer monitor positioned on top of it; or a tower case, which stands vertically, and usually sits beside the monitor or on a lower shelf or the floor. Most cases come equipped with a case fan, which is extremely critical for keeping the computer components cool when in use. **Laptop** computers combine the casing in a flat rectangular casing that is attached to the hinged or foldable monitor. **Palm computers** and **personal digital assistants** also have a protective outer plastic and metal case with an embedded liquid crystal display screen.

Central Processing Unit Sometimes conceptualized as the "brain" of the computer, the **central processing unit** (CPU) is the computer component that actually **executes**, calculates, and processes the binary computer code (comprised of various configurations of 0s and 1s) instigated by the **operating system** (OS) and other **applications** on the computer. It serves as the command center that directs the actions of all other computer components, and manages both incoming and outgoing data that are processed across components. Common CPUs include the Pentium, K6, PowerPC, and Sparc models.

The CPU contains specific mechanical units, including registers, arithmetic and logic units, a floating point unit, control circuitry, and **cache memory**. Together, these inner components form the computer's central processor. Registers consist of data-storing circuits that are processed by the adjacent arithmetic and logic units or the floating point unit. Cache memory is extremely quick memory that holds whatever data and code is being used at any one time. The CPU uses the cache to store in-process data so that it is quickly retrieved as needed. The CPU is protected by a heatsink, a copper or aluminum metal block that cools the processor (often with the help of a fan) to prevent overheating.

The speed and power of a CPU used to be measured in megahertz and was written as a value in MHz (e.g., 400 MHz, meaning the **microprocessor** ran at 400 MHz, executing 400 million cycles per second). Now it is more common to see the speed measured in **gigahertz** (1 GHz is equal to 1,000 MHz); thus, a CPU that operates at 4 GHz is a thousand times faster than an older one set at 4 MHz. The more cycles a processor can engage in per second, the faster computer programs can run.

In recent years, processor manufacturers, such as Intel, have moved to multicore microprocessors, which are chips that combine two or more processors. In fact, multiple microprocessors have become a standard in personal and professional level computers. "Minicomputers, which were traditionally made from off-the-shelf logic or from gate arrays, have been replaced by servers made using microprocessors. **Mainframes** have been almost replaced with multiprocessors consisting of small numbers of off-the-shelf microprocessors. Even high-end **supercomputers** are being built with collections of microprocessors" (Hennessy & Patterson, 2006, p. 3).

Motherboard The **motherboard** has been called the "central nervous system" of the computer, and is a key foundational component because all other components are connected to it in some way (either directly via local sockets, attached directly to it, or connected via cables). This includes **universal serial bus** (**USB**) controllers, Ethernet network controllers, integrated graphics controllers, and so forth. The essential structures of the motherboard include the major chipset, Super Input/Output hip, BIOS **read-only memory** (ROM), **bus** communications pathways, and a variety of sockets that allow components to plug into the board. The chipset (often a pair of chips), determines the computer's CPU type and memory. It also houses the north bridge and south bridge controllers that allow the buses to transfer data from one to another.

Power Supply The **power supply** is a critical component of any computer, because it provides the essential electrical energy needed to allow a computer to operate. The power supply unit converts the 240-V AC main power provided via the power cable from the wall socket the computer is plugged into, into low-voltage DC power. Computers are dependent on a reliable steady supply of DC power to function properly. The more devices and programs used on a computer, the higher the power supply should be to avoid damage and malfunctioning. Power supplies normally range from 160 to 700 W, with an average of 300 to 400 W. Most contemporary power supply units come equipped with at least one fan to cool the unit under heavy use. The power supply is controlled by pressing the on and off switch, and the reset switch (which restarts the system) of a computer.

Laptop and other portable computing machines, such as electronic readers and tablet computers, are equipped with a rechargeable battery power supply and the standard plug-in variety.

Hard Disk This component is so named because of the rigid hard disks that reside in it, which are mounted to a spindle that is spun by a motor when in use. Drive heads (most computers have two or more heads) produce a magnetic field through their transducers that magnetizes the disk surface as a voltage is applied to the disk. The hard disk acts as a permanent data storage area that holds the **gigabytes** or even terabytes worth of data, information, documents, and programs saved on the computer, even when the computer is shut off. Disk drives are not infallible, however, making the need to back up important data imperative.

The computer writes binary data to the **hard drive** by magnetizing small areas of its surface. Each drive head is connected to an actuator that moves along the disk to hover over any point on the disk surface as it spins. The parts of the hard disk are encased in a sealed unit. The hard drive is managed by a disk controller, which is a circuit board that controls the motor and actuator arm assembly. The hard drive produces the voltage waveform that contacts the heads to write and read data, and handles communications with the motherboard. The hard drive is usually located within the computer's hard outer casing. Some people also attach a second hard drive externally, to increase available memory or to backup data.

Main Memory or Random Access Memory **Random access memory** (RAM) is considered to be "volatile" memory because it is a temporary storage system that allows the processor to access program codes and data while working on a task. RAM memory is lost once the system is rebooted, shut off, or loses power.

The memory is actually situated on small chip boards, which sport rows of pins along the bottom edge, and are plugged into the motherboard of the computer. These memory chips contain complex arrays of tiny memory circuits that can be either set by the CPU during write operations (puts them into storage) or read by the CPU during data retrieval. The circuits store the data in binary form as either low (on) voltage stage, expressed as a 0, or high (off) voltage stage, expressed as a 1. All of the work being done on a computer resides in this RAM memory until it is saved onto the hard drive or other storage drive. Computers generally come with 2 GB of RAM or more, and may offer more RAM via graphics cards and other expansion cards.

A select portion of the RAM is called the **main memory**, which serves the **hard disk**, and facilitates interactions between the hard disk and central processor. Main memory is provided by dynamic RAM and is attached to the processor using specific addresses and data buses.

Synchronous or static dynamic RAM is "much faster than conventional (**non-synchronous**) memory because it can synchronize itself with a microprocessor's bus" (Null & Lobur, 2006, p. 8).

ROM ROM is essential permanent or semipermanent nonvolatile memory that stores saved data and is critical in the working of the computer's OS and other activities. ROM is primarily stored in the motherboard but may also be available through the graphics card, other expansion cards, and peripherals. In recent years, rewriteable ROM chips have become available that may include other forms of ROM, such as programmable ROM; erasable ROM; electrically erasable programmable ROM; and a **flash memory** (a variation of electrically erasable programmable ROM).

BIOS Input/Output System This is a specific type of ROM used by the computer when it first boots up, to establish basic communication between the processor, motherboard, and other components. It is often called boot firmware, which controls the computer from the time it is switched on until the primary OS (e.g., Windows, OS X, or Linux) takes over. Then firmware initializes the hardware and boots (loads and executes) the primary OS.

Virtual Memory This special type of memory is stored on the hard disk to provide temporary data storage so data can be swapped in and out of the RAM as needed. This is particularly handy when working with large data-intensive programs, such as games and multimedia.

Integrated Drive Electronics Controller This component is the primary interface for the hard drive, **compact disc read-only memory (CD)-ROM**, or **digital video disc (DVD)** drive, and the floppy disk drive.

Peripheral Component Interconnection Bus This component is important for connecting additional plug-in components to the computer, because it uses a series of slots on the motherboard that allow **peripheral component interconnection card** plug-in.

Small Computer System Interface This component provides the means to attach additional devices, such as scanners and extra hard drives, to the computer.

DVD/CD drive The CD-ROM drive reads and records data to portable CDs, using a laser diode to emit an infrared light beam that reflects onto a track on the CD using a mirror positioned by a motor. The light reflected on the disc is directed by a system of lens to a photo detector that converts the light pulses into an electrical signal that is then decoded by the drive electronics to the motherboard. Both **CD-R (recordable)** and **CD-RW (recordable and rewritable)** drives are common. The same principle applies to **DVD-R** and **DVD-RW** discs. A DVD drive can do everything a CD drive can do, plus it can play, and if it is a recordable unit record, onto blank DVDs.

Flash or USB Drive This is a portable memory device that uses electrically erasable programmable ROM to provide fast permanent memory.

Modem The **modem** is a component that can either be situated externally (external modem) or internally (internal modem) and enables internet connectivity via a cable connection through network adaptors situated within the computer apparatus.

Connection Ports All computers have connection ports made to fit different types of plug-in devices. The ports include monitor cable port, keyboard and mouse ports, network cable port, microphone/speaker/auxiliary input ports, USB ports, and printer ports (small computer system interface or parallel). These ports allow data to move to and from the computer via peripheral or storage devices. Specific ports include the following:

Parallel: connects to a printer

Serial: connects to an external modem

USB: connects to a myriad of plug-in devices, such as portable flash drives, digital cameras, MP3 players, graphics tablets, and light pens, using a plug and play connection (the ability to add devices automatically)

FireWire (IEEE 1394): often used to connect digital-video devices to the computer

Ethernet: connects networking apparatus, such as Internet and modem cables

Graphics Card Most computers come equipped with a graphics accelerator card slotted in the microprocessor of a computer to process image data and output it to the monitor. These in situ graphic cards provide satisfactory graphics quality for two-dimensional art and general text and numerical data. However, if a user intends to create or view three-dimensional images or is an active game user, one or more enhancement graphics cards are often installed.

Video Adapter Cards This component provides video memory, a video processor, and a digital-to-analog converter that works with the CPU to output higher-quality video images to the monitor.

Sound Card The **sound card** converts digital data into an analog signal that is then outputted to the computer's speakers or headphones. The reverse is also accomplished, by inputting a signal from a microphone or other audio recording equipment, which then converts the analog signal to a digital signal.

Bit This is the smallest possible chunk of data memory used in computer processing, exhibited as either a 1 or a 0, making up the **binary system** of the computer.

Byte A **byte** is a chunk of memory that consists of eight **bits**, and is considered to be the best way to indicate computer memory or storage capacity. In modern computers, bytes are reflected as **megabytes (MB)**; gigabytes (GB), which equals 1,000 MB; or **terabytes (TB)**, which equals one trillion or 1,000 GB. Box 3-2 discusses storage capacities.

Software

Software are the application programs developed to facilitate various user functions, such as writing, artwork, organizing meetings, surfing the internet, communicating

BOX

3-2

Storage Capacities

Dee McGonigle and Kathleen Mastrian

Storage and memory capacities are evolving. There have been great leaps in data storage. It all begins with the bit, the basic unit of data storage, composed of zeros and ones or binary digits (bit). A byte is generally considered to be equal to 8 bits. The files on a computer are stored as binary files. The software that is used translates these binary files into words, numbers, pictures, images, or video. Using this binary code in the binary numbering system, measurement is counted by factors of two, such as 1, 2, 4, 8, 16, 32, 64, and 128. To add confusion, the multiples of the binary system in computer usage are prefixed based on the metric system. Therefore, a kilobyte (KB) is actually two to the 10th power (2^{10}) or 1,024 bytes, but is typically considered to be 1,000 bytes. This is why one sees 1,024 or multiples of that number instead of an even 1,000 mentioned at times in relation to kilobytes.

In the early 1980s, kilobytes were the norm as far as computer capacity and 128 KB machines were launched for personal use. The next couple of decades have seen advanced computing power and storage capacity. As capabilities soared so did the ability to save and store what was used and created. Megabytes (MB) emerged, which are actually 1,048,576 bytes but are considered to be 1 million bytes. The next leap was one that some people could not even imagine. Gigabytes (GB) emerged; they are actually 1,073,741,824 bytes but are considered to be 1 billion bytes. Some experts are very concerned that valuable bytes are lost when these measurements are rounded, whereas the hard drive manufacturers are using the decimal system so their capacity is expressed as an even billion bytes per gigabyte.

The next advancements are moving into terabytes (TB), petabytes (PB), **exabytes (EB), zettabytes (ZB),** and **yottabytes (YB)**. Term storage capacity is as follows:

TB	1,000 GB
PB	1,000,000 GB
EB	1,000 PB
ZB	1,000 EB
YB	1,000 ZB

To put all of this in perspective, Williams (n.d., para. 5) writes about the data powers of 10:

2	kilobytes: A typewritten page
2	megabytes: A high resolution photograph
10	megabytes: A minute of high-fidelity sound **OR** a digital chest X-ray
50	megabytes: A digital mammogram
1	gigabyte: A symphony in high-fidelity sound **OR** a movie at TV quality
1	terabyte: All the X-ray films in a large technological hospital

Continues

BOX *(Continued)*

3-2

2 petabytes: All U.S. academic research libraries

5 exabytes: All words ever spoken by human beings

We have not even addressed ZB and YB. Stay tuned. . .

Reference

Williams, R. (n.d.). *Data powers of ten.* Retrieved from http://www.cch.kcl.ac.uk/ legacy/teaching/avmmet/data-powers-of-ten.html

with others, and so forth. For this overview, software has been divided into four categories: (1) OS software, (2) **productivity software**, (3) creativity software, and (4) communication software.

User friendliness is a critical condition for effective software adoption. "End user performance is likely to be facilitated by user friendliness of software packages" (Mahmood, 2003, p. 71). The easier and more intuitive a software package seems to be to a user influences their perception of how clear the package is to understand and to use. The rapid evolution of hardware mentioned previously has been equally matched by the phenomenal development in software over the past three or four decades.

Commercial Software Several large commercial software companies, such as Apple, Microsoft, IBM, and Adobe, dominate market shares in software sales, and have done so since the advent of the personal computer. Licensed software has evolved over time; hence, most have a long version history. Many software packages, such as **office suites**, are expensive to purchase; hence, there is a digital divide as far as access and affordability goes across societal spheres, especially when viewed from a global perspective.

Open Source Software The **open source** movement began several years ago, but recently has become a powerful movement that is changing the software production and consumer market. In addition to commercially available software, there is a growing number of open source software being developed in all four of the categories addressed in this chapter. Open source is a very unique movement begun by developers who wished to offer their creations to others "for the good of the community" and encouraged them to do the same. Users who modify or contribute to the evolution of the software are obligated to share their new code, but essentially, the software is free to all. Open Office and Koffice are both examples of open source productivity software.

OS Software The OS is the most important software on any computer. It is the very first program to load on computer start up, and is fundamental for the operation of all other software and the computer hardware. Examples of commonly used operating systems include the Microsoft Windows family, Linux, Mac OS X, and Unix. The OS manages both the hardware and software and provides a reliable consistent interface for the software applications to work with the computer's hardware. An OS must be both powerful and flexible to adapt to the myriad of types of software available, made by a variety of development companies. New versions of the major OSs are equipped to deal with multiple users and handle multitasking with ease. For instance, a user can work on a word processing document, while listening for an email received signal, have a web browser window open to look for references on the internet as needed, listen to music in the CD drive, and download a file all at the same time. OS tasks can be summarized into six basic processes:

- Memory management
- Device management
- Processor management
- Storage management
- Application interface
- **User interface** (usually a **graphical user interface** [GUI])

OSs should be convenient to use, easy to learn, reliable, safe, and fast. OSs should be easy to design, implement, and maintain, and flexible, reliable, error-free and efficient. For example, Silbershatz, Baer Galvin, and Gagne (2004) described how the Windows OS has been designed with the following goals from Microsoft:

- **Portability:** the OS can be moved from one hardware architecture to another with little changes needed
- **Security:** the OS incorporates hardware protection for virtual memory, and software protection mechanisms for OS resources
- **POSIX** compliance: applications designed to follow the POSIX (IEEE 1003.1) standard can be compiled to run on Windows without changing the source code
- Multiprocessor support: the OS is designed for symmetrical multiprocessing
- **Extensibility:** provided by using a layered architecture with a protected executive layer for basic system services, several server subsystems that operate in user mode, and a modular structure that allows additional environmental subsystems to be added without affecting the executive layer
- International support: the Windows OS supports different locales via the national language support API
- **Compatibility** with MS-DOS and MS-Windows applications

Productivity Software Productivity software, such as office suites, is the most common software used both in the workplace and on personal computers. Several software companies produce these multiple program software, which usually combines **word processing**, **spreadsheets**, **databases**, **presentation**, web development, and email programs all bundled together.

The intent of office suites is generally to provide all of the basic programs that an office or knowledge worker needs to do their work. The bundled programs within the suite are organized to be compatible with one another; are designed to look similar to one another for ease of use; and provide a powerful array of tools for data manipulation, information gathering, and knowledge generation. Some office suites add other programs, such as database creation software, mathematical editors, drawing, and desktop **publishing** programs. Table 3-1 provides a summary

TABLE 3-1
Office Suite Software Features and Examples

| | OFFICE SUITE SOFTWARE | |
Program	Application	Examples
Word processing	Composition, editing, formatting, and producing text documents	Microsoft Word, Open Office Writer, KOffice KWord, Corel WordPerfect or Corel Write, Apple Pages
Spreadsheets	Grid-based documents in ledger format; organizes numbers and text; calculates statistical formulae	Microsoft Excel, Open Office Calc, Koffice Kspread, Corel Quattro Pro, Apple Numbers
Presentations	Slideshow software, usually used for business or classroom presentations using text, images, graphs, media	Microsoft Power Point, Open Office Impress, Koffice KPresenter, Corel Show, Apple Keynote
Databases	Database creation for text and numbers	Microsoft Access (in elite packages), Open Office Base, Koffice Kexi, Corel Calculate, Corel Paradox
E-mail	Integrated e-mail program to send and receive electronic mail	Microsoft Outlook, Corel WordPerfect Mail, Mozilla Thunderbird
Drawing	Graphics and diagram drawing	Open Office Draw, Corel Presentation Graphics, Koffice Kivio, Karbon, Krita
Math formulas	Inserts math equations in word processing and presentation work	Open Office Math, Koffice KFormula
Desktop publishing	Page layouts and publication ready documents	Microsoft Publisher (in elite packages), Apple Pages

of common programs included in five of the most popular office suites: Microsoft Office, Open Office, KOffice, Corel WordPerfect Suite, and Apple iWork (for Mac computers). Of these five, Open Office (for Windows, Linux, Solaris, Mac OS X, FreeBSD, and HP-UX OSs) and Koffice (for Linux environments but also being developed for Windows and Mac OS X platforms) are open source, free software.

Creative Software Creative software includes programs that allow users to draw, paint, render, record music and sound, and incorporate digital video and other multimedia in professional aesthetic ways to share and convey information and knowledge (Table 3-2).

Communication Software Networking and communication software enable users to dialogue, share, and network with other users via the exchange of email or **instant messages,** by accessing the **World Wide Web**, or by engaging in virtual meetings using **conferencing software** (Table 3-3).

TABLE 3-2
Creative Software Features and Examples

CREATIVE SOFTWARE	
Program and Application	**Software Examples**
Raster graphics programs Draw, paint, render, manipulate and edit images, fonts, and photographs to create pixel-based (dot points) digital art and graphics.	Adobe Photoshop and Fireworks, Ulead PhotoImpact, Corel Draw, Painter, and Paint Shop Pro, GIMP (open source), KOffice's Krita (open source)
Vector graphics programs Mathematically rendered, geometric modeling is applied through shapes, curves, lines, points and manipulated for shape, color, size. Ideal for printing and three-dimensional (3D) modeling.	Adobe Flash, Freehand, and Illustrator, CorelDraw and Designer, Open Office Draw (open source), Mirosoft Visio, Xara Xtreme, Koffice Karbon14 (open source)
Desktop publishing programs Page layout and publishing preparation for printed and web documents, such as magazines, journals, books, newsletters, brochures	Adobe InDesign, Corel PageMaker, Microsoft Publisher, Scribus (open source), QuarkXPress, Apple Pages (note that many of the graphics programs can also be used for DTP)
Web design programs Create, edit, update web pages using specific codes, such as XML, CSS, HTML, and JAVA	Adobe Dreamweaver, Coffee Cup, Microsoft FrontPage, Nvu (open source), W3C's Amaya (open source)
Multimedia programs Combines text, audio, images, animation, and video into interactive content for electronic presentation.	Adobe Flash, Microsoft Movie Maker, Apple QuickTime and FinalCut Studio, Corel VideoStudio, Ulead VideoStudio, Real Studio, CamStudio (open source), Audacity (open source)

TABLE 3-3
Communication Software Features and Examples

COMMUNICATION SOFTWARE	
E-mail client Allows user to read, edit, forward, and send email messages to other users via an Internet connection. The software can be resident on the computer or accessed via the World Wide Web	**Resident programs** Microsoft Outlook and Outlook Express, Eudora, Pegasus, Mozilla Thunderbird, Lotus Notes **Web-based programs** Gmail, Yahoo Mail, Hotmail
Internet browsers Enables user to access, browse, download, upload, and interact with text, audio, video, and other web-based documents	Mozilla Firefox, Microsoft Internet Explorer, Google Chrome, Apple Safari, Opera, Microbrowser (for mobile access)
Instant messaging (IM) Real-time text messaging between users, can attach images, videos, and other documents via personal computer, cell phone, hand-held devices	MSN Instant Messenger, Microsoft Live Messenger, Yahoo Messenger, Apple iChat
Conferencing Enables user to communicate in a virtual meeting room setting to share work, discussions, planning, using an intranet or Internet environment; can exhibit files, video, screenshots of content	Adobe Acrobat Connect, Microsoft Live Meeting or Meeting Space, GotoMeeting, Meeting Bridge, Free Conference, RainDance, WebEx

Acquisition of Data and Information (Input Components)

Input devices include the keyboard; mouse; joysticks (usually used for playing computer games); game controllers or pads; web cameras (webcams); stylus (often used with tablets or personal digital assistants); image scanners for copying a digital image of a document or picture; or other plug and play input devices, such as a digital camera, digital video recorder (camcorder), MP3 player, electronic musical instrument, or physiologic monitor (Figure 3-1). These devices are the origin or medium used to input text, visual, audio, or multimedia data into the computer system for viewing, listening, manipulating, creating, or editing. The two primary input devices on a computer are the keyboard and mouse.

Keyboard

Computer **keyboards** are very similar to old typewriter keyboards, and usually serve as the prime input device that enables the user to type words, numbers, and commands into the computer's programs. Standard computer keyboards have 101 keys, and are organized to facilitate Latin-based languages using a **QWERTY** layout (so named because these letters are on the first six keys in the first row of letters).

FIGURE

3-1   Computer System

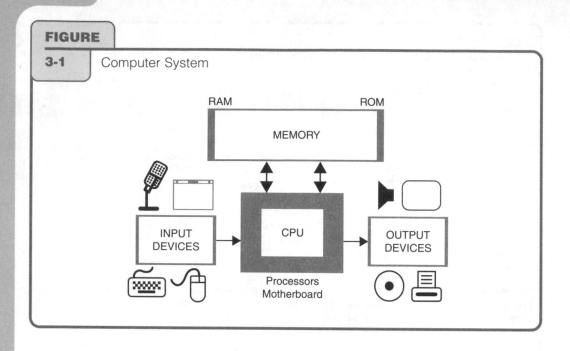

Select keys are used as command keys, particularly the control (CTRL), alternate (Alt), delete (Del), and shift keys, which can all be used to activate useful commands. The escape (ESC) key allows the user instantly to exit a process or program. The F keys, F1 through F12, are function keys. These are used in different ways by particular programs. If a program instructs the user to click on the "F8" key, they would do so by clicking F8. The print screen (PrtSc) key sends a graphical picture or screenshot of a computer screen to the clipboard. This copied screenshot can then be pasted in any graphic program that can work with bitmap files.

Mouse

The **mouse** is the second most common input device, manipulated by the user's hand to point, click, and move objects around on the computer screen. A mouse can come in a number of different configurations including a standard mechanical trackball serial mouse, bus mouse, PS/2 mouse, USB connected mouse, optical lens mouse, cordless mouse, and optomechanical mouse.

Processing of Data and Information (throughput/processing components)

All of the hardware discussed in Section 1 of this chapter is involved in the **throughput** or **processing** of inputted data and in the preparation of output data and information. Specific software is used, depending on the application and data involved. One key hardware component, the computer **monitor**, is a unique example of a visible throughput component because it is the part of the computer focused on the most when users are working on a computer. Inputted data can be visualized and accessed by manipulating the mouse and keyboard input devices, but it is the monitor that receives the user's attention. The monitor is critical for the efficient rendering during this part of the cycle, because it facilitates user access and control of the data and information.

Monitor

The monitor is the visual display that serves as the landscape for all interactions between user and machine. It typically resembles a television screen, and comes in various sizes (usually ranging from 15–21 inches) and configurations. Monitors are either cathode ray tube, which is the conventional monitor with a large section behind the screen, or thinner, flatscreen liquid crystal display devices. Some computer monitors also have a touchscreen that can serve as an input device when the user touches key areas of the screen.

Monitors vary in refresh rate (usually measured in **megahertz**) and in dot pitch. Both of these characteristics are important for user comfort. The faster the refresh rate, the cleaner and clearer the image on the screen because the monitor refreshes the screen contents more frequently. For instance, a monitor with a 100 MHz refresh rate refreshes the screen contents 100 times per second. The higher the dot pitch factor, the smaller the dots that make up the screen image, meaning it provides a more detailed display on the monitor, which also facilitates clarity and ease of viewing.

If equipped with a touchscreen, a monitor can also serve as an input device when activated by a stylus or finger pressure. Some might also consider the monitor to be an output device, because access to inputted and stored documents is often performed via the screen (e.g., reading a document that is stored on the computer or viewable from the Internet).

Dissemination (Output Components)

Output devices carry data in a usable form through exit devices in or attached to a computer. Common forms of output include printed documents; audio or video files; physiologic summaries; scan results; or saved files on portable disc drives, such as a CD, DVD, flash drives, or external hard drive. Output devices literally put data and information at a user's fingertips, which can be used to develop knowledge and even wisdom. The most commonly used output devices include printers, speakers, and portable disc drives.

Printer

Printers are external components that can be attached to a computer using a printer cord that is secured into the computer's printer port. Printers enable users to print a hard paper copy of documents that are housed on the computer.

The most common printer types are the ink jet and the laser printer. Inkjets are more economic to use, with quite good quality, and apply ink to paper using a jetspray mechanism. Laser printers produce publisher-ready quality printing if combined with good quality paper but cost more to print. Both types of printers can print in black and white or in color.

Speakers

All computers have some sort of speaker set up, usually small speakers embedded in the monitor; case; or if a laptop, close to the keyboard. Often, external speakers are added to a computer system by the user, using speaker connectors for enhanced sound and a more enjoyable listening experience.

WHAT IS THE RELATIONSHIP OF COMPUTER SCIENCE TO KNOWLEDGE?

Scholars and researchers are just beginning to understand the effect that computer systems, architecture, applications, and processes have on the potential for knowledge acquisition and development. Users who have access to contemporary computers equipped with full Internet access have resources at their fingertips that were only dreamed of before the 21st century. Entire library collections are accessible, with many documents available in full printable form. Users are able to contribute to the development of knowledge and through the use of productivity, creativity, and communication software. Using the World Wide Web interface, users are also able to disseminate knowledge on a grand scale with other users. The deluge of information available via computers must be mastered and organized by the user for knowledge to emerge. Discernment and the ability to critique and filter this information must also be present to facilitate the further development of wisdom.

The development of an understanding of computer science principles as they apply to technology used in nursing can facilitate optimal usage of the technology for knowledge development in the profession. The maxim that "knowledge is power" and that the skillful use of computers is at the heart of this power is a presumption. "The computer literate nurse will have knowledge, and as a result, power and influence. Society has accepted computers as standard elements, and as such, computers will continue to shape nurses' psychological, social, economic, and political existence in innumerable ways. Nursing, in order to interface with other spheres of society, must be computer literate. In short, society has accepted computer technology as a means to enhance life; so must nursing" (Richards, 2001, p. 9). Once nurses become comfortable with various technologies, they can shape them, refine them, and apply them in new and different ways, just as they have always adapted earlier equipment and technologies.

HOW DOES THE COMPUTER SUPPORT COLLABORATION AND INFORMATION EXCHANGE?

Computers can be linked to other computers through networking software and hardware to promote communication, information exchange, work sharing, and collaboration. **Networks** can be local or organizationally based, joined together into a local area network; or on a wider area scope (e.g., a city or district) using a metropolitan area network; or from an even greater distance (e.g., a whole country or continent, or the Internet itself) using a wide area network configuration (Sarkar, 2006). Network interface cards are used to connect a computer and its modem to a network.

Networks within health care can manifest in several different configurations, including client-focused networks, such as in telenursing, e-health, and client support networks; work-related networks including virtual work and virtual social networks; and learning and research networks as in communities of practice. These trends are still in their infancy in most nursing work environments (and personal lives) but they are predicted to be a strong trend in the future. "As the Net generation grows in influence, the trend will be toward networks, not hierarchies, toward open collaboration rather than authority; toward consensus rather than arbitrary edict. The communication support provided by networks and information systems will also alter patterns of social interaction within a healthcare organization. This technology provides a medium for greater accessibility to shared information and support for rich interpersonal exchange and collaboration across departmental boundaries" (Richards, 2001, p. 10).

Virtual social networks are another form of professional network that have expanded phenomenally since the advent of the Internet and other computer software and hardware. "Electronic media do more than just expand access to vast bodies of information. They also serve as a convenient vehicle for building virtual social networks for creating shared knowledge through collaborative learning and problem solving. Cross pollination of ideas through worldwide connectivity can boost creativity synergistically in the co-construction of knowledge" (Bandura, 2002, p. 4). Nursing-related virtual social networks provide a cyberspace for nurses to make contacts, share information and ideas, and build a sense of community.

Social communication software are used to provide a dynamic virtual environment, and often virtual social networks provide communicative capabilities through posting tools, such as blogs, forums, and wikis; email for sharing ideas on a smaller scale; collaborative areas for interaction, creating, and building digital artifacts or planning projects; navigation tools for moving through the virtual network landscape; and profiles to provide a space for each member to disclose personal information with others. Nurses who have to engage in shift-work often find that virtual social networks can provide a sense of connection with other professionals that is available around the clock. Because time is often a factor in any social interchange, virtual communication often offers an alternative for practicing nurses who can access information and interchange at any time of day. With active participation, the interchanges and shared information and ideas of the network can culminate into valuable social and cultural capital, available to all members. Often, nursing virtual social networks are created for the purpose of exchanging ideas on practice issues and best practices; to become more knowledgeable about new trends, research, and innovations in health care; or to participate in advocacy, activist, and educational initiatives.

Through the use of portable disc devices, such as flash drives, CDs, and DVDs, people can share information, documents, and communications by exchanging files. Since the advent of the Internet in the mid 1980s, the World Wide Web has evolved to become a viable and user-friendly way for people to collaborate and exchange information, projects, and other knowledge-based files, such as websites, email, social networking applications, and web conferencing logs. See Box 3-3 for information on Web 2.0.

BOX 3-3

Web 2.0 Tools

Dee McGonigle, Kathleen Mastrian, and Wendy Mahan

Web 2.0, the new World Wide Web tools, enables users to collaborate, network socially, and disseminate knowledge with other users on a scale that was once not even comprehensible. These programs promote data and information exchange, feedback, and knowledge development and dissemination.

To facilitate a selective review of the Web 2.0 tools available, they have been categorized into three areas: (1) tools for creating and sharing information, (2) tools for collaborating, and (3) tools for communicating. Examples of tools for creating and sharing information include blogs, podcasts, Flickr, YouTube, Hellodeo, jing, Screencast-o-matic, Facebook, MySpace, and MakeBeliefsComix. Examples of tools for collaborating with others include Google Docs, Zoho, wikis, Del.icio.us, and Gliffy. Finally, some tools for communicating with others include Adobe Connect, Vyew, Skype, Twitter, and Instant Messaging.

Through the use of the creating and sharing information tools there has been an explosion of social networking on the Web. YouTube has promoted the "broadcast

Continues

yourself" proliferation. One can launch a video onto YouTube that is shared with others over the Web. Similarly, Flickr allows one to upload and tag personal photos to share either privately or publicly. Facebook and MySpace both promote socializing on the Web. Facebook is a social utility and MySpace is a place for friends according to each of their websites. Other tools let one create and share recorded messages, diagrams, screen captures, and even custom comic strips.

Collaborating over the Web has become easier. It is a way of life for many. Google Docs and Zoho allow one to create online and share and collaborate in real time. Wikis are server-based software programs that enable one to generate and edit webpage content using any browser. Del.icio.us is a social bookmarking manager that uses tags to identify or describe the bookmarks that can be shared with others.

Communicating with others includes audio and video conferencing in real time. Adobe Connect is a comprehensive Web communications solution. It is a fee-based service that does provide a free trial. One should read all of the documentation on their site before downloading, installing, and using this software. Vyew is free, always-on collaboration plus live Web conferencing. Skype allows one to make calls in audio only or with video. One can download Skype for free but depending on the type of calls made, fees or charges could be assessed. One should read through all of the information before downloading, installing, and using this software. Twitter allows one to answer the question "what are you doing" in 140 characters or less. Although Twitter can be used to keep the friends in one's network updated on daily activities, it can also be used for other purposes, such as asking questions or expressing thoughts. In addition, Twitter can be accessed by cell phones, so one can stay in touch on the go.

Along with all of the advantages and intellectual harvesting capabilities from the use of these tools come security issues. Wagner (2007) warns the user to "bear in mind before you jump in that you're giving information to a third-party company to store" (para. 5). He also states that "you should talk to your company's legal and compliance offices to be sure you're obeying the law and regulations with regard to managing company's information" (para. 5). One suggestion that he offers is that if you do not want to involve a third party, "Wikis provide a good alternative for organizations looking to maintain control of their own software. Organizations can install wiki software on their own, internal servers" (para. 6).

This new wave of Web-based tools presents the ability to interact, exchange, collaborate, communicate, and share in ways that have only begun to be envisioned. As the tools and their innovative uses continue to increase, users need to stay vigilant to handle the associated security challenges. These Web 2.0 tools are providing a new cyber playground that is only limited by one's own imaginations and intelligence. We encourage you to explore these tools. Refer to this book's companion website http://go.jblearning.com/mcgonigle for more information.

Reference

Wagner, M. (2007). *Nine easy web-based collaborative tools*. Retrieved from
http://www.forbes.com/2007/02/26/google-microsoft-bluetie-ent-tech-cx_mw_
0226smallbizresource.html

WHAT IS THE HUMAN–TECHNOLOGY INTERFACE?

In the context of using a computer system, the human–technology interface is facilitated by the input and output devices discussed previously in this chapter. Specifically, the keyboard, mouse, monitor, laserpen, joystick, stylus, or game pads and controls, and other USB or plug and play devices, such as **MP3** players, digital cameras, digital camcorders, musical instruments, and hand-held smaller computers, such as personal digital assistants, are all viable devices for interfacing with a computer.

The GUI afforded by the OS of a computer provides the on-screen environment for direct interaction between the user and the computer. The typical GUI provided by Windows or Mac OS X provides a user-friendly desktop metaphor interface that is made up of the input and output devices and icons that represent files, programs, actions, and processes. These interface icons can be activated by clicking the mouse buttons to perform various actions, such as provide information, execute functions, open and manipulate folders (directories), select options, and so forth.

Although these aspects of a computer system may be taken for granted, they are critical in facilitating a sense of comfort and competency in users of the system. This is particularly critical in nursing, when computers are used in the context of nursing care. One question that arises is, do nurses control these information technology tools, or do the "tools" shape the activities, decisions, and attention of the nurses as users of technology? Both possibilities can be answered in the affirmative to some extent, but the former is the safest situation for nursing care. If the nurse user needs to focus on the software or hardware because of difficult programs, confusing GUI schema, or sheer complexity in the programming, the provision of client care is going to suffer. It is critical that software and hardware used in the nursing milieu be expertly designed to facilitate nursing care in a user-friendly, intuitive way. This is one reason that informatics experts, called nurse informaticians, are being placed in positions of authority to facilitate the adoption of computer systems within nursing care environments. It is essential that the activities of the staff nurses are reflected well within the software that is used in the care setting. If nurses are knowledgeable about computers and related technologies, they will be able to provide meaningful data and information about how computer systems best work within their particular care areas.

In an ideal world, nurses would be able effectively to use and interact with computer technologies to enhance patient care. They would understand computer science and how to harness its capabilities to benefit the profession and ultimately their patients.

SUMMARY

The field of computer science is one of the fastest growing disciplines. Astonishing innovations in computer hardware, software, and architecture have occurred over the past few decades and there are no indications that this trend will stop anytime soon. Computers have developed in speed, accuracy, and efficiency, yet also cost less and have reduced physical size. These trends are predicted to continue. Current computer hardware and software offer vital and valuable tools for both nurses and clients to engage in on-screen and on-line activities that provide rich access to data and information. The productivity, creative, and communicative software tools can also enable nurses to work with computers to further foster knowledge acquisition and development. Wide access to vast stores of information and knowledge shared by others also facilitates the emergence of wisdom in users, which can be applied to nursing in meaningful and creative ways. It is imperative that nurses become discerning yet skilled users of computer technology to apply the principles of nursing informatics to practice, and to contribute to the profession's ever growing body of knowledge.

LOOKING TO THE FUTURE

The coming trends in wearable technology, smaller and faster hand-held and portable computer systems, and high-quality voice-activated inventions will further facilitate the use of computers in nursing practice and professional development. The field of computer science will continue to contribute to the evolving art and science of nursing informatics. New trends promise to bring wide-sweeping and it is hoped positive changes to the practice of nursing. Computers and other technologies have the potential to support a more client-oriented healthcare system where clients truly become active participants in their own healthcare planning and decisions. Mobile health technology, tele-nursing, sophisticated electronic health records, and next generation technology are predicted to contribute to high-quality nursing care and consultation within healthcare settings, including patients' homes and communities.

Computers will become more powerful yet more compact, which will contribute to the development of several technologic initiatives that are still in their infancy. The following include some of these initiatives. These predicted innovations are only some of the many computer and technologic applications being developed. As nurses gain proficiency in capitalizing on the creative, time-saving, and interactive capabilities emerging from information technology research, the field of nursing informatics will grow in similar proportions.

Voice-Activated Communicators

Voice activated communicators are already being developed by companies, such as Vocera Communications. These new technologies will permit nurses and other healthcare professionals to use wireless, hands-free devices to communicate with each other, and to record data. This can promote this technology, which promises to become a user-friendly and cost-effective way to increase clinical productivity.

Game and Simulation Technology

Game and simulation technology promises to offer realistic, innovative ways to teach nursing content in general, including nursing informatics concepts and skills. The same technology that powers video games can be used to create dynamic educational interfaces to help student nurses learn about pathophysiology, care guidelines, medication usage, and a host of other topics. These applications can also be very valuable for client education and health promotion materials. The "serious games" industry is just beginning to develop. Video game producers are now looking beyond mere entertainment to address public and private policy, management, and leadership issues and topics, including those related to health care. For example, the Games for Health Project, initiated by the Robert Wood Johnson Foundation (2006), is working on developing best practices to support innovation in healthcare training, messaging, and illness management.

Virtual Reality

Virtual reality is another technologic breakthrough that will become common in nursing education and professional development. Virtual reality is a three-dimensional computer generated "world" where a person (with the right equipment) can move about and interact as if he or she were actually in the visualized location. The person's senses are immersed in this virtual reality world using special gadgetry, such as head-mounted displays, data gloves, joysticks, and other hand tools. The equipment and special technology provides a sense of presence that is lacking in multimedia and other complex programs.

Mobile Devices

Mobile devices will be used more by nurses both at the point-of-care and in planning, documenting, interacting with the healthcare team, and research. "There are strong indicators that nursing is ready to move quickly to adopt this new technology and utilize it to its full potential at the point-of-care. We anticipate the rate of adoption for mobile information systems within nursing to be rapid, and it will ultimately equal and perhaps exceed that of physicians. Mobile Nursing Informatics will be at the core of nursing in the 21st century. Ready access to data and analytical tools will fundamentally change the way practitioners of the health sciences conduct research, and approach and solve problems" (Suszka-Hildebrandt, 2000, p. 3).

WORKING WISDOM

Since the beginning of the profession, nurses have applied their ingenuity, resourcefulness, and professional awareness of what works to adapt technology and objects to support nursing care, usually with the intent to promote efficiency but also client comfort and healing. This resourcefulness could also be applied effectively to the adaptation of information technology within the care environment, to ensure that the technology truly does serve clients and nurses, and the rest of the interdisciplinary team.

Consider this question: "How can you develop competency in using the various computer hardware and software not only to promote efficient nursing care, and develop yourself professionally, but also to further the development of the profession's body of knowledge?"

APPLICATION SCENARIO

Dan P. is a first year student in graduate studies in nursing. In the past, he has learned to use his family's personal computer to surf the World Wide Web, exchange email with friends, and play some computer games. However, he now realizes that the computer is a vital tool for his academic success and has saved up enough money to purchase a laptop computer. He has decided on a Pentium CPU system with 400 GB of ROM and 2 GB of RAM. Now he wishes to choose appropriate software for his system. He is on a limited budget, but wants to make the most of his investment.

Which of the four categories of software discussed in this chapter would benefit Dan the most in his studies (OS, productivity, creativity, or communication)? Dan definitely needs an OS, this is critical. He would also directly benefit from productivity software and at least connective email and web browser software from the communication group so he can access the Internet for research and collaborating with peers and communicating with his teachers.

How could Dan afford to install software from all four groups on his new laptop? If Dan accessed some open source software (e.g., Open Office for his productivity software) he could save money to put toward **creativity software**.

THOUGHT-PROVOKING Questions **www**

1. How can knowledge of computer hardware and software help nurses to participate in information technology adoption decisions in the practice area?
2. How can new computer software help nurses engage in professional development, collaboration, and knowledge dissemination activities at their own pace and leisure?

For a full suite of assignments and additional learning activities, use the access code located in the front of your book to visit this exclusive website: http://go.jblearning.com/mcgonigle. If you do not have an access code, you can obtain one at the site.

www

Internet and Software Resources

BBC Absolute Beginner's Guide to using your computer. A WebWise Guide. http://www.bbc.co.uk/webwise/abbeg/abbeg.shtml

BBC's Computer Tutor: The BBC's guide to using a computer. http://www.bbc.co.uk/computertutor/computertutorone/index.shtml

References

Bandura, A. (2002). Growing primacy of human agency in adaptation and change in the electronic era. *European Psychologist, 7*(1), 2–16.

Evans, D. (2010). *Introduction to computing: Explorations in language, logic, and machines.* University of Virginia. Retrieved from http://www.computingbook.org

Hennessy, J., & Patterson, D. (2006). *Computer architecture: A quantitative approach* (4th ed.). San Francisco, CA: Morgan Kaufmann.

Intel Corporation. (2008). *Concealing complexity.* Technology and Research. Retrieved from http://techresearch.intel.com/articles/Exploratory/1430.htm

Mahmood, M. (2003). *Advanced topics in end user computing.* Hershey, PA: Idea Group Inc.

Null, L., & Lobor, J. (2006). *The essentials of computer organization and architecture* (2nd ed.). Sudbury, MA: Jones & Bartlett Publishing.

Richards, J. A. (2001). Nursing in a digital age. *Nursing Economic$, 19*(1), 6–12.

Robert Woods Johnson Foundation. (2006). *Games for health.* Retrieved from http://www.gamesforhealth.org/index3.html

Sarkar, N. (2006). *Tools for teaching computer networking and hardware concepts.* Hershey, PA: Idea Group Inc.

Silbershatz, A., Baer Galvin, P., & Gagne, G. (2004). *Operating system concepts* (7th ed.). Hoboken, NJ: John Wiley & Sons.

Suszka-Hildebrandt, S. (2000). *Mobile information technology at the point-of-care.* PDA Cortex. Retrieved from http://www.rnpalm.com/mitatpoc.htm

CHAPTER 4

Introduction to Cognitive Science and Cognitive Informatics

Dee McGonigle and Kathleen Mastrian

1. Describe cognitive science.
2. Assess how our minds process and generate information and knowledge.
3. Explore cognitive informatics.
4. Examine artificial intelligence and its relationship to cognitive science and computer science.

www

Key Terms

www

Artificial intelligence
Brain
Cognitive informatics
Cognitive science
Computer science
Connectionism
Decision making
Empiricism
Epistemology
Intelligence
Intuition
Knowledge
Logic
Memory
Mind
Neuroscience
Perception
Problem solving
Psychology
Rationalism
Reasoning
Wisdom

INTRODUCTION

Cognitive science is the fourth of four basic building blocks used to understand informatics. Section I began by examining nursing science, information science and computer science and how each relates to and helps one understand the concept of informatics. This chapter explores the building blocks of cognitive science, **cognitive informatics** (CI), and **artificial intelligence** (AI).

Throughout the centuries, cognitive science has intrigued philosophers and educators alike. Beginning in Greece, the ancient philosophers sought to comprehend how the **mind** works and the nature of **knowledge**. This age-old quest for unraveling the processes inherent in the working **brain** has been under study by the greatest minds. However, it was only about 50 years ago that computer operations and actions were linked to cognitive science, theories of the mind, intellect, or brain. This led to the expansion of cognitive science to examine the complete array of cognitive processes from lower-level perceptions to high-level critical thinking, logical analysis, and reasoning. The focus of this chapter is the impact on nursing informatics (NI). This section provides the reader with an introduction and overview of cognitive science, nature of knowledge, wisdom, and AI as they apply to the Foundation of Knowledge model and NI. The applications to NI include problem solving, decision support systems, usability issues, user-centered interfaces and systems, and the development and use of terminologies.

COGNITIVE SCIENCE

The interdisciplinary field of cognitive science studies the mind, **intelligence**, and behavior from an information processing perspective. According to Wikipedia (2007), "The term cognitive science was coined by Christopher Longuet-Higgins in his 1973 commentary on the Lighthill report, which concerned the then-current state of artificial intelligence research" (para. 1). The Cognitive Science Society and the Cognitive Science Journal date back to 1980 (Cognitive Science Society, 2005). Their interdisciplinary base arises from **psychology**, philosophy, **neuroscience**, **computer science**, linguistics, biology, and physics and covers **memory**, attention, perception, reasoning, language, mental ability, and computational models of cognitive processes and the nature of the mind, knowledge representation, language, problem solving, decision making, and the social factors influencing the design and use of technology. Simply defined, cognitive science is the study of the mind and how information is processed in the mind. As described in the Stanford Encyclopedia of Philosophy,

> The central hypothesis of cognitive science is that thinking can best be understood in terms of representational structures in the mind and computational procedures that operate on those structures. While there is much disagreement about the nature of the representations and computations that constitute thinking, the central hypothesis is general enough to encompass the current range of thinking in cognitive science, including connectionist theories which model thinking using artificial neural networks (2010, para. 9).

Connectionism is a component of cognitive science that uses computer modeling through artificial neural networks to explain human intellectual abilities. Neural networks can be thought of as interconnected simple processing devices or simplified models of the brain and nervous system that consist of a considerable number of elements or units (analogs of neurons) linked together in a pattern of connections (analogs of synapses). A neural network that models the entire nervous system would have three types of units: (1) input units (analogs of sensory neurons), which receive information to be processed; (2) hidden units (analogs to all of the other neurons, not sensory or motor), which work in between input and output units; and (3) output units (analogs of motor neurons), where the outcomes or results of the processing are found.

Connectionism is rooted in how computation occurs in the brain and nervous system or biologic neural networks. On its own, a neuron has minimal computational capacity, but when interconnected with other neurons they have immense computational power. The connectionism system or model learns by modifying the connections linking the neurons. Just as neurons form elaborate information processing networks, artificial neural networks are unique computer programs that model or simulate their biologic analogs.

The mind is frequently compared to a computer and experts in computer science strive to understand how the mind processes data and information, whereas experts in cognitive science model human thinking using artificial networks provided by computers. Some refer to the latter as AI. How does the mind process all of the inputs received? What and how are things stored or placed into memory, accessed, augmented, changed, reconfigured, and restored? Cognitive science provides the scaffolding for the analysis and modeling of complicated, multifaceted human performance and has a tremendous effect on the issues impacting informatics. The end user is the focus because the concern is with enhancing the performance in the workplace; in nursing, the end user could be the actual clinician in the clinical setting, and cognitive science can enhance the integration and implementation of the technologies being designed to facilitate this knowledge worker with the ultimate goal of improving patient care. Technologies change rapidly, and this evolution must be harnessed for the clinician at the bedside. To do this at all levels of nursing practice, one must understand the nature of knowledge, the information and knowledge needed, and how the nurse processes this information and knowledge in the situational context.

SOURCES OF KNOWLEDGE

Just as philosophers have questioned the nature of knowledge, they have also strived to determine how it arises, because the origins of knowledge can help one understand its nature. How do people come to know what they know about themselves, others, and their world? There are many viewpoints on this issue, both scientific and nonscientific.

Holt (2006) stated that "There are two competing traditions concerning the ultimate source of our knowledge: **empiricism** and **rationalism**" (para. 3). Empiricism is based on knowledge being derived from experiences or senses, whereas rationalism contends that "some of our knowledge is derived from reason alone and that reason plays an important role in the acquisition of all of our knowledge" (para. 5). Empiricists do not recognize innate knowledge, whereas rationalists believe that reason is more essential in the acquisition of knowledge than the senses.

There are three sources of knowledge: (1) instinct, (2) reason, and (3) intuition. Instinct is when one reacts without reason, such as when a car is heading toward someone and he jumps out of the way instinctively. Instinct is found in humans and animals, whereas reason and intuition are found only in humans. Reason "Collects facts, generalizes, reasons out from cause to effect, from effect to cause, from premises to conclusions, from propositions to proofs" (Sivananda, 2004, para. 4). **Intuition** is a way of acquiring knowledge that cannot be obtained by inference, deduction, observation, reason, analysis, or experience. Intuition was termed by Aristotle as "A leap of understanding, a grasping of a larger concept unreachable by other intellectual means, yet fundamentally an intellectual process" (Shallcross & Sisk, 1999, para. 4).

Some believe that knowledge is acquired through perception and logic. **Perception** is the process of acquiring knowledge about the environment or situation by obtaining, interpreting, selecting, and organizing sensory information from seeing, hearing, touching, tasting, and smelling. **Logic** is "[a] science that deals with the principles and criteria of validity of inference and demonstration: the science of the formal principles of **reasoning**" (Merriam-Webster, 2007, para. 1). Acquiring knowledge through logic requires reasoned action to make valid inferences.

The sources of knowledge provide a variety of inputs, throughputs, and outputs through which knowledge is processed. No matter how one believes knowledge is acquired, it is important to be able to explain or describe those beliefs, communicate those thoughts, enhance shared understanding, and discover the nature of knowledge.

NATURE OF KNOWLEDGE

Epistemology is the study of the nature and origin of knowledge—what it means to know. Everyone has a conception of what it means to know based on their own perceptions, education, and experiences; knowledge is a part of life that continues to grow with the person. Thus, a definition of knowledge is somewhat difficult to agree on because it reflects the viewpoints, beliefs, and understandings of the person or group defining it. Some people believe that it is a sequential process resembling a pyramid with data on the bottom, rising to information, then knowledge, and finally wisdom. Others believe that knowledge arises from interactions and experience with the environment, and still others think that it is religiously or culturally bound. It is thought to be an internal process derived through thinking and cognition or an external process from senses, observations, studies, and interactions. Descartes' important premise "called 'the way of ideas' represents the attempt in epistemology to provide a foundation for our knowledge of the external world (as well as our knowledge of the past and of other minds) in the mental experiences of the individual" (Encyclopedia Britannica, 2007, para. 4). For the purpose of this text, knowledge is defined as the awareness and understanding of a set of information and ways that information can be made useful to support a specific task or arrive at a decision; it abounds with others' thoughts and information or is information that is synthesized so that relationships are identified and formalized.

HOW KNOWLEDGE AND WISDOM ARE USED IN DECISION MAKING

The reason for collecting and building data, information, and knowledge is to be able to make informed, judicious, prudent, and intelligent decisions. When one considers the nature of knowledge and its applications, one must also examine the concept of wisdom. **Wisdom** has been defined as knowledge applied in a practical way or translated into actions; to use knowledge and experience to heighten common sense and insight to exercise sound judgment in practical matters; sometimes thought of as the highest form of common sense resulting from accumulated knowledge or erudition (deep, thorough learning) or enlightenment (education that results in understanding and the dissemination of knowledge); it is the ability to apply valuable and viable knowledge, experience, understanding, and insight while being prudent and sensible; is focused on our own minds; the synthesis of our experience, insight, understanding, and knowledge; the appropriate use of knowledge to solve human problems. It is knowing when and how to apply knowledge. The **decision-making** process revolves around knowledge and wisdom. It is through efforts to understand the nature of knowledge and its evolution to wisdom that one can conceive of, build, and implement informatics tools that enhance and mimic the mind's processes to facilitate decision making and job performance.

COGNITIVE INFORMATICS

Wang (2003) describes (CI) as an emerging transdisciplinary field of study that bridges the gap of understanding how information is processed in the mind and in the computer. Computing and informatics theories can be applied to help understand the information processing of the brain, and cognitive and neurologic sciences can likewise be applied to build better and more efficient computer processing systems. Wang suggests that the common issue among the human knowledge sciences is developing an understanding of natural intelligence and human problem solving. Pacific Northwest National Laboratory (PNNL), operated for the US Department of Energy (2008), suggests the disciplines of neuroscience, linguistics, AI, and psychology comprise this field. It defines CI as "the multidisciplinary study of cognition and information sciences, which investigates human information processing mechanisms and processes and their engineering applications in computing" (para. 1). CI helps to bridge this gap by systematically exploring the mechanisms of the brain and mind and exploring specifically how information is acquired, represented, remembered, retrieved, generated, and communicated. This dawning of understanding can then be applied and modeled in AI situations resulting in more efficient computing applications. Wang explains further:

> Cognitive informatics attempts to solve problems in two connected areas in a bidirectional and multidisciplinary approach. In one direction, CI uses informatics and computing techniques to investigate cognitive science problems, such as memory, learning and reasoning; in the other direction, CI uses cognitive theories to investigate the problems in informatics, computing, and software engineering. (p. 120)

CI and Nursing Practice

According to Mastrian (2008), the recognition of the potential application of principles of cognitive science to NI is relatively new. The traditional and widely accepted definition of NI advanced by Graves and Corcoran (1989) is that NI is a combination of nursing science, computer science, and information science used to describe the processes nurses use to manage data, information, and knowledge in nursing practice. Turley (1996) proposed the addition of cognitive science to the mix as nurse scientists strived to capture and explain the influence of the human brain on data, information, and knowledge processing and how these in turn affect nursing decision making. The need to include cognitive sciences is imperative as one attempts to model and support nursing decision making in complex computer programs.

In 2003, Wang proposed the term CI as a branch of information and computer sciences that investigates and explains information processing in the human brain. The science of CI grew out of interest in AI as computer scientists developed computer programs that mimic the information processing and knowledge generation functions of the human brain. CI bridges the gap between artificial and natural intelligence and enhances the understanding of how information is acquired, processed, stored, and retrieved so that these functions can be modeled in computer software.

What does this have to do with nursing? At its very core, nursing practice requires **problem solving** and decision making. Nurses help people manage their responses to illnesses and identify ways that they can maintain or restore their health. Nurses must first recognize that there is a problem to be solved, identify the nature of the problem, pull information from knowledge stores that is relevant to the problem, decide on a plan of action, implement the plan, and evaluate the effectiveness of the interventions. When one has practiced the science of nursing for some time, one tends to do these processes automatically; it is instinctively known what needs to be done to intervene in the problem. What happens, however, if faced with a situation or problem with which one has no experience on which to draw? The ever increasing acuity and complexity of patient situations coupled with the explosion of information in health care has fueled the development of decision support software for nursing. This software models the human and natural decision making processes of professionals in an artificial program. These systems can help decision makers to consider the consequences of different courses of action before implementing the action. They also provide stores of information that the user may not be aware of and can use to choose the best course of action and ultimately make a better decision in unfamiliar circumstances.

Decision support programs continue to evolve as research in the fields of cognitive science, AI, and CI is continuously generated and then applied to the development of these systems. One must embrace, not resist, these advances as support and enhancement of the practice of nursing science.

WHAT IS AI?

The field of AI deals with the conception, development, and implementation of informatics tools based on intelligent technologies. This field captures the complex processes of human thought and intelligence. Herbert Simon believes that the field of AI could have two functions: "One is to use the power of computers to augment human thinking, just as we use motors to augment human or horse power. The other is to use a computer's artificial intelligence to understand how humans think. In a humanoid way" (Association for the Advancement of Artificial Intelligence [AAAI], 2007a, para. 1). According to the AAAI (2007b), AI is the "scientific understanding of the mechanisms underlying thought and intelligent behavior and their embodiment in machines" (para. 2). John McCarthy, one of the men credited with founding the field of AI in the 1950s, stated that AI "is the science and engineering of making intelligent machines, especially intelligent computer programs. It is related to the similar task of using computers to understand human intelligence, but AI does not have to confine itself to methods that are biologically observable" (AAAI, 2007b, para. 4). Lamont (2007) interviewed Ray Kurzweil, a visionary who defined AI as "the ability to perform a task that is normally performed by natural intelligence, particularly human natural intelligence. We have in fact artificial intelligence that can perform many tasks that used to require—and could only be done by—human intelligence" (para. 6). The intelligence factor is extremely important in AI and has been defined by McCarthy as "the computational part of the ability to achieve goals in the world. Varying kinds and degrees of intelligence occur in people, many animals and some machines" (AAAI, 2007b, para. 4).

The challenge of this field rests in capturing, mimicking, and creating the complex processes of the mind in informatics tools, including software, hardware, and other machine technologies with the goal that the tool be able to initiate and generate its own mechanical thought processing. The brain's processing is highly intricate and complicated. This complexity is reflected in Cohn's (2006) comment that "Artificial intelligence is 50 years old this summer, and while computers can beat the world's best chess players, we still can't get them to think like a 4-year-old" (para. 1). AI uses cognitive science and computer science to replicate and generate human intelligence. This field will continue to evolve and produce artificially intelligent tools to enhance personal and professional lives.

SUMMARY

Cognitive science is the interdisciplinary field that studies the mind, intelligence, and behavior from an information processing perspective. CI is a field of study that bridges the gap of understanding how information is processed in the mind and in the computer. Computing and informatics theories can be applied to help understand the information processing of the brain, and cognitive and neurologic sciences can likewise be applied to build better and more efficient computer processing systems. AI is the field that deals with the conception, development, and implementation of informatics tools based on intelligent technologies. This field captures the complex processes of human thought and intelligence. AI uses cognitive science and computer science to replicate and generate human intelligence. The sources of knowledge, nature of knowledge, and rapidly changing technologies must be harnessed by clinicians to enhance their bedside care. Therefore, we must understand the nature of knowledge, the information and knowledge needed, and how nurses process this information and knowledge in their own situational context. The reason for collecting and building data, information, and knowledge is to be able to build wisdom, the ability to apply valuable and viable knowledge, experience, understanding, and insight while being prudent and sensible; it is focused on our own minds, the synthesis of our experience, insight, understanding, and knowledge. Nurses must use their wisdom and make informed, judicious, prudent, and intelligent decisions while enacting care. Cognitive science, CI, and AI will continue to evolve to help build knowledge and wisdom.

THOUGHT-PROVOKING Questions

WWW

1. How would you describe CI? Reflect on a plan of care that you have developed for a patient. How could CI be used to create tools to help with this important work?

2. Think of a clinical setting with which you are familiar and envision AI tools. Are there any current tools in use? What tools would enhance practice in this setting and why?

For a full suite of assignments and additional learning activities, use the access code located in the front of your book to visit this exclusive website: **http://go.jblearning.com/mcgonigle**. If you do not have an access code, you can obtain one at the site.

WWW

References

Association for the Advancement of Artificial Intelligence. (2007a). AI overview. Retrieved from http://www.aaai.org/AITopics/ html/ overview.html

Association for the Advancement of Artificial Intelligence. (2007b). Cognitive science. Retrieved from http://www.aaai.org/ aitopics/pmwiki/pmwiki.php/AITopics/Cognitive Science

Cognitive Science Society. (2005). CSJ archive. Retrieved from http://www.cogsci.rpi.edu/CSJarchive/1980v04/index.html

Cohn, D. (2006). AI reaches the golden years. Retrieved from http://www.wired.com/news/technology/0,71389-0.html

Encyclopedia Britannica. (2007). Epistemology. Retrieved from http://www.britannica.com/eb/article-247960/epistemology

Holt, T. (2006). Sources of knowledge. Retrieved from http://www. theoryofknowledge.info/sourcesof knowledge.html

Graves, J., & Corcoran, S. (1989). The study of nursing informatics. Image: Journal of Nursing Scholarship, 21(4), 227–230.

Lamont, I. (2007). The grill: Ray Kurzweil talks about 'augmented reality' and the singularity. Retrieved from http://www.computerworld.com/action/article.do?command=viewArticleBasic&articleId=306176

Mastrian, K. (February, 2008). Invited editorial: cognitive informatics and nursing practice. Online Journal of Nursing Informatics, 12(1). Retrieved from http://ojni.org/12_1/ kathy.html

Merriam-Webster Online Dictionary. (2007). Logic. Retrieved from http://www.m-w.com/cgi-bin/netdict?logic

Pacific Northwest National Laboratory (US Department of Energy). (2008). Cognitive informatics. Retrieved from http://www.pnl.gov/coginformatics/

Shallcross, D. J., & Sisk, D. A. (1999). What is intuition? In T. Arnold (Ed.), Hyponoesis glossary: Intuition. Retrieved from http://www. hyponoesis.org/html/glossary/intu_n.html

Sivananda, S. (2004). Four sources of knowledge. Retrieved from http://www.dlshq.org/messages/knowledge.htm

Stanford Encyclopedia of Philosophy. (2010). Cognitive science. Retrieved from http://plato.stanford.edu/entries/cognitive-science/

Turley (1996). Toward a model for nursing informatics. Image: Journal of Nursing Scholarship 28(4), 309–313.

Wang, Y. (2003). Cognitive informatics: A new transdisciplinary research field. Brain and Mind, 4(2), 115–127.

Wikipedia. (2007). Cognitive science. Retrieved from http://en.wikipedia.org/wiki/Cognitive_science

CHAPTER 5

Ethical Applications of Informatics

Kathleen Mastrian, Dee McGonigle, and Nedra Farcus

Objectives

1. Recognize ethical dilemmas in nursing informatics.
2. Examine ethical implications of nursing informatics.
3. Evaluate professional responsibilities for the ethical use of healthcare informatics technology.
4. Explore the ethical model for ethical decision making.
5. Analyze practical ways of applying the ethical model for ethical decision making to manage ethical dilemmas in nursing informatics.

WWW

Key Terms

WWW

Alternatives
Antiprinciplism
Autonomy
Beneficence
Bioethics
Bioinformatics
Care ethics
Casuist approach
Confidentiality
Consequences
Courage
Decision making
Decision support
Duty
Ethical decision making
Ethical dilemma
Ethical, social, and legal
  implications
Ethicist
Ethics
Eudaemonistic
Fidelity
Good
Harm
Justice
Liberty
Moral dilemmas
Moral rights
Morals

Continues

INTRODUCTION

Those who followed the actual events of Apollo 13, or who were entertained by the movie (Howard, 1995), watched the astronauts try against all odds to bring their crippled spaceship back to Earth. The speed of their travel was incomprehensible to most viewers, and the task of bringing the spaceship back to Earth seemed nearly impossible. They were experiencing a crisis never imagined by the experts at NASA, and they made up their survival plan moment by moment. What brought them back to Earth safely? Surely, credit must be given to the technology and the spaceship's ability to withstand the trauma it experienced. What is most amazing, however, are the traditional nontechnologic tools, skills, and supplies that were used in new and different ways to stabilize the spacecraft's environment and keep the astronauts safe while traveling toward their uncertain future.

This sense of constancy in the midst of change serves to stabilize experience in many different life events and contributes to the survival of crisis and change. This rhythmic process is also vital to the healthcare system's stability and survival in the presence of the rapidly changing events of the Knowledge Age. No one can dispute the fact that the Knowledge Age is changing health care in ways that will not be fully recognized and understood for years. The change is paradigmatic and every expert who addresses this change reminds healthcare professionals of the need to go with the flow of rapid change or be left behind.

As with any paradigm shift, a new way of viewing the world brings with it some of the enduring values of the previous worldview. As health care journeys into the brave new world of digital communications, it brings some familiar tools and skills recognized in the form of **values**, such as **privacy**, **confidentiality**, autonomy, and nonmaleficence. Although these basic values remain unchanged, the **standards** for living out these values will take on new meaning as health professionals are confronted with new and different moral dilemmas brought on by technologic tools for information management and knowledge development. Ethical decision-making frameworks will remain constant, but the context for examining these moral issues or ethical dilemmas will become increasingly complex.

This chapter provides some familiar ethical concepts to consider on the challenging journey into the increasingly complex future of healthcare informatics. Ethics and bioethics are briefly defined and the evolution of ethical approaches from the Hippocratic ethic era through principlism and to the current antiprinciplism movement of ethical **decision making** are examined. New and challenging ethical dilemmas are surfacing in the venture into the unfolding era of healthcare informatics. Also presented are some of the more recent literature related to these issues. The reader is challenged to think constantly and carefully about ethics as they become involved in healthcare informatics and to stay abreast of new developments in ethical approaches.

ETHICS

Ethics is a process of systematically examining varying viewpoints related to moral questions of right and wrong. **Ethicists** have defined the term in a variety of ways, with each reflecting a basic theoretical philosophic perspective. Beauchamp and Childress (1994) refer to ethics as a generic term for various ways of understanding and examining the moral life. Ethical approaches to this examination may be normative, presenting standards of right or **good** action; descriptive, reporting what people believe and how they act; or explorative, analyzing the concepts and methods of ethics. Husted and Husted (1995) emphasize a practice-based ethics, stating "ethics examines the ways men and women can exercise their power in order to bring about human benefit—the ways in which one can act in order to bring about the conditions of happiness" (p. 3). Velasquez, Andre,

Shanks, and Myer (1987) posed the question, What is ethics?, and answered this question with the following two-part response: "First, ethics refers to well-based standards of right and wrong that prescribe what humans ought to do, usually in terms of **rights**, obligations, benefits to society, fairness, or specific virtues" (para. 10); and "Secondly, ethics refers to the study and development of one's ethical standards" (para. 11). Regardless of the theoretical definition, common characteristics regarding ethics are its dialectical, goal-oriented approach to answering questions that have the potential for multiple acceptable answers.

BIOETHICS

Bioethics is defined as the study and formulation of healthcare ethics. Bioethics takes on relevant ethical problems experienced by healthcare providers in the provision of care to individuals and groups. Husted and Husted (1995) state the fundamental background of bioethics that forms its essential nature is "1. The nature and needs of humans as living, thinking beings; 2. The purpose and function of the healthcare system in a human society; and 3. An increased cultural awareness of human beings' essential moral status" (p. 7). Bioethics arose in the 1970s as health care began to change its focus from a mechanistic approach of treating disease to a more holistic approach of treating people with illnesses. As technology advanced, recognition and acknowledgment of rights and the needs of individuals and groups receiving this high-tech care also increased.

ETHICAL DILEMMAS AND MORALS

Ethical dilemmas arise when moral issues raise questions that cannot be answered with a simple, clearly defined rule, fact, or authoritative view. **Morals** refer to social convention about right and wrong human conduct that is so widely shared that it forms a stable (although usually incomplete) communal consensus (Beauchamp & Childress, 1994). **Moral dilemmas** arise with uncertainty, as is the case when the evidence one is confronted with indicates an action is morally right and other evidence indicates that this action is also morally wrong. **Uncertainty** is stressful and in the face of inconclusive evidence on both sides of the dilemma, causes the person to question what he or she should do. There are times when the individual concludes that based on his or her moral beliefs, he or she cannot act. Uncertainty also arises from unanticipated effects or unforeseeable behavioral responses to actions or the lack of action. Adding uncertainty to the situational factors and personal beliefs that must be considered creates a need for an ethical decision-making model to help one choose the best action.

ETHICAL DECISION MAKING

Ethical decision making refers to the process of making informed choices about ethical dilemmas based on a set of standards differentiating right from wrong.

The decision making reflects an understanding of the principles and standards of ethical decision making, and philosophic approaches to ethical decision making, and it requires a systematic framework for addressing the complex and often controversial moral questions.

As the high-speed era of digital communications progresses, the rights and the needs of individuals and groups will be of the utmost concern to all healthcare professionals. The changing meaning of communication alone will bring with it new concerns by healthcare professionals for protecting patients' rights of confidentiality, privacy, and autonomy. Systematic and flexible ethical decision-making abilities will be essential for all healthcare professionals. The concept of nonmaleficence, or do no **harm**, will be broadened to include those individuals and groups one may never see in person, but with whom one will enter into a professional relationship of trust and care. Mack (2000) discussed the popularity of individuals seeking information online instead of directly from their healthcare providers and the effects this has on patient–provider relationships. He is emphatic in his reminder that, "organizations and individuals that provide health information on the Internet have obligations to be trustworthy, provide high-quality content, protect users' privacy, and adhere to standards of best practices for online commerce and online professional services in healthcare" (p. 41). Makus (2001) suggests that both autonomy and justice are enhanced with universal access to information, but that tensions may be created in patient–provider relationships as a result of this access to outside information. Healthcare workers need to realize that they are no longer the sole providers and gatekeepers of health-related information and that they should embrace information empowerment and suggest websites to patients that contain reliable, accurate, and relevant information (Resnick, 2001). It is clear that patients' increasing use of the Internet for healthcare information may prompt entirely new types of ethical issues, such as who is responsible if a patient is harmed as a result of following online health advice. Derse and Miller (2008) discuss this issue extensively and conclude that there is a clear line between information and practice. Practice occurs when there is direct or personal communication between the provider and the patient, when the advice is tailored to the patient's specific health issue, and when there is a reasonable expectation that the patient will act in reliance on the information.

A summit sponsored by the Internet Healthcare Coalition (www.ihealthcoalition.org) in 2000, developed the E-Health Code of Ethics, which includes eight standards for the ethical development of health-related Internet sites: (1) candor, (2) honesty, (3) quality, (4) informed consent, (5) privacy, (6) professionalism, (7) responsible partnering, and (8) accountability. For more information about each of these standards, access the full discussion of the E-Health code of ethics (http://www.ihealthcoalition.org/ehealth-code/). It is important to realize that the standards for ethical development of health-related Internet sites are voluntary;

there is no overseer perusing these sites and issuing safety alerts for users. Although there are sites that carry a specific symbol indicating that they have been reviewed and are trustworthy (HONcode and Trust-e), the healthcare provider cannot control what patients are accessing or their perceptions of and action related to the health information they find online. See Research Brief on a study of consumer perceptions of health information on the web.

THEORETICAL APPROACHES TO HEALTHCARE ETHICS

Theoretical approaches to healthcare ethics have evolved in response to societal changes. In a 30-year retrospective article for the *Journal of the American Medical Association*, Pellegrino (1993) traced the evolution of healthcare ethics from the Hippocratic ethic through principlism and into the current antiprinciplism movement. The Hippocratic tradition emerged from relatively homogenous societies where beliefs were similar and most societal members shared common values. The emphasis was on **duty**, virtue, and gentlemanly conduct.

Principlism arose as societies became more heterogeneous and members began experiencing a diversity of incompatible beliefs and values. Principlism emerged as a foundation for ethical decision making. Principles were expansive enough to be shared by all rational individuals, regardless of their background and individual beliefs. This approach continued into the 1900s and was popularized by two bioethicists, Beauchamp and Childress (1977, 1994), in the last quarter of 20th century. Principles are considered as broad guidelines that provide guidance or direction but leave substantial room for case-specific judgment. From principles, one can develop more detailed rules and policies. Beauchamp and Childress (1994) proposed four principles: (1) respect for autonomy, (2) nonmaleficence, (3) beneficence, and (4) justice. **Nonmaleficence** asserts an obligation not to inflict harm intentionally and forms the framework for the standard of due care to be met by any professional. Obligations of nonmaleficence are obligations of not inflicting harm and not imposing risks of harm.

Research Brief

Using an online survey of 1,227 randomly selected respondents, Bodkin and Miaoulis (2007) sought to describe the characteristics of information seekers on eHealth websites, the types of information they seek, and their perceptions of the quality and ethics of the websites. Of the respondents, they found that 74% had sought health information on the Web with women accounting for 55.8% of the health information seekers. A total of 50% of the seekers were between 35 and 54 years of age. Nearly two thirds of the users began their searches using a general search engine rather than a health-specific site, unless they were seeking information related to symptoms or diseases. Top reasons for seeking information were related to diseases or symptoms of medical conditions, medication information, health news, health insurance, locating a doctor, and Medicare or Medicaid information. The level of education of information seekers was related to the ratings of website quality in that more educated seekers found health information websites more understandable, but were more likely to perceive bias in the website information. The researchers also found that the ethical codes for eHealth websites seem to be increasing consumers trust in the safety and quality of information found on the Web, but that most consumers are not comfortable purchasing health products or services online.

SOURCE: Bodkin, C., & Miaoulis, G. (2007). eHealth information quality and ethics issues: an exploratory study of consumer perceptions. *International Journal of Pharmaceutical and Healthcare Marketing, 1*(1), 27-42. Retrieved from ABI/INFORM Global (Document ID: 1515583081).

Negligence, a departure from the standard of due care toward others, includes intentionally posing risks that are unreasonable and unintentionally but carelessly imposing risks. **Autonomy** refers to the individual's freedom from controlling interferences by others and from personal limitations that prevent meaningful choices, such as adequate understanding. Two conditions are essential for autonomy: **liberty**, the independence from controlling influences; and the individual's capacity for intentional action. **Beneficence** refers to actions performed that contribute to the welfare of others. There are two principles of beneficence: positive beneficence requires the provision of benefits, and utility requires that benefits and drawbacks be balanced. One must avoid negative beneficence, which occurs when there are constraints on activities that, even though might not be unjust, could in some situations cause detriment or harm to others. **Justice** refers to the fair, equitable, and appropriate treatment in light of what is due or owed to a person. Distributive justice refers to fair, equitable, and appropriate distribution in society determined by justified norms that structure the terms of social cooperation. Beauchamp and Childress also suggest three types of rules for guiding actions (rules are more restrictive in scope than principles and are more specific in content). Substantive rules are rules of **truth** telling, confidentiality, privacy, **fidelity**, and those pertaining to the allocation and rationing of health care, omitting treatment, physician-assisted suicide, and informed consent. Authority rules are those rules regarding who may and should perform actions. Procedural rules establish procedures to be followed.

The **antiprinciplism** movement has emerged with the expansive technologic changes and the tremendous rise in ethical dilemmas accompanying these changes. Opponents of principlism include those who claim that its principles do not represent a theoretical approach and those who claim that its principles are too far removed from the concrete particularities of everyday human existence; the principles are too conceptual, intangible, or abstract; or they disregard or do not take into account a person's psychological factors, personality, life history, sexual orientation, or religious, ethnic, and cultural background. Different approaches to making ethical decisions are next briefly explored, providing the reader with an understanding of the varied methods professionals may use to arrive at an ethical decision.

The **casuist approach** to ethical decision making grew out of the concern for more concrete methods of examining ethical dilemmas. Casuistry is a case-based ethical reasoning method that analyzes the facts of a case in a sound, logical, and ordered or structured manner. The facts are compared to decisions arising out of consensus in previous paradigmatic or model cases. One casuist proponent, Jonsen (1991), prefers particular and concrete paradigms and analogies over the universal and abstract theories of principlism.

The Husted bioethical decision-making model centers on the healthcare professional's implicit agreement with patient or client (Husted & Husted, 1995), and is based on six contemporary bioethical standards: (1) autonomy, (2) freedom, (3) veracity, (4) privacy, (5) beneficence, and (6) fidelity.

The **virtue ethics** approach emphasizes the virtuous character of individuals who make the choices. A **virtue** is any characteristic or disposition desired in others or oneself. It comes from the Greek word *aretai*, meaning excellence, and it refers to what one expects of oneself and others. Virtue ethicists emphasize the ideal situation and attempt to identify and define ideals. Virtue ethics dates back to Plato and Socrates. When asked "whether virtue can be taught or whether virtue can be acquired in some other way, Socrates answers that if virtue is knowledge, then it can be taught. Thus, Socrates assumes that whatever can be known can be taught" (Scott, 2002, para. 9). The cause of any moral weakness was not a matter of character flaws but of ignorance. A person acts immorally because he does not know what is really good for him or her. A person can be overpowered by immediate pleasures and forget to consider the long-term **consequences**. Plato emphasized that to lead a moral life and not succumb to immediate pleasures and gratification one must have a moral vision. He identified four cardinal virtues: (1) **wisdom**, (2) **courage**, (3) **self-control**, and (4) justice. Aristotle's **Nicomachean** principles (Aristotle, 350 BC) also contribute to virtue ethics. Virtues are connected to will and motive because the intention is what determines if one is or is not acting virtuously. Ethical considerations, according to his **eudaemonistic** principles, address the question, "What is it to be an excellent person?" For Aristotle this ultimately means acting in a temperate manner according to a rational mean between extreme possibilities.

Virtue ethics has seen a recent resurgence (Healthcare Ethics, 2007). Two of the most influential moral and medical authors, Pellegrino and Thomasma (1993), have maintained that virtue theory should be related to other theories within comprehensive philosophy of the health professions. They argued that moral events are composed of four elements (the agent, the act, the circumstances, and the consequences) and that a variety of theories must be interrelated to account for different facets of moral judgment.

Care ethics is responsiveness to the needs of others that dictates providing care, preventing harm, and maintaining relationships. This viewpoint has been in existence for some time. Engster (n.d.) states that "Carol Gilligan's In a Different Voice (1982) established care ethics as a major new perspective in contemporary moral and political discourse" (p. 2). The relationship between care and virtue is complex and Benjamin and Curtis (1992) base their framework on care ethics; they propose that "critical reflection and inquiry in ethics involves the complex interplay of a variety of human faculties, ranging from empathy and moral imagination on the one hand to analytic precision and careful reasoning on the other" (p. 12). Care ethicists are less guided by rules and focus on the needs of others and one's responsibility to meet those needs. The central focus is responsiveness to the needs of others that dictates providing care, preventing harm, and maintaining relationships. As opposed to the aforementioned theories that focused on the individual's rights, an ethic of care emphasizes a personal part of an interdependent relationship that affects how decisions are made. In this theory, the specific situation and context in which the person is embedded becomes a part of the decision-making process.

The consensus-based approach to bioethics was proposed by Martin (1999), who claims that American bioethics harbors a variety of ethical methods that emphasize different ethical factors, including principles, circumstances, character, interpersonal needs, and personal meaning. Each method reflects an important aspect of ethical experience, adds to the others, and enriches the ethical imagination. Thus, working with these methods provides the challenge and the opportunity necessary for the perceptive and shrewd bioethicist to transform them into something new with value through the process of building ethical consensus. Diverse ethical insights can be integrated to support a particular bioethical decision, and that decision can be understood as a new, ethical whole.

APPLYING ETHICS TO INFORMATICS

With the Knowledge Age has come global closeness or the ability to reach around the globe instantaneously through technology. Language barriers are being broken through technologic translators to enhance interaction and exchange of data and information. Informatics practitioners are bridging continents, and international panels, committees, and organizations are beginning to establish standards and rules for the implementation of informatics. This international perspective must be taken into consideration as informatics dilemmas are ethically examined, because they will influence the development of ethical approaches that begin to accept that one is working within international networks and must recognize, respect, and regard the diverse political, social, and human factors within informatics ethics.

The ethical approaches can be used to help healthcare professionals make ethical decisions in all areas of practice. The focus of this text is on informatics. Informatics theory and practice has continued to grow at a rapid rate and is infiltrating every area of professional life. New applications and ways of performing skills are being developed daily. Therefore, education in informatics ethics is extremely important.

Typically, situations are analyzed using past experience and in collaboration with others. Each situation warrants its own deliberation and unique approach, because each individual patient seeking or receiving care has his or her own preferences, quality of life, and healthcare needs in a situational milieu framed within financial, provider, setting, or institutions, and social context issues. Clinicians must take into consideration all of these factors when making ethical decisions.

The use of expert systems, **decision support** tools, evidence-based practice, and artificial intelligence in the care of patients provides challenges as to who should use these tools, how they are implemented, and how they are tempered with clinical judgment. All clinical situations are not the same, and even though the result of interacting with these systems and tools is enhanced information and knowledge, the clinician must weigh this information in light of the patient's unique clinical circumstances including their beliefs and wishes. Our patients demand access to quality care and the information necessary to control their lives. Clinicians need to analyze and synthesize the parameters of each distinctive situation using a specific decision-making framework that helps them make the best decisions. Getting it right the first time has a tremendous impact on expected patient outcomes. The focus should remain on patient outcomes while the informatics tools available are ethically incorporated.

Facing ethical dilemmas on a daily basis and struggling with unique client situations cause many clinicians to question their own actions and the actions of their colleagues and patients. One must realize that colleagues and patients may reach very different decisions, but that does not mean anyone is wrong. Instead, everyone reaches their ethical decision based on their own review of the situational facts and understanding of ethics. As one deals with diversity among patients, colleagues, and administrators, one must constantly strive to use ethical imaginations to reach ethically competent decisions. Balancing the needs of society, his or her employer, and patients could cause the clinician continually to face ethical challenges. Society expects judicious use of finite healthcare resources. Employers have their own policies, standards, and practices that at times can inhibit the practice of the clinician. Each patient is unique and has life experiences that affect his or her healthcare perspective, choices, motivation, and adherence. Combine all of this with the challenges of informatics, and it is clear that the evolving healthcare arena calls for an informatics-competent, politically active, consumer-oriented, business-savvy, ethical clinician to rule this ever-changing landscape known as health care.

The goal of any ethical system should be that a rational, justifiable decision was reached. Ethics is always there to help one decide what is right. Indeed, the measure of an adequate ethical system or theory or approach is in part its ability to be useful in novel contexts. A comprehensive, robust theory of ethics should be up to the task of addressing a broad variety of new applications and challenges at the intersection of informatics and health care.

The information concerning an ethical dilemma must remain in the context of the dilemma to be useful. **Bioinformatics** could gather, manipulate, classify, analyze, synthesize, retrieve, and maintain databases related to ethical cases, the effective reasoning applied to various ethical dilemmas, and the resulting ethical decisions. This would be potent but the resolution of dilemmas cannot be had from just examining relevant cases from this database. Clinicians must assess each situational context, the patient's specific situation and needs, and make their ethical decisions based on all of the information they have at hand.

Ethics is exciting, and competent clinicians need to know about ethical dilemmas and solutions in their professions. Ethicists have been thought of as experts in the arbitrary, ambiguous, and ungrounded judgments of other people. Ethicists know that they make the best decision they can based on the situation and stakeholders at hand. Just as clinicians try to make the best healthcare decisions with and for their patients, ethically they must do the same. One must critically think through the situation to arrive at the best decision.

To make ethical decisions about informatics technologies and patients' intimate healthcare data and information, one must be informatics competent. To the extent that information technology is reshaping healthcare practices or promises to improve patient care, then healthcare professionals must be trained and be competent in the use of these tools. This competency needs to be evaluated by instruments developed by professional groups or societies; this will help with consistency and quality. For the healthcare professional to be a patient advocate, it is necessary for the professional to understand how information technology impacts the patient and the subsequent delivery of care. Information science and its effect on health care are both interesting and important. It follows that information technology and its **ethical, social, and legal implications** should be incorporated into all levels of professional education. The need for confidentiality was perhaps first articulated by Hippocrates, so if anything is different it is in the ways it can be violated. It might be that the use of computers for clinical decision support and data mining in research raise new ethical issues. Ethical dilemmas associated with the integration of informatics must be examined to provide an ethical framework that considers all of the stakeholders. Patients' rights must be protected in the face of a healthcare provider's duty to his or her employer and society at large when initiating care and assigning finite healthcare resources. An ethical framework is necessary to help guide healthcare providers in reference to the ethical treatment of electronic data and information during all stages of collection, storage, manipulation, and dissemination. These new approaches and means come with their own ethical dilemmas. Often they are dilemmas not yet faced on the cutting edge of these technologies.

Just as processes and models are used to diagnose and treat patients in practice, a model in the analysis and synthesis of ethical dilemmas or cases can also be applied. The ethical model for ethical decision making (Box 5-1) facilitates the ability to analyze the dilemma and synthesize the information into a plan of action (McGonigle, 2000). It is based on the letters in the word ethical. Each letter guides and prompts one to think critically (think and rethink) through the situation presented. The model is a tool because, in the final analysis, it allows one objectively to ascertain the essence of the dilemma and develop a plan of action.

BOX

5-1

Ethical Model for Ethical Decision Making

*E*xamine the ethical dilemma (conflicting values exist).
*T*horoughly comprehend the possible alternatives available.
*H*ypothesize ethical arguments.
*I*nvestigate, compare, and evaluate the arguments for each alternative.
*C*hoose the alternative you would recommend.
*A*ct on your chosen alternative.
*L*ook at the ethical dilemma and examine the outcomes while reflecting on the
  ethical decision.

APPLYING THE ETHICAL MODEL

Examine the ethical dilemma

- Use your problem-solving, decision-making, and critical-thinking skills.
- What is the dilemma you are analyzing? Collect as much information about the
  dilemma as you can, making sure to gather the relevant facts that clearly iden-
  tify the dilemma. You should be able to describe the dilemma you are analyz-
  ing in detail.
- Ascertain exactly what must be decided.
- Who should be involved in the decision-making process for this specific case?
- Who are the interested players or stakeholders?
- Reflect on the viewpoints of these key players and their value systems.
- What do you think each of these stakeholders would like you to decide as a
  plan of action for this dilemma?
- How can you generate the greatest good?

Thoroughly comprehend the possible alternatives available

- Use your problem-solving, decision-making, and critical-thinking skills.
- Create a list of the possible alternatives. Be creative when developing your
  alternatives. Be open minded; there is more than one way to reach a goal.
  Compel yourself to discern at least three alternatives.
- Clarify the alternatives available and predict the associated consequences,
  good and bad, of each potential alternative or intervention.
- For each alternative, ask the following questions
  - Do any of the principles or rules, such as legal, professional, or organiza-
    tional, automatically nullify this alternative?
  - If this alternative is chosen, what do you predict as the best-case and
    worst-case scenarios?
  - Do the best-case outcomes outweigh the worst-case outcomes?
  - Could you live with the worst-case scenario?

Continues

- Will anyone be harmed? If so, how will they be harmed?
- Does the benefit obtained from this alternative overcome the risk of potential harm that it could cause to anyone?

Hypothesize ethical arguments

- Use your problem-solving, decision-making, and critical-thinking skills.
- Determine which of the five approaches apply to this dilemma.
- Identify the moral principles that can be brought into play to support a conclusion as to what ought to be done ethically in this case or similar cases.
- Ascertain whether the approaches generate converging or diverging conclusions about what ought to be done.

Investigate, compare, and evaluate the arguments for each alternative

- Use your problem-solving, decision-making, and critical-thinking skills.
- Appraise the relevant facts and assumptions prudently.
- Is there ambiguous information that must be evaluated?
- Are there any unjustifiable factual or illogical assumptions or debatable conceptual issues that must be explored?
- Rate the ethical reasoning and arguments for each alternative in terms of their relative significance.
    - 4 = extreme significance
    - 3 = major significance
    - 2 = significant
    - 1 = minor significance
- Compare and contrast the alternatives available against the values of the key players involved.
- Reflect on these alternatives:
- Does each alternative consider all of the key players?
- Does each alternative take into account and reflect an interest in the concerns and welfare of all of the key players?
- Which alternative will produce the greatest good or the least amount of harm for the greatest number of people?
- Refer to your professional codes of ethical conduct. Do they support your reasoning?

Choose the alternative you would recommend

- Use your problem-solving, decision-making, and critical-thinking skills.
- Make a decision about the best alternative available.
- Remember the Golden Rule—does your decision treat others as you would want to be treated?
- Does your decision take into account and reflect an interest in the concerns and welfare of all of the key players?
- Does your decision maximize the benefit and minimize the risk for everyone involved?

Continues

- Become your own critic; challenge your decision as you think others might. Use the ethical arguments you predict they would use and defend your decision.
- Would you be secure enough in your ethical decision-making process to see it aired on national television or sent out globally over the Internet?
- Are you secure enough with this ethical decision that you could have allowed your loved ones to observe your decision-making process, your decision, and its outcomes?

Act on your chosen alternative

- Use your problem-solving, decision-making, and critical-thinking skills.
- Formulate an implementation plan delineating the execution of the decision.
- This plan should be designed to maximize the benefits and minimize the risks.
- This plan must take into account all of the resources necessary for implementation, including personnel and money.
- Implement the plan.

Look at the ethical dilemma and examine the outcomes while reflecting on your ethical decision

- Use your problem-solving, decision-making, and critical-thinking skills.
- Monitor the implementation plan and its outcomes. It is extremely important to reflect on specific case decisions and evaluate their outcomes in order to develop your ethical decision-making ability.
- If new information becomes available, the plan must be reevaluated.
- Monitor and revise the plan as necessary.

Source: The ethical model for ethical decision making was developed by Dr. Dee McGonigle and is the property of Educational Advancement Associates (EAA). The permission for its use in this text has been granted by Mr. Craig R. Goshow, Vice President, EAA.

CASE ANALYSIS DEMONSTRATION

The following case study helps one to apply the ethical model. Review the model and then read through the case. Try to apply the model to this case or follow along as the model is implemented. The reader is challenged to determine their decision in this case and then compare and contrast their response with the decision the authors reached. There are several more case studies presented for practice in implementing the ethical model for ethical decision making on this book's companion website (http://nursing.jbpub.com/informatics).

Case Study

Allison is a charge nurse on a busy medical–surgical unit. She is expecting the clinical instructor from the local university at 2:00 pm to review and discuss potential patient assignments for the nursing students scheduled for the following day. Just as the university professor arrives, one of the patients on the unit develops a crisis requiring Allison's attention. To expedite the student nurse assignments for the following day, Allison gives her electronic medical record access password to the instructor.

Examine the Ethical Dilemma

Allison made a commitment to meet with the university instructor to develop student assignments at 2:00 PM. The patient emergency that developed prevented Allison from living up to that commitment. Allison had an obligation to provide patient care during the emergency and a competing obligation to the professor. She solved the dilemma of competing obligations by providing her electronic medical record access password to the university professor. By sharing her password, Allison most likely violated hospital policy related to the **security** of healthcare information. She may also have violated the American Nurses Association code of ethics in that nurses must judiciously protect information of a confidential nature. Because the university professor was also a nurse and had a legitimate interest in the protected healthcare information, there might not be a code of ethics violation.

Thoroughly Comprehend the Possible Alternatives Available

The possible **alternatives** available include the following: (1) Allison could have asked the professor to wait until the patient crisis was solved; (2) Allison could have delegated another staff member to assist the university professor; or (3) Allison could have logged on to the system for the professor.

Hypothesize Ethical Arguments

The utilitarian approach applies to this situation. An ethical action is one that provides the greatest good for the greatest number; the principles are beneficence and nonmaleficence. The rights to be considered are as follows: right of the individual to choose for himself or herself (autonomy); right to truth (**veracity**); right of privacy (ethical right to privacy avoids conflict and like all rights promotes harmony); right not to be injured; and right to what has been promised (fidelity). Does the action respect the **moral rights** of everyone? The principles to consider are autonomy, veracity, and fidelity. As for the fairness or justice, how fair is an action? Does it treat everyone in the same way, or does it show favoritism and discrimination? The principles to consider are justice and distributive justice. Thinking about the common good assumes one's own good is inextricably linked to good of the community; community members are bound by pursuit of common values and goals and ensure that the social policies, social systems, institutions, and environments on which one depends are beneficial to all. Examples are affordable health care, effective public safety, a just legal system, and an unpolluted environment. The principle of distributive justice is considered. Virtue assumes there are certain ideals toward which one should strive that provide for the full development of humanity. Virtues are attitudes or character traits that enable one to be and to act in ways that develop the highest potential; examples are honesty, courage, compassion, generosity, fidelity, integrity, fairness, self-control, and prudence. Like habits, they become a characteristic of the person. The virtuous person is the ethical person. Ask yourself, what kind of person should I be? What will promote the development of character within myself and my community? The principles considered are fidelity, veracity, beneficence, nonmaleficence, justice, and distributive justice.

In this case, there is a clear violation of institutional policy designed to protect the privacy and confidentiality of medical records. However, the professor had a legitimate interest in the information and a legitimate right to the information. Allison trusted that the professor would not use the system password to obtain information outside the scope of the legitimate interest. However, Allison cannot be sure that the professor would not access inappropriate information. Further, Allison is responsible for how her access to the electronic system is used. Balancing the rights of everyone—the professor's right to the information, the patients' rights to expect that their information is safeguarded, and the right of the patient in crisis to expect the best possible care—is important and is the crux of the dilemma. Does the patient care obligation outweigh the obligation to the professor? Yes, probably. Allison did the right thing by caring for the patient in crisis. By giving out her system access password, Allison compromised the rights of the other patients on the unit to expect that their confidentiality and privacy would be safeguarded.

Virtue ethics suggests that individuals use power to bring about human benefit. One must consider the needs of others and the responsibility to meet those needs. Allison has to provide care, prevent harm, and maintain professional relationships all at the same time.

Allison may want to effect a long-term change in hospital policy for the common good. It is reasonable to assume that this is not an isolated incident and that the problem may recur in the future. Can institutional policy be amended to include professors in the access to medical records system? As suggested in the Health Insurance Portability and Accountability Act (HIPAA) administrative guidelines, the professor could receive the same staff training regarding appropriate and inappropriate use of access and sign the agreement to safeguard the records. If the institution has tracking software, the access could be monitored to watch for inappropriate use.

Identify the moral principles that can be brought into play to support a conclusion as to what ought to be done ethically in this case or similar cases. The International Council of Nurses (2006) code of ethics states that "The nurse holds in confidence personal information and uses judgment in sharing this information" (p. 4). The code also states, "The nurse uses judgment in relation to individual competence when accepting and delegating responsibilities" (p. 5). Both of these statements apply to the current situation.

Ascertain whether the approaches generate converging or diverging conclusions about what ought to be done. From the analysis, it is clear that the best immediate solution is to delegate assisting the professor with assignments to another nurse on the unit.

Investigate, Compare, and Evaluate the Arguments for Each Alternative

Review and think through the items listed in Table 5-1.

TABLE 5-1
Detailed Analysis of Alternative Actions

Alternative	Good Consequences	Bad Consequences	Do Any Rules Nullify	Expected Outcome	Potential Benefit > Harm
1. Wait until crisis was solved	No policy violation Patient rights safeguarded	Not the best use of the professor's time	No	Best: Crisis will require a short time Worst: Crisis may take a long time	Patient rights protected Collegial relationship jeopardized Patient rights may take precedence
2. Delegate to another staff member	No policy violated	Other staff may be equally busy or might not be as familiar with all patients	No	Best: Assignments will be completed Worst: May not have benefit of expert advice	Confidentiality of record is assured May compromise student learning Patient rights may take precedence
3. Log on to the system for the professor	Professor can begin making assignments	May still be a violation of policy regarding system access	Rules regarding access to medical record	Best: Assignments can be completed Worst: Abuse of access to information	Potential compromise of records Patient in crisis is cared for

Choose the Alternative You Would Recommend

The best immediate solution is to delegate another staff member to assist the professor. The best long-tem solution is to change the hospital policy to include access for professors, as described.

Act on Your Chosen Alternative

Allison should delegate another staff member to assist the professor in making assignments.

Look at the Ethical Dilemma and Examine the Outcomes While Reflecting on the Ethical Decision

As already indicated in the alternative analyses, delegation may not be an ideal solution because the staff nurse who is assigned to assist the professor may not possess the same extensive information about all of the patients as the charge nurse. It is, however, the best immediate solution to the dilemma and certainly safer than compromising computer system integrity. As noted, Allison may want to pursue a long-term solution to a potentially recurring problem by helping the professor gain legitimate access to the computer system with the professor's own password. This way the system administrator may have the ability to track who used the system and what types of information were accessed during use.

This case analysis demonstration provides the authors' perspective of this case and the ethical decision they made. If the reader's decision varied, what was the basis for the difference of opinion? If one worked through the model, a different decision might be reached given one's individual background and perspective. This does not make the decision right or wrong. A decision should reflect the best decision one can make given a review, reflection, and critical thinking about this specific situation. There are six additional cases provided in the online Learner's Manual for review. Apply the model for each case study and discuss these with colleagues or classmates.

NEW FRONTIERS IN ETHICAL ISSUES

The expanding use of new information technologies in healthcare will bring about new and challenging ethical issues. Consider that patients and health care providers no longer have to be in the same place for a quality interaction. How then does one deal with licensing issues if the electronic consultation takes place across a state line? Derse and Miller (2008) describe a second opinion medical consultation on the Internet where the information was provided to the referring physician and not the patient, thus avoiding the licensing issue. Consider the ethical issues created by genomic databases or by sharing information in a health information exchange to promote population health. Alpert (2008) asks, "Is it wise to put genomic sequence data into electronic medical records that are poorly protected, that cannot adhere well to Fair Information Practice Principles for privacy, and that can potentially be seen by tens of thousands of people/entities, when it is clear that we do not understand the functionally of the genome and likely will not for several years?" (p. 382). Further, how does one really obtain informed consent for such data collection, when how the data will ultimately be used is not known, but clearly it will be important to health research uses that are beyond the immediate medical care of the patient. Angst (2009) asks whether public good outweighs individual interests because the information contained in these databases is important to developing new understandings and creating new knowledge by matching data in aggregated pools. "Thus, science adds meaning and context to data, but to what extent do we agree to make the data available such that this discovery process can take place, and are the impacts of discovery great enough to justify the risks?" (p. 172) Further, if a voluntary system where patients can opt out of such data collection is adopted, then are health care disparities related to incomplete electronic health records created?

In an ideal world, healthcare professionals must not be affected by conflicting loyalties; nothing should interfere with judicious, ethical decision making. As the technologically charged waters of health care are navigated, one must hone a solid foundation of ethical decision making and practice it consistently.

SUMMARY

As science and technology advance, and policy makers and healthcare providers continue to shape healthcare practices including information management, it is paramount that ethical decisions are made. Healthcare professionals are typically honest, trustworthy, and ethical and understand that they are duty bound to focus on the needs and rights of their patients. At the same time, their day-to-day work is conducted in a world of changing healthcare landscapes consisting of new technologies, diverse patients, varied healthcare settings, and changing policies set by their employers, insurance companies, and providers. Healthcare professionals need to juggle all of these balls, often resulting in far too many gray areas or ethical decision-making dilemmas with no clear correct course of action. Patients rely on the ethical competence of their healthcare providers, believing that their situation is unique and will be respected and evaluated based on their own needs, abilities, and limitations. The healthcare professional cannot allow conflicting loyalties to interfere with judicious, ethical decision making. Just as in the opening example of the Apollo mission, it is uncertain where this technologically heightened information era will lead, but if with a solid foundation of ethical decision making, duties and rights will be judiciously and ethically fulfilled.

THOUGHT-PROVOKING Questions

WWW

1. Identify moral dilemmas in healthcare informatics that would best be approached with the use of an ethical decision-making framework.
2. Discuss the evolving healthcare ethics traditions within their social and historical context.
3. Differentiate among the theoretical approaches to healthcare ethics as they relate to the theorists' perspectives of individuals and their relationships.
4. Select one of the healthcare ethics theories and support its use in examining ethical issues in healthcare informatics.
5. Select one of the healthcare ethics theories and argue against its use in examining ethical issues in healthcare informatics.

For a full suite of assignments and additional learning activities, use the access code located in the front of your book to visit this exclusive website: **http://go.jblearning.com/mcgonigle.** If you do not have an access code, you can obtain one at the site.

WWW

References

Alpert, S. (2008). Privacy issues in clinical genomic medicine, or Marcus Welby, M.D., meets the $1000 Genome. *Cambridge Quarterly of Healthcare Ethics, 17*(4), 373-384. Retrieved from Health Module (Document ID: 1880623501).

Angst, C. (2009). Protect my privacy or support the common-good? Ethical questions about electronic health information exchanges. *Journal of Business Ethics: Supplement, 90,* 169-178. Retrieved from ABI/INFORM Global (Document ID: 2051417481).

Aristotle. (350 BC). *Nichomachean ethics. Book I.* (W. D. Ross, Trans.). Retrieved from http://www.constitution.org/ari/ethic_00.htm

Beauchamp, T. L., & Childress, J. F. (1977). *Principles of biomedical ethics.* New York, NY: Oxford University Press.

Beauchamp, T. L., & Childress, J. F. (1994). *Principles of biomedical ethics* (4th ed.). New York, NY: Oxford University Press.

Benjamin, M., & Curtis, J. (1992). *Ethics in nursing* (3rd ed.). New York, NY: Oxford University Press.

Derse, A., & Miller, T. (2008). Net effect: professional and ethical challenges of medicine online. *Cambridge Quarterly of Healthcare Ethics, 17*(4), 453–464. Retrieved from Health Module (Document ID: 1540615461).

ehealth code. (n.d.). Retrieved from http://www.ihealthcoalition.org/ehealth-code/

Engster, D. (n.d.). Can care ethics be institutionalized? Toward a caring natural law theory. Retrieved from http://www.csus.edu.org/wpsa/pisigmaalphaaward.pdf

Healthcare Ethics. (2007). Virtue ethics. Retrieved from http://www.ascensionhealth.org/ethics/public/issues/virtue.asp

Howard, R. (Director). (1995). Apollo 13 [Motion picture]. Universal City, CA: MCA Universal Studios.

Husted, G. L., & Husted, J. H. (1995). *Ethical decision-making in nursing* (2nd ed.). New York, NY: Mosby.

International Council of Nurses (ICN). (2006). The ICN code of ethics for nurses. Retrieved from http://www.icn.ch/icncode.pdf

Jonsen, A. R. (1991). Casuistry as methodology in clinical ethics. *Theoretical Medicine 12,* 295–307.

Mack, J. (2000). Patient empowerment, not economics, is driving E-health: Privacy and ethics issues need attention too! *Frontiers of Health Services Management, 17*(1), 39–43; discussion 49–51. Retrieved from ABI/INFORM Global (Document ID: 59722384).

Makus, R. (2001). Ethics and Internet healthcare: An ontological reflection. *Cambridge Quarterly of Healthcare Ethics, 10*(2), 127-136. Retrieved from Health Module (Document ID: 1409693941).

Martin, P. A. (1999). Bioethics and the whole: Pluralism, consensus, and the transmutation of bioethical methods into gold. *Journal of Law, Medicine & Ethics, 27*(4), 316–327.

McGonigle, D. (2000). The ethical model for ethical decision making. *Inside Case Management, 7*(8), 1–5.

Pellegrino, E. D. (1993). The metamorphosis of medical ethics: A thirty-year retrospective. *JAMA, 269,* 1158–1162.

Pellegrino, E., & Thomasma, D. (1993). The virtues in medical practice. New York, NY: Oxford University Press.

Resnik, D. (2001). Patient access to medical information in the computer age: Ethical concerns and issues. *Cambridge Quarterly of Healthcare Ethics, 10*(2), 147–154; discussion 154–156. Retrieved from Health Module (Document ID: 1409693961).

Scott, A. (2002). Plato's Meno. Retrieved from http://www.angelfire.com/md2/timewarp/ plato.html

Velasquez, M., Andre, C., Shanks, T., & Myer, M. (for the Markkula Center for Applied Ethics). (1987). What is ethics? Retrieved from http://www.scu.edu/SCU/Centers/Ethics/practicing/decision/whatisethics.shtml

Perspectives on Nursing Informatics

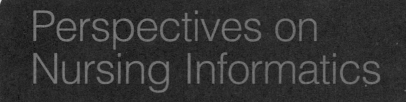

Nursing informatics (NI) is the synthesis of nursing science, information science, computer science, and cognitive science for the purpose of managing and enhancing healthcare data, information, knowledge, and wisdom to improve patient care and the nursing profession. In Section I the reader learned about the four sciences of NI, also referred to as the four building blocks, and the ethical application of these sciences to manage patient information. Nursing knowledge workers must be able to understand the evolving specialty of NI to harness and use the tools available for managing the vast amount of healthcare data and information. It is essential that NI capabilities be appreciated, promoted, expanded, and advanced to facilitate the work of the nurse, improve patient care, and enhance the nursing profession.

Section II presents the perspectives of nursing experts on NI. Chapter 6 is an overview of NI. In Chapter 7, the reader learns about the development of standardized terminologies in NI. Chapter 8 explores NI roles, competencies, and skills. Chapter 9 reviews the information and knowledge needs of nurses in the 21st century. Legislative aspects of NI including an overview of the HIPAA and the HITECH Acts are presented in Chapter 10. Professional development and collaboration tools are presented in Chapter 11, providing insights into the power of informatics to facilitate professional growth. Although some of the information presented by the expert contributing authors may seem duplicated in these chapters, it is important to expose readers to the various perspectives about NI as provided by the NI experts who contributed their wisdom to this section.

In the Chapter 6 overview of NI, interrelationships among major NI concepts are discussed. As data are transformed into information and information into knowledge, increasing complexity and interrelationships ensue. The boundaries between concepts can be blurred, and feedback loops from one concept level to another occur. Structured languages and human–computer interaction concepts, which are critical elements for NI, are noted. Taxonomies and other current structured languages for nursing are listed. Human–computer interaction concepts are briefly defined and discussed because they are critical to the success of informatics solutions. Last and importantly, the construct of decision making is added to the traditional nursing metaparadigms: nurse, person, health, and environment. Decision making is not only at the crux of nursing practice in all settings and roles, but it is a fundamental concern of NI. The work of nursing is centered in the concepts of NI: data, information, knowledge, and wisdom. Information technology per se is not the focus; it is the information that the technology conveys that is central. NI is no longer the domain of experts in the field. More interestingly, one does not need technology to perform informatics. The centerpiece of informatics is the manipulation of data, information, and knowledge, especially related to decision making in any aspect of nursing or in any setting. In a way, nurses are all already informatics nurses.

In Chapter 7, "Developing Standardized Terminologies to Support Nursing Practice," different approaches to terminology development are discussed. Standardized nursing terminologies (and the structures and systems that support their implementation and use) are merely a means to an end; they do not obviate the need to think and work creatively, to do right by the people in our care, and to continue to advance nursing.

Chapter 8, "Nursing Informatics Roles, Competencies, and Skills," discusses NI as a relatively new nursing specialty that combines the building block sciences covered in Section I. Combining these sciences results in nurses being able to care for their patients effectively and safely because the information that they need is readily available. Nurses have been actively involved in NI since computers were introduced into health care. With the advent of electronic health records, it became apparent that nursing needed to develop its own language. NI was instrumental in assisting in nursing language development. The healthcare industry employs the largest number of knowledge workers. This has resulted in the realization that healthcare administrators must begin to change the way they look at their employees. Nurses and physicians are bright, highly skilled, and dedicated to giving the best patient care. Administrators who tap into this wealth of knowledge find that patient care becomes safer and more efficient. NI is governed by standards established by the American Nurses Association and is a very diverse field, which results in many nurse informaticist specialists becoming focused on one segment of NI. Although NI is a recognized specialty area of practice, all nurses will be expected to have some knowledge of the field. NI competencies have been developed to ensure that all entry level nurses are ready to enter a field that is becoming more technologically advanced. The competencies may also be used to determine the educational needs of currently practicing nurses. Nurse informatics specialists no longer have to enter the field as a result of on-the-job exposure, but can now obtain an advanced degree in NI at many well-established universities throughout the country. NI has grown tremendously as a specialty since its inception and is predicted to continue growing.

Chapter 9, "Information and Knowledge Needs of Nurses in the 21st Century," states that the core concepts and competencies of informatics are particularly well suited to a model of interprofessional education. Ideally, when emulating clinical settings, informatics knowledge should be integrated with the processes of interprofessional teams and decision making. Because simulation laboratories are becoming increasingly common fixtures in the delivery of health-related professional education, they provide a perfect opportunity to incorporate the electronic health records applications. The learning laboratory for nursing education will then more closely approximate the information technology–enabled clinical settings that are emerging. A presumption is often made that future graduates will be more computer literate than nurses currently in practice. Although this may be true, computer literacy or comfort does not equate to an understanding of the facilitative and transformative role of information technology. It is essential that the future curricula of basic nursing programs embed the concepts of the role of information technology in supporting clinical care delivery.

Equally important in informatics practice is a thorough understanding of current legislation and regulations that shape 21st century practice. Chapter 10 provides insights into HIPAA rules and an overview of the rules associated with technology implementation as defined by the HITECH Act. The information provided in this text reflects current rules that were in effect at the time of publication. The reader should follow the rules development and evolution of informatics legislation at the U.S. Department of Health and Human Services website (www.hhs.gov) for the most current information related to health information management.

Most nurses have yet to embrace the notion of informatics and understand its meaning and relevance to their work and to their professional development. In Chapter 11, the reader learns more about the power of informatics tools to develop a professional ePortfolio and to help network with other professionals to build and share professional knowledge.

There is an emerging global focus on information technology to support clinical care and on the potential benefits for clinicians and patients. Anticipate that in the future, nurses will have the computing power to aggregate and transform additional multidimensional data and information sources (e.g., historical, multisensory, experiential, genetic) into a clinical information system to engage with individuals, families, and groups in ways not yet imagined. Every nurse's practice will make contributions to new nursing knowledge in these dynamically interactive clinical information system environments. Afforded with the right tools to support the management of data, complex information processing, and ready access to knowledge, the core concepts and competencies associated with informatics will be embedded in the practice of every nurse, whether administrator, researcher, educator, or practitioner. Information technology is not a panacea, but it provides the profession with unprecedented capacity to generate and disseminate new knowledge more rapidly.

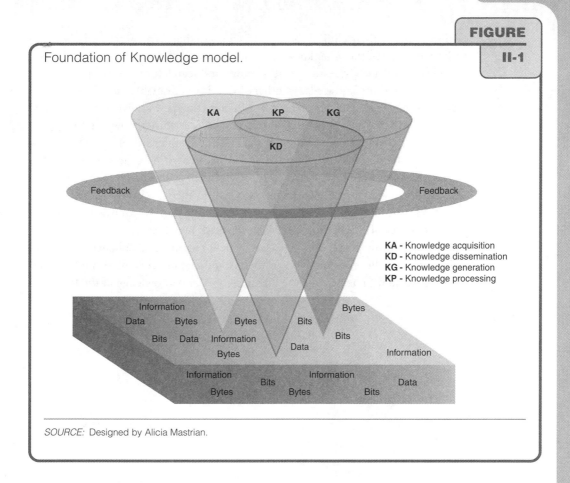

FIGURE

II-1

Foundation of Knowledge model.

KA
KP
KG
KD

Feedback   Feedback

KA - Knowledge acquisition
KD - Knowledge dissemination
KG - Knowledge generation
KP - Knowledge processing

Information
Data   Bytes   Bytes   Bits   Bytes
        Bits   Data   Information   Bits
                    Bytes   Data   Information
            Information   Information   Data
                    Bytes   Bits   Bytes   Bits

SOURCE: Designed by Alicia Mastrian.

The material within this book is placed within the context of the Foundation of Knowledge model (Figure II-1) to meet the needs of healthcare delivery systems, organizations, patients, and nurses. Through involvement in NI and learning about this evolving specialty, one will be able to use the current theories, architecture, and tools, while beginning to challenge what is known. This questioning and search for what could be will provide the basis for the future landscape of nursing. By using the Foundation of Knowledge model as an organizing framework for this text, the authors have attempted to capture this process. In this section, the reader learns about NI. Those readers who are beginning their education will consciously focus on input and knowledge acquisition, trying to glean as much information and knowledge as possible. As these readers become more comfortable in their clinical setting and with nursing science, they will begin to take over some of the other knowledge functions. Experienced nurses, also known as "seasoned nurses," question what is known and search for ways to enhance their knowledge and the knowledge of others. What is not available must be created. It is through these leaders, researchers, or clinicians that new knowledge is generated and disseminated and nursing science advanced. Sometimes, however, to keep up with the explosion of information in nursing and health care, one must continue to rely on the knowledge generated and disseminated by others. In this sense, nurses are committed to lifelong learning and the use of knowledge in the practice of nursing science. How one interacts within their environment and applies what is learned depends on placement in the Foundation of Knowledge model.

The reader of this section is challenged to ask how they can (1) apply knowledge gained from the practice setting to benefit patients and enhance one's practice; (2) help colleagues and patients understand and use current technology; and (3) use wisdom to help create the theories, tools, and knowledge of the future.

CHAPTER 6

Overview of Nursing Informatics

Ramona Nelson and Nancy Staggers

Objectives

1. Define nursing informatics and key terminology.
2. Explore nursing informatics metastructures, concepts, and tools.
3. Analyze the sciences underpinning nursing informatics and their relationship to nursing informatics practice.
4. Describe phenomena of nursing.

Key Terms WWW

Data
Decision support system
Ergonomics
Expert system
Human–computer
   interaction
Informatics nurse
Informatics nurse specialist
Informatics solution
Information
Knowledge
Nanotechnology
Nursing informatics
Usability
Wisdom

INTRODUCTION

Nurses in all settings and areas of practice are considered knowledge workers. The foundations of **nursing informatics** (NI) conceptualize the process of knowledge generation in nursing. The conceptual framework underpinning the science and practice of NI centers on the concepts of data, information, knowledge, and wisdom. These salient concepts are described in this chapter.

The following quote was crafted by a panel of NI experts as they revised the metastructures portion of the American Nurses Association's (ANA) scope and standards for NI:

> Nursing informatics (NI) is a specialty that integrates nursing science, computer science, and information science to manage and communicate data, information, knowledge and wisdom in nursing practice. NI supports consumers, patients, nurses, and other providers in their decision-making in all roles and settings. This support is accomplished through the use of information structures, information processes, and information technology.
>
> The goal of NI is to improve the health of populations, communities, families, and individuals by optimizing information management and communication. These activities include the design and use of **informatics solutions** and/or technology to support all areas of nursing, including, but not limited to, the direct provision of care, establishing effective administrative

systems, designing useful decision support systems, managing and delivering educational experiences, enhancing life-long learning, and supporting nursing research. (ANA, 2008, p. 1)

Within the scope and standards document the term "individuals refer to patients, healthcare consumers and any other recipient of nursing care or informatics solutions. The term patient refers to consumers in both a wellness and illness model" (ANA, 2008, p. 1).

The authors thank Paulette Fraser, MS, RN, BC, for her work as co-leader of the metastructures section of the ANA's 2007 revision of the Scope and Standards for Nursing Informatics Practice.

The following passage is reprinted with permission of the ANA. Boldface type has been applied to key terms, and figure and table numbers have been changed to correspond to this chapter.

The conceptual framework for NI is based on work by Graves and Corcoran (1989), who provided the initial definition and description of data, information, and knowledge as these terms apply to the science and practice of NI. Nelson (1989, 2002) and (Joos, 2010) added the concept of wisdom and reconceptualized how these concepts interrelate. In addition, the discussion of the definition and goal of nursing presented in the Scope and Standards of Practice evolved from work by Staggers and Thompson (2002). NI is one example of a discipline-specific informatics practice within the broader category of health informatics. NI has become well established within nursing since its recognition as a specialty for registered nurses by the ANA in 1992. It focuses on the representation of nursing data, information, knowledge, and wisdom and the management and communication of nursing information within the broader context of health informatics. NI (1) provides a nursing perspective, (2) illuminates nursing values and beliefs, (3) denotes a practice base for nurses in NI, (4) produces unique knowledge, (5) distinguishes groups of practitioners, (6) focuses on the phenomena of interest for nursing, and (7) provides needed nursing language and word context to health informatics (Brennan, 2003).

METASTRUCTURES, CONCEPTS, AND TOOLS OF NI

To understand the foundations of NI one must begin by exploring, its metastructures, sciences, concepts, and tools. Metastructures are overarching concepts used in theory and science. Also of interest are the sciences underpinning NI, concepts and tools from information science and computer science, **human–computer interaction** (HCI) and ergonomics concepts, and the phenomena of nursing.

Metastructures: Data, Information, Knowledge, and Wisdom

In the mid 1980s Blum (1986) introduced the concepts of data, information, and knowledge as a framework for understanding clinical information systems and their impact on health care. He did this by classifying the then current clinical information systems by the three types of objects that these systems processed: data, information, and knowledge. He noted that the classification was artificial with no clear boundaries; however, increasing complexity between the concepts existed. In 1989, Graves and Corcoran built on this work when they published their seminal work describing the study of NI using the concepts of data, information, and knowledge. The article contributed two broad principles to NI that are acknowledged here: a definition of NI that has been widely accepted in the field; and an information model that identified data, information, and knowledge as key components of NI practice. The Graves model is presented in Figure 6-1.

Graves and Corcoran (1989) drew from Blum (1986) to define the three concepts as follows: (1) **data** are discrete entities described objectively without interpretation; (2) **information** is data that are interpreted, organized, or structured; and (3) **knowledge** is information that is synthesized so that relationships are identified and formalized. Drawing on this work, Nelson (1989, 2002) defined **wisdom** as the appropriate application of knowledge to the management and solution of human problems.

Data, which are processed to create information and then knowledge, may be obtained from individuals, families, communities, and populations and the environment in which they exist. Data, information, knowledge, and wisdom are of concern to nurses in all areas of practice. For example, data derived from direct care of an individual may then be compiled across persons and aggregated for decision-making by nurses, nurse administrators, or other health professionals.

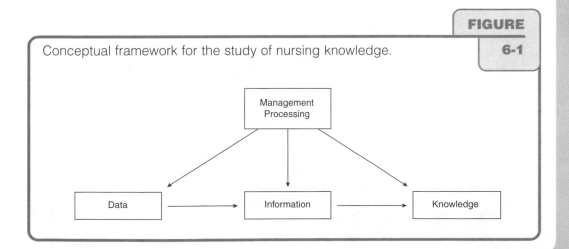

FIGURE 6-1

Conceptual framework for the study of nursing knowledge.

Further aggregation may address communities and populations. Nurse-educators may create case studies using these data, and nurse-researchers may access aggregated data for systematic study.

As an example, an instance of vital signs for an individual's heart rate, respiration, temperature, and blood pressure can be considered a set of data elements. A serial set of vital signs taken over time, placed into a context, and used for longitudinal comparisons is considered information. That is, a dropping blood pressure and increasing heart rate, respiratory rate, and fever in an elderly, catheterized person are recognized as being abnormal for this person. The recognition that the person may be septic and therefore may need certain nursing interventions reflects information synthesis (knowledge) based on nursing knowledge and experience.

Figure 6-2 builds on the work of Graves and Corcoran (1989) by adding the concept of wisdom and reconfiguring the interrelationships between and among

FIGURE

6-2   The relationship of data, information, knowledge, and wisdom.

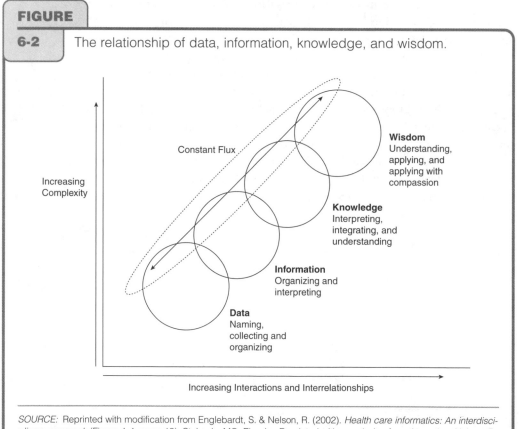

SOURCE: Reprinted with modification from Englebardt, S. & Nelson, R. (2002). *Health care informatics: An interdisciplinary approach* (Figure 1-4, page 13). St. Louis, MO: Elsevier, Reprinted with permission from the author, Nelson, R. (note Elsevier no longer owns the copyright).

the concepts. As data are transformed into information and information into knowledge, each level increases in complexity and requires greater application of human intellect. The X-axis in Figure 6-2 represents interactions within and between the concepts as one moves from data to wisdom; the Y-axis represents the increasing complexity of the concepts' increasing interrelationships.

Wisdom is knowing when and how to apply knowledge to deal with complex problems or specific human need (Nelson & Joos, 1989; Nelson, 2002). Although knowledge focuses on what is known, wisdom focuses on the appropriate application of that knowledge. For example, a knowledge base may include several options for managing an anxious family, whereas wisdom would guide the decisions about which of these options are most appropriate within a specific family. As this example demonstrates, the scope of NI is based on the scope of nursing practice and nursing science with a concentration on data, information, knowledge, and wisdom. It is not limited by current technology. If the study of NI was limited to what the computer can process, the study of informatics could not fully appreciate or support the full scope and complexity of nursing practice. NI must consider how nurses impact technology and how technology impacts nursing. An understanding of this interaction makes it possible to understand how nurses create knowledge and how they make use of that knowledge in their practices.

The appropriate use of knowledge involves the integration of empirical, ethical, personal, and aesthetic knowledge in the process of implementing actions. The individual must apply a high level of empirical knowledge in understanding the current situation; apply a professional value system in considering possible actions, be able to predict the potential outcome of these actions with a high level of accuracy, and then to have the will power to carry out the selected action in the current environment. An example of applied wisdom demonstrating this integration in NI is the appropriate use of information management and technological tools to support effective nursing practice.

The addition of wisdom raises new and important research questions. This addition challenges the discipline to develop tools and processes for classifying, measuring, and coding wisdom as it relates to nursing, NI, and informatics education. These research avenues help clarify the relationships between wisdom and the intuitive thinking of expert nurses. Such research is invaluable in building information systems to support expert healthcare practitioners and to support the decision process of more novice nurses.

Two interrelated forces have encouraged expansion of the NI model to include wisdom. First, the initial work was limited to the types of objects processed by automated systems in the mid-1980s. However, NI is now concerned with the use of information technology to improve the access and quality of health care that is delivered to individuals, families, and communities. Addition of the concept of wisdom expands the focus of the model from the technology and the processing of objects to include interaction of the human with the technology and resultant outcomes.

The previous ANA Scope and Standards of Practice (2001) had considered the inclusion of the concept of wisdom as too controversial. However, with the recognition of this concept in the 2008 ANA Scope and Standards of Practice, nurses are now demonstrating the practical application of the concept to the practice of NI. For example, Schleyer and Beaudry (2009) described how the data-to-wisdom continuum applies to informatics in telephone triage nursing practice. Another example from acute care is a statement by Troy Seagondollar posted on the NI list-serv ni-wg on Friday November 19, 2010, at 11:27 am:

> I recently had the honor of being part of a group focused on advancing the utility of the Plan of Care in an EHR. The ultimate goal was to create a Data entry system that followed each disciplines work flow, presented the Information in contextual format, and enhanced interdisciplinary/multidisciplinary Knowledge exchange about what was being worked on and how each individual added value to the patient-centered goal. All of this was created using a foundation of evidenced-based content that could be referenced to, electronically, thus increasing the Wisdom of the whole care team.
>
> If every Informatics Nurse on this list-serv could form a group and begin formulating similar Plans of Care, there would be no argument about whether or not the Plan of Care, coordinated by nursing, should be included in the Stage 2 Meaningful Use criteria as a way to advance health care in America. We as a group would already hold the evidence in hand. Case closed. (Source: Troy Seagondollar, RN-BC, MSN, Informatics Certified Informatics Nurse, with permission.)

More formally, the philosophical underpinnings and validity of the concept of wisdom in the data-information-knowledge-wisdom framework are discussed in more detail by Matney, Brewster, Sward, Cloyes and Staggers (2011). Essentially, two perspectives in philosophy, postpositivism, and hermeneutics together support the addition of wisdom in the framework for NI.

Sciences Underpinning NI

A significant contribution of Graves and Corcoran (1989) was a description and definition of NI that was widely accepted in the field in the 1990s. It stated that NI is a combination of nursing science, information science, and computer science to manage and process nursing data, information, and knowledge to facilitate the delivery of health care. The central notion was that the application of these three core sciences was what made NI unique and differentiated it from other informatics specialties.

In addition to these three core sciences, other sciences may be required to solve informatics issues. James Turley (1996) expanded the model of NI to include cognitive science. Certainly the cognitive aspect of humans is a critical piece for the **informatics nurse specialist** (INS) and the **informatics nurse** (IN) to understand. However, other sciences may be equally as critical depending on the issue at hand. For example, if the INS is dealing with a systems implementation in an institution, an understanding of organizational theory may be germane to successful implementation (Staggers & Thompson, 2002). As science evolves, it may be necessary to include other core sciences in future models.

Although the core sciences are foundational to the work of NI, the practice of the specialty is considered an applied science rather than a basic science. The combination of sciences creates a unique blend that is greater than the sum of its parts, a unique combination that creates the definitive specialty of NI. Further, informatics realizes its full potential within health care when it is grounded within a discipline; in this case, the discipline is nursing. Computer and information science applied in isolation have less impact than if applied within a disciplinary framework. Through application, the science of informatics can solve critical healthcare issues of concern to a particular discipline.

Structured Language as a Tool for NI

Many of the tools used by the IN and INS are based on metastructures and concepts that incorporate knowledge from nursing and other health and information sciences. Nursing knowledge is gained by the ability to extract data that specifically defines nursing phenomena. Many different languages and ways of organizing data, information, and knowledge exist based on different concepts.

The creation of nursing taxonomies and nomenclatures has occurred over the past years allowing these iterations to occur. The ANA has formalized the recognition of these languages and vocabularies through a review process of the Committee on Nursing Practice Information Infrastructure (CNPII). Box 6-1 lists the ANA-approved nursing languages (as of August 2010) and provides a Web site for each approved language (http://www.nursingworld.org/MainMenuCategories/The PracticeofProfessionalNursing/NursingStandards/Recognized-Nursing-Practice-Terminologies.aspx).

At a higher level of structure, several resources have been developed to facilitate interoperability among different systems of concepts and nomenclature. For instance, the Systemized Nomenclature of Medicine (SNOMED CT) is considered a universal healthcare terminology and messaging structure. In nursing, SNOMED enables terminology from one system to be mapped to concepts from another (e.g., North American Nursing Diagnosis Association (NANDA), Nursing Intervention Classification (NIC), and Nursing Outcome Classification (NOC). On a

ANA-Recognized Terminologies that Support Nursing Practice (August 2010)

1. NANDA: Nursing Diagnoses, Definitions, and Classification, 1992
   Website: www.nanda.org

2. Nursing Interventions Classification System (NIC) 1992
   Website: www.nursing.uiowa.edu/excellence/nursing_knowledge/clinical_
   effectiveness/index.htm
   (NIC/NOC can be obtained from the same source)

3. Clinical Care Classification (CCC) 1992
   Formerly Home Health Care Classification (HHCC)
   Website: www.sabacare.com

4. Omaha System, 1992
   Website: www.omahasystem.org

5. Nursing Outcomes Classification (NOC) 1997
   Sue Moorehead, PhD, RN, Center Director
   Website: www.nursing.uiowa.edu/excellence/nursing_knowledge/clinical_
   effectiveness/index.htm
   (NIC/NOC can be obtained from the same source)

6. Nursing Management Minimum Data Set (NMMDS) 1998
   Website: http://www.nursing.umn.edu/ICNP/USANMMDS/home.html

7. PeriOperative Nursing Data Set (PNDS) 1999
   Website: www.aorn.org or www.aorn.org/PracticeResources/PNDSAnd
   StandardizedPerioperativeRecord/

8. SNOMED CT, 1999
   Website: www.ihtsdo.org/snomed-ct/

9. Nursing Minimum Data Set (NMDS) 1999
   Website: http://www.nursing.umn.edu/ICNP/USANMDS/home.html

10. International Classification for Nursing Practice (ICNP®) 2000
    Website: http://www.icn.ch/icnp.htm

11. ABC Codes, 2000
    WebSite: www.abccodes.com
    Prepared from information located at http://www.nursingworld.org/
    MainMenuCategories/ThePracticeofProfessionalNursing/Nursing
    Standards/Recognized-Nursing-Practice-Terminologies.aspx.

12. Logical Observation Identifiers Names and Codes (LOINC®) 2002
    WebSite: http://loinc.org

13. Retired Data Sets
    Patient Care Data Set (PCDS) 1998

larger scale, the Unified Medical Language System of the National Library of Medicine (UMLS) http://www.nlm.nih.gov/research/umls) incorporates the work of over 100 vocabularies, including SNOMED (http://www.nlm.nih.gov/research/umls/metaa1.html). The INS must be aware of these tools, and may be called on to understand the concepts of one or more languages, the relationships between related concepts, and integration into existing vocabularies for a given organization.

The importance of languages and vocabularies cannot be overstated. The INS must seek a broader picture of the implications of their work, and the uses and outcomes of languages and vocabularies for end users. For instance, nurses working in mapping a home care vocabulary with an intervention vocabulary must see beyond the technical aspect of the work. They must understand that there may be a case manager for a multisystem health organization or a home care agency who is developing knowledge of nursing acuity and case mix based on the differing vocabularies that they have integrated. The INS must envision the differing functions that may be used with the data, information, and knowledge that have been created.

Concepts and Tools from Information Science and Computer Science

Computer science focuses on the study of the theoretical foundations of computation processes and of practical techniques for their application in computer systems. Information science is an interdisciplinary science concerned with the collection, classification, manipulation, storage, retrieval, and dissemination of information. Informatics tools and methods from computer and information sciences are considered fundamental elements of NI, including information technology, information structures, information management, and information communication.

Information technology includes computer hardware, software, communication, and network technologies, derived primarily from computer science. The other three elements are derived primarily from information science. Information structures organize data, information, and knowledge for processing by computers. Information management is an elemental process within informatics in which one is able to file, store, and manipulate data for various uses. Information communication processes enable systems to send data, and to present information in a format that improves understanding. The use of information technology distinguishes informatics from more traditional methods of information management. Thus, NI incorporates the four previously mentioned additional elements from computer and information science. Underlying all of these are HCI concepts, discussed next.

HCI and Related Concepts

HCI, usability, and ergonomics concepts are of fundamental interest to the INS. Essentially, HCI deals with people, software applications, computer technology, and the ways they influence each other (Dix, Finlay, Abowd, & Beale, 2004). Elements of HCI are rooted in psychology, social psychology, and cognitive science. However, the design, development, implementation, and evaluation of applications derive from applied work in computer science; the specific discipline at hand (in this case nursing); and information science. For example, an INS assesses an application before purchase to determine whether the application design complements the way nurses cognitively process medication orders.

A related concept is "**usability**," which deals with specific issues of human performance during computer interactions for specific tasks within a particular context (Dix et al., 2004). Usability issues address the efficiency and effectiveness of an application. For example, an INS might study the ease of learning an application, the ease of using an application, or the speed of task completion and errors that occurred during application use when determining which system or application would be best used on a nursing unit.

The term "**ergonomics**" typically is used in the United States to describe the design and implementation of equipment, tools, and machines related to human safety, comfort, and convenience. Commonly, the term "ergonomics" refers to attributes of physical equipment or to principles of arrangement of equipment in the work environment. For instance, an INS may have a role in ensuring that good ergonomics principles are used in an intensive care unit to select and arrange various devices to support workflow for cross-disciplinary providers and patients' families.

HCI, usability, and ergonomics are related concepts typically subsumed under the rubric of human factors or how humans and technology relate to each other. The overall goal is better design for software, devices, and equipment to promote optimal task completion in various contexts or environments. Optimal task completion includes the concepts of efficiency and effectiveness, including considerations about the safety of the user. It is essential that the INS understand these concepts to be able to develop effective strategies to select, implement, and evaluate information structures and informatics solutions.

The importance of human factors in health care was elevated with the Institute of Medicine's 2001 report (2001). Before this, HCI and usability assessments and methods were being incorporated into health at a glacial speed. In the past 5 years the number of HCI and usability publications in health care has increased substantially. Vendors have installed usability laboratories and incorporated usability testing of their products into their systems lifecycles. The Food and Drug Administration (FDA) has mandated usability testing as part of their approval process for any new devices (Medical Devices Today, 2007). Thus, HCI and usability are critical concepts for INs and INSs to understand. Numerous usability methods and tools are available (e.g., heuristics [rules of thumb], naturalistic observation, and think-aloud protocols). Readers are referred to HCI references and Chapter 5 to learn more about these methods.

Phenomena of Nursing

The metaparadigm of nursing comprises four key concepts: (1) nurse, (2) person, (3) health, and (4) environment. Nursing actions are based on interrelationships between the concepts and are related to the values nurses hold relative to them. Nurses make decisions about interventions from their unique perspectives. Decision making is the process of choosing among alternatives. The decisions that nurses make can be characterized by both the quality of decisions and the impact of the actions resulting from those decisions. As knowledge workers, nurses make numerous decisions that affect the life and well-being of individuals, families, and communities. The process of decision making in nursing is guided by the concept of critical thinking. Critical thinking is the intellectually disciplined process of actively and skillfully using knowledge to conceptualize, apply, analyze, synthesize, or evaluate data and information as a guide to belief and action (Scriven & Paul, 1997).

Clinical wisdom is the ability of the nurse to add experience and intuition to a situation involving the care of a person (Benner, Hooper-Kyriadkidis, & Stannard, 1999). Wisdom is demonstrated in informatics by the ability of the INS to evaluate the documentation drawn from a health information system (HIS) and the ability to adapt or change the system settings or parameters to improve the workflow of the clinical nurse.

Nurses' decision making is described as an array of decisions that include specific behaviors and cognitive processes surrounding a cluster of issues. For example, nurses use data transformed into information to determine interventions for persons, families, and communities. Nurses make decisions about potential problems presented by an individual and about appropriate recommendations for addressing those problems. They also make decisions in collaboration with other healthcare professionals, such as physicians, pharmacists, or social workers. Decisions also may occur within specific environments, such as executive offices, classrooms, and research laboratories.

An information system collects and processes data and information. Decision-support systems are computer applications designed to facilitate human decision-making processes. Decision-support systems are typically rule-based, using a specified knowledge base and a set of rules to analyze data and information and provide recommendations. Other decision-support systems are based on knowledge models induced directly from data, regression, or classification models that predict characteristics or outcomes. Recommendations take the form of alerts (i.e., calling user attention to abnormal laboratory results or potential adverse drug events) or suggestions (e.g., appropriate medications, therapies, or other actions) (Haug, Gardner, & Evans, 1999).

An **expert system** is a type of **decision support system** that implements the knowledge of one or more human experts without human intervention. For example, an insulin pump that senses the patient's blood glucose level and administers insulin based on that data is a form of expert system. Whereas control systems implement decisions without involvement of a user, decision support systems merely provide recommendations and rely on the wisdom of the user for appropriate application of these provided recommendations. Within informatics there is always a tension between what decisions should be automated and what decisions require human intervention. The relationships among these concepts and information, decision support, and expert systems are represented in Figure 6-3.

An INS must be able to navigate the complexity of the relationships between the following elements and understand how they facilitate decision making:

- Data, information, knowledge, and wisdom
- Nursing science, information science, computer science, and other sciences of interest to the issue at hand (e.g., cognitive science)
- Nurse, person, health, and environment
- Information structures, information technology, managing and communicating information

FIGURE 6-3   Levels and types of automated systems.

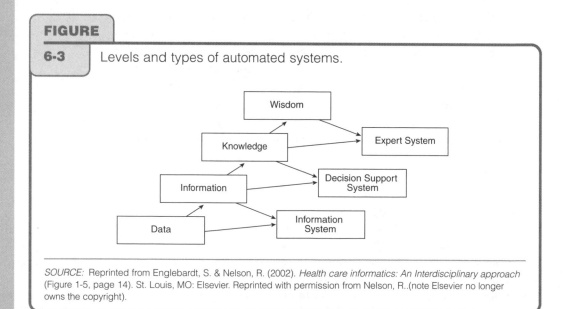

SOURCE: Reprinted from Englebardt, S. & Nelson, R. (2002). *Health care informatics: An Interdisciplinary approach* (Figure 1-5, page 14). St. Louis, MO: Elsevier. Reprinted with permission from Nelson, R..(note Elsevier no longer owns the copyright).

THE FUTURE OF NI

The future of NI will impact and be impacted by several driving trends. These include (1) changes in society, such as the aging population, the AIDS epidemic, or the increased use of participatory and mobile technology; (2) changes in health care delivery including the changing and expanding role of nursing within healthcare delivery; and (3) changes in technology, such as **nanotechnology**, which promises to redefine the composition of nearly every man-made material and drastically alter biomedical applications (Alivisatos, 2001).

All of these changes will drive increased saturation of informatics concepts and solutions into mainstream nursing and healthcare practices. As informatics solutions become as common a tool as the stethoscope, every nurse to be safe and effective will need to incorporate informatics concepts into all aspects of practice. One example is the increased recognition of the concept of wisdom as a key concept for NI. Its more detailed definition and measurement will be a part of the future practice of all nursing.

SUMMARY

This chapter outlines the foundations of NI. The following definition for NI is offered: NI is a specialty that integrates nursing science, computer science, and information science to manage and communicate data, information, knowledge, and wisdom in nursing practice. Interrelationships among major NI concepts are discussed. As data are transformed into information and information into knowledge, and knowledge is applied through wisdom to ensure appropriate, effective, and compassionate nursing care increasing complexity and interrelationships ensue. The boundaries between concepts can be blurred and feedback loops from one concept level to another occur. These major concepts can be related to types of systems including information, expert, and decision-support systems. The following sciences for NI are provided: nursing, computer, and information science. Other sciences are used as required by the issue at hand. Critical elements for NI are noted; they include structured languages and HCI concepts. Taxonomies and other current structured languages for nursing are listed. HCI concepts are briefly defined and discussed because they are critical to the success of informatics solutions.

Finally, in an ideal world, the authors would like to see the following:

- Patients would be truly active participants in managing their health. The use of technology, such as personal health records and automated monitoring devices, along with the implementation of participatory medicine will make that possible.
- Safe care where over 100,000 patients do not die each year from medical error. Improved use of technology, such as decision-support systems and alerts, will make that possible.

- Health care that can be afforded by all. An increased use of prevention strategies and efficiencies gained from technology will make that possible.
- A working environment for all nurses where data, information, and knowledge are effectively managed to ensure wisdom guides all nursing decisions.

THOUGHT-PROVOKING Questions

WWW

1. How is the concept of wisdom in NI like or unlike professional nursing judgment?

2. Can you create examples of how expert systems (not decision-support but true expert systems) can be used to support nursing practice?

3. How would you incorporate the data-to-wisdom continuum into a job description for a NI specialist?

4. If computer and information science are foundational to NI, should computer and information literacy be a requirement in all nursing programs at all levels?

5. Can any aspect of nursing wisdom be automated?

6. The chapter states that research will be invaluable in building information systems to support expert healthcare practitioners and support the decision process of more novice nurses. What is the significance of this statement to the study of HCI in NI?

For a full suite of assignments and additional learning activities, use the access code located in the front of your book to visit this exclusive website: http://go.jblearning.com/mcgonigle. If you do not have an access code, you can obtain one at the site.

WWW

References

Alivisatos, A. P. (2001). Less is more in medicine: Sophisticated forms of nanotechnology will find some of the first real-world applications in biomedical research, disease diagnosis and possibly therapy. *Scientific American, 285*(3), 66–73.

American Nurses Association (ANA). (2008). *Nursing informatics: Scope & standards of practice.* Springfield, MD: Nursesbooks.org

Benner, P., Hooper-Kyriadkidis, P., & Stannard, D. (1999). *Clinical wisdom and interventions in critical care: A thinking-in-action approach.* Philadelphia, PA: W.B. Saunders.

Blum, B. (1986). *Clinical information systems.* New York, NY: Springer-Verlag.

Brennan, R. (2003). *One size doesn't fit all—Pedagogy in the online environment: Vol. 1.* Adelaide, Australia: National Centre for Vocational Education Research. Retrieved from http://www.ncver.edu.au/research/proj/nr0F05e.htm

Dix, A., Finlay, J., Abowd, G., & Beale, R. (2004). Human–computer interaction. Harlow, England: Pearson, Prentice Hall.

Graves, J., & Corcoran, S. (1989). The study of nursing informatics. *Image, 21*(4), 227–230.

Haug, P., Gardner, R., & Evans, S. (1999). Hospital-based decision support. In E. S. Berner (Ed.), *Clinical decision support systems: Theory and practice* (pp. 77–104). New York, NY: Springer-Verlag.

Institute of Medicine. (2001). *Crossing the quality chasm: A new health system for the 21st century.* Washington, DC: National Academies Press.

Joos, I., Nelson, R., & Smith, M. (2010). *Introduction to computers for healthcare professional* (5th ed.). Sudbury, MA: Jones and Bartlett Publishers.

Matney, S., Brewster, P., Sward, K., Cloyes, K., & Staggers, N. (March, 2011). Philosophical approaches to the data-information-knowledge-wisdom framework. *Advances in Nursing Science, 34* (1).

Medical Devices Today. (2007). *New usability standard aims to help firms institute human factors programs.* Retrieved from http://www.medicaldevicestoday.com/2007/04/new_usability_s.html

Nelson, R., & Joos, I. (Fall, 1989). On language in nursing: From data to wisdom. Pennsylvania League for Nursing *PLN Vision* (p. 6).

Nelson, R. (2002) Major theories supporting health care informatics. In S. Englebardt & R. Nelson (Eds.), *Health care informatics: An interdisciplinary approach* (pp. 3–27). St. Louis, MO: Mosby-Year Book.

Schleyer, R., & Beaudry, S. (2009) Data to wisdom: Informatics in telephone triage nursing practice. *AAACN Viewpoint, 31*(5), 1, 10–3.

Scriven, M., & Paul, R. (1997). *A working definition of critical thinking.* Retrieved from http://lonestar.texas.net/~mseifert/crit2.html

Staggers, N., & Thompson, C. B. (2002). The evolution of definitions for nursing informatics: A critical analysis and revised definition. *Journal of the American Medical Informatics Association (JAMIA), 33*(1), 75–81.

Turley, J. (1996). Toward a model for nursing informatics. *Image: Journal of Nursing Scholarship, 28*(4), 309–313.

CHAPTER 7

Developing Standardized Terminologies to Support Nursing Practice

Nicholas Hardiker

Objectives

1. Explore the need for consistent terminology in nursing.
2. Describe the different approaches to terminology development.
3. Assess initiatives seeking to exploit commonalities among terminologies and to ensure appropriate implementation and consistent use.

WWW

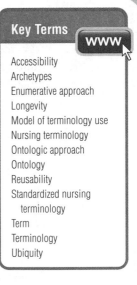

Key Terms **WWW**

Accessibility
Archetypes
Enumerative approach
Longevity
Model of terminology use
Nursing terminology
Ontologic approach
Ontology
Reusability
Standardized nursing
  terminology
Term
Terminology
Ubiquity

INTRODUCTION

Agreement on the consistent use of a term, such as "impaired physical mobility," allows that term to be used for a number of purposes: to provide continuity of care from care provider to care provider, to ensure care quality by facilitating comparisons between care providers, or to identify trends through data aggregation. Since the early 1970s there has been a concerted effort to promote consistency in nursing terminology. Work continues, driven by the following increasing demands placed on health-related information and knowledge:

- **Accessibility**: It should be easy to access the information and knowledge needed to deliver care or manage a health service.
- **Ubiquity**: With changing models of healthcare delivery, information and knowledge should be available anywhere.
- **Longevity**: Information should be usable beyond the immediate clinical encounter.
- **Reusability**: Information should be useful for a range of purposes.

Without consistent terminology, nursing runs the risk of becoming invisible; it will remain difficult to quantify nursing, the unique contribution and impact of nursing will go unrecognized, and the nursing component of electronic health record systems will remain at best rudimentary. Not least, without consistent terminology the nursing knowledge base will suffer, in terms of development and in terms of access, thereby delaying the integration of evidence-based health care into nursing practice. External pressures compound the problem. For example, in the United States, the Health Information Technology for Economic and Clinical Health (HITECH) Act, signed in January 2009, provides a financial incentive for the use of electronic health records; similar steps are being taken in other regions. The HITECH Act mandates that electronic health records are used in a meaningful way; this is problematic without consistent terminology (see Chapter 10 for more information on the HITECH Act). Finally, the current and future landscape of information and communication technologies (e.g., connection anywhere, borderless communication, Web-based applications, collaborative working, disintermediation and reintermediation, consumerization, ubiquitous advanced digital content [van Eecke, da Fonseca Pinto, & Egyedi, 2007]) and their inevitable infiltration into health care will only serve to reinforce the need for consistent nursing terminology while providing an additional sense of urgency. This chapter explains what is meant by a standardized nursing terminology and lists several examples. It describes in detail the different approaches taken in the development of two example terminologies. It presents, in the form of an international technical standard, a means of ensuring consistency among the plethora of contemporary standardized nursing terminologies, with a view to harmonization and possible convergence. Finally, it provides a rationale for the shared development of models of terminology use; models that embody both clinical and pragmatic knowledge to ensure that contemporary nursing record systems reflect the best available evidence and fit comfortably with routine practice.

STANDARDIZED NURSING TERMINOLOGIES

A **term** at its simplest level is a word or phrase used to describe something concrete (e.g., leg) or abstract (e.g., plan). **A nursing terminology** is a body of the terms used in nursing. There are many nursing terminologies, formal and informal. Nursing terminologies allow one consistently to capture, represent, access, and communicate nursing data, information, and knowledge. A **standardized nursing terminology** is a nursing terminology that is in some way approved by an appropriate authority (de jure standardization) or by general consent (de facto standardization).

In North America, one such authority is the American Nurses Association (ANA) (2007), which operates a process of de jure standardization through its committee for nursing practice information infrastructure (CNPII) (http://www.nursingworld.org/npii/). Although in 2010 there were many more nursing terminologies in use around the world, in that year CNPII recognized the following seven active (i.e., not retired) nursing terminologies (so-called "interface terminologies"):

1. Clinical Care Classification (CCC) (http://www.sabacare.com): The clinical care classification (CCC) system consists of two interrelated terminologies that cover nursing diagnoses, nursing outcomes, nursing interventions, and nursing actions. The two terminologies are linked by a common framework of care components.

2. International Classification of Nursing Practice (ICNP) (http://www.icn.ch/pillarsprograms/international-classification-for-nursing-practicer/): a compositional nursing terminology developed by the International Council of Nurses that covers nursing phenomena (i.e., diagnoses), nursing actions, and nursing outcomes. Seeks to support the development of local terminologies and facilitate cross-mapping among terminologies.

3. North American Nursing Diagnosis Association International (NANDA-I) (http://www.nanda.org):—NANDA International maintains an agreed set of nursing diagnoses organized as a multiaxial taxonomy of domains and classes.

4. Nursing Intervention Classification (NIC) (http://www.nursing.uiowa.edu/excellence/nursing_knowledge/clinical_effectiveness/nic.htm): The nursing interventions classification (NIC) is terminology that covers interventions performed by nurses and other providers. In common with NANDA, NIC interventions are organized into classes and domains.

5. Nursing Outcomes Classification (NOC) (http://www.nursing.uiowa.edu/excellence/nursing_knowledge/clinical_effectiveness/noc.htm):—The nursing outcomes classification (NOC) is a terminology that covers patient–client outcomes, presented as an alphabetical list.

6. Omaha Home Health Care System (http://www.omahasystem.org): the problem classification scheme, the intervention scheme, and the problem rating scale for outcomes. These components provide both a terminology and a framework for documentation.

7. Perioperative Nursing Data Set (PNDS) (http://www.aorn.org/PracticeResources/PNDSAndStandardizedPerioperativeRecord/): In contrast to the other terminologies listed here, which are intended for use in any setting and for any specialty, the perioperative nursing data set (PNDS) is a terminology that covers specifically the perioperative patient experience in terms of nursing diagnoses, nursing interventions, and nurse-sensitive patient outcomes.

In 2010 the CNPII had also recognized the retired nursing terminology patient care data set along with three multidisciplinary terminologies: (1) alternative billing codes (ABC) (http://www.alternativelink.com); (2) logical observation identifiers names and codes (LOINC) (http://loinc.org/); and (3) systematic nomenclature of medicine clinical terms (SNOMED CT) (http://www.ihtsdo.org/snomed-ct/).

Finally, CNPII recognized two data element sets: nursing minimum data set (NMDS) and nursing management minimum data set (NMMDS). Work on a standardized data element set for nursing, which in the United States began in the 1980s with the nursing minimum data set NMDS (Werley & Lang, 1988), provided an additional catalyst for the development of many of the aforementioned nursing terminologies that could provide values (e.g., chronic pain) for particular data elements in the nursing minimum data set NMDS (e.g., nursing diagnosis). The data element sets provide a framework for the uniform collection and management of nursing data; the use of a standardized nursing terminology to represent that data serves further to enhance consistency.

APPROACHES TO NURSING TERMINOLOGY

From relatively humble beginnings, nursing terminologies have evolved significantly over the past several decades in line with best practices in terminology work, from simple lists of words or phrases to large, complex so-called "ontologies" (descriptions of entities within a domain and the relationships between them). This evolution has been facilitated by advances in knowledge representation (e.g., the refinement of the description logic that underpins many contemporary ontologies) and in their accompanying technologies (e.g., automated reasoners that can check consistency and identify equivalence) and subsumption (i.e., subclass–superclass) relationships within those ontologies. The following section expands on two of the terminologies listed previously: NANDA and ICNP. These terminologies have been selected as examples to demonstrate the relative extremes of the terminologic evolutionary path. No assumption should be made that either of the example terminologies is better than or worse than the other. Nor should any assumption be made that either of these terminologies is better than or worse than any other terminology. The examples merely represent different approaches that serve to complement one another, affording an opportunity for synergism.

Enumerative Approach

With the **enumerative approach**, words or phrases are represented in a list or a simple hierarchy. In NANDA, a nursing diagnosis has an associated name or label and a textual definition (NANDA International, 2008). Each nursing diagnosis may have a set of defining characteristics and related or risk factors. These additional features do not constitute part of the core terminology. Instead, they are intended to be used as an aid to diagnosis. NANDA's multiaxial taxonomy (i.e., Taxonomy II) organizes nursing diagnoses into classes and domains. Although Taxonomy II provides an organizational framework for NANDA nursing diagnoses, it makes no attempt to organize nursing diagnoses among themselves (i.e., there are no hierarchical relationships among NANDA nursing diagnoses). Furthermore, there are no associative relationships apart from the implicit and global sibling relationship (i.e., every nursing diagnosis appears at the same level of indentation in the list, and there is no means to identify equivalent nursing diagnoses). However, what NANDA may lack in terms of hierarchical sophistication, it makes up for in terms of simplicity and potential ease of implementation and use.

Ontologic Approach

The **ontologic approach** is compositional in nature and a partial representation of the entities within a domain and the relationships that hold between them. ICNP takes the ontologic approach, a different approach than NANDA. ICNP is described as a unified nursing language system. It seeks to provide a resource that can be used to develop local terminologies and to facilitate cross-mapping between terminologies to compare and combine data from different sources; the existence of a number of overlapping but inconsistent standardized nursing terminologies is problematic in terms of data comparison and aggregation.

ICNP version 2 is an example of ontology. The core of ICNP is represented in the Web ontology language (OWL), a recommendation of the World Wide Web Consortium (W3C) and a de facto standard language for representing ontologies (McGuiness & van Harmelen, 2004). The ICNP ontology comprises OWL classes and OWL properties. Classes are organized into taxonomy. Properties link individuals (i.e., members of classes) together. A simplified graphic representation of chronic confusion showing the hasOnset property and the relationship that holds between individuals in the confusion and chronic classes is shown in Figure 7-1.

FIGURE 7-1

Simplified OWL representation of chronic confusion. Squares represent classes, while circles represent individuals with classes. The arrow represents a relationship along the has Onset property.

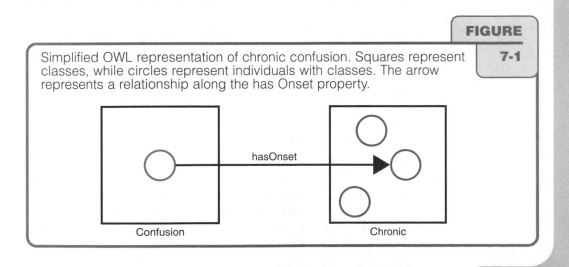

Confusion   hasOnset   Chronic

Because it is underpinned by description logic, OWL permits the use of automated reasoners that can check consistency, identify equivalence, and support classification within the ICNP ontology. The result is a rigorously and predictably defined multiple hierarchy. The compositional nature of the ICNP ontology makes it well suited to support the development of local terminologies; the rich hierarchy (and the opportunity for automated reasoning) makes it well suited to support cross-mapping between terminologies. However, ICNP is computer-based; it may be more powerful than NANDA, but in its raw form it may also be more difficult to implement and use.

EXPLOITING COMMONALITY AMONG NURSING TERMINOLOGIES

There are many differences between NANDA and ICNP. However, they both purport at least to represent nursing diagnoses (ICNP also represents nursing actions and nursing outcomes); and they are both recognized by the American Nurses Association (ANA) (through CNPII) as interface terminologies that support nursing practice.

Indeed, there are many differences between the broader set of standardized nursing terminologies in terms of scale, scope, structure, and intended use. However, as with NANDA and ICNP there are many similarities, particularly concerning content. These similarities have been exploited in the development of an international technical standard: ISO 18104:2003 health informatics—integration of a reference terminology model for nursing (International Organization for Standardization, 2003). ISO 18104:2003, in routine revision at the time of writing, was developed through a consensus process that considered a number of standardized nursing terminologies to determine a model or schema that could outline the basic form of nursing statements (i.e., a reference terminology model for nursing).

At the heart of the standard are two models: a model for nursing diagnosis and a model for nursing action. A graphic representation of the model for statements that describes nursing diagnoses is presented in Figure 7-2. According to this model, for a statement to be considered a valid nursing diagnosis, its decomposition must at minimum comprise both a focus and a judgment. For example, impaired physical mobility is considered a valid nursing diagnosis because its decomposition comprises the focus physical mobility and the judgment impaired.

A graphic representation of the model for statements that describe nursing actions is presented in Figure 7-3. As in the previous model, according to this model, for a statement to be considered a valid nursing action, its decomposition must as a minimum comprise both an action (e.g., monitoring) and a target (e.g., blood glucose, as in the case of monitoring blood glucose).

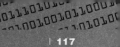

FIGURE 7-2

Model for nursing diagnosis.

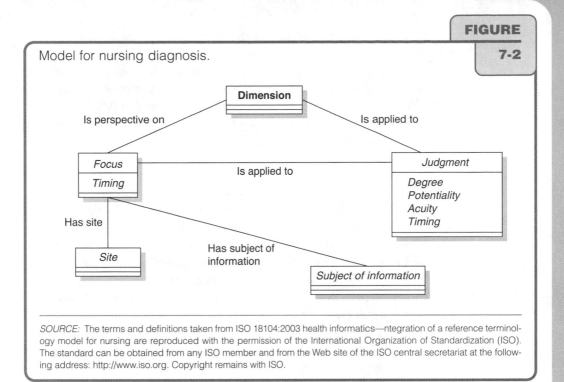

SOURCE: The terms and definitions taken from ISO 18104:2003 health informatics—ntegration of a reference terminology model for nursing are reproduced with the permission of the International Organization of Standardization (ISO). The standard can be obtained from any ISO member and from the Web site of the ISO central secretariat at the following address: http://www.iso.org. Copyright remains with ISO.

FIGURE 7-3

Model for nursing action.

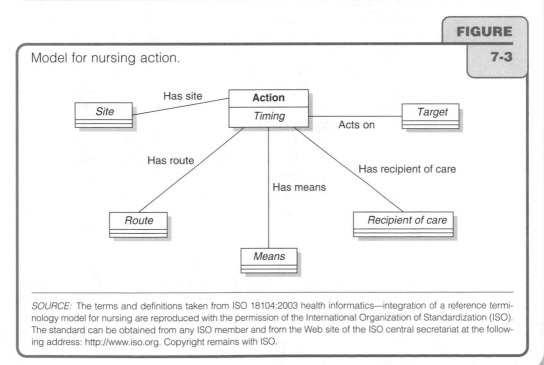

SOURCE: The terms and definitions taken from ISO 18104:2003 health informatics—integration of a reference terminology model for nursing are reproduced with the permission of the International Organization of Standardization (ISO). The standard can be obtained from any ISO member and from the Web site of the ISO central secretariat at the following address: http://www.iso.org. Copyright remains with ISO.

One of the main purposes cited by ISO 18104:2003 is to facilitate the systematic evaluation and refinement of existing terminologies, discovering anomalies within nursing terminologies through noncompliant decompositions. Another purpose is to support the generation, in regular form, of composite nursing statements, ensuring consistency in emerging terminologies. It is hoped that the standard will facilitate the harmonization or convergence of standardized nursing terminologies across the world.

USING NURSING TERMINOLOGIES

The discussion thus far has focused predominantly on the developmental aspects of standardized nursing terminologies. However, if these terminologies are to fulfill their various roles, they must be used. As standardized nursing terminologies increase in complexity, however, they become more difficult to implement; they may be computer-based but they are far from plug-and-play.

This final section describes attempts to ease the burden of implementation through the development of models of terminology use. Terminologies help to convey the understanding of the world. Models of terminology use help to structure information for particular purposes. For example, a restaurant menu lists all of the dishes one might wish to order; this represents the terminology. The menu organizes the dishes in a way that encourages one to select dishes, and allows one to select dishes according to a shared view of the world (e.g., appetizer, followed by main course, followed by dessert); this represents the **model of terminology use**. The menu encourages one to make use of the terminology while delivering it in a way that fits with the task at hand.

A **terminology** or **ontology** describes how general entities (i.e., classes, such as leg) are represented and how those representations relate to each other. In contrast, a model of terminology use describes how particular entities (i.e., individual entities, such as John's leg) are represented and how those representations relate to each other. A model of terminology use may have an informational facet (e.g., relating to a record structure or message) or an operational facet (e.g., relating to a pick list for data entry or query reports).

In a particular context of use and at a particular point in time, it may not be natural for users to view particular data items in the form of a terminology or ontology; indeed, this would rarely be the case. A model of terminology use seeks to organize data items in a way that fits with that context at that time.

Previously the onus had been on the developers of end-user applications to determine their own models of terminology use. The nursing terminologies were standardized, but the models of terminology use were not. These were often embedded within applications, and it would not be possible to share the valuable clinical and pragmatic knowledge they contained. There had been much duplication of effort, with the developers of end-user applications and their prospective users working toward the same goal, but in parallel streams. This situation provided a major motivation for further standards development, standards that might support the shared development of shareable models of terminology use. Examples of a shareable model of terminology use include archetypes, care information models, clinical statements, templates, clinical elements, and detailed clinical models. Archetypes are used as an example to illustrate the common principles that underpin many of these initiatives.

An **archetype** is "a computable expression of a domain content model in the form of structured constraint statements, based on a reference (information) model" (Beale & Heard, 2007, p. 8). In routine general clinical practice, a blood pressure observation usually comprises, at a minimum, a systolic blood pressure and a diastolic blood pressure. Without an explicit model of terminology use, these either remain as separate terms in a terminology or ontology, or they need to be linked together within individual end-user applications. Archetypes capture this knowledge along with appropriate terminologic bindings and other nonterminologic details, such as associated units (e.g., mm Hg, minimum value = 0). Thus, archetypes provide a means of defining explicitly clinical and pragmatic knowledge apart from the applications that might use it.

SUMMARY

This chapter describes the need for and motivation behind the development of standardized terminologies for nursing. It describes different approaches to terminology development and introduces initiatives that seek to exploit commonalities among today's terminologies and to ensure their appropriate implementation and consistent use. The results of contemporary terminology work are encouraging. However, further work is needed to harmonize standardized nursing terminologies and to scale up and mainstream the development and implementation of models of terminology use.

In an ideal world, one would see standardized nursing terminologies and the structures and systems that support their implementation and use merely as means to an end, as tools to support good nursing practice and good patient care. Standardized nursing terminologies are important. However, they do not obviate the need to think and work creatively, to do right by the people in our care, and to continue to advance nursing.

THOUGHT-PROVOKING Questions

1. What do you believe are the advantages and disadvantages of having a single shared consensus-driven model of terminology use?
2. How can a single agreed-upon model of terminology use (with linkages to a single terminology) help to integrate knowledge into routine clinical practice?

For a full suite of assignments and additional learning activities, use the access code located in the front of your book to visit this exclusive website: **http://go.jblearning.com/mcgonigle.** If you do not have an access code, you can obtain one at the site.

References

American Nurses Association (ANA). (2007). *Nursing practice information infrastructure.* Retrieved from http://www.nursingworld.org/npii/

Beale, T., & Heard, S. (Eds.). (2007). *Archetype definitions and principles. Revision 1.0. [online].* The openEHR Foundation. Retrieved from http://svn.openehr.org/specification/TRUNK/publishing/architecture/am/archetype_principles.pdf

International Organization for Standardization. (2003). *International standard ISO 18104:2003 health informatics—integration of a reference terminology model for nursing.* Geneva, Switzerland: International Organization for Standardization.

McGuiness, D. L., & van Harmelen, F. (Eds.). (2004). *OWL Web ontology language overview [online].* World Wide Web Consortium. Retrieved from http://www.w3.org/TR/owl-features

NANDA International. (2008). *Nursing diagnoses: Definitions & classification 2009–2011 edition.* Indianapolis: Wiley-Blackwell.

van Eecke, P., da Fonseca Pinto, P., & Egyedi, T., for the European Commission. (2007). *EU study on the specific policy needs for ICT standardisation. [Final report].* Retrieved from http://ec.europa.eu/enterprise/ict/policy/doc/2007-ict-std-full-rep.pdf

Werley, H. H., & Lang, N. M. (Eds.). (1988). *Identification of the nursing minimum data set.* New York, NY: Springer Publishing Company.

CHAPTER 8

Nursing Informatics Roles, Competencies, and Skills

Julie A. Kenney and Ida Androwich

Objectives **WWW**

1. Provide an overview of nursing informatics' historical development.
2. Explore the concept of nurses as knowledge workers.
3. Discuss the evolving roles and competencies of nursing informatics practice.

Key Terms **WWW**

Advocate/policy
  developer
Certification
Cognitive activity
Consultant
Continuous learner
Core sciences
Data
Data gatherer
Decision support/
  outcomes manager
Educator
Entrepreneur
Industrial Age
Informatics
Informatics innovator
Informatics nurse specialist
Information
Information Age
Information user
Interdisciplinary knowledge
  team
Knowledge
Knowledge builder
Knowledge user
Knowledge worker

Continues

INTRODUCTION

The world has witnessed an unprecedented number of technologic advances during the last 100 years. The early 20th century witnessed the invention of the car and the airplane. These modes of transportation drastically changed how people work and play. The entertainment world was dramatically altered by the invention of radio and television. The introduction of the computer altered the way **data** and **information** are viewed and used and changed the way business is conducted. The computer is now changing nursing and health care.

Nurses have historically gathered and interpreted data. Florence Nightingale is credited as one of the first statisticians to collect and use data to change the way she cared for her patients. While serving in the Crimean War, she began to gather data regarding the conditions in which patients were living and the diseases they contracted and from which they expired. These data were later used to improve patient conditions at both city and military hospitals (O'Connor & Robertson, 2003).

Today, nurses are able to access information quickly and easily. Accessing information via the Internet or the electronic health record

(EHR) allows the nurse to provide the best possible patient care. Genomic health care and the interaction between genetic factors and the environment require new understanding of the types of information needed to make decisions, characterized as a "data tsunami" (Bakken, Stone, & Larson, 2008).

Nursing recognized early on that computers would change health care and became actively involved in shaping how computers were used in health care. The American Nurses Association (ANA) first recognized nursing informatics (NI) as a specialty in 1992 (Saba & McCormick, 2006; ANA, 2008). The introduction of this specialty has spurred the development of many informatics jobs, organizations, and publications. Nurses now have the ability to further their education by attending informatics conferences, reading journals, obtaining certificates and advanced degrees, and participating in numerous hospital-based and national and international informatics committees and groups.

WHAT IS NI?

Definitions

The term "**informatics**" was derived from the French term informatique, which means to refer to the computer milieu (Saba, 2001). The Health Information and Management Systems Society (HIMSS) defines informatics as "the discipline concerned with the study of information and manipulation of information via computer-based tools" (2006, p. 44). The definition for **medical informatics** was the first connection between informatics and health care. Medical informatics is described as collected informational technologies that affect the medical decisions made regarding patient care (Hannah, Ball, & Edwards, 2006).

NI has been defined numerous times over the years. A classic and one of the most widely cited definitions was by Graves and Corcoran (1989). Their definition moved away from the earlier definitions that tended to put a greater emphasis on technology and toward a more conceptually based definition. Graves and Corcoran define NI as a "combination of computer science, information science and nursing science designed to assist in the management and processing of nursing data, information and **knowledge** to support the practice of nursing and the delivery of nursing care" (p. 227). In 2008, ANA published an updated NI definition and an updated scope and practice. The ANA definition of NI is

> Nursing Informatics is a specialty that integrates nursing science, computer science, and information science to manage and communicate data, information, knowledge, and wisdom in nursing practice. (It) supports consumers, patients, nurses, and other providers in their decision making in all roles and

settings. This support is accomplished through the use of information, structures, information processes, and information technology (ANA, p. 1).

An excellent philosophic overview of the concept of NI is found in Matney, Brewster, Sward, Cloyes, and Staggers (2010). They believe that the foundational concepts of NI, data, information, knowledge, and wisdom, can clarify the aims of NI and that use of the data, information, knowledge, and wisdom framework can promote a foundation for "linking theory and practice." Staggers and Thompson (2002) believe that there are too many definitions for NI, causing the specialty to grow without a solid foundation. They believe that without this foundation it is difficult to build a solid informatics practice or the needed educational base for this specialty practice. Staggers and Thompson performed a critical analysis of the definitions, which resulted in a new definition as follows:

> Nursing informatics is a specialty that integrates nursing science, computer science, and information science to manage and communicate data, information, and knowledge in nursing practice. Nursing informatics facilitates the integration of data, information, and knowledge to support patients, nurses, and other providers in their decision making in all roles and settings. This support is accomplished through the use of information structures, information processes, and information technology (p. 260).

One theme that flows throughout these definitions is the combining of nursing, computer, and information science. The ANA (2008) calls these the **core sciences** of NI. These core sciences differentiate NI from other informatics specialties. NI may incorporate other sciences to solve informatics issues. An example is an informatics nurse who is working on a system implementation project. This informatics nurse needs to be able to apply the three core sciences, and organizational science and change management, to the project. The ANA points out that even though NI is based on science, it is an applied science and not a basic science. In this text, the contributions of cognitive science to informatics are also emphasized (see Chapter 4).

A second theme that flows through these definitions is the use of data, information, and knowledge by an informatics nurse. Graves and Corcoran (1989) and the ANA (2008) both believe that data, information, and knowledge are key components of NI practice. Data is defined by Graves and Corcoran as a single entity that has been described objectively and not interpreted. An example of data is a single blood pressure reading. Information is defined as data that have been interpreted, organized, or structured. An example of information is a nurse beginning to notice trends in the patient data. Knowledge is defined as information that has been synthesized so that relationships are identified and formalized (ANA, 2008). An example of this is realizing that the increased temperature, heart, and respiratory rate and the dropping blood pressure are probably the result of sepsis, which requires certain medical treatments for the patient to improve. Wisdom has been added to the newest ANA definition of NI. Wisdom is "the appropriate use of knowledge to manage and solve human problems" (ANA, p. 5). Wisdom is when the Nursing Informatics Specialist (INS) applies knowledge appropriately to deal with a complex problem or specific human need. In the previous example of sepsis, the NIS would review the data; come to the realization that the patient was most likely septic; and then based on the current situation, work with the physician to determine the best course of action for the patient's care. Data, information, knowledge, and the core sciences, when combined, represent the foundation of NI practice.

History

To understand NI, one must understand its history. Health care began to use computers in the 1950s. Computers, in this era, were typically used in the business office to track financial aspects of health care (Saba & McCormick, 2006). In the 1970s, nursing began to realize the importance of computers to the nursing profession and became involved in the design, purchase, and implementation of information systems (IS) (Saba & McCormick). In the 1980s, medical informatics and NI specialties emerged. The personal computer was introduced, which allowed for flexibility in how these clinical systems were used. It also brought to everyone's attention that not just NISs, but all healthcare personnel, need to know about these systems (Hannah et al., 2006; Saba & McCormick). The first **certification** examination for NI was taken in 1995 (Saba & McCormick). The post-2000 era saw an unprecedented explosion in the number and sophistication of both computer hardware and software. Electronic patient records became an integral part of clinical IS. Telemedicine became possible and was recognized as a specialty in the late 1990s (Saba & McCormick). NI has experienced rapid growth in the last 40 years, and it does not seem to be slowing. It will be interesting to see what happens over the next 40 years.

Goal of NI

In 2008, the ANA updated the Scope and Standards of Nursing Informatics Practice. The ANA lists the goal of NI as: "The goal of NI is to improve the health of populations, communities, families, and individuals by optimizing information management and communication" (p. 1).

THE NURSE AS A KNOWLEDGE WORKER

It has been established that nurses use data and information. This information is then converted to knowledge. The nurse then acts on this knowledge by initiating a plan of care, updating an existing one, or maintaining status quo. Does this use of knowledge make the nurse a **knowledge worker**? This section focuses on the definition of a knowledge worker and the history of the term and how it is used in health care and business. This chapter examines how nursing relates to the term "knowledge worker" and the effect a knowledge worker has on health care.

Definitions

Knowledge can be defined as "the distillation of information that has been collected, classified, organized, integrated, abstracted, and value added" (HIMSS, 2006, p. 49). A worker is "one that works especially at manual or industrial labor or with a particular material" (Merriam-Webster, 2011). The term "knowledge worker" was first coined by Peter Drucker in his 1959 book, *Landmarks of Tomorrow* (Drucker, 1994). Knowledge work is defined as nonrepetitive, nonroutine work that entails a significant amount of **cognitive activity** (Sorrells-Jones & Weaver, 1999a). Drucker (1994) describes a knowledge worker as one who has advanced formal education and is able to apply theoretical and analytical knowledge. According to Drucker, the knowledge worker must be a **continuous learner** and a specialist in a field. McCormick (2009) estimates that a knowledge worker spends at least 50% of his or her work time searching for and evaluating information. Androwich (2010) concludes that it is important to understand that there is a dual role for accessing and using information (content) in health care. In the first instance, when the nurse is caring for an individual patient, evidenced-based information (content) and patient data need to be available at the point-of-care to inform the present patient encounter. In the second instance, patient data that are entered by the nurse in the process of documentation need to be entered in such a manner that they are able to be aggregated to inform future patient encounters.

Knowledge Worker Concept

The world is transitioning from the **Industrial Age** to the **Information Age** (Snyder-Halpern, Corcoran-Perry, & Narayan, 2001; Sorrells-Jones & Weaver, 1999a). The early 1900s workforce consisted predominantly of farmers. After World War I, the workforce began to become predominantly industrial. This occurred when many farmers and domestic help moved to the cities to take jobs at factories. The industrial worker is slowly being replaced by the **technologist** (Drucker, 1994). The technologist is adept at using both mind and hand. Many industrial workers are finding it more and more difficult to obtain jobs because they do not have the educational base or mind set required of knowledge workers (Drucker). The technologist is no longer trained on the job as were the industrial workers, which can cause significant problems for the industrial worker who does not have the education required to transition to a knowledge worker position (Drucker; Sorrells-Jones & Weaver).

Knowledge workers are innovators, and the work they produce is the foundation for organizational sustainability and growth. Knowledge workers are specialized, have advanced education, and typically have a high degree of autonomy and control over their own work environments (Davenport, Thomas, & Cantrell, 2002; Sorrells-Jones & Weaver, 1999a). Knowledge workers are most efficient when they are working in a multidisciplinary team. The teams are typically composed of members whose knowledge bases are complementary. The team members possess problem-solving and decision-making skills and advanced interpersonal skills. All members of the team are considered equal and are there to contribute their expertise. Leadership shifts and changes as the team tackles different parts of the project, with the topic expert taking the lead. A well-functioning team consistently outperforms an individual (Sorrells-Jones & Weaver, 1999b). Many of these teams become focused and passionate about the project.

A key impediment to an effective team is a lack of understanding between team members and a lack of respect for each other's knowledge and experience (Sorrells-Jones & Weaver, 1999a). Another barrier to the efficient multidisciplinary team is the individual knowledge worker who does not want to give up his or her own identity even though he or she may be swayed by other professional opinions. Professionals have a more difficult time adjusting to working in a team than do nonprofessionals. Professionals fail very few times in their lives, which results in their not being able to learn from their failures (Sorrells-Jones & Weaver, 1999b). Knowledge workers tend to be resistant to change, and as a result they dig in their heels and refuse to adapt to changes that management has implemented to improve the work process or work flow (Davenport et al., 2002).

Companies that employ knowledge workers have had to change their management structure to support the knowledge workers. Management no longer commands but inspires workers to produce the best product (Drucker, 1992). These companies have come to the realization that the machines are unproductive without the knowledge of a knowledge worker. Loyalty is no longer purchased with a paycheck, but is earned by giving knowledge workers the ability to use their knowledge effectively and innovatively (Drucker, 1992). The physical environment and workplace arrangements have been adjusted to maximize the work flow of the knowledge workers (Davenport et al., 2002). Many of these changes have occurred in the business world but have been slow to be adopted in health care.

Knowledge Workers and Health Care

The healthcare industry is firmly rooted in the Industrial Age. This results in an industry that is not conducive to support the knowledge workers that represent most of the workforce (Sorrells-Jones & Weaver, 1999a; Wickramasinghe & Ginzberg, 2001). Sorrells-Jones & Weaver (1999a) state that "healthcare institutions are among the most rigidly bureaucratic and hierarchical, discipline-fragmented organizations in the U.S." (p. 16). This is evidenced by multiple administrative levels that manage a single function unit. Corporate values reflect the desire for employees to be loyal and compliant, to avoid risk, and to see failure as negative instead of positive. Senior leadership keeps information tightly controlled and fails to see the need to bring in external intelligence and influence. Rewards are based on individual rather than team performance and a significant pay difference exists between those at the top and those who produce the product (Weaver & Sorrells-Jones, 1999).

Health care is in the process of transitioning from the Industrial Age to the Information Age. This transition is challenging because of the success healthcare institutions have had using current management methods. This success will make it difficult to abandon the old in order to learn the new. A new philosophy that recognizes that employees are mature, self-reliant, independent-thinking adults who function as partners in carrying out the work of the organization is needed. The organization needs to view the (knowledge worker) employee as an asset and supply the resources, tools, information, and power they need to self-manage their work. Innovation needs to be supported, especially when it meets the customers' needs, desires, and wishes (Weaver & Sorrells-Jones, 1999).

Currently, there is a healthcare management trend to use flatter management styles with fewer layers of administration. Organizations are beginning to switch to a clinical product or service line format. This format is typically designed with the physician as the content expert and the nurse as the patient care expert. Unfortunately, this format does not represent a significant change from the way things are currently done (Weaver & Sorrells-Jones, 1999). Management needs to understand and support the knowledge work and nonknowledge work that is performed daily in health care. Both types of work are integral to caring for patients safely. Organizations must switch from measuring the number of tasks completed to measuring the outcomes obtained by knowledge workers (Sorrells-Jones & Weaver, 1999b). This trend is becoming more evident with the posting of hospital report cards that demonstrate how effectively the hospital is caring for certain types of patients.

Nurses as Knowledge Workers

The question to ask is, "Are nurses knowledge workers?" As shown in Table 8-1, when nursing characteristics are compared to the characteristics of a knowledge worker, nursing does meet the criteria of a knowledge worker. Nursing entails a significant amount of knowledge and nonknowledge work. Knowledge work includes such things as interpreting trends in laboratories and symptoms. Nonknowledge work includes such items as calling the laboratory to check on laboratory results

TABLE 8-1

A Comparison of Knowledge Worker Characteristics and
Nursing Characteristics

Knowledge Worker Characteristics	Nursing Characteristics
Advanced formal education	• All nurses have college degrees ranging from AND to PhD
Able to apply theoretical and analytical knowledge	• Nurses are educated on nursing theory and how to apply it in patient situations
Continuous learner	• Obtain advanced degrees • Attend seminars • Earn contact hours
Specialized	• Nursing specialties are as numerous as medical specialties
Innovator	• Nurses become innovative when they do not have proper equipment to care for the patients or they feel that current products are inadequate
Team member	• Have been a member of the interdisciplinary team for a significant amount of time

or making beds. Nurses, on a daily basis, rely on their extensive clinical information and specialized knowledge to implement and evaluate the processes and outcomes related to patient care (Snyder-Halpern et al., 2001).

Snyder-Halpern et al., 2001, have identified the following four tasks associated with human information processing: (1) data gathering, (2) information use, (3) creative application of knowledge to clinical practice, and (4) generation of new knowledge. These four tasks are associated with four roles that nursing takes on as a knowledge worker. These roles are the **data gatherer**, **information user**, **knowledge user**, and **knowledge builder**.

Nurses are data gatherers by nature. Nurses collect and record objective clinical data on a daily basis. These include such things as patient history information, vital signs, and patient assessment data. Data gatherers transition to information users. This transition occurs when nurses begin to interpret the data that they have collected and recorded. The information users then structure the clinical data into information that can be used to guide patient care decisions (Snyder-Halpern et al., 2001). An example of this is when the nurse notices that the patient's blood pressure has been elevated. Information users transition to knowledge users when they begin to notice trends in a patient's clinical data and determine if the clinical data fall within or outside of the normal data range. Nurses transition from knowledge users to knowledge builders when they examine clinical data and trends across groups of patients. These trends are interpreted and compared to current scientific data to determine if these data would improve the nursing knowledge domain. An example of the transition to knowledge builder is an observation of medication compliance rates over a specified time period for patients diagnosed with chronic high blood pressure, and then comparing these rates to evidence-based literature to determine if this information improves the nursing knowledge base (Snyder-Halpern et al.).

Snyder-Halpern et al., 2001, found that as nurses assumed each of these roles, nurses required different types of decision support processes to support their knowledge needs. The data gatherer requires a system that captures and stores data accurately and reliably and allows the data to be readily accessed. Most current healthcare decision support systems (DSSs) support the nurse in this role. The information user role requires a system that can transform clinical data into a format that allows for easy recognition of patterns and trends. These data recognize the trend and display it for the nurse, who in turn uses it to adjust the plan of care for the patient. The information user role is generally well supported by current DSSs. The knowledge user role is the least supported role, and many systems are currently looking at ways to support nurses in this role. One advantage of these DSSs is their ability to bring knowledge to nurses so that they do not have to retrieve the information themselves, which allows them to adjust the patient's plan of care in a more efficient and timely manner. The knowledge builder role is typically seen in conjunction with the nurse **researcher** role and quality management roles. These roles typically look at aggregated data that have been captured over time and from numerous patients and are then compared to clinical variables and interventions, which then results in the development of new domain knowledge (Snyder-Halpern et al., 2001). The knowledge needs of nurses will continue to improve as the systems improve.

The Challenge of Nurses as Knowledge Workers

For nurses to be treated as knowledge workers, nurses must first be recognized as knowledge workers (Snyder-Halpern et al., 2001). Nurses have been part of the interdisciplinary team for years, but are nurses ready to become part of the **interdisciplinary knowledge team**? Nursing may be ready to take that step, but are other members of the healthcare team ready to acknowledge nurses as a respected member of the team (Sorrells-Jones & Weaver, 1999a)? One reason that acceptance may be difficult is the fact that nurses tend to be the least educated member of the interdisciplinary knowledge team. Another reason is that nurses, historically, have had a difficult time being an active member of the interdisciplinary team (Sorrells-Jones & Weaver, 1999b). Nursing still has a long way to go before being accepted as an equal participant in the interdisciplinary knowledge team.

For nurses to be an accepted member of the interdisciplinary knowledge team, a major attitude change toward nursing needs to take place. In addition, nurses must become better educated and more involved in the interdisciplinary knowledge team.

THE KNOWLEDGE NEEDS AND COMPETENCIES OF NURSES

In the early days of medicine, all medical knowledge fit into a single volume. Today, the amount of information available is vast and expanding exponentially, which makes the healthcare industry the most knowledge-intense environment (Snyder-Halpern, Corcoran-Perry, & Narayan, 2001). Computers, technology, and the informatics fields are assisting healthcare workers in dealing with this information explosion.

Knowledge Needs

Nurses deal with a vast amount of information and knowledge every day, which they use to care for their patients. Nurses rely on an extensive amount of clinical information and specialized knowledge to evaluate the processes they have implemented and measure the corresponding outcomes (Snyder-Halpern, Corcoran-Perry, & Narayan, 2001). Nurses rely on their own knowledge, but there are times when this is not adequate and they must access information to provide safe patient care. A national survey was conducted and found that consulting a peer was the most frequent way that information was obtained. The survey also found that most of those surveyed did not use information resources to gather practice information, and that only approximately 25% had been trained on how to use an electronic database (Barton, 2005). If a peer does not have the information the nurse is seeking, the nurse turns to a hospital policy, a journal, a textbook, a drug book, an online resource, the EHR, or many other possible sources.

For this information to be beneficial to the nurse and the patient, it must be reliable and credible. The resource must be easily accessible and packaged in such a way that the nurse is able to find the necessary information quickly and with a minimal amount of difficulty. One way this can be accomplished is by implementing a DSS, which is designed to support nurses in their decision-making activities. DSSs may be incorporated into the EHR.

Nursing Informatics Competencies

One challenge that health care is currently facing is the vast differences in computer literacy and information management skills that healthcare workers possess (McNeil, Elfrink, Beyea, Pierce, & Bickford, 2006). Barton (2005) believes that new nurses should have the following critical skills: use e-mail, operate Windows applications, search databases, and know institution-specific nursing software used for charting and medication administration. These skills should not be limited to just new nurses but should be required of all nurses and healthcare workers.

Staggers, Gassert, and Curran (2001) believe that nursing students and practicing nurses should be educated on core NI competencies. Many authors have devised lists of NI competencies, but none agree on how to incorporate this information into curricula or educate practicing nurses. Information technology and informatics concepts need to be incorporated into nursing school curriculum, but progress has been slow. In the 1980s, a nursing group of the International Medical Informatics Association convened to develop the first level of nursing competencies. While developing these competencies, the nursing group found that nurses fell in to one of the following three categories: (1) user, (2) developer, or (3) expert. These categories have since been expanded.

Staggers et al. (2001) decided that the NI competencies developed in the 1980s were inadequate and needed to be updated. Staggers et al. reviewed 35 NI competency articles and 14 job descriptions, which resulted in 1,159 items that were sorted into three broad categories: (1) computer skills, (2) informatics knowledge, and (3) informatics skills.

These items were placed in a database where redundant items were removed. When this process was completed, 313 items remained. When these items were then further subdivided, Staggers and colleagues, along with the American Medical Informatics Association (AMIA) work group, realized that these competencies were not universal to all nurses, and before it could be determined if the competency was an NI competency, nursing skill levels needed to be defined. This group determined that practicing nurses fell into the following four categories: (1) beginning nurse, (2) experienced nurse, (3) **informatics nurse specialist**, and (4) **informatics innovator**. Each of these skill levels needed to be defined before Staggers et al. (2001) could determine which level was the most appropriate for that skill set. Table 8-2 provides the definition criteria of each skill level. Once the levels were defined, the group determined that 305 items were NI competencies and placed them into appropriate categories.

Staggers, Gassert, and Curran (2002) conducted a Delphi study to validate the placement of the competencies into the correct skill level. Of the 305 original competencies identified, 281 achieved an 80% approval rating for both importance as a competency and placement in the correct practice level. They stress that this is a comprehensive list and that for a nurse to enter a skill level, that nurse does not have to have mastered every item listed in the skill level. To access the entire list of competencies by skill level, visit http://www.nurs.utah.edu/informatics/competencies.htm. See Table 8-3 for a modified version of the list.

In 2004, a group of nurses came together after attending a national informatics conference to ensure that nursing was equally recognized in the national

TABLE 8-2
Definitions of Four Levels of Practicing Nurses

Beginning Nurse

- Has basic computer technology skills and information management skills
- Uses institution's information systems and the contained information to manage patients

Experienced Nurse

- Proficient in a specialty
- Highly skilled in using computer technology skills and information management skills to support his or her specialty area of practice
- Pulls trends out of data and makes judgments based on this information
- Uses current systems, but will collaborate with informatics nurse specialist regarding concerns or suggestions provided by staff

Informatics Nurse Specialist

- RN with advanced education who possesses additional knowledge and skills specific to computer technology and information management
- Focuses on nursing's information needs, which include education, administration, research, and clinical practice
- Application and integration of the core informatics sciences: information, computer, and nursing science
- Uses critical thinking, process skills, data management skills, systems life cycle development, and computer skills

Informatics Innovator

- Conducts informatics research and generates informatics theory
- Vision of what is possible
- Keen sense of timing to make things happen
- Creative in developing solutions
- Leads the advancement of informatics practice and research
- Sophisticated level of skills and understanding in computer technology and information management
- Cognizant of the interdependence of systems, disciplines, and outcomes, and is able to finesse situations to obtain the best outcome

SOURCE: Staggers, N., Gassert, C., & Curran, C. (2001). Informatics competencies for nurses at four levels of practice. *Journal of Nursing Education, 40*(7), 303–316.

informatics movement. They were called the Technology Informatics Guiding Education Reform (TIGER) team. This group determined that using informatics was a core competency for all healthcare workers. They also determined that many nurses lack information technology skills, which limits their ability to access evidence-based information that could be incorporated into their daily practice. This group is currently working on a plan to incorporate informatics courses into all levels of nursing education, and then they will examine how to get the infor-

---

TABLE 8-3
Nursing Informatics Competencies by Skill Level

Beginning Nurse

- Uses e-mail
- Uses Internet to locate and download information of interest
- Uses computerized patient monitoring systems
- Identifies the basic components of a computer system
- Recognizes that a computer program has limitations due to its design and capacity of the computer

Experienced Nurse

- Defines the impact of computerized information management on the role of the nurse
- Applies monitoring system appropriately according to the data needed
- Performs basic troubleshooting in applications
- As a clinician, participates in the selection process, design, implementation, and evaluation of systems
- Assesses the accuracy of health information on the Internet

Informatics Nurse Specialist

- Demonstrates fluency in informatics and nursing terminologies
- Implements and evaluates application/system training programs for users and clients
- Determines projected impacts to users and organizations when changing to computerized information management
- Applies human factors and ergonomics to the design of the computer screen, location and design of devices, and design of software
- Consults in the design or enhancements to integrated patient information, management, educational, or research systems

Informatics Innovator

- Develops models for simulation purposes
- Evaluates the performance and impact of information management technologies on clinical practice, education, administration, and/or research
- Develops new methods of organizing data to enhance research capacities
- Applies advanced analysis and design concepts to the system life cycle process
- Applies sophisticated educational design and research evaluation concepts to the use of innovative computer-based education techniques

---

NOTE: A complete list of NI competencies is available at http://www.nurs.utah.edu/informatics/competencies.htm

SOURCE: Staggers, N., Gassert, C., & Curran, C. (2002). A Delphi study to determine informatics competencies for nurses at four levels of practice. *Nursing Research, 51*(6), 383–390.

---

mation out to practicing nurses who are not currently enrolled in an academic program (TIGER Initiative, 2006). Many of the items identified as lacking in both nursing students and practicing nurses are items that Staggers et al. (2002) determined to be NI competencies. To learn more about the **TIGER initiative**, please visit http://www.tigersummit.com/.

WHAT IS NURSING INFORMATICS SPECIALTY PRACTICE?

NI is an established and ever-evolving profession that began when computers were introduced into health care. Those choosing NI as a career find it full of numerous and varied opportunities. Until recently, most nurse informaticists entered the field by showing an understanding and enthusiasm for working with computers. Now, nurses have many educational opportunities available to become formally trained in the field of NI. This section of the chapter explores the scope and standards of NI, NI roles, education and specialization, rewards of working in the field, and organizations and professional journals of the NIS.

Nursing Contributions to Healthcare Informatics

Nursing has been involved in the purchase, design, and implementation of IS since the 1970s (Saba & McCormick, 2006). One of the first health IS vendors studied how nurses managed patient care and realized that nursing activity was the core of patient activity and needed to be the foundation of the health IS. Nursing informaticians have been instrumental in developing, critiquing, and promoting standard nursing terminologies to be used in the health IS. Nursing is involved heavily in the design of educational materials for practicing nurses, student nurses, other healthcare workers, and patients. Computers have revolutionized the way individuals accesses information and have revolutionized educational and social networking processes.

Scopes and Standards

NI is important to nursing and health care because it focuses on representing nursing data, information, and knowledge. NI does the following for health informatics (ANA, 2008; Brennan, 1994):

- Provides a nursing perspective
- Showcases nursing values and beliefs
- Provides a foundation for nurses in NI
- Produces unique knowledge
- Distinguishes groups of practitioners
- Emphasizes the interest for nursing
- Provides needed nursing language and word context

In 2008, ANA published a revised Scope and Standards of Nursing Informatics Practice. The publication includes the INS standards of practice and the INS standards of professional performance. The three overarching standards of practice are (ANA, p. 33)

1. Incorporate theories, principles, and concepts from appropriate sciences into informatics practice.

2. Integrate ergonomics and human–computer interaction (HCI) principles into informatics solution design, development, selection, implementation, and evaluation.
3. Systematically determine the social, legal, and ethical impact of an informatics solution within nursing and health care.

The standards of practice and professional performance for an INS are listed in Box 8-1.

Nursing Informatics Roles

NI has become a viable and essential nursing specialty with the introduction of computers and the EHR to health care. Many nurses entered the NI field because

BOX
8-1

Informatics Nurse Specialist Standards of Practice and Performance

Standards of Practice
Standard 1: Assessment
Standard 2: Problem and Issues Identification
Standard 3: Outcomes Identification
Standard 4: Planning
Standard 5: Implementation
Standard 5A: Coordination of Activities
Standard 5B: Health Teaching and Heath Promotion and Education
Standard 5C: Consultation
Standard 6: Evaluation

Standards of Professional Performance
Standard 7: Education
Standard 8: Professional Practice Evaluation
Standard 9: Quality of Practice
Standard 10: Collegiality
Standard 11: Collaboration
Standard 12: Ethics
Standard 13: Research
Standard 14: Resource Utilization
Standard 15: Advocacy
Standard 16: Leadership

SOURCE: American Nurses Association (ANA). (2008). *Nursing informatics: Scope and standards of practice.* Silver Spring, MD: Author.

of their natural curiosity and their dedication to being a lifelong learner. Nurses who enter this field may have done so by accident because they were comfortable working with computers and their coworkers used them as a resource for computer-related questions. The introduction of the EHR has strained clinicians to learn this new technology and incorporate it into their already busy days. It has been estimated that nurses spend as little as 15% of their days with their patients and as much as 50% of their day documenting (HIMSS Nursing Informatics Awareness Task Force, 2007). Assisting nurses to incorporate this new technology into their daily workflow is one of many challenges that the INS may tackle. The roles that the INS may engage in are numerous. One position that nurses do quite well in is the role of the **project manager**, which is a result of their ability to manage multiple complex situations at one time (HIMSS Nursing Informatics Awareness Task Force). Because of the breadth of the NI field, many INSs find that they need to further specialize. The following list includes some typical INS positions. This list is far from comprehensive, because this field changes as rapidly as does technology (ANA, 2008; Thede, 2003). For a listing of NI positions with job descriptions, visit http://www.amia.org/mbrcenter/wg/ni/roles.asp.

Project Manager—In the project manager role, the NIS is responsible for the planning and implementing of an informatics project. The NIS uses communication, change management, process analysis, risk assessment, scope definition, and team building. This role acts as the liaison between clinicians, management, IS, vendors, and all other interested parties.

Consultant—The NI who takes on the **consultant** role provides expert advice, opinions, and recommendations based on their area of expertise. Flexibility, good communication skills, excellent interpersonal skills, and extensive clinical and informatics knowledge are highly desirable skill sets needed by the NI consultant.

Educator—The success or failure of an informatics solution can be directly related to the education that was provided. The NIS who chooses the **educator** role develops and implements educational materials and educational sessions and provides education about the system to new employees or during an implementation or an upgrade.

Researcher—The researcher role entails conducting research to create new informatics knowledge. Research may range from basic informatics research to developing clinical decision support tools for nurses.

Product Developer—An NIS in the **product developer** role participates in the design, production, and marketing of new informatics solutions. An understanding of business and nursing is essential in this role.

Decision Support/Outcomes Manager—Nurses assuming the role of **decision support/outcomes manager** uses tools to maintain data integrity and reliability. Contributing to the development of a nursing knowledge base is an integral component of this role.

Advocate/Policy Developer—INSs are a key to developing the infrastructure of health policy. Policy development on a local, national, and international level is an integral part of the **advocate/policy developer** role.

Clinical Analyst/System Specialist—INSs may work at varying levels and serve as a link between nursing and information services.

Entrepreneur—Those involved in the **entrepreneur** role analyze nursing information needs and develop and market solutions.

Specialty Education and Certification

Many nurses who entered into NI did so without any formal education. These nurses were the unit resource for computer or program questions. Many of these nurses acquired their skills with on-the-job training or by attending classes. This still holds true today, but now there are formal ways of acquiring these skills. The informatics nurse has a bachelor of science in nursing and additional knowledge and expertise in the informatics field (ANA, 2008). The INS holds an advanced degree or a post-master's certificate and is prepared to assume roles requiring this advanced knowledge. INSs may attend informatics conferences and obtain contact hours or continuing education units. See Box 8-2 for a list of colleges and universities that offer advanced degrees or certificates in NI. This is not a comprehensive list; new programs are continually being developed. Local colleges and universities should be researched to see which may have informatics programs.

Nurses who choose to specialize in NI have two certifications available to them. The first is through the American Nurses Credentialing Center. The Center's examination is specific for the informatics nurse. The applicant must be a licensed registered nurse with at least 2 years of recent experience and have a baccalaureate degree in nursing. The applicant must have completed 30 contact hours of continuing education in informatics. The applicant must meet one of the following criteria: (1) 2,000 hours practicing as an informatics nurse, (2) 1,000 hours practicing as an informatics nurse and 12 semester hours of graduate academic credit toward a NI degree, or (3) completion of a NI degree that included at least 200 supervised practicum hours. For further information on this certification examination, visit http://www.nursecredentialing.org/NurseSpecialties/Informatics.aspx. This website includes the aforementioned criteria and information about test eligibility, fees, examination context, examination locations, study materials, and practice tests.

The second certification examination is sponsored by HIMSS. Candidates who successfully pass this examination carry the designation of certified professional in healthcare information and management systems. This examination is open to any candidate who is involved in healthcare informatics. Candidates must hold

Formal Nursing Informatics Educational Programs

Graduate Degree Programs

Duke University: http://nursing.duke.edu/modules/son_academic/index.php?id=101

Excelsior College: https://www.excelsior.edu/Excelsior_College/School_Of_Nursing/MS_in_Nursing_Degree/NURSING_INFORMATICS

Loyola University Chicago: http://www.luc.edu/nursing/graduate_hsm.shtml

New York University: http://www.nyu.edu/nursing/academicprograms/masters/programs/informatics.html

Northeastern University: http://www.healthinformatics.neu.edu/

University of Alabama at Birmingham: http://main.uab.edu/shrp/default.aspx?pid=77369

University of Colorado at Denver: http://www.ucdenver.edu/academics/colleges/nursing/programs-admissions/masters-programs/ms-program/specialties/healthcareinformatics/Pages/default.aspx

University of Iowa: http://www.nursing.uiowa.edu/excellence/nursing_knowledge/nursing_informatics/CenterforNursingInformatics_000.htm

University of Kansas: http://www2.kumc.edu/son/academicinformation/nursing informatics.html

University of Maryland: http://nursing.umaryland.edu/academic-programs/grad/masters-degree/ms-academic-program/informatics

University of North Carolina at Chapel Hill: http://nursing.unc.edu/degree/msn/hcs.html

University of Pittsburgh: http://www.unmc.edu/nursing/programs.htm

University of Utah: http://nursing.utah.edu/programs/masters/specialty/informatics/index.html

University of Washington: http://www.son.washington.edu/portals/cipct/

Vanderbilt University: http://www.nursing.vanderbilt.edu/msn/ni.html

Certificate Programs

Indiana University: http://nursing.iupui.edu/continuing/informatics.shtml

Loyola University Chicago: http://www.luc.edu/nursing/cert_informatics.shtml

Northeastern University: http://www.healthinformatics.neu.edu/

University of Iowa: http://informatics.grad.uiowa.edu/health-informatics/curriculum

positions in the following fields: administration/management, clinical IS, e-health, IS, or management engineering. Candidates may include any of the following: chief executive officers, chief information officers, chief operating officers, senior executives, senior managers, IS technical staff, physicians, nurses, consultants, attorneys, financial advisors, technology vendors, academicians, management engineers, and students. Candidates must meet the following criteria to be eligible to sit for the examination: a baccalaureate degree plus 5 years of associated information and management systems experience, three of those years in health care; or a graduate degree plus 3 years of associated information and management systems experience, two of those years in health care. The information discussed in this text and additional information about the examination can be found by visiting http://www.himss.org/ASP/certification_cphims.asp.

Rewards of NI Practice

NI is a nursing specialty that does not focus on direct patient care but instead focuses on how to improve patient care and safety and on improving the workflow and work processes of nurses and other healthcare workers. The INS is instrumental in designing the electronic healthcare records that healthcare workers use on a daily basis. The INS is responsible for designing tools that allow healthcare workers to access patient information more efficiently than they have been able to in the past. Watching these changes take place brings great satisfaction to the INS.

Change is a factor that an INS deals with on a daily basis. This is probably the most difficult aspect of the position because people deal with change differently. Understanding change and how it affects people allows the INS to develop strategies to allow healthcare workers to accept changes and become proficient in informatics solutions that have been implemented. Seeing the change adopted with a minimal amount of discord is very rewarding to the INS.

The INS participates in informatics organizations that allow INSs to network and share experiences with each other. This allows them to bring these new solutions back to their respective organizations and improve informatics issues. Attending professional conferences allows the INS to stay abreast of changes in the industry. Continuing education allows the INS to improve a process or workflow within the hospital or to change the way a system upgrade is rolled out.

NI Organizations and Journals

One of the first informatics organizations founded was the Healthcare Information and Management Systems Society (HIMSS). HIMSS, celebrating its 50th year in 2011, was founded in 1961 with offices throughout the United States and Europe. HIMSS currently represents 20,000 individuals and 300 corporations. HIMSS offers local and national chapters. HIMSS has many associated work groups; one of them is a NI work group. HIMSS is well known for its development of industry-wide policies and its educational and professional development initiatives, which all lead to the goal of ensuring safe patient care. HIMSS offers many advantages for its members, such as numerous weekly and monthly publications, and a scholarly journal, *The Journal of Healthcare Information Management*. There are many educational programs offered, including virtual expos, which allow participants to experience the expo without having to travel. These educational opportunities allow participants to network with colleagues and peers, which is a valuable asset in this field. To find out more about HIMSS, visit their homepage at http://www.himss.org/ASP/index.asp.

The American Medical Informatics Association (AMIA) was founded in 1990 when three health informatics associations merged. AMIA currently has over 3,000 members who reside in 42 countries. AMIA focuses on the development and application of biomedical and healthcare informatics. Members include physicians, nurses, dentists, pharmacists, health information technology professionals, and biomedical engineers. AMIA offers many benefits to its members, such as weekly and monthly publications and a scholarly journal, *JAMIA—The Journal of the American Medical Informatics Association*. Members may join a working group that is specific to their specialty, including a NI work group. AMIA offers multiple educational opportunities and many opportunities for networking with colleagues. To view this information and to see other AMIA offerings visit http://www.amia.org/ index.asp (AMIA, 2010).

The American Nursing Informatics Association (ANIA) was established in 1992 to provide an opportunity for southern California informatics nurses to meet. It has since grown to a national organization whose members include healthcare professionals who work with clinical IS, educational applications, data collection/research applications, administrative/DSS, and those who have an interest in the field of NI. In 2009, ANIA merged with the Capital Area Roundtable on Informatics in Nursing (CARING) and is now called ANIA-CARING. Membership benefits include the following:

- Access to a network of over 3,200 informatics professionals in 50 states and 34 countries
- Reduced rate at the annual conference
- Active e-mail list
- Quarterly newsletter indexed in CINAHL and Thomson
- Job bank with employee-paid postings
- Toll free number for contact with ones CARING Board
- Reduced rate for *CIN: Computers, Informatics, Nursing*
- Annual ANIA-CARING event during AMIA and annual dinner during SINI July
- Membership in the Alliance for Nursing Informatics
- Web-based meetings
- In-person meetings and conferences nationally and worldwide

To view this information and learn more about ANIA-CARING, visit http://www.ania-caring.org (ANIA-CARING, 2010).

The Alliance of Nursing Informatics (ANI) is a collaboration of NI groups that represents over 3,000 nurses and 20 distinct NI groups in the United States. The membership represents local, national, and international NI members and groups. These individual groups have developed organizational structures and have established programs and publications. ANI functions as the link between NI organizations and the general nursing and healthcare communities. ANI provides the united voice of NI. To view this information and learn more about ANI visit http://www. allianceni.org (Alliance of Nursing Informatics, 2010).

These groups have been instrumental in establishing the informatics community. There are many informatics groups that have not been covered here. For additional groups, please see Box 8-3 for a list of organizations and the publications produced by each group.

BOX 8-3

Nursing Informatics Websites and Corresponding Journals

Alliance for Nursing Informatics
Website: www.allianceni.org

American Health Information Management Association
Website: www.ahima.org
Journal: *Journal of AHIMA & Perspectives in Health Information Management* (online)

American Medical Informatics Association
Website: www.amia.org
Journal: *JAMIA—Journal of the American Medical Informatics Association*
NI website: http://www.amia.org/mbrcenter/wg/ni

American Nursing Informatics Association
Website: www.ania.org
Resources link: http://www.ania.org/Resources.htm
Journal: *CIN: Computers, Informatics, Nursing*

Capital Area Roundtable on Informatics in Nursing
Website: www.caringonline.org
Newsletter: *CARING*, available at http://www.caringonline.org/mc/page.do?orgId=car&site
    PageId= 27887

Health Information and Management Systems Society
Website: www.himss.org
Chapter websites: http://www.himss.org/ASP/chaptersHome.asp
Journal: *The Journal of Healthcare Information Management*
NI website: http://www.himss.org/asp/topics_nursingInformatics.asp

International Medical Informatics Association
Website: www.imia.org
Journal: *International Journal of Medical Informatics*
NI website: http://www.imia.org/ni

Online Journal of Nursing Informatics
Website: http://www.ojni.org

SUMMARY

Nursing informatics is an emerging nursing specialty that combines nursing science, information science, and computer science. Informatics practices support nurses to care for their patients effectively and safely as the information that they need is made more readily available. Nurses have been actively involved in this field since computers were introduced to health care. With the advent of EHRs, it became apparent that nursing needed to develop its own terminology; NI has been instrumental in this process.

The healthcare industry employs the largest number of knowledge workers. Healthcare administrators now realize that they must begin to change the way that they view their employees. Nurses and physicians are bright, highly skilled, and dedicated to giving the best patient care. Administrators who tap into this wealth of knowledge will begin to find they have happier employees and find that patient care will become safer and more efficient.

NI is a specialty governed by standards that have been established by the ANA. NI is a very diverse field, which results in many INSs becoming specialized in one segment of the field. NI is a recognized specialty, but it affects all nurses. **Nursing informatics competencies** have been developed to ensure that all entry-level nurses are ready to enter a field that is becoming more technologically advanced. The competencies may be used to determine the educational needs of current staff members. The growth of the NI field has resulted in the formation of numerous NI organizations or subgroups of the medical informatics organizations. Nurses no longer have to enter the field by chance but can obtain an advanced degree in NI at many well-established universities throughout the country. The INS may continue learning by attending the numerous conferences offered. NI has grown tremendously as a specialty since its inception, with the expectation of continued growth. It will be interesting to see where technology takes health care in the future.

THE FUTURE OF NURSING INFORMATICS

NI is in its infancy, as is the technology that the INS uses on a daily basis. NI will continue to influence development of the EHR. The EHR will continue to improve and will one day accurately capture the care nurses give to their patients. This is a formidable challenge because much of the care provided by nurses is intangible. The EHR will provide data to the INS to be used to improve nursing workflow and determine if current practices are the most efficient and beneficial to the patient. Nursing and health care are on a rollercoaster ride that looks to prove very interesting. New technology is being introduced at a breakneck speed and nursing and health care must be ready to ride this rollercoaster. Programs need to be developed to keep nurses and healthcare workers abreast of the new technologic changes as they occur. Educating new and current nurses presents a significant challenge to the INS. The INS's future looks very promising and rewarding.

It is likely that in the future all healthcare providers will be educated in informatics. All healthcare providers need basic informatics skills, such as using search engines to find information about a specific topic. All healthcare providers need to be able to attend classes to improve their computer literacy. Those entering the nursing field need a general knowledge of computer capabilities. There are many new trends, such as Web 2.0, increased attention to evidence-based practice, and a better understanding of genomics, that will impact care delivery, and NI nurses need to lead these efforts to improve care (Baaken et. al., 2008). Change plays a significant part in health care today and those interested in NI must embrace change. They must also be good at enticing others to embrace change. NI candidates must realize that with change comes resistance. They must also be ready to leave the bedside because nurses entering into this field will no longer be working at the bedside. NI is a very challenging but very rewarding field. In an ideal world, all healthcare agencies will employ at least one NIS, and all nurses will embrace the knowledge worker title.

THOUGHT-PROVOKING Questions

www

1. A hospital is looking to implement an EHR. It has been suggested that an INS be hired. This position does not involve direct patient care and the administration is struggling with how to justify the position. How can this position be justified?
2. This chapter discusses the fact that nurses are knowledge workers. How does nursing move from measuring the tasks completed to measuring the final outcome of the patient?

For a full suite of assignments and additional learning activities, use the access code located in the front of your book to visit this exclusive website: **http://go.jblearning.com/mcgonigle.** If you do not have an access code, you can obtain one at the site.

www

References

Alliance of Nursing Informatics. (2010). *Homepage.* Retrieved from http://http://www.allianceni.org

American Medical Informatics Association. (2010). *Homepage.* Retrieved from http://www.amia.org

American Nurses Association. (2008). *Nursing informatics: Scope and standard of practice.* Silver Spring, MD: Nursesbooks.org.

American Nursing Informatics Association and Capital Area Roundtable on Informatics in Nursing. (2010). *Homepage.* Retrieved from http://www.ania-caring.org/mc/page.do?sitePageId=104292&orgId=car

Androwich, I. (2010). Paper presented at Delaware Valley Nursing Informatics Annual Meeting, Malvern, PA, June, 2010.

Bakken, S., Stone, P., & Larson, E. (2008). A nursing informatics research agenda for 2008-2018: Contextual influences and key components. *Nursing Outlook, 56*(5), 206–214.

Barton, A. J. (2005). Cultivating informatics competencies in a community of practice. *Nursing Administration Quarterly, 29*(4), 323–328.

Brennan, P. F. (1994). On the relevance of discipline to informatics. *Journal of the American Medical Informatics Association, 1*(2), 200–201.

Davenport, T. H., Thomas, R., & Cantrell, S. (2002). The mysterious art and science of knowledge worker performance. *MIT Sloan Management Review, 44*(1), 23–30.

Drucker, P. F. (1992). The new society of organizations. *Harvard Business Review, 70*(5), 95–104.

Drucker, P. F. (1994). The age of social transformation. *The Atlantic Monthly, 274*(5), 52–80.

Graves, J. R., & Corcoran, S. (1989). The study of nursing informatics. *IMAGE: Journal of Nursing Scholarship, 21*(4), 227–231.

Hannah, K. J., Ball, M. J., & Edwards, M. J. A. (2006). *Introduction to nursing informatics* (3rd ed.). New York, NY: Springer.

Health Information and Management Systems Society (HIMSS). (2006). *HIMSS dictionary of healthcare information technology terms, acronyms and organizations.* Chicago, IL: Healthcare Information and Management Systems Society.

Health Information and Management Systems Society (HIMSS). (2010). *CPHIMS: HIMSS CPHIMS certification.* Retrieved from http://www.himss.org/ASP/certification_cphims.asp

Health Information and Management Systems Society (HIMSS). (2010). *Homepage.* Retrieved from http://www.himss.org

HIMSS Nursing Informatics Awareness Task Force. (2007). An emerging giant: Nursing informatics. *Nursing Management, 13*(10), 38–42.

Matney, S., Brewster, P., Sward, K., Cloyes, K., & Staggers, N. (2010). Philosophical approaches to the nursing informatics data-information-knowledge-wisdom framework. *Advances in Nursing Science, 34* (1), 6–18.

McCormick, J. (2009). Preparing for the Future of Knowledge Work: A Day in the Life of the Knowledge Worker. *Infomanagment Direct* Online. May 14, 2009. Retrieved from http://www.information-management.com/infodirect/2009_121/knowledge_worker_information_management_ecm_content_management-10015405-1.html?pg=1

McNeil, B. J., Elfrink, V., Beyea, S. C., Pierce, S., & Bickford, C. J. (2006). Computer literacy study: Report of qualitative findings. *Professional Nursing, 22*(1), 52–59.

Merriam-Webster Online. (2011). Retrieved from http://mw1.merriam-webster.com/dictionary/worker

O'Connor, J. J., & Robertson, E. F. (2003). Florence Nightingale biography. Retrieved from http://www-history.mcs.st-andrews.ac.uk/history/Printonly/Nightingale.html

Saba, V. K. (2001). Nursing informatics: Yesterday, today, and tomorrow. *International Nursing Review, 48*(3), 177–187.

Saba, V. K., & McCormick, K. A. (Eds.). (2006). *Essentials of nursing informatics* (4th ed.). New York, NY: McGraw-Hill.

Snyder-Halpern, R., Corcoran-Perry, S., & Narayan, S. (2001). Developing clinical practice environments supporting the knowledge work of nurses. *Computers in Nursing, 19*(1), 17–26.

Sorrells-Jones, J., & Weaver, D. (1999a). Knowledge workers and knowledge-intense organizations, Part 1: A promising framework for nursing and healthcare. *Journal of Nursing Administration, 29*(7/8), 12–18.

Sorrells-Jones, J., & Weaver, D. (1999b). Knowledge workers and knowledge-intense organizations, Part 3: Implications for preparing healthcare professionals. *Journal of Nursing Administration, 29*(10), 14–21.

Staggers, N., Gassert, C., & Curran, C. (2001). Informatics competencies for nurses at four levels of practice. *Journal of Nursing Education, 40*(7), 303–316.

Staggers, N., Gassert, C., & Curran, C. (2002). A Delphi study to determine informatics competencies for nurses at four levels of practice. *Nursing Research, 51*(6), 383–390.

Staggers, N., & Thompson, C. B. (2002). The evolution of definitions for nursing informatics. *Journal of the American Medical Informatics Association, 9*(3), 255–261.

Thede, L. Q. (2003). *Informatics and nursing: Opportunities & challenges* (2nd ed.). Philadelphia, PA: Lippincott Williams & Wilkins.

The TIGER Initiative. (2006). *Welcome to TIGER!* Retrieved from http://www.tigersummit .com

Weaver, D., & Sorrells-Jones, J. (1999). Knowledge workers and knowledge-intense organizations, Part 2: Designing and managing for productivity. *Journal of Nursing Administration, 29*(9), 19–25.

Wickramasinghe, N., & Ginzberg, M. J. (2001). Integrating knowledge workers and the organization: Role of IT. *International Journal of Health Care Quality Assurance, 14*(6), 245–253.

CHAPTER 9

Information and Knowledge Needs of Nurses in the 21st Century

Lynn M. Nagle

1. Define nursing informatics.
2. Describe the goal of nursing informatics.
3. Describe how clinical information technologies are and will impact nursing practice.
4. Explore how nurses can create and derive clinical knowledge from information systems.
5. Speculate on the future of nursing in the context of health informatics.

Key Terms

www

Clinical
decision support
Clinical information system
Evidence-based practice
International Classification
of Nursing Practice
Nursing informatics
Nursing knowledge
Research utilization

www

INTRODUCTION

The information and knowledge informing the 21st century of healthcare delivery has been growing at an unprecedented pace in recent years. Research in particular has propelled the understanding of the efficacy of various clinical practices, treatment regimes, and interventions. Extended and expanded access to clinical research findings and decision support tools has been significantly influenced by the advent of computerization and the Internet. Indeed, the conduct of research itself has been accelerated by virtue of ubiquitous computing. Working in environments of increasingly complex clinical care and contending with the management of large volumes of information, nurses need to avail themselves of the technologic tools that can support quality practice that is optimally safe, informed, and knowledge based. Although the increased deployment of information technologies within healthcare settings presumes that nurses and other health professionals are proficient in the use of computing devices, the processes and potential outcomes associated with informatics are yet to be fully realized or understood. Nurses need to participate in the creation of those possibilities.

This chapter defines and addresses the goal of informatics as it relates to nursing. More specifically, benefits to be derived from the creation of a culture of knowledge-based nursing practice that is enabled and advanced through the use of information and communication technologies is described. The author also addresses some of the challenges associated with the attainment of this goal, but also the opportunities for nurses to create and derive knowledge from emerging health information technologies. Finally, the author provides a contemplative view of the future for nurses and informatics.

Case Study:
Casting to the Future

In the year 2025, nursing practice enabled by technology has created a professional culture of reflection, critical inquiry, and interprofessional collaboration. Nurses use technology at the point of care in all clinical settings (e.g., primary care, acute care, community, and long-term care) to inform their clinical decisions and effect the best possible outcomes for their clients. Information is gathered and retrieved via human–technology biometric interfaces including voice, visual, sensory, gustatory, and auditory interfaces, continuously monitoring physiologic parameters for potentially harmful imbalances. Longitudinal records are maintained for all citizens from their initial prenatal assessment to death; all life-long records are aggregated into the knowledge bases of expert systems. These systems are providing the basis of the artificial intelligence being embedded in emerging technologies. Smart technologies and invisible computing are ubiquitous in all sectors where care is delivered. Clients and families are empowered to review and contribute actively to their record of health and wellness. Invasive diagnostic techniques are obsolete, nanotechnology therapeutics are the norm, and robotics supplement or replace much of the traditional work of all health professions. Nurses provide expertise to citizens to help them effectively manage their health and wellness life plans, and navigate access to appropriate information and services.

INFORMATICS DEFINED

Although varied and evolving over the years, the most commonly applied definitions of **nursing informatics** (NI) describe it as the intersection of computer, information, and nursing science (Graves & Corcoran, 1989; Staggers & Thompson, 2002). In 2009, the International Medical Informatics Association—Nursing Interest Group created a revised definition of NI to reflect the global nature of contemporary practice: "Nursing informatics science and practice integrates nursing, its information and knowledge and their management with information and communication technologies to promote the health of people, families and communities world wide." (para. 2)

Nonetheless, readers may still find Staggers and Thompson's (2002) definitional review particularly helpful in understanding the different foci of those most widely cited in years past. They suggested that previous definitions were primarily one of three orientations: (1) information technology, (2) conceptual, or (3) role focused. Building on the work of others (Graves & Corcoran, 1989; Hannah, Ball, & Edwards, 1984; Schwirian, 1986; Turley, 1996), they attempted to capture all of these elements in advancing the following definition:

> A specialty that integrates nursing science, computer science, and information science to manage and communicate data, information, and knowledge in nursing practice. NI facilitates the integration of data, information, and knowledge to support patients, nurses, and other providers in their decision-making in all roles, and settings. This support is accomplished through the use of information structures, information processes, and information technology (p. 260).

In general, this definition reflects the work of nurse informaticists, the emergence of patients as active participants in their own care, and the key concepts intersecting nursing and informatics (Staggers & Thompson, 2002). Nurses in identified informatics roles typically focus their efforts on articulating meaningful clinical nursing data and information structures that can be codified and processed; identifying the information processes associated with nurses' work; and determining ways in which information and communication technologies can be most effectively used to support the capture, retrieval, and use of data, information, and knowledge. However, for nurses in other roles, the term "informatics" still remains substantively obscure and misunderstood, if at all, as does the relevance and importance of the associated work.

WHAT IS THE GOAL OF INFORMATICS?

Although already in use for a number of decades, the term "informatics" is typically viewed by the broader nursing community as the use of computers by nurses. But informatics experts are quick to identify that computer literacy is but one dimension of the latter. Hence, one might surmise that the goal of informatics is even less understood and in greater need of clear articulation. According to Staggers and Thompson (2002), the goal of NI is

> to improve the health of populations, communities, families, and individuals by optimizing information management and communication. This includes the use of information and technology in the direct provision of care, in establishing effective administrative systems, in managing and delivering educational experiences, in supporting lifelong learning, and in supporting nursing research. (p. 260)

This goal statement reflects the breadth of the potential impact on nurses no matter what their specific role or practice setting. One might also consider that with minor modifications this statement could be applied to the broader concept of health informatics. To this end, there are some nurse authors beginning to deemphasize the notion of NI and discussing the role of nurses and their work processes in the context of health informatics (Hannah, 1995). Health informatics has been described as "knowledge of health services delivery, technology, applications, information, methodologies, and data management processes" (Kathryn Hannah cited in Thede, 2006, p. 244). The umbrella of health informatics suggests that the informatics work being done by nurses must fit within the context of the whole system. Furthermore, nurses in informatics roles are contributing to the foundation of information technology solutions and clinical processes that will support and inform interprofessional care that is client rather than discipline centric.

More timely access to data and information, clinical and financial, has been identified as a necessity in the climate of healthcare delivery in the 21st century (Hannah, 1995). Health service organizations, societies, and governments throughout the industrialized world are obsessed with ensuring that healthcare delivery is safer, knowledge-based, cost effective, seamless, and timely. Beyond these deliverables are also expectations of improved efficiency and quality, and the active engagement of consumers in their care. In particular, given the evolving emphasis on such issues as chronic disease management and aging at home, the goal of informatics needs to encompass the use of technologies to empower citizens to manage more effectively their own health and wellness.

A current challenge within the nursing profession is the pending human resource crisis and dire projections of imminent shortages. Consequently, nursing's focus on Information Technology (IT) has been elevated as a central means by which nurses can be sufficiently supported in their work environments. Most importantly, IT has the potential to reduce the waste of valuable nursing resources by reducing the time spent in the "care and feeding" of patient records. Having more time for direct client care that is supported by ready access to information and knowledge translates into the provision of safer, quality care. Nurses need to be appropriately equipped with the tools to manage data, information, and knowledge effectively and efficiently. The work of nurse informaticists has become germane to the future of all nurses' work.

HEALTH INFORMATION TECHNOLOGIES IMPACTING NURSING

Nurses fall into the category of knowledge workers. Studies have identified that depending on the setting, nurses spend between 25% and 50% of their day managing and recording clinical information and seeking knowledge to inform their practice (Gugerty et al., 2007). Nurses gather atomic-level data (e.g., blood pressure, pulse, blood glucose, pallor); aggregate data to derive information (e.g., impending shock); and apply knowledge (e.g., lowering head of bed to minimize the potentially deleterious effects of impending shock). Over the years, these data have been recorded into individuals' hard copy health records, chronicling findings, actions, and outcomes; this is data and information forever lost unless extracted for research purposes.

As the evidence to support nursing practice continues to be uncovered by researchers and integrated into healthcare delivery, attention must be given to the tools that afford ready and easy access to same. It could be suggested that as knowledge workers, nurses are also, albeit unwittingly, informaticians to a large extent. With the advent of **clinical information systems** (CIS), specifically electronic documentation and clinical decision support (CDS) applications, every nurse has the capacity to contribute to the advancement of nursing knowledge on many levels. Imagine the use of IT solutions not only to capture discrete, quantifiable data, but also the nurse's experiential and intuitive personal knowledge not typically captured in paper records. Further, add to that family history, culture, environment and social factors, past experiences, and perspectives from patients and families into the mix; the possibilities for generating new understandings within populations and across the life span and care continuum are endless.

The impact of CISs on the practice of nursing is just beginning to be explicated because the opportunities to study wholly computerized clinical environments have been limited to date. As yet, the evidence that CISs actually improve nursing efficiency has been inconclusive. Poissant, Pereira, Tamblyn, and Kawasumi (2005) found that bedside terminals and central station desktops resulted in a 24% reduction in the time nurses spent on documentation activities. However, surveys of nurses' perceptions and attitudes toward CISs have suggested that although the quality of documentation may improve, there is an increase in the time associated in completing computer-related tasks (DesRoches, Donelan, Buerhaus, & Zhonghe, 2008; Kossman & Scheidenhelm, 2008). Others have not found a significant time savings for nurses using specific CIS applications (Franklin, O'Grady, Donyai, Jacklin, & Barber, 2007; Asaro & Boxerman, 2008; Hakes & Whittington, 2008). A 2005 Health Information Management Systems Society survey of nurses (n = 1,760) revealed that most nurses believe that CISs improve patient safety (86%) and facilitate interdisciplinary collaboration (69%) and independent decision making (72%) (Dykes et al., 2005). These findings are reflective of what promises to be a growing trend in clinical settings as the sophistication and functionality of CISs continue to advance. However, more research is needed to understand the full extent of the impact of the current and future CISs on nursing practice.

NURSES CREATING AND DERIVING NEW KNOWLEDGE

Nursing Data Standards

There are major efforts underway, internationally through the International Council of Nurses', **International Classification of Nursing Practice** (International Council of Nurses, 2010), and many others among and within countries, where nurses are attempting to standardize the language of nursing practice (Hannah, White, Nagle, & Pringle, 2009). These efforts are particularly important in the face of CISs, because the capacity to have consistent nomenclatures that reflect the practice of nurses is now possible. Standardized language nets the profession and health care delivery systems, the capability to capture, codify, retrieve, and analyze the impact of nursing care on client outcomes. For example, with the use and documentation of standardized client assessments, including risk measures, interventions based on best practices, and consistently measured outcomes within different care settings and across the continuum of care, there will be an ability to demonstrate more clearly the contributions and impact of nursing care from the analysis of CIS outputs. Additionally, clinical outcomes can be further understood in the context of care environments, particularly implications related to the availability of human and material resources to support care delivery. The standardization of clinical inputs and outputs into CISs will eventually provide a rich knowledge base from which practice and research can be enhanced, and inform better administrative and policy decisions (Nagle, White, & Pringle, 2010). Although significant progress has been made in this work, it is still in its early days.

Integrated Decision Support Tools

CDS tools have evolved beyond the previously prevailing notion of accessible reference texts and written resource materials, such as policies and procedures. In the world of clinical computing, the capability to link various information sources and present a clinician with immediate guidance and support has begun to net benefits for safer care and improved clinical outcomes. Osheroff and colleagues (2007) defined CDS as tools that "provide clinicians, staff, patients, or other individuals with knowledge and person-specific information, intelligently filtered or presented at appropriate times, to enhance health and health care" (p. 141).

Most available CDS for nursing practice, although promising, are simplistic and in early development. Typically, CDS includes such tools as (1) computerized alerts and reminders (e.g., medication due, patient has an allergy, potassium level abnormal); (2) clinical guidelines (e.g., best practice for prevention of skin breakdown); (3) online information retrieval (e.g., CINAHL, drug information); (4) clinical order sets and protocols; and (5) online access to organizational policies and procedures. In the future, these tools may be expanded to include applications with embedded case-based reasoning.

Nursing Knowledge in Evolution

Many renowned nurse authors have described the knowledge used by nurses (Benner, 1983; Carper, 1978; Schultz & Meleis, 1988). According to Carper (1978), "nursing . . . depends on the scientific knowledge of human behavior in health and in illness, the esthetic perception of significant human experiences, a personal understanding of the unique individuality of the self and the capacity to make choices within concrete situations involving particular moral judgments" (p. 22).

In the context of nursing practice supported by CISs, nurses will eventually have access to evidence and knowledge derived from large aggregates of clinical data including nursing interventions and resultant outcomes. Experiential evidence provides practice guidelines and directives to ensure concurrence with optimal clinical decisions and actions. To illustrate, consider this example: A nurse assesses a stroke patient for signs of skin breakdown, photographs and documents early ulcerations, and submits the photos and documentation to CIS. The nurse receives an option to review the best practices for care of the patient and to submit consult to a wound management specialist. Ongoing clinical findings, treatment, and response are logged and aggregated with similar cases contributing to the knowledge base related to nursing and care of the integumentary system.

The informational elements of CISs can also be designed to include specifics about individuals' multicultural practices and beliefs. Consider the situation where a client expresses concerns about her prescribed dietary treatment and expresses a preference for a female care provider. With a query to the CIS for the client's history and sociocultural background, the nurse derives an explanation from the patient's religious and cultural background, and makes a notation to highlight and carry this information forward for any future admissions. Future systems may also be designed to provide access to standards of ethical practice, and online access to experts in the field of moral reasoning to guide clinical interactions and decision-making.

In each and every instance of interacting with the CIS, nurses add further to these repositories of knowledge on the basis of their daily clinical challenges and queries. The continued expansion and aggregation of knowledge about clients and populations, their personal, cultural, physical, and clinical presentations, and individuals' experiences and the guidance received from others, enhance the delivery of personalized, knowledge-based care.

Generating Nursing Knowledge

Graves and Corcoran (1989) suggested that **nursing knowledge** is "simultaneously the laws and relationships that exist between the elements that describe the phenomena of concern in nursing (factual knowledge) and the laws or rules that the nurse uses to combine the facts to make clinical nursing decisions" (p. 230). In their view, not only does knowledge support decision making, but it also leads to new discoveries. Thus, one might think about the future creation of nursing knowledge as being the discovery of new laws and relationships that can continue to advance nursing practice.

New technologies have made the capture of multifaceted data and information possible through the use of such technologies as digital imaging (e.g., photography to support wound management). Now part of the clinical record, such images add a new dimension to the assessment, monitoring, and treatment of illness and the maintenance of wellness. Beyond the use of computer keyboards, input devices are being integrated with CISs and used to gather data and information for the following clinical and administrative purposes:

- Biometrics (e.g., facial recognition, security)
- Voice and video recordings (e.g., client interviews and observations, diagnostic procedures, ultrasounds)
- Voice-to-text files (e.g., voice recognition for documentation)
- Medical devices, (e.g., infusion pumps, ventilators, hemodynamic monitors)
- Bar-code technologies (e.g., medication administration)
- Telehomecare monitoring (e.g., for use in diabetes and other chronic disease management)

These are but a few of the emerging capabilities that allow for numerous data inputs to be transposed, combined, analyzed, and displayed to provide information and views of clinical situations currently not possible in a world dominated by hard copy documentation. With the use of information and communication technologies to support the capture and processing (i.e., interpretation, organization, and structuring) of all relevant clinical data, relationships can be identified and formalized into new knowledge. This transformational process is at the core of generating new nursing knowledge at a rate never experienced before, and in the context of current research paradigms, the same relationships would likely take years to uncover.

As CISs advance, nurses will eventually become generators of new knowledge by virtue of designs that embed machine learning and case-based reasoning methods within their core functionality. This functionality will be made possible only through national and international adoption of standardized nursing language, as previously described. Imagine the power of having access to systems that aggregate the same data elements and information garnered from multiple clinical situations and provide a probability estimate of the likely outcome for individuals of a certain age, with a specific diagnosis and comorbid conditions, medication profile, symptoms, and interventions. How much more rapidly would an understanding of the efficacy of clinical interventions be elucidated? Historically, some knowledge might have taken years of research to discover (e.g., that long-standing practices are sometimes more harmful than beneficial). A case in point is the long-standing practice of instilling endotracheal tubes with normal saline before suctioning (O'Neal, Grap, Thompson, & Dudley, 2001). Based on the evidence gathered through several studies, there is now awareness of the potentially deleterious effects of this practice. Conceivably, a meta-analysis approach to clinical studies will be expedited by converging large clinical data repositories across care settings, reflecting the collective contributions of health professionals and longitudinal outcomes for individuals, families, and populations.

Nurses need to be engaged in the design of CIS tools that support access to and the generation of nursing knowledge. Of particular importance to the future design of CIS is the adoption of clinical data standards. Although beyond the scope of this chapter, there has been at least two decades of work effort directed to the articulation of standardized data elements that reflect nursing practice. The profession has been steadily moving toward consensus on the adoption of data standards, and recent work suggests that significant strides have been achieved (Bickford & Hunter, 2006; Delaney, 2006; Hannah et al., 2009). Consider that as CISs are widely implemented, as standards for nursing documentation and reporting are adopted, and as healthcare IT solutions continue to evolve, the potential to synthesize findings from a variety of methods and world views becomes much more probable.

CHALLENGES IN GETTING THERE

Leadership

The field of nurse leaders in health informatics has markedly grown in the past two decades. However, a significant knowledge gap must be addressed within the nursing leadership community. Many nurse leaders need to acquire a new set of skills and knowledge to understand and advance the adoption of information tools and technologies to support the delivery of clinical care. For several years, nurse informaticians have advocated for the need for all nursing leaders to become knowledgeable and engaged in setting the direction for informatics in the profession (Nagle, 2005; Pringle & Nagle, 2009; Simpson, 2000). Strategies include the following: (1) identify the informatics education needs of nurse leaders, (2) develop mentorship programs for the acquisition of informatics leadership skills, and (3) ensure enrollment of nurse leaders as sponsors for electronic health records initiatives.

Clinical Practice

Despite valiant efforts to implement comprehensive CIS throughout North American healthcare settings, there are still many provider organizations with limited online functionality available to nurses. As indicated by numerous studies and reports of the state of IT adoption, many providers are still in the early phases of acquisition and implementation (Eggert & Protti, 2006). Ironically, this is probably good news for nursing. There is an opportunity for nurses to immerse themselves in the developmental work of IT solutions to support practice.

Over the years, nurses have been on the receiving end of systems that either did not add value to their work or by virtue of poor design created additional work. Now is the opportunity to avoid future installations of IT solutions that do nothing to benefit and support the clinical practice of nurses and healthcare teams. It behooves nurses to be engaged in the acquisition, design, implementation, and evaluation of CIS to ensure the realization of benefits for clinical care and outcomes.

It is equally important to consider that because of the average age of most practicing nurses, many have yet to develop a comfort level with the use of computers in their work settings. To minimize the anxiety associated with expected IT use, particular attention needs to be given to the issue of computer literacy. If nurses lack a solid footing in computer use, expectations for integration of informatics is difficult to realize. Strategies for nurses include the following: (1) be encouraged and supported to participate in the acquisition, design, implementation, and evaluation phases of CIS; (2) demand the adoption of IT solutions that support the delivery of safe, quality care; and (3) be provided with material and people resources to support their acquisition of informatics competencies.

Education

Over the years, numerous efforts have been undertaken to identify the core informatics competencies needed by nurses. These efforts have encompassed attempts to articulate core competencies for all nurses, from novice to expert (Hebert, 2000) and competencies for informatics experts (Hersh, 2006). In recognizing NI as a specialty, the American Nurses Association (2001) has articulated scope and standards of NI practice. What remains clear is that although progress has been made in the preparation of NI experts, there is still much work to be done at the grassroots level of nursing education.

Recent studies of schools of nursing indicate that few basic nursing education programs have embedded the concepts and processes associated with informatics within the core curricula (Carty & Rosenfeld, 1998; Nagle & Clarke, 2004). The primary obstacles to realizing curricula with embedded informatics concepts include a lack of faculty capacity; constraints of clinical practice environments (e.g., lack of student access to CISs); and limited funding. These barriers need to be addressed to ensure that graduates of the future are prepared for settings using information technology to support clinical care.

The core concepts and competencies of informatics are particularly well suited to a model of interprofessional education. Ideally, when emulating clinical settings, informatics knowledge should be integrated with the processes of interprofessional teams and decision making. Because simulation laboratories are becoming increasingly common fixtures in the delivery of health professional education, they provide a perfect opportunity to incorporate Electronic Health Records (EHR) applications including access to CDS. The learning laboratory will then more closely approximate the IT-enabled clinical settings that are emerging.

A presumption is often made that future graduates will be more computer literate than nurses currently in practice. Although this is likely true, computer comfort does not equate to an understanding of the facilitative and transformative role that IT will have in the future. It is essential that the future curricula of basic nursing programs embed the concepts of the role of information technology in supporting clinical care delivery. Strategies include the following: (1) need to share prototypes of informatics integration among schools of nursing, (2) consider interprofessional education opportunities in addressing informatics concepts and competencies, (3) nursing faculty need to be obligated and supported in the attainment of basic informatics competencies, (4) seek and allocate funding for the development of innovative curricular models and associated technologic support, and (5) incorporate accreditation criteria that necessitate an integration of informatics core concepts and competencies in all basic nursing programs.

IN AN IDEAL WORLD

The ideal is a nursing practice that has wholly integrated informatics and nursing education that is driven by the use of information and knowledge from a myriad of sources, creating practitioners whose way of being is grounded in informatics. Nursing research is dynamic and an enterprise in which all nurses are engaged by virtue of their use of technologies to gather and analyze findings that inform specific clinical situations. In every practice setting, the contributions of nurses to health and well-being of citizens will be highly respected and parallel, if not exceed, the preeminence granted physicians.

THE FUTURE

The future holds a landscape yet to be understood as technology evolves with a rapidity and unfolding that is rich with promise and potential peril. It is anticipated that in the future, there will be the computing power to aggregate and transform additional multidimensional data and information sources (e.g., historical, multisensory, experiential, and genetic sources) into CIS. With the availability of such rich repositories, there will be opportunities further to enhance the training of health professionals, advance the design and application of CDSs, deliver care that is informed by the most current evidence, and engage with individuals and families in ways yet unimagined.

The basic education of all health professions will evolve over the next decade to incorporate core informatics competencies. In general, the clinical care environments will be connected, and information will be integrated across disciplines to the benefit of care providers and citizens alike. The future of health care will be highly dependent on the use of CIS and CDS to achieve the global aspiration of safer, quality care for all citizens.

SUMMARY

This chapter advances a view that every nurse's practice will make contributions to new nursing knowledge in dynamically interactive CIS environments. The core concepts and competencies associated with informatics will be embedded in the practice of every nurse, whether administrator, researcher, educator, or practitioner. Informatics will be prominent in the knowledge work of nurses, yet it will be a subtlety because of its eventual fulsome integration with clinical care processes. Clinical care will be substantially supported by the capacity and promise of technology today and tomorrow.

Most importantly, readers need to contemplate a future without being limited by the world of practice as it is known today. Information technology is not a panacea, but it will provide the profession with unprecedented capacity more rapidly to generate and disseminate new knowledge. Realizing the possibilities necessitates that all nurses understand and leverage the informatician within and contribute to the future.

THOUGHT-PROVOKING Questions   WWW

1. What are the possibilities to accelerate the generation and uptake of new nursing knowledge?
2. What should be the areas of priority for the advancement of informatics in nursing?

For a full suite of assignments and additional learning activities, use the access code located in the front of your book to visit this exclusive website: **http://go.jblearning.com/mcgonigle**. If you do not have an access code, you can obtain one at the site.

References

American Nurses Association. (2001). *Scope and standards of nursing informatics practice.* Washington, DC: Author.

Asaro, P.V., & Boxerman, S. B. (2008). Effects of computerized provider order entry and nursing documentation on workflow. *Journal of the American Medical Informatics Association, 14*(4), 415–423.

Benner, P. (1983). Uncovering the knowledge embedded in clinical practice. Image: The Journal of Nursing Scholarship, 15(2), 36–41.

Bickford, C. J., & Hunter, K. M. (2006). Theories, models, and frameworks. In V. K. Saba & K. A. McCormick (Eds.), *Essentials of nursing informatics* (4th ed., pp. 265–278). New York, NY: McGraw Hill.

Carper, B. A. (1978). Fundamental patterns of knowing in nursing. *Advances in Nursing Science, 1*(1), 13–23.

Carty, B., & Rosenfeld, P. (1998). From computer technology to information technology. Findings from a national study of nursing education. *Computers in Nursing, 16*(5), 259–265.

Delaney, C. W. (2006). Nursing minimum data set systems. In V. K. Saba & K. A. McCormick (Eds.), *Essentials of nursing informatics* (4th ed., pp. 249–261). New York, NY: McGraw Hill.

DesRoches, C. K., Donelan, P., Buerhaus, P., & Zhonghe, L. (2008). Registered nurses' use of electronic health records: Findings from a national survey. *Medscape Journal of Medicine, 10*(7), 164–173.

Dykes, P., Cashen, M., Foster, M., Gallagher, J., Kennedy, M., MacCallum, R., . . . Whetstone, S. (2005). Surveying acute care providers in the U.S. to explore the impact of HIT on the role of nurses and the interdisciplinary communication in acute care settings. *Journal of Healthcare Information Management, 20*(2), 36–44.

Eggert, C., & Protti, D. (2006). Clinical electronic communications: A new paradigm that is here to stay? *Electronic Healthcare, 5*(2), 88–96.

Franklin, B. D., O'Grady, K., Donyai, P., Jacklin, A., & Barber, N. (2007). The impact of a closed-loop electronic prescribing and administration system on prescribing errors, administration errors, and staff time: A before and after study. *Quality and Safety in Health Care, 16*(4), 279–284.

Graves, J. R., & Corcoran, S. (1989). The study of nursing informatics. *Image: The Journal of Nursing Scholarship, 21*(4), 227–231.

Gugerty, B., Maranda, M. J., Beachley, M., Navarro, V. B., Newbold, S., Hawk, W, Karp, J., Koszalka, M., Morrison, S., Poe, S. & Wilhelm, D. (2007). Challenges and opportunities in documentation of the nursing care of patients. Baltimore: Documentation Work Group, Maryland Nursing Workforce Commission. Retrieved from http://www.mbon.org/commission2/documentation_challenges.pdf

Hakes, B., & Whittington, J. (2008). Assessing the impact of an electronic medical record on nurse documentation time. *Computers Informatics Nursing, 26*(4), 234–241.

Hannah, K. J. (1995). Transforming information: Data management support of healthcare reorganization. *Journal of the American Medical Informatics Association, 2*(3), 147–155.

Hannah, K. J., Ball, M. J., & Edwards, M. J. A. (1984). Introduction to nursing informatics. New York, NY: Springer-Verlag.

Hannah, K.J., White, P., Nagle, L.M., & Pringle, D.M. (2009). Standardizing nursing information in Canada for inclusion in electronic health records: C-HOBIC. *Journal of the Americas Medical Informatics Association, 16*(4), 524–530.

Hersh, W. (2006). Who are the informaticians? What we know and should know. *Journal of the American Medical Informatics Association, 13*(2), 166–170.

Kossman, S. P., & Scheidenhelm, S. L. (2008). Nurses' perceptions of the impact of electronic health records on work and patient outcomes. *Computers Informatics Nursing, 26*(2), 69–77.

International Council of Nurses (2010). ICNP Version 2.0. Retrieved from http://www.icn.ch/pillars programs/international-classification-for-nursing-practicer/.

International Medical Informatics Association—Nursing Informatics Special Interest Group (2009). Definition. Retrieved from http://www.imiani.org/index.php.

Nagle, L. M. (2005). Dr. Lynn Nagle and the case for nursing informatics. *Canadian Journal of Nursing Leadership, 18*(1), 16–18.

Nagle, L. M., & Clarke, H. F. (2004). Assessing informatics in Canadian schools of nursing. Proceedings 11th World Congress on Medical Informatics. San Francisco. [CD].

Nagle, L.M., White, P., & Pringle, D. (2010). Realizing the benefits of standardized measures of clinical outcomes. *Electronic Healthcare, 9*(2), e3–e9.

O'Neal, P. V., Grap, M. J., Thompson, C., & Dudley, W. (2001). Level of dyspnea experienced in mechanically ventilated adults with and without saline instillation prior to endotracheal suctioning. *Intensive Critical Care Nursing, 17*(6), 356–363.

Osheroff, J. A., Teich, J. M., Middleton, B., Steen, E. B., Wright, A., & Detmer, D. E. (2007). A roadmap for national action on clinical decision support. *Journal of the American Medical Informatics Association, 14*(2), 141–145.

Poissant, L.J., Pereira, R., Tamblyn, R., & Kawasumi, Y. (2005). The impact of electronic health records on time efficiency of physicians and nurses: A systematic review. *Journal of the American Medical Informatics Association, 12*(5), 505–516.

Pringle, D., & Nagle, L.M. (2009). Leadership for the information age: The time for action is now. *Canadian Journal of Nursing Leadership, 22*(1), 1–6.

Schultz, P. R., & Meleis, A. I. (1988). Nursing epistemology: Traditions, insights, questions. *Image: The Journal of Nursing Scholarship, 20*(4), 217–221.

Schwirian, P. (1986). The NI pyramid: A model for research in nursing informatics. *Computers in Nursing, 4*(6), 134–136.

Simpson, R. L. (2000). Need to know: Essential survival skills for the information age. *Nursing Administration Quarterly, 25*(1), 142–147.

Staggers, N., & Thompson, C. B. (2002). The evolution of definitions for nursing informatics: A critical analysis and revised definition. *Journal of the American Medical Informatics Association, 9*(3), 255–261.

Thede, L. Q. (2006). Top drawer. *Computers, Informatics, Nursing, 24*(5), 243–245.

Turley, J. (1996). Toward a model for nursing informatics. *Image: Journal of Nursing Scholarship, 28,* 309–313.

CHAPTER 10

Legislative Aspects of Nursing Informatics: HITECH and HIPAA

Kathleen M. Gialanella

Objectives

1. Describe the purposes of the Health Information Technology for Economic and Clinical Health (HITECH) Act of 2009
2. Explore how the HITECH Act is enhancing the security and privacy protections of the Health Insurance Portability and Accountability Act (HIPAA) of 1996.
3. Determine how the HITECH Act and its impact on HIPAA apply to nursing practice.

WWW

Key Terms WWW

Access
Agency for Healthcare
  Research and Quality
American National
  Standards Institute
American Recovery and
  Reinvestment Act
Centers for Medicare and
  Medicaid Services
Certified EHR technology
Civil monetary penalties
Compliance
Confidentiality
Consequences
Electronic health record
Enterprise Integration
Entity
Gramm-Leach-Bliley Act
Health disparities
Health information
  technology
Health Insurance
  Portability and
  Accountability Act
Health Level 7
Healthcare-associated
  infections

Continues

INTRODUCTION

The federal Health Information Technology for Economic and Clinical Health Act of 2009 (Leyva & Leyva, 2011) (HITECH Act), enacted February 17, 2009, is part of the **American Recovery and Reinvestment Act** (ARRA). The ARRA, also known as the "Stimulus" law, was enacted to stimulate various sectors of the US economy during the most severe recession this country has experienced since the Great Depression of the late 1920s and early 1930s. The **health information technology** (HIT) industry was one area where lawmakers saw an opportunity to stimulate the economy and improve the delivery of health care at the same time. This explains why the title of the HITECH Act contains the phrase "for Economic and Clinical Health."

The ARRA is a lengthy piece of legislation organized into two major sections: Division A and Division B. Each Division contains several Titles. Title XIII of Division A of the ARRA is the HITECH Act. It addresses the development, adoption, and implementation

Key Terms Continued

International Standards
   Organization
Meaningful use
National Institute of
   Standards and
   Technology
Office of Civil Rights
Office of the National
   Coordinator for Health
   Information Technology
Open systems
   interconnection
Patient-centered care
Policy
Privacy
Protected health information
Qualified EHR
Rights
Sarbanes-Oxley Act
Security
Standard
Standards-developing
   organizations
Treatment payment
   operations

of HIT policies and **standards** and provides enhanced **privacy** and **security** protections for patient information, an area of the law that is of paramount concern in nursing informatics. Title IV of Division B of the ARRA is considered part of the HITECH Act. It addresses Medicare and Medicaid HIT and provides significant financial incentives to healthcare professionals and hospitals that adopt and engage in the "**meaningful use**" of **electronic health record** (EHR) technology.

This chapter presents an overview of the HITECH Act, including the Medicare and Medicaid HIT provisions of the law. Nurses need to be familiar with the goals and purposes of this law, how it enhances the security and privacy protections of the **Health Insurance Portability and Accountability Act** (HIPAA) of 1996, and how it otherwise impacts nursing practice in the emerging EHR age. The concepts of "meaningful use" and "**certified EHR technology**" also are explored in this chapter.

OVERVIEW OF THE HITECH ACT

At the time the HITECH Act was enacted, it was estimated that less than 8% of US hospitals used a basic EHR system in at least one of their clinical units, and less than 2% of US hospitals had an EHR system in all of their clinical settings (Ashish, 2009). Not surprisingly, the cost of an EHR system has been a major barrier to widespread adoption of this technology in most healthcare facilities. The HITECH Act seeks to change that by providing each person in the United States with an EHR. In addition, a nationwide HIT infrastructure will be developed so that access to a person's EHR will be readily available to every healthcare provider who treats the patient, no matter where the patient may be located at the time treatment is rendered.

Definitions

There are some important definitions in the HITECH Act that anyone involved in nursing informatics should know. These include the following:

- "Certified EHR Technology"—which means an EHR that meets specific governmental standards for the type of record involved, whether it is an ambulatory EHR used by office-based healthcare practitioners or an inpatient EHR used by hospitals. The specific standards that are to be met for any such EHRs are set forth in federal regulations;

- "**Enterprise Integration**"—which means "the electronic linkage of healthcare providers, health plans, the government and other interested parties, to enable the electronic exchange and use of health information among all the components in the health care infrastructure;"
- "**Healthcare Provider**"—which includes hospitals, skilled nursing facilities, nursing homes, long term care facilities, home health agencies, hemodialysis centers, clinics, community mental health centers, ambulatory surgery centers, group practices, pharmacies and pharmacists, laboratories, physicians, therapists, etc.;
- "**Health Information Technology**" (HIT)—which means "hardware, software, integrated technologies or related licenses, intellectual property, upgrades, or packaged solutions sold as services that are designed for or support the use by healthcare entities or patients for the electronic creation, maintenance, access, or exchange of health information;" and
- "**Qualified Electronic Health Record**"—which means "an electronic record of health-related information on an individual." A "qualified" EHR contains a patient's demographic and clinical health information, including medical history and a list of health problems, and is capable of providing support for clinical decisions and entry of physician orders. It must also have the capacity "to capture and query information relevant to health care quality" and "exchange electronic health information with, and integrate such information from other sources" (Readthestimulus.org, 2009, pp. 32–35).

Purposes

The HITECH Act established the **Office of the National Coordinator for Health Information Technology** (ONC) within the US Department of Health and Human Services (HHS). The ONC is headed by the National Coordinator, who is responsible for overseeing the development of a nationwide HIT infrastructure that supports the use and exchange of information to achieve the following:

1. Improve healthcare quality by enhancing coordination of services between and among the various healthcare providers a patient may have, fostering more appropriate healthcare decisions at the time and place of delivery of services, and preventing medical errors and advancing the delivery of **patient-centered care**
2. Reduce the cost of health care by addressing inefficiencies, such as duplication of services within the healthcare delivery system, and by reducing the number of medical errors
3. Improve people's health by promoting prevention, early detection, and management of chronic diseases

4. Protect public health by fostering early detection and rapid response to infectious diseases, bioterrorism, and other situations that could have a widespread impact on the health status of many individuals
5. Facilitate clinical research
6. Reduce **health disparities**
7. Better secure patient health information

Improving healthcare quality has been an ongoing challenge in this country. According to the **Agency for Healthcare Research and Quality** (AHRQ), quality health care is care that is "safe, timely, patient centered, efficient, and equitable" (AHRQ, 2009, p. 1). AHRQ, an agency within HHS, has been releasing a National Healthcare Quality Report (NHQR) every year since 2003 and the current report, not unlike previous reports, finds the quality of health care in this country "suboptimal" (AHRQ, p. 2). The NHQR discussed the need for HIT to support the goal of improving quality of care.

> Providers need reliable information about their performance to guide improvement activities. Realistically, HIT infrastructure is needed to ensure that relevant data are collected regularly, systematically, and unobtrusively while protecting patient privacy and confidentiality . . . Systems need to generate information that can be understood by endusers and that are interoperable across different institutions' data platforms . . .
>
> Quality improvement typically requires examining patterns of care across panels of patients rather than one patient at a time...Ideally, performance measures should be calculated automatically from health records in a format that can be easily shared and compared across all providers involved with a patient's care (AHRQ, p. 13).

The prevalence of **healthcare-associated infections** serves as an excellent example of how use of EHR technology and a nationwide HIT infrastructure can play a significant role in addressing healthcare quality issues. According to the NHQR, "wound infections are a common occurrence following surgery, but hospitals can reduce the risk of these health care-associated infections by making sure patients receive an appropriate antibiotic within an hour before their procedures" (AHRQ, 2009, p. 110). The Centers for Medicare and Medicaid Services (CMS) already has the capacity to track Medicare patients who receive this prophylactic treatment and the rate of postsurgical wound infections for those patients who do and do not receive the treatment. Imagine being able to track this issue for all surgical patients and developing evidence-based care plans to ensure that all patients within the infrastructure receive the same quality of care. This is just one of many examples in which the end result is better patient outcomes.

EHR technology also will make it easier for all providers involved in a patient's care to readily access that patient's complete and current healthcare record, thereby allowing providers to make well-informed, efficient, and effective decisions about a patient's care at the time those decisions need to be made. This is of tremendous benefit to the patient and promotes a higher level of patient-centered care. It also allows effective coordination of care between and among all providers involved in the patient's care, including doctors, nurses, therapists, nutritionists, hospitals, nursing homes, rehabilitation facilities, home health agencies, laboratories, and other diagnostic centers, thereby assuring the continuum of patient care.

Imagine how much easier it would be for a patient with a rare form of cancer to obtain a second oncologist's opinion before beginning a course of treatment. The patient's complete record, including the results of numerous diagnostic tests conducted at multiple sites, such as bloodwork, biopsies, radiographs, and scans, would be readily available to the second oncologist. Imagine how much easier it would be for a patient with end-stage renal disease, who is receiving outpatient hemodialysis several times a week, to receive appropriate treatment if he or she is suddenly hospitalized or would like to take a vacation out of state. Imagine how much easier it would be for nurses to complete a medication reconciliation for a newly admitted patient. The possibilities are endless and the savings realized from enhancing quality, avoiding duplication of services, and streamlining delivery of patient care are obvious.

Reducing healthcare errors has been another ongoing challenge in this country. Healthcare providers strive to meet the standard of care and avoid harm to patients. Patients have a right to receive appropriate care, but that does not always happen. Ten years ago the Institute of Medicine's Committee on the Quality of Health Care in America undertook a comprehensive literature review and summarized the results of more than 40 studies about healthcare errors in its seminal report, *To Err Is Human: Building a Safer Health System* (Institute of Medicine, 2000). That report concluded that approximately 44,000–98,000 people in this country die each year as a result of healthcare errors. Many thousands more who do not die are seriously injured. In addition to the human pain and suffering associated with healthcare errors, the monetary costs associated with these types of errors are substantial. Although some progress in reducing healthcare errors has been made since the release of *To Err Is Human*, there still is substantial work to be done. It is anticipated that a nationwide HIT infrastructure will contribute to a reduction in healthcare errors by providing mechanisms to assist with the prevention of errors and to provide timely warnings of the possibility of a repetitive error that may affect many patients.

Containing and reducing healthcare costs in this country, where more than $2 trillion is spent each year (Keehan, Sisko, & Truffler, 2008), is another daunting challenge. Using EHR technology and a nationwide HIT infrastructure to improve quality and reduce errors within the healthcare delivery system is one way to address this challenge. Imagine the billions of dollars that can be saved just by reducing the estimated 1.7 million cases of healthcare-associated infections contracted by patients in United States hospitals each year (AHRQ, 2009, p. 108).

Promoting prevention, early detection, and management of chronic diseases is another purpose of the HITECH Act. The delivery of health care in this country traditionally has been based on a disease model rather than a wellness model. Having an EHR for each individual could help with the necessary transition as providers and their patients become more aware of the variables that positively or negatively impact health. The ability to identify appropriate choices to promote wellness and either prevent illness and injury or detect and manage chronic diseases sooner will be enhanced.

Chronic diseases are of major concern to this country, not only because of the impact they have on an individual, but also because of the tremendous cost associated with providing treatment for patients with these conditions. Adult-onset diabetes, for example, has reached epidemic proportions. A national HIT infrastructure will help providers better identify those patients who are at risk for developing the disease and provide treatment strategies to avoid it. For those patients who develop the disease, their providers will be able to diagnose the condition much sooner and manage it more effectively because of the vast resources that a national HIT infrastructure can provide.

Improving public health is another purpose of the HITECH Act. The recent H1N1 flu pandemic is illustrative of how a national HIT infrastructure can protect public health by fostering early detection and rapid response to infectious diseases, bioterrorism, and other situations that could have a widespread impact on the health status of many individuals and groups.

The impact that a national HIT infrastructure will have on clinical research is self-evident. Once the infrastructure becomes operational, the amount of data that will become readily available for clinical research will increase exponentially compared to what is available today. The ability of researchers to conduct studies and provide clinicians with the most current evidence-based practice will be of tremendous benefit to patients everywhere.

Reducing health disparities is another purpose of the HITECH Act. According to the AHRQ (2010), "Health care disparities are differences or gaps in the care experienced by one population compared with another population" (p. 1).

Detailed information about healthcare disparities can be found at the website for the Office of Minority Health and Health Disparities at www.cdc.gov/omhd. The AHRQ routinely examines the issue of disparities in health care and reports its findings to the public. AHRQ's current report, the *National Healthcare Disparities Report of 2009*, confirms that some Americans continue to receive inferior care because of such factors as race, ethnicity, and socioeconomic status. This report found disparities

- Across all dimensions of healthcare quality: effectiveness, patient safety, timeliness, and patient centeredness.
- Across all dimensions of access to care: facilitators and barriers to care and health care utilization.
- Across many levels and types of care: preventive care, treatment of acute conditions, and management of chronic diseases.
- Across many clinical conditions: cancer, diabetes, end stage renal disease, heart disease, HIV disease, mental health and substance abuse, and respiratory diseases.
- Across many care settings: primary care, home health care, hospice care, emergency department, hospitals, and nursing homes.
- Within many subpopulations: women, children, older adults, residents of rural areas, and individuals with disabilities and other special health care needs (AHRQ, 2010, p. 2).

All patients, regardless of race, ethnicity, or socioeconomic status should receive care that is effective, safe, and timely. With the national HIT infrastructure contemplated by the HITECH Act, such disparities are bound to decrease. The ability to monitor for disparities and promote the delivery of appropriate care to all patients will be enhanced. Clinicians will be prompted to base their treatments on appropriate factors and avoid biased care.

Perhaps the most important task facing the National Coordinator during the development and implementation of a nationwide HIT infrastructure is ensuring the security of the patient health information within that system. The ability to secure and protect confidential patient information has always been of paramount importance to clinicians who view it as an ethical and legal obligation of practice. Patients value their privacy and they have a right to expect that their confidential health information will be properly safeguarded. Nurses have been complying with the regulatory requirements of HIPAA for years and the HITECH Act has enhanced the security and privacy protections each patient has a right to expect under HIPAA (Box 10-1). The specific changes are discussed in greater detail later in this chapter.

Overview of the Health Insurance Portability and Accountability Act of 1996

Dee McGonigle, Kathleen Mastrian, and Nedra Farcus

HIPAA was signed into law by President Clinton in 1996. Hellerstein (1999) summarized the intent of the act as follows: to curtail healthcare fraud and abuse, enforce standards for health information, guarantee the security and privacy of health information, and ensure health insurance portability for employed persons. Consequences were put into place for institutions and individuals who violate the requirements of this act. For this text, we concentrate on the health information security and privacy aspects of HIPAA, which are outlined as follows:

> The privacy provisions of the federal law, the Health Insurance Portability and Accountability Act of 1996 (HIPAA), apply to health information created or maintained by healthcare providers who engage in certain electronic transactions, health plans, and healthcare clearinghouses. The Department of Health and Human Services (HHS) has issued the regulation, "Standards for Privacy of Individually Identifiable Health Information," applicable to entities covered by HIPAA. The Office for Civil Rights (OCR) is the Departmental component responsible for implementing and enforcing the privacy regulation. (See the Statement of Delegation of Authority to the Office for Civil Rights, as published in the Federal Register on December 28, 2000 (U.S. Department of Health and Human Services, 2006, para. 1).

Guaranteeing the security and privacy of health information has been the focus of numerous debates. Comprehensive standards for the implementation of this portion of the act eventually were finalized, but the process to adopt final standards took years. In August of 1998, the US Department of Health and Human Services (HHS) released a set of proposed rules addressing health information management. Proposed rules specific to health information privacy and security were released in November of 1999. The purpose of the proposed rules was to balance patients' rights to privacy and providers' needs for access to information (Hellerstein, 2000).

One of the biggest stumbling blocks to implementation of comprehensive standards for privacy was the associated cost. The administrative simplification portion of HIPAA calling for standardized forms for claims, medical records, laboratory reports, insurance forms, and so forth was expected to save up to $250 billion after the initial conversion costs. Compliance with the proposed security and privacy rules was projected to be $6.7 billion by HHS. Not everyone agreed with the HHS estimate; a study conducted by Blue Cross/Blue Shield and reported by Egger (2000) projected the costs would be closer to $43 billion over 5 years. An overview of the proposed standards helps to illustrate why implementation was estimated to be so costly.

Hellerstein (2000) summarized the proposed privacy rules. The rules do the following:

- Define protected health information as "information relating to one's physical or mental health, the provision of one's health care, or the payment for that health

Continues

care, that has been maintained or transmitted electronically and that can be reasonably identified with the individual it applies to" (Hellerstein, 2000, p. 2).

- Propose that authorization by patients for release of information is not necessary when the release of information is directly related to treatment and payment for treatment. Specific patient authorization is not required for research, medical or police emergencies, legal proceedings, and collection of data for public health concerns. All other releases of health information require a specific form for each release and only information pertinent to the issue at hand is allowed. All releases of information must be formally documented and accessible to the patient on request.
- Establish patient ownership of the healthcare record and allow for patient-initiated corrections and amendments.
- Mandate administrative requirements for the protection of healthcare information. All healthcare organizations are required to have a privacy official and an office to receive privacy violation complaints. A specific training program for employees that includes a certification of completion and a signed statement by all employees that they will uphold privacy procedures must be developed and implemented. All employees must re-sign the agreement to uphold privacy every 3 years. Sanctions for violations of policy must be clearly defined and applied.
- Mandate that all outside entities that conduct business with healthcare organizations (e.g., attorneys, consultants, auditors) must meet the same standards as the organization for information protection and security.
- Allow protected health information to be released without authorization for research studies. Patients may not access their information in blinded research studies because this access may affect the reliability of the study outcomes.
- Propose that protected health information may be deidentified before release in such a manner that the identity of the patient is protected. The healthcare organization may code the deidentification so that the information can be reidentified once it has been returned.
- Apply only to health information maintained or transmitted by electronic means.

As the concern mounted but deadlines loomed, the healthcare arena prepared to comply with the requirements of the law. The administrative simplification portion of this law is intended to decrease the financial and administrative burdens by standardizing the electronic transmission of certain administrative and financial transactions. This section also addresses the security and privacy of healthcare data and information for the covered entities of healthcare providers who transmit any health information in electronic form in connection with a covered transaction, health plans, and healthcare clearinghouses. For more information, visit http://aspe.os.dhhs.gov/admnsimp/ (US Department of Health and Human Services, 2007a).

The privacy requirements went into effect on April 14, 2003, and limit the release of protected health information without the patient's knowledge and consent. Covered entities must comply with the requirements. Among the necessary rules they must comply with, they must dedicate a privacy officer, adopt and implement privacy

Continues

procedures, educate their personnel, and secure their electronic patient records. Most individuals are familiar with the need to notify patients of their privacy rights, having signed forms on interacting with healthcare providers.

According to the HHS (2002), there are certain rights provided to patients by the privacy rule. Some of the rights include the following: the right to request restrictions to access of the health record; the right to request an alternate method of communication with a provider; the right to receive a paper copy of the notice of privacy practices; the right to file a complaint if one believes his or her privacy rights were violated; the right to inspect and copy one's health record; the right to request an amendment to the health record; and the right to see an account of disclosures of one's health record. This places the burden on the healthcare system and not the patient.

On October 16, 2003, the electronic transaction and code set standards became effective. This does not require electronic transmission but mandates that if transactions are conducted electronically, they must comply with the required federal standards for electronically filed healthcare claims. "The Secretary has made the **Centers for Medicare & Medicaid Services (CMS)** responsible for enforcing the electronic transactions and code sets provisions of the law" (Guidance on Compliance with HIPAA Transactions and Code Sets, 2003, para. 3).

The security requirements went into effect on April 21, 2005, and require the covered entities to put safeguards that protect the confidentiality, integrity, and availability of protected health information when stored and transmitted electronically into place. According to Savage (2006), "After HIPAA's security requirements went into effect, many organizations in the healthcare industry continue to improve their security" (para. 5). Some have had to engage in enormous amounts of resource expenditures involving people, time, and money. Savage states that "While the HIPAA rules have driven security improvements, their lack of specifics and a dearth of enforcement leaves much room for interpretation, making compliance hard to gauge" (para. 5). Because it is believed that the pursuit of a perfect security system is a wild goose chase, the journey should be reflective of the needs of the organization and their unique requirements in relation to their obligations to the patients they serve while addressing the demands of HIPAA. The safeguards that are addressed are administrative, physical, and technical. The administrative safeguards refer to the documented formal policies and procedures that are used to manage and execute the security measures. They govern the protection of healthcare data and information and the conduct of the personnel. The physical safeguards refer to the policies and procedures that must be in place to limit physical access to electronic information systems. Technical safeguards are the policies and procedures used to control access to healthcare data and information. Safeguards need to be in place to control access whether the data and information are at rest, residing on a machine or storage medium, being processed, or in transmission, such as being backed up to storage or disseminated across a network.

References

Egger, E. (2000). HIPAA offers hospitals the good, the bad, and the ugly. *Health Care Strategic Management, 18*(4), 1, 21–23.

Continues

BOX *(Continued)*

10-1

Guidance on compliance with HIPAA transactions and code sets. (2003). Retrieved from http://www.dmh.ca.gov/hipaa/Transactions_and_Code_Sets.asp

Hellerstein, D. (1999). *HIPAA's impact on healthcare. Health Management Technology.* Retrieved from http://findarticles.com/p/articles/mi_m0DUD/is_3_20/ai_54396227

Hellerstein, D. (2000). *HIPAA and health information privacy rules: Almost there. Health Management Technology.* Retrieved from http://findarticles.com/p/articles/mi_m0DUD/is_4_21/ai_61523494

Savage, M. (2006). *Security news: Perfect HIPAA security impossible, experts say.* Retrieved from http://searchsecurity.techtarget.com/originalContent/0,289142,sid14_gci1268986,00.html

US Department of Health and Human Services. (2002). *Federal Register, Part V, Department of Health and Human Services: Standards for privacy of individually identifiable health information; Final rule.* Retrieved from http://www.hhs.gov/ocr/hipaa/privrulepd.pdf

US Department of Health and Human Services. (2006). *Medical privacy—National standards to protect the privacy of personal health information.* Retrieved from http://www.hhs.gov/ocr/hipaa/bkgrnd.html

US Department of Health and Human Services. (2007a). *Administrative simplification in the health care industry.* Retrieved from http://aspe.os.dhhs.gov/admnsimp

How a National HIT Infrastructure Is Being Developed

Developing a national HIT infrastructure is an enormous and extremely complex undertaking that requires extensive financial, technologic and human resources. The HITECH Act established the ONC and HSS appointed a National Coordinator, who is responsible for the development of the infrastructure. The HITECH Act also established two committees within the ONC: the HIT Policy Committee and the HIT Standards Committee.

The Policy Committee is responsible for making recommendations to the Coordinator about how to implement the requirements of the HITECH Act, such as the technologies to use in the infrastructure. The Policy Committee has a total of 20 members, one of whom must be a member from a labor organization and two of whom must be healthcare providers. At least one of the healthcare providers must be a physician. There is no specific requirement that a nurse be on the Policy Committee. A complete list of the Policy Committee members is available at www.healthit.hhs.gov.

The Standards Committee is responsible for recommending standards by which health information is to be electronically exchanged. The HITECH Act does not designate the number of members to be on the committee; however, its members include healthcare providers, ancillary healthcare workers, consumers of health care, and others. Again, there is no specific requirement that a nurse be on the Standards Committee and a complete list of the Standards Committee members is available at www.healthit.hhs.gov.

The HITECH Act also made provisions to foster "meaningful public input" in the development of a national HIT infrastructure. Both the Policy Committee and the Standards Committee hold public meetings and anyone interested in this process can participate. A schedule of meetings, committee agendas, and the transcripts of past meeting are posted at www.healthit.hhs.gov.

The National Coordinator has several duties. He or she decides whether to endorse the recommendations of the Policy and Standards Committees and acts as a liaison among the Committees and various federal agencies involved in the process of developing a national HIT infrastructure. He or she consults with these other agencies, including the **National Institute of Standards and Technology**, and along with those agencies updates the Federal HIT Strategic Plan (US Department of Commerce, 2011). The Federal HIT Strategic Plan was published in June 2008, before enactment of the HITECH Act, and can be accessed at http://www.hhs.gov/healthit/resources/HITStrategicPlan.pdf.

The HITECH Act also provides significant monetary incentives for providers who engage in meaningful use of health information technology. "Meaningful use" is defined as "using electronic health records (EHRs) in a meaningful manner, which includes, but is not limited to electronically capturing health information in a coded format, using that information to track key clinical conditions, communicating that information to help coordinate care, and initiating the reporting of clinical quality measures and public health information" (CMS, 2010, para. 3).

Monetary incentives are available to clinicians and facilities which implement EHR systems that meet the specific standards. Providers that fail to adopt such systems within a specified time frame may be subject to significant governmental penalties.

HOW THE HITECH ACT CHANGED HIPAA

HIPAA Privacy and Security Rules

Nurses have been complying with HIPAA for years. HIPAA was enacted by the federal government for several purposes, including better portability of health insurance as a worker moved from one job to another; deterrence of fraud, abuse, and waste within the healthcare delivery system; and simplification of the administrative functions associated with the delivery of health care, such as reimbursement claims sent to Medicare and Medicaid. Simplification of administrative functions entailed the adoption of electronic transactions that included sensitive healthcare information. To protect the privacy and security of health information, two sets of federal regulations were implemented. The "Privacy Rule" became effective in 2003 and the "Security Rule" became effective in 2005. Many practitioners that refer to HIPAA are not referring to the comprehensive federal statute enacted in 1996. Rather, they are referring to the "Privacy Rule" and the "Security Rule," the federal regulations that were adopted years after HIPAA became law.

Under the Privacy Rule, patients have a right to expect privacy protections that limit the use and disclosure of their health information. Under the Security Rule, providers are obligated to safeguard their patients' health information from improper use or disclosure, maintain the integrity of the information, and ensure its availability. Both rules apply to **protected health information** (PHI), defined as any physical or mental health information created, received, or stored by a "covered **entity**" that can be used to identify an individual patient, regardless of the form of the health information (i.e., it can be electronic, hand-written, or verbal) (Vllex, 2011). Covered entities include hospitals and other healthcare providers that transmit any health information electronically, and health insurance companies and healthcare clearinghouses (Vllex).

Clinicians have become very knowledgeable about the requirements of the Privacy and Security Rules. They are familiar with their obligations to protect patient information and the **rights** afforded to their patients under these regulations. Patients are entitled to a notice of privacy practices from their healthcare provider. Inpatients are entitled to opt out of the facility's directory, thereby protecting disclosure of information that they are even a patient in the facility. Under certain circumstances, patients must authorize disclosure of their PHI before it can be released by the provider. Patients can request and obtain access to their own healthcare records and may request that corrections and additions be made to their records. Providers must consider a patient's request to amend a healthcare record, but they are not required to make such an amendment if the request is unwarranted. Unauthorized access or use or any loss of healthcare information must be disclosed to any patient affected by the breach. Patients may request an accounting of anyone who accessed their healthcare information and the provider is required to provide that information in a timely manner. Finally, patients have a right to complain if they perceive that the privacy or security of their healthcare information has been compromised in some way. Such complaints can be made directly to the provider or to the **Office of Civil Rights** (OCR).

The OCR, part of HHS, is responsible for enforcing HIPAA. It provides significant information and guidance to clinicians who must comply with the Privacy and Security Rules. It has been tracking complaints and investigating violations since 2003. Guidance and information about the complaint process and the violations that the OCR has handled are available on its website at www.hhs.gov/ocr/privacy/hipaa. One such violation involved the case of a nurse practitioner who had privileges within a healthcare system. She accessed her ex-husband's medical records without his authorization by using the system-wide EHRs. A complaint was filed and the OCR investigated the matter. The OCR resolved the complaint with the healthcare system. As a result, the healthcare system curtailed the nurse practitioner's access to its EHRs and it required her to undergo remedial training. In addition, it reported the nurse practitioner to her professional board (US Department of Health and Human Services, Office of Civil Rights, n.d.)

Compliance with the Privacy and Security Rules is mandatory for all covered entities and the HITECH Act extends compliance with these requirements directly to other entities that are "business associates" of a covered entity. Requirements include that there be privacy and information security officials to protect health information and that any complaints be handled appropriately. Sanctions must be imposed if there has been a violation of HIPAA. The Privacy and Security Rules also mandate that certain physical and technical safeguards be implemented for PHI and require entities to conduct periodic training of all staff to ensure compliance with these safeguards. Most entities adhere to industry standards and provide their personnel with yearly training. In addition, entities are to conduct regular audits to ensure compliance and any breaches in the privacy or security of PHI must be remedied immediately. It is important to avoid a security incident, defined as "the attempted or successful unauthorized access, use, disclosure, modification, or destruction of information or interference with system operations in an information system" (US Department of Human Services, CMS, 2008, p. 1). Such incidents trigger certain notification requirements.

The HITECH Act Enhanced HIPAA Protections

The HITECH Act has had a significant impact on HIPAA's Privacy and Security Rules in the following ways:

- HHS is to provide annual guidance about how to secure health information.
- Notification requirements in the event of a breach in the security of health information have been enhanced.
- HIPAA requirements now apply directly to any business associates of a covered entity.
- The rules that pertain to providing an accounting to patients who want to know who accessed their health information have changed.
- Enforcement of HIPAA has been strengthened.

These measures are being implemented to provide further assurance that health information will be protected as the country transitions to a nationwide HIT infrastructure (Box 10-2).

BOX

10-2

Other Organizations Assisting HIPAA

Dee McGonigle, Kathleen Mastrian, and Nedra Farcus

There are other organizations assisting in HIPAA implementation. The **American National Standards Institute** (ANSI) X12N and Health Level 7 (HL7) standards organizations worked together to develop an electronic standard for claims attachments to recommend to HHS (Spencer and Bushman, 2006, para. 2). The American National Standards Institute (ANSI, n.d.) was founded in 1918 and has served as the coordinator of the United States voluntary standards and conformity assessment system (para. 1). ANSI provides a forum where the private and public sectors can cooperatively work together toward the development of voluntary national consensus standards and the related compliance programs (para. 2). HL7 (n.d.) is one of several American National Standards Institute–accredited **Standards-Developing Organizations** (SDOs) operating in the healthcare arena (para. 1). It states that its mission is that HL7 provides standards for interoperability that improve care delivery, optimize workflow, reduce ambiguity, and enhance knowledge transfer among all of our stakeholders, including healthcare providers, government agencies, the vendor community, fellow SDOs and patients (para. 5). HL7 was initially associated with HIPAA in 1996 through the creation of a claims attachments special interest group charged with standardizing the supplemental information needed to support healthcare insurance and other e-commerce transactions. The initial deliverable of this group was six claim attachments. This special-interest group is currently known as the Attachment Special Interest Group. As the attachment projects continue, they are slated to include skilled nursing facilities, home health care, preauthorization, and referrals.

The Level Seven in Health Level Seven's name means the

> highest level of the **International Standards Organization**'s (ISO) communications model for **Open Systems Interconnection** (OSI) application level. The application level addresses definition of the data to be exchanged, the timing of the interchange, and the communication of certain errors to the application. The seventh level supports such functions as security checks, participant identification, availability checks, exchange mechanism negotiations and, most importantly, data exchange structuring. (HL7, n.d., para. 5)

The OSI was an attempt to standardize networking by the ISO. HL7 addresses the distinct requirements of the systems in use in hospitals and other facilities, is more concerned with application than the other levels, and user authentication and privacy are considered (Webopedia, 2008). The lower levels address hardware, software, and data reformatting. The HL7 mission is supported through two separate groups, the Extensible Markup Language (XML) special interest group and the structured documents technical committee. The XML special interest group makes recommendations on use of XML standards for all of HL7's platform- and vendor-independent healthcare specifications (HL7, n.d., para. 21). XML

Continues

began as a simplified subset of the standard generalized markup language; XML's major purpose is to facilitate the exchange of structured data across different information systems, especially via the Internet. It is considered an extensible language because it permits its users to define their own elements allowing customization to enable purpose-specific development. The structured documents technical committee supports the HL7 mission through development of structured document standards for health care (HL7, para. 21). HL7 also organizes, maintains, and sustains a repository for the vocabulary terms used in its messages to provide a shared, well-defined, and unambiguous knowledge of the meaning of the data transferred.

ISO (2008a) is a network of the national standards institutes of 157 countries, on the basis of one member per country, with a Central Secretariat in Geneva, Switzerland, that coordinates the system (para. 1). ISO is

> a non-governmental organization: its members are not, as is the case in the United Nations system, delegations of national governments. Nevertheless, ISO occupies a special position between the public and private sectors. This is because, on the one hand, many of its member institutes are part of the governmental structure of their countries, or are mandated by their government. On the other hand, other members have their roots uniquely in the private sector, having been set up by national partnerships of industry associations. (ISO, 2008a, para. 2)

This placement enables them to become a bridging organization where they can reach agreement on solutions that meet both the requirements of business and the broader needs of society, consumers, and users. These international agreements become standards that use the prefix ISO followed by the number of the standard. An example is the health informatics, health cards, numbering system, and registration procedure for issuer identifiers, ISO 20302:2006, which is designed to confirm, via a numbering system and registration procedure, the identities of both the healthcare application provider and the health card holder so that information may be exchanged by using cards issued for healthcare service (ISO, 2008b, para. 12). ISO provides standards for interoperability that improve care delivery, optimize workflow, reduce ambiguity, and enhance knowledge transfer among all of their stakeholders, including healthcare providers, government agencies, the vendor community, fellow SDOs, and patients. The standards are used on a voluntary basis because ISO has no power to force enactment.

It is evident that all of these organizations have guidelines, standards, and rules to help healthcare entities collect, store, manipulate, dispose of, and exchange secure PHI. Many SDOs work to help develop standards. HIPAA guarantees the security and privacy of health information and curtails healthcare fraud and abuse while enforcing standards for health information.

UNITED STATES AND BEYOND

Health care was not the only focus of United States legislative acts. One often sees "GLBA" and "SOX" when searching for information on HIPAA. The **Gramm-Leach-Bliley Act** (GLBA) is federal legislation in the United States to control how financial

Continues

institutions handle the private information they collect from individuals. The **Sarbanes-Oxley (SOX) Act** is legislation put in place to protect shareholders and the public from deceptive accounting practices in organizations.

There are privacy and data regulations being established around the world, such as the Data Protection Act 1998 in the United Kingdom (Ministry of Justice, 2008); the Dutch Data Protection Authority (2007), which released privacy legislation guidelines on publishing personal data on the Internet; and Finland's Personal Data File Act 1988 and Personal Data Act 1999 (Data Protection Board, n.d.). New Zealand's Health Information Privacy Code 1994 had amendment number six come into effect in November of 2007; this amendment covered such things as definitions of ethics committee, hospital, health, or disability services, health professional body, registered health professional, and health practitioner (Privacy Commissioner, 2007). Argentina's Privacy and Data Protection (2007) states that it is the first Latin American country to be awarded the status of "adequate country" from the point of view of European Data Protection authorities, and this breakthrough is expected to encourage other countries in the region to work toward improving data protection rights for individuals (Privacy and Data Protection, 2007, para. 7). In Canada, the Personal Information Protection and Electronic Documents Act received royal assent in 2000 (Office of the Privacy Commissioner of Canada, 2004). Safe Harbor deals with the transfer of personal data from the European Union to the United States; the regulations in Article 25 and 26 of the European Data Protection Directive serve as a basis. According to these regulations, transferring data to third countries is in principle only possible if these countries guarantee an adequate level of protection as required by the Directive (Federal Commissioner for Data Protection and Freedom of Information, n.d., para. 1). It is quite evident that privacy and security have become global concerns.

Avoiding security incidents has become tantamount. Providers must protect their information and prevent unauthorized persons from accessing, using, disclosing, changing, or destroying a patient's health information, or otherwise interfering with the operations of a health information system, such as an EHR. To facilitate a provider's ability to do this, the HITECH Act requires HHS to provide annual guidance to secure health information. PHI can be "secured" or "unsecured." PHI is considered unsecured if the provider does not follow the guidance provided by HHS for implementing technologies and methodologies that make PHI "unusable, unreadable, or indecipherable to unauthorized individuals (US Department of Health and Human Services, 2009). PHI can be secured through encryption, shredding, and other forms of complete destruction, or electronic media sanitation.

The distinction between secured and unsecured PHI is important because providers that have a breach in the privacy or security of PHI must adhere to certain notification requirements depending on the type of PHI affected by the breach. The HITECH Act enhanced the breach notification requirements of HIPAA. If the PHI is unsecured the provider must take certain steps to notify those individuals who have been affected. Providers can avoid these onerous breach notification requirements if the PHI is secured in accordance with the specifications of HHS.

A breach is considered discovered as soon as an employee other than the individual who committed the breach knows or should have known of the breach, such as unauthorized access or even an unsuccessful attempt to access information. For example, if a nurse knows that a colleague has accessed or attempted to access the record of a patient for whom the colleague is not providing care (e.g., the nurse practitioner who accessed her ex-husband's EHR, as discussed previously), the nurse's employer is deemed to have discovered the breach as soon as the nurse learned of it. The discovery of a breach triggers the beginning of the time frame in which the provider has to fulfill the notification requirements. A provider must fulfill these requirements within a reasonable period of time and under no circumstances may a provider take more than 60 days from discovery of the breach. It is easy to understand why providers require their employees to report knowledge of such breaches immediately to the privacy or information security officer. A provider's failure to adhere to the breach notification requirements could result in OCR sanctions, including monetary penalties.

Whenever a breach involves unsecured PHI, covered entities are responsible to alert each individual impacted by mail, or email if preferred by the individual. If there is insufficient contact information for 10 or more patients, the provider is required to place conspicuous postings on the home page of its website or in major print or broadcast media (without identifying patients). A toll free telephone number must be provided so that affected individuals can call for information about the breach. For breaches involving unsecured PHI of more than 500 individuals, a "prominent media outlet" must also be notified. Notice must also be given to HHS and HHS will post the information on its public website (US Department of Health and Human Services, 2009). It is easy to see why providers want to avoid these requirements by making sure their PHI is secured. Having to post such notices undermines the trust that exists between healthcare providers and the patients and communities they serve.

The HITECH Act has improved privacy and security of patient health information by applying the requirements of HIPAA directly to the business associates of covered entities. In the past, it was up to the covered entity to enter into contracts with its business associates to ensure compliance with HIPAA. Now business associates are responsible for their own compliance. An example of such a business associate is a HIT company hired by a hospital to implement or upgrade an EHR system. The technology company has access to the hospital's EHR system and must **comply** with the HIPAA Privacy and Security Rules just as covered entities must comply. This includes being subject to enforcement by the OCR for any violations.

Existing accounting rules are enhanced under the HITECH Act, giving patients the right to **access** their EHR and receive an accounting of all disclosures. Before the HITECH Act, HIPAA regulations provided an exception to the accounting requirements. Providers and other covered entities were not required to include in the accounting any disclosures that were made to facilitate the **treatment** of patients, the **payment** for services, or the **operations** of the entity. This is commonly known at the "TPO exception." This exception ended in January 2011 for providers that recently implemented new EHR systems. For those providers with EHR systems that were implemented before the HITECH Act, the TPO exception ends in January 2014. It is easy to understand why this exception is ending. As all providers implement comprehensive EHR systems, it will be very easy to generate an electronic record with an accounting of anyone who accessed a patient's record.

Finally, the HITECH Act strengthens the enforcement of HIPAA. HHS can conduct audits, which will be even easier to accomplish once there is a nationwide HIT infrastructure. In addition, stiffer **civil monetary penalties** (CMP) for violations of HIPAA became effective as soon as the HITECH Act became law in February 2009. CMPs are divided into three tiers. A Tier 1 CMP, in which the covered entity had no reason to know of a violation, is $100 per incident up to a cap of $25,000 per year. A Tier 2 CMP, in which the covered entity had reasonable cause to know of a violation, is $1,000 per incident up to a cap of $100,000 per year. A Tier 3 CMP, in which the covered entity engaged in willful neglect that resulted in a breach, is $10,000 per incident up to a cap of $250,000 per year. In addition, the HITECH Act gives authority to impose an additional CMP of $50,000 to $1.5 million if the covered entity does not properly correct a violation. Criminal penalties also can be imposed when warranted. It is imperative that providers avoid these penalties.

Before enactment of the HITECH Act, the federal government alone enforced HIPAA. Now, State Attorneys General can play a significant role in the enforcement and prosecution of HIPAA violations. Once the HITECH Act became law, State Attorneys General were authorized to pursue civil claims for HIPAA violations and collect up to $25,000 plus attorneys fees. As of 2012, individuals who are damaged by such violations will be able to share in any monetary awards obtained by these state officials.

IMPLICATIONS FOR NURSING PRACTICE

Being Involved and Staying Informed

The development and implementation of a nationwide EHR system holds great promise for nursing practice and nursing informatics. The profession of nursing will benefit from the many enhancements such an infrastructure has to offer, including the ability to improve the delivery of nursing care and the quality of that care, the ability to make more efficient and timely nursing care decisions for patients, the ability to avoid errors that may harm patients, and the ability to promote health and wellness for the patients they serve. On a broader scale, nurse researchers will have the ability more readily to access data that can be used to continue to foster evidence-based practice. The possibilities seem endless. For those who devote their professional careers to nursing informatics or plan to do so, the opportunities abound. There is much work to be done as this country transitions to a nationwide HIT infrastructure and there are monetary incentives available from the government for adopting systems that comply with the "meaningful use" requirement.

What also is important to keep in mind is that all nurses need to be engaged in this process, whether they treat patients, are managers within healthcare organizations, teach, develop computer programs, or help create institutional or governmental policies. Nurses, as the end-users of developing technologies, cannot afford to be left behind in these exciting times. Their voices must be heard, whether it is within the facility where they work as changes to the EHR system are contemplated, or whether it is in the public **policy** arena. How often are nurses the last to know that a new EHR system has been adopted by their hospital? How many times have nurses been trained to use a system that would have benefited from their input before it was implemented or even purchased? Nurses often are not invited to the table when entities make decisions about informatics, so nurses should not be afraid to ask to be included, whether it is to be heard within the workplace or within the governmental agencies that are overseeing the changes that are taking place.

Even nurses who do not get involved in the process need to stay current with the rapid changes that are taking place. Information about federal initiatives is available from the ONC and the OCR. Both offices are housed within HHS and are excellent resources for additional information about the HITECH Act and HIPAA. Regulations to implement the HITECH Act and enhance the HIPAA protections required by it are being proposed and adopted at a rapid pace. The ONC can be accessed at www.hhs.gov/healthit. The OCR can be accessed at www.hhs.gov/ocr/privacy/hipaa. State resources also are available.

Protecting Yourself

Nurses who strive to protect the privacy and security of patient information are protecting themselves from ethical lapses and violations of law. The American Nurses Association Code of Ethics for Nurses with Interpretive Statements mandates that nurses protect a patient's rights to privacy and **confidentiality**.

> Associated with the right to privacy, the nurse has a duty to maintain confidentiality of all patient information. The patient's well-being could be jeopardized and the fundamental trust between patient and nurse destroyed by unnecessary access to data or by the inappropriate disclosure of identifiable patient information. The rights, well-being, and safety of the individual patient should be the primary factors in arriving at any professional judgment

concerning the disposition of confidential information received from or about the patient, whether oral, written or electronic. The standard of nursing practice and the nurse's responsibility to provide quality care require that relevant data be shared with those members of the health care team that have a need to know. Only information pertinent to a patient's treatment and welfare is disclosed, and only to those directly involved with the patient's care. When using electronic communications, special effort should be made to maintain data security (American Nurses Association, 2010, p. 6).

The similarities between these ethical obligations and the legal requirements of HIPAA and other federal and state privacy and confidentially laws are readily apparent to nurses. By complying with their ethical code, nurses were complying with the Privacy and Security Rules before they were required to do so. Since the adoption of the HIPAA Privacy and Security Rules, and now with the passage of the HITECH Act, it is more important than ever for nurses to understand their obligations in this area and avoid the pitfalls of any violations.

In addition to the sanctions imposed by the OCR, violations can lead to disciplinary actions by employers and professional licensing boards, and litigation. Such actions can have a serious negative impact on the nurse's reputation and financial well-being. If a nurse is terminated for invading a patient's privacy or breaching the confidentiality of a patient's information, some state laws require reporting the information to prospective employers of the nurse and other laws require reporting to the State Board of Nursing. State Boards of Nursing have the authority to publicly discipline a nurse who has engaged in professional misconduct by invading a patient's privacy, which includes inappropriately accessing a patient's EHR, and breaching confidentiality of patient information, such as allowing or tolerating unauthorized access to a patient's EHR. These types of situations can also cause patients to file complaints with the OCR and lawsuits against the offenders. Nurses must be ever mindful of their obligations to report a breach in the privacy or security of PHI to their employers, even if it entails reporting a colleague.

Finally, some view the EHR as a convenient method for employers to monitor the performance of its nurses. It is undisputed that an EHR system provides a wealth of information that can be, and often is required to be, monitored. Audits are required to make sure there are not any breaches in the system's security. Audits are not necessarily required to determine, for example, which nurses are failing to timely complete the hospital's documentation requirements; which nurses are improperly altering (attempting to correct) the record; or which nurses are dispensing more pain medication than the average. Nurses have been challenged by employers who allege failure to document, improper or false documentation, and suspected diversion of narcotics. These types of situations are unsettling and may be on the rise as more and more providers adopt or augment EHR systems. Thus, it behooves every nurse who works with such a system to obtain proper training and to know the policies and procedures that pertain to its use.

SUMMARY

The HITECH Act and the HIPAA Privacy and Security Rules are intended to enhance the rights of individuals. These laws provide patients with greater access and control over their PHI. They can control its uses, dissemination, and disclosures. Covered entities must not only establish a required level of security for PHI but also sanctions for employees who violate the organization's privacy policies and administrative processes for responding to patient requests regarding their information. Therefore, they must be able to track the PHI and note access from both a perspective of what information was accessed and also by whom and any disclosures. Finally, readers should recognize that there is global awareness of the need for privacy protections for personal information or PHI. Over the next few years, international efforts will accelerate, enhancing international data exchange.

THOUGHT-PROVOKING Questions   WWW

1. Why is it important to establish patient ownership of the healthcare record?
2. What are the potential negative **consequences** of the right of amendment and correction of healthcare records by patients?
3. One of the largest problems with healthcare information security has always been inappropriate use by authorized users. How do HIPAA and the HITECH Act help to curb this problem?
4. How do you envision **Health Level 7**, HIPAA, and the HITECH Act evolving in the next decade?
5. Imagine that you are the designated privacy officer in a healthcare institution. What types of monitoring procedures would you develop?
6. If you were the privacy officer, what would you include in your sanctions for violations policy?
7. As privacy officer, how would you address the following:
   a. Tracking each point of access of the patient's database including who entered the data.
   b. Nurses in your hospital have an access code that only gives them access to their unit's patients. A visitor accidently comes to the wrong unit looking for a patient and asks the nurse to find out what unit the patient is on.
   c. Encouraging nurses to report privacy and security breaches.

For a full suite of assignments and additional learning activities, use the access code located in the front of your book to visit this exclusive website: http://go.jblearning.com/mcgonigle. If you do not have an access code, you can obtain one at the site.

WWW

References

Agency for Healthcare Research and Quality. (2009). *National Healthcare Quality Report (NHQR) 2009: Crossing the quality chasm: A new healthcare system for the 21st century.* Washington, DC: National Academies Press.

Agency for Healthcare Research and Quality. (2010). *2009 National Healthcare Disparities Report.* Retrieved from http://www.ahrq.gov/qual/nhdr09/nhdr09.pdf

American National Standards Institute (ANSI). (n.d.). *ANSI: A historical overview.* Retrieved from http://ansi.org/about_ansi/introduction/history.aspx?menuid=1

American Nurses Association. (2010). *Code of Ethics for Nurses with Interpretive Statements.* Retrieved from http://www.nursingworld.org/MainMenuCategories/EthicsStandards/CodeofEthicsfor Nurses/Code-of-Ethics.aspx

Ashish, J. (2009). Use of electronic health records in U.S. hospitals. *New England Journal of Medicine, 360*(16), 1628-1638.

Centers for Medicare and Medicaid Services. (2010). *Meaningful use.* Retrieved from https://www .cms.gov/EHRIncentivePrograms/30_Meaningful_Use.asp

Data Protection Board. (n.d.). *Legislation for the protection of privacy.* Retrieved from http://www .tietosuoja.fi/27305.htm

Dutch Data Protection Authority (DPA). (2007, December). *Dutch DPA publication of personal data on the Internet.* Retrieved from http://www.dutchdpa.nl/downloads_overig/en_20071108_rechtsnoeren _internet.pdf?refer=true&theme=purple

Egger, E. (2000). HIPAA offers hospitals the good, the bad, and the ugly. *Health Care Strategic Management, 18*(4), 1, 21–23.

Federal Commissioner for Data Protection and Freedom of Information. (n.d.). *Safe harbor.* Retrieved from http://www.bfdi.bund.de/cln_007/nn_671558/EN/EuropeanInternationalAffaires/Artikel/ SafeHarbor.html

Fifteenth National HIPAA Summit: Special Edition. (2007). *Healthcare privacy and security training and professional certification.* Retrieved from http://www.hipaasummit.com/past15/index.html

Final Rule. Retrieved from http://edocket.access.gpo.gov/2009/pdf/E9-20169.pdf

Guidance on compliance with HIPAA transactions and code sets. (2003). Retrieved from http://www .dmh.ca.gov/hipaa/Transactions_and_Code_Sets.asp

Hagland, M. (1998). The gap: HIPAA and secure IT. *Health Management Technology, 19*(6), 24–26, 28, 30.

Health Level Seven (HL7). (n.d.). *What is HL7?* Retrieved from http://www.hl7.org/

Hellerstein, D. (1999). *HIPAA's impact on healthcare. Health Management Technology.* Retrieved from http://findarticles.com/p/articles/mi_m0DUD/is_3_20/ai_54396227

Hellerstein, D. (2000). *HIPAA and health information privacy rules: Almost there. Health Management Technology.* Retrieved from http://findarticles.com/p/articles/mi_m0DUD/is_4_21/ai_61523494

Institute of Medicine. (2000). *To err is human: Building a safer health system.* Washington, DC: National Academies Press.

International Standards Organization (ISO). (2008a). *About ISO.* Retrieved from http://www.iso.org/iso/about.htm

International Standards Organization (ISO). (2008b). *Health informatics.* Retrieved from http://www.iso.org/iso/iso_catalogue/catalogue_tc/catalogue_detail.htm?csnumber=35376

Keehan, S., Sisko, A.Q., & Truffler, C. (2008). Health spending projections through 2017: The baby-boom generation is coming to Medicare. *Health Affairs, 27*(2), 145-155.

Leyva, C., & Leyva, D. (2011). *HITECH Act.* Retrieved from http://www.hipaasurvivalguide.com/hitech-act-text.php

Ministry of Justice. (2008). *Data sharing and protection.* Retrieved from http://www.justice.gov.uk/whatwedo/datasharingandprotection.htm

Office of the Privacy Commissioner of Canada. (2004). *Privacy legislation.* Retrieved from http://www.privcom.gc.ca/legislation/02_06_07_e.asp

Pretzer, M. (1999). The clock is ticking on patient privacy. *Medical Economics, 76*(2), 29–30, 32.

Privacy and Data Protection. (2007). *Data protection in Argentina.* Retrieved from http://www.proteccion dedatos.com.ar

Privacy Commissioner. (2007). *Health information privacy code.* Retrieved from http://www.privacy.org.nz/health-information-privacy-code

Readthestimulus.org. (2009). *Committee Print, January 16, 2009.* Retrieved from http://readthestimulus.org/ec-health_001_xml.pdf

Savage, M. (2006). *Security news: Perfect HIPAA security impossible, experts say.* Retrieved from http://searchsecurity.techtarget.com/originalContent/0,289142,sid14_gci1268986,00.html

Spencer, J., & Bushman, M. (2006). *HIPAAdvisory: The next HIPAA frontier: Claims attachments.* Retrieved from http://www.hipaadvisory.com/action/tcs/nextfrontier.htm

US Department of Commerce. (2011). *National Institute of Standards and Technology (NIST).* Retrieved from http://www.nist.gov/index.html

US Department of Health and Human Services. (2002). *Federal Register, Part V, Department of Health and Human Services: Standards for privacy of individually identifiable health information; Final rule.* Retrieved from http://www.hhs.gov/ocr/hipaa/privrulepd.pdf

US Department of Health and Human Services. (2006). *Medical privacy—National standards to protect the privacy of personal health information.* Retrieved from http://www.hhs.gov/ocr/hipaa/bkgrnd.html

US Department of Health and Human Services. (2007a). *Administrative simplification in the health care industry.* Retrieved from http://aspe.os.dhhs.gov/admnsimp

US Department of Health and Human Services. (2007b). *Security standard overview.* Retrieved from http://www.cms.hhs.gov/SecurityStandard

US Department of Health and Human Services, CMS, (2008). *CMS information security incident handling and breach analysis/notification process.* Retrieved from https://www.cms.gov/information security/downloads/incident_handling_procedure.pdf

US Department of Health and Human Services. (2009). *Federal Register: 45 CFR Parts 160 and 164: Breach Notification for Unsecured Protected Health Information; Interim*

US Department of Health and Human Services, Office of Civil Rights. (n.d.). *Health information privacy: All case examples.* Retrieved from http://www.hhs.gov/ocr/privacy/hipaa/enforcement/examples/allcases.html#case1

Vllex. (2011). *45 CFR 160.103—Definitions.* Retrieved from http://cfr.vlex.com/vid/160-103-definitions-19933565

Webopedia. (2008). *The 7 layers of the OSI model.* Retrieved from http://www.webopedia.com/quick_ref/OSI_Layers.asp

Weil, S. (2004). *HIPAA security rule.* Retrieved from http://www.securityfocus.com/infocus/1764

CHAPTER 11

Professional Development and Collaboration Tools

Glenn Johnson and Jeff Swain

Objectives

1. Describe an e-portfolio.
2. Distinguish between social networking and professional networking.
3. Examine the e-portfolio process.

WWW

Key Terms **WWW**

E-portfolio
Evidence
Privacy
Professional networking
Reflective commentary
Social networking
Web publishing

INTRODUCTION

Web-based electronic portfolios (**e-portfolios**) have fast become a popular and powerful way for students in postsecondary educational programs to demonstrate not only what they know but also what they can do with what they know. For reasons that become apparent in development, the process of creating a meaningful e-portfolio is as important as the presentation of the final e-portfolio product. This process involves synthesizing and then purposefully presenting **evidence** of the learning and experiences that an individual has accumulated both inside and outside of the classroom. The purpose and the audience of a professional e-portfolio are also important considerations. An e-portfolio might focus on what was learned in a single course, another might span an entire program of study, or chronicle an entire career. The audience may also change. An e-portfolio may be required for review by faculty, might be used by advisors or mentors, or could be shared with prospective employers. Once completed, today's Internet-based technology infrastructure allows for convenient and efficient sharing of a variety of media types—how the e-portfolio is put together depends on the author's purpose and audience.

WHAT IS AN ELECTRONIC PORTFOLIO?

Today's information technology infrastructure allows users easily to build Web-based collections that include evidence of knowledge and skills. Users can upload artifacts that represent evidence of their learning experiences both inside and out-side of the classroom. E-portfolios may also contain a blog element where students reflect on their total experience and demonstrate growth in their areas of study.

E-portfolios can be built using a range of different technologies. Some individuals use PowerPoint presentations to capture and present evidence. Web-based e-portfolios are built using common **Web publishing** tools to create Web pages, which are then published on the Internet (Penn State, 2010). In addition, there is an increasing number of institutional e-portfolio systems that users can log into that allow them to upload, enter, and share information or evidence related to their experiences. Examples of such systems include the following:

Association for Authentic, Experiential and Evidence-Based Learning:
　http://www.aaeebl.org
Digication: http://www.digication.com
Epsilen: http://www.epsilen.com/Epsilen/Public/Home.aspx
Facebook: http://www.facebook.com
iWebfolio: http://www.iwebfolio.com
LiveText: http://www.livetext.com
MySpace: http://www.myspace.com
PebblePAD: http://www.pebblepad.com
TaskStream: https://www.taskstream.com/pub
TypePad: http://www.typepad.com

E-PORTFOLIOS IN POSTSECONDARY EDUCATION

As an instructional strategy, portfolios have been around for a long time. Instructionally portfolios, whether electronic or paper based, require students to demonstrate or provide evidence that they have attained specific learning outcomes. For instance, in the arts portfolios have been used to demonstrate the depth and breadth of the work of an artist. Although performance-based programs of study are more likely to be familiar with the concept of demonstrating what a student knows and can do, other areas of study have also begun to adopt this method of assessment.

Portfolios can be particularly helpful in areas where higher-level thinking and analysis are essential. For instance, being a good nurse is more than being able to get high scores on examinations. Nurses need to be able to collect information, analyze the information presented, relate it to past experience, apply related knowledge, and evaluate various options, and from this present a diagnosis and a plan of action. In short, nurses need to be able to think critically and make informed decisions. In learning to become a nurse, portfolios can be used to capture, support, and improve this type of thinking as it develops.

Like the artist, a nursing student can connect, share, and present cases and findings and include with this evidence the **reflective commentary** that serves to unveil how he or she arrived at a decision, what information or experiences were vital, and how his or her action plan evolved. However, from the variety of evidence that an individual might use to represent themselves, what should one select and how should this be shared?

SOCIAL NETWORKING VERSUS PROFESSIONAL NETWORKING

New opportunities to share information via social networks have grabbed the headlines. But to what degree does **social networking** serve the same purpose as an e-portfolio? How do online profiles differ from what is included in an e-portfolio?

Since their inception in 2004, the rise of social networking tools, such as Facebook (http://www.facebook.com) and Twitter (http://twitter.com), has been phenomenal. In 2007, Facebook reported over 30 million users, over 40 billion page views every month, and is reportedly the top photo-sharing site on the Web (Locke, 2007). Twitter has over 100 million users and adds approximately 300,000 new users daily (Roumen, 2010). What makes these sites so attractive? Web-based applications, such as Facebook, allow users to connect and share information in ways that they had never been able to before. Users develop online profiles that contain information they select to share with others. Using simple online utilities, users easily connect and share their profile, communicating with friends over the Internet. Virtual groups of users with similar profiles are created connecting users with others who have similar interests. Twitter, a micro-blogging platform, allows users to create interpersonal networks for socializing, support, and information sharing. The power of such tools as Twitter lies in their being lightweight, updates are limited to 140 characters or less, and one can update their status from any device that has an internet connection or text messaging capabilities.

Are Networked Communities Changing How People Communicate?

The popularity of social and mobile networking applications is one indication of how new Web-based technologies are changing communication preferences. The Web is no longer a destination place and instead has become a vehicle of communication where individuals use application software ("apps") installed or downloaded, to connect with others. Individuals act as their own portal and can connect from anywhere with their various communities. This makes it difficult to separate out various communities and social networks. Where once it was relatively easy to separate out work relationships from friends and family, networked communities tend to overlap, thus blurring the boundaries between them and creating phenomena known as "networked individualism" where each individual acts as a switchboard between networks (Wellman et al., 2003). The phenomenon of overlapping networks means that the unintended audience is almost always greater than the intended one. A status update that may be construed as harmless and funny to one's friends could be taken an entirely different way by family or colleagues. This is not to say networked communities are harmful or bad. Rather, the benefit far exceeds the negative. However, the immediacy and the permanence of the updates shared mean that one must think about the impact beyond the intended audience in ways never before required.

The Social Networking Dilemma

Whereas professional e-portfolios have a specific goal in mind, information use within a Facebook or MySpace profile may or may not target a specific purpose. For many, the social aspects of connecting with others are simply a fun activity. However, a social dilemma results from the openness required to make social networks fun, the accessibility of personal information about someone. For some, differentiating between what is "fun personal information" and what is "professional personal information" is easy for owners to delineate. For viewers, however, this differentiation may not be so clear cut. Photos or journal entries that may be viewed as seemingly innocent by one may be interpreted entirely differently by another audience. What for some might be a simple distinction, for others the inherent biases and judgments that blur this distinction are naturally going to occur.

To offset this conundrum, several professional versions of networking sites have emerged including Linkedin, Naymz, and Ying. The sites are used to maintain and establish a network of professional contacts for the purposes of sharing information, creating business opportunities, and finding employment. Linkedin (http://linkedin.com) has over 75 million members in over 200 counties, including the CEO of every Fortune 500 company (http://press.linkedin.com). Networked communities of practice have developed for professionals (Box 11-1).

E-PORTFOLIO FOR PROFESSIONAL DEVELOPMENT

Using an e-portfolio to support **professional networking** involves a predetermined and focused purpose. The purpose may be to foster better communication between oneself and a mentor. The purpose may be to establish how what a nurse is doing fits into the goals of the institution or perhaps an institution for which the individual would like to work. A professional e-portfolio is evidence based and uses this evidence to make a case that highlights one's capacity not only to perform but also to grow and develop professionally within one's chosen field.

BOX

11-1

Communities of Practice

Developing and sustaining communities of practice (CoP) in the work environment are beyond the main scope of this book. However, educators need to understand how the effective collaboration skills that learners acquire in learning communities during their formal education may promote the development of CoPs in students' future professional lives. The following is a brief overview of this important and emerging trend for work in the knowledge era.

Wenger (n.d.) defines a CoP as follows: "Communities of practice are groups of people who share a concern or a passion for something they do and learn how to do it better as they interact regularly" para. 3). He suggests that CoPs have three important characteristics: (1) the domain, (2) the community, and (3) the practice. Wenger defines a domain as a shared interest about which people are passionate and possess some competence related to the domain. The community aspect relates to the joint activities that are undertaken by the group to build relationships and knowledge about the domain. The practice denotes that the members of the community are practitioners of something and through the CoP develop and share resources, knowledge, and solutions to problems. The recent improvement of Internet-based communications technologies has the potential to promote the global expansion of CoPs.

Nursing is a profession that is particularly suited to the development of CoPs, especially in light of the new knowledge generated and disseminated every day. The many nursing List-Servs are evidence of the growing practice of sharing knowledge in a CoP. Caring, a nursing informatics organization, has a very active List-Serv where members post questions to other members and request information and experiences related to informatics. For example, a member of the list might ask others about their experiences related to a specific issue in implementing a Bar Code Medication Administration system, or about training procedures for implementing an electronic medical record. One of the difficulties with a List-Serv as a CoP is that the discussion is not moderated; many threads could be running simultaneously. An example of a well-organized and global CoP is the Cochrane Collaboration (http://www.cochrane.org/) an international organization that promotes and supports collaboration among healthcare professionals to develop evidence-based practice recommendations for health care interventions. A nursing practice council within a health care organization is also an example of a CoP. In the future, it is hoped that the use of CoPs in nursing will grow beyond knowledge sharing and promote more knowledge discovery and sense making.

SOURCE: Wenger, E. (2006). Communities of practice: A brief introduction. Retrieved from http://www.ewenger.com/theory/communities_of_practice_intro.htm

THE E-PORTFOLIO PROCESS

The four steps involved in developing an e-portfolio are recursive in nature in that during the process one can backtrack to fill in missing pieces or re-evaluate earlier decisions that were made. The four steps are (1) collect, (2) select, (3) reflect, and (4) connect.

Collect

Evidence should demonstrate what a person knows, what they can do, or the values that they hold as being important. When it comes to developing e-portfolios, it is important to think of evidence in very broad terms. This evidence might include the results of what someone has learned in courses that they have taken, especially in terms of demonstrating a new skill or increased knowledge of a subject. More importantly, evidence can come from experiences that take place outside of the classroom. For instance, someone may have been involved in an internship or clinical observation where they have had the opportunity to connect what they learned in the classroom with how this is applied in a real world setting. Not only is this experience valuable but it represents their understanding of how this knowledge can be applied; thus, it enhances others' perception of the depth of what they know.

Resumes are evidence documents. They are very important and every professional should have an updated copy available. However, they only list an individual's experiences or accomplishments. E-portfolios, however, go beyond the resume to emphasize personal attributes that are very important in the nursing profession. These attributes include, but are not limited to, interpersonal skills, leadership skills, appreciation of diversity, ability to work in a team, and self-sufficiency. These attributes are difficult if not impossible to feature in a resume. By using reflective commentary that accompanies evidence of an individual's involvement, these attributes and values can become the highlights of an e-portfolio.

Select

Everyone has their own unique pool of evidence from which to pull, and over time this evidence pool can become quite large. What will someone choose to feature and why? Putting together a professional e-portfolio requires that two intertwining questions related to purpose and audience be addressed.

What is the purpose? What is it that someone is attempting to gain by putting an e-portfolio together? Is the purpose related to personal development (i.e., feedback and advice about the professional direction that is being taken)? Is the purpose to connect with colleagues? An individual may be interested in using her e-portfolio to find a job or gain admission into a graduate program. Each of these purposes addresses a different audience, which in turn informs the careful selection of what evidence to feature (Figure 11-1).

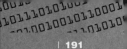

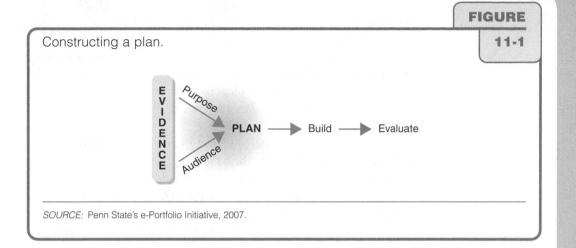

FIGURE 11-1

Constructing a plan.

SOURCE: Penn State's e-Portfolio Initiative, 2007.

Although an e-portfolio can link to everything that a person has accomplished, this may not be the best strategy. Instead, it is essential that an individual consider their audience and establish a plan that enables them to select the most appropriate pieces of evidence for their particular purpose and audience. A helpful way to start is to select the top five pieces of evidence that support their plan. Next, they should consider why they selected these pieces of evidence. What it is about each piece of evidence that makes it representative of who they are, what they know, what they can do, and what they value as important.

Reflect

Reflection and reflective commentary take an e-portfolio to the next level. This may be included in a single reflective statement or it can be attached to the evidence throughout an e-portfolio. Reflective comments should open up a window into why an individual thinks this evidence is important, the ways in which the individual values what they have learned, or why they think it is important for their profession. For instance, they may present an experience where they were challenged to provide assistance. Describing this experience would be important; however, their reflective comments can extend this description—they can talk about the alternatives that they considered as the basis for how they made their decision to provide the type of assistance they provided and the manner in which it was provided. By itself, a description of this experience is good. With reflective comments, readers have a much more thorough perception of and insight into an individual's professional thinking. This is where having a blog element as part of an e-portfolio becomes extremely powerful.

Unlike static Web pages, a blog page is a space designed to be interactive. The blog owner posts commentary, thoughts, and experiences for others to read and comment. Regular entries on a blog give others a reason to return to one's e-portfolio site over and over again. It is an opportunity to share one's perspective on topics of interest and critical to the chosen field. A blog is a place where conversation happens. It provides a nice counter-balance to the static Web pages, such as a resume and project pieces.

Most blogging platforms allow users to select from a range of templates that include a blogging element along with static Web pages. Such platforms as WordPress, MoveableType, and Google are free for at least the basic service enabling the user to create a dynamic e-portfolio without having to build Web pages. Most platforms allow entries to be in both text and multimedia format so it is the perfect place for personal expression. A blog is quickly becoming a standard part of an e-portfolio.

Connect (Connections) and Feedback

The connection and feedback step is important to validate the assertions someone makes about what it is they know, understand, or value. Individuals may choose to receive feedback from those who are close to them and from here reach out to others who may provide different perspectives. For instance, if one was thinking about using their e-portfolio to apply for a position, they may want to start by first getting feedback from friends and family. They might share their e-portfolio with a mentor or faculty, raising the bar by getting professionally grounded feedback before they share their e-portfolio with a prospective employer.

E-Portfolio Process—Summary Comments

With this process in mind, one might think about the process of developing a professional e-portfolio as boiling down to the telling of a rather simple story, a story that has three parts: looking back, looking around, and looking ahead. The reader should think of their own evidence pool as they answer these questions:

1. Looking back: What have you done? In what have you been involved? Where have you been? With whom have you worked? How did this help get you where you are today?
2. Looking around: In what are you currently involved? Why are you doing this? What are you getting out of it?
3. Looking ahead: Where would you like to be in 2 years? Where would you like to be in 5 years? Why do you feel this way? What makes you think your goals are realistic?

CHALLENGES AND ISSUES: PRIVACY AND SECURITY

The ease and popularity that both Web-based social networking and professional e-portfolio tools bring to users also raises several challenges and issues. Never before has information been so accessible or personal. For this reason, issues related to **privacy** and security need to be addressed. What might be appropriate socially can be deadly in a professional context.

What Kind of Personal Information Should Be Available About Someone?

Is the personal information one finds by searching the Internet for their own name unsettling? Give it a try and see what results. An e-portfolio is one place that an individual has control over what personal information is included. How personal an individual wants this to be is up to the individual. What contact information should be included? Usually an e-mail address is all that is required. Those creating an e-portfolio should look for mechanisms that allow them to restrict access to certain pages they deem personal. When publishing in open Web space, users likely have to engineer this themselves, whereas these capabilities are built into larger online e-portfolio systems. In any case, users should get feedback from family, colleagues, or other professionals to help gauge whether an e-portfolio is or is not personal enough.

How Much Information Should Be Revealed?

Especially true in the nursing profession, patient client identity is critical. Although one might write about an experience or relate an observation, this should be done in a manner that does not include any personal information about patients or clients. Including personal information is not only a violation of a patient's right to privacy, but it demonstrates a lack of ethical judgment on the part of the e-portfolio creator.

SUMMARY—WHY CREATE AN E-PORTFOLIO?

Although academic institutions may use e-portfolios for assessment of student learning, for the individual, e-portfolios are all about opportunity. This opportunity might be to support a working relationship with a mentor, network with other professionals, or to help represent certain qualities and characteristics to prospective employers. In any of these cases, having gone through the process of developing an e-portfolio requires critical examination of what qualities make an individual who they are and why these qualities are important to them and their profession. It is important for every professional to have a foundational understanding of where they are in their career trajectory and how this fits their long-term professional goals.

Practically speaking, e-portfolios are efficient. When introducing oneself in an e-mail message, a self-starting individual who has taken the initiative to develop and publish an e-portfolio can add this line to their message: "Here is a link to my e-portfolio." The recipient can click on this link, which automatically opens that individual's e-portfolio in a Web browser. Metaphorically, they have just walked into the recipient's office with information that features who they are, what they know, what they can do, and what they value as important. They have just walked in with what could be a multimedia showcase of their qualities. The Internet is a very powerful communication medium, and individuals with professional e-portfolios are simply taking advantage of this fact. To find information about how e-portfolios are developed and used, visit Penn State University's e-portfolio support Web site at http://portfolio.psu.edu.

WHAT THE FUTURE HOLDS

The e-portfolio phenomenon is not going to go away. Academic and business leaders predict a continued growth in global educational initiatives that cross both academic and professional bounds (Economist Intelligence Unit, 2008). E-Portfolios are increasingly a critical component in making that happen. It is often one of the first things colleges and corporations look for when they are interested in a candidate.

There are significant initiatives underway both in the United States and in Europe. For example, the state of Minnesota allocates e-portfolio space to each of its citizens to "reach their career and education goals" (eFolio Minnesota, 2007, para. 1). The state of Indiana announced Indiana@Work, which provides free e-portfolio space to those who apply (Indiana@Work, 2004). In Europe, goals established at professional meetings include an e-portfolio for all European citizens by the year 2010 under the justification that, "In the context of a knowledge society, where being information literate is critical, the portfolio can provide an opportunity to demonstrate one's ability to collect, organize, interpret and reflect on documents and sources of information" (European Institute for E-Learning, 2007, para. 1).

Web-based technologies will continue to evolve to find better ways to support an individual's ability to articulate personalized representations of who they are and what they are doing. The questions themselves have not changed. The ability to support this thinking process and the sharing of results with others through electronic portfolios will become more commonly available.

In an ideal world, e-portfolios will become vibrant, dynamic articulations of one's accomplishments that celebrate one's life.

THOUGHT-PROVOKING Questions

WWW

1. What would be the top five pieces of evidence that you would select to be featured in your own portfolio? Why did you select these pieces of evidence? What was it about them that made you think they would represent who you are?

2. Some institutions that require students to develop e-portfolios as a part of their program of study also may use this evidence of student learning to evaluate the program quality or generate evidence for accreditation reports. What do you think should be the driving purpose behind requiring e-portfolios—professional development planning or institutional evaluation? What are the merits of each approach?

For a full suite of assignments and additional learning activities, use the access code located in the front of your book to visit this exclusive website: http://go.jblearning.com/mcgonigle. If you do not have an access code, you can obtain one at the site.

WWW

References

Economist Intelligence Unit. (2008). *The future of higher education: How technology will shape learning.* Retrieved from http://www.nmc.org/pdf/Future-of-Higher-Ed-(NMC) .pdf

eFolio Minnesota. (2007). Welcome. Retrieved from http://www.efoliominnesota.com

European Institute for E-Learning. (2007). Why do we need an ePortfolio? Retrieved from http://www .eife-l.org/publications/eportfolio

Indiana@Work. (2004). State launches new online career development, job search tool. Retrieved from http://www.insideindianabusiness.com/newsitem.asp?id=12497

Locke, L. (2007). The future of Facebook. Time. Retrieved from http://www.time.com/time/business/ article/0,8599,1644040,00.html

Penn State's e-Portfolio Initiative. (2010). Retrieved from http://portfolio.psu.edu

Roumen, M. (2010). Statistic video: The state of the internet. Retrieved from http://www.viralblog .com/social-media/statistic-video-the-state-of-the-internet/

Wellman, B., Quan-Hasse, A., Boase, J., Chen, W., Hampton, K., Isla de Diaz, I., & Miyata, K. (2003). The social affordances of the internet for networked individualism. Retrieved from http://jcmc .indiana.edu/vol8/issue3/wellman.html

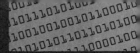

SECTION **III**

Nursing Informatics Administrative Applications: Precare and Care Support

Nursing informatics (NI) and information technology (IT) have invaded nursing, and some nurses are happy with the capabilities afforded by this specialty. Others, however, remain convinced that changes wrought by IT are nothing more than a nuisance. In the past, nursing administrators have found the implementation of technology tools to be an expensive venture with minimal rewards. This is likely related to their lack of knowledge about NI, which caused nursing administrators to listen to vendors or other colleagues; in essence, it was decision making based on limited and biased information. There were at least two reasons for the experience of limited rewards. One was the failure to include nurses in the testing and implementation of products designed for nurses and nursing tasks. Second, the new products they purchased had to interface with old, legacy systems and were not at all compatible or seemed compatible until the glitches arose. The glitches caused frustration for clinicians and administrators alike. They purchased tools that should have made the nurses happy, but instead all they did was grumble. The good news is that approaches have changed as a result of the difficult lessons learned from the early forays into technology tools. Nursing personnel are involved both at the agency level and the vendor level, in the decision making and development of new systems and products charged with enhancing the practice of nursing. Older legacy systems are being replaced with newer systems that have more capacity to interface with other systems. Nurses and administrators have become more astute in the realm of NI, but there is still a long way to go. Chapter 12 introduces the system development life cycle, used to make important and appropriate organizational decisions for technology adoption.

Administrators need information systems that facilitate their administrative role, and they particularly need systems that provide financial, risk management, quality assurance, human resources, payroll, patient registration, acuity, communication, and scheduling functions. The administrator must be open to learning about all of the tools available. One of the most important tasks that an administrator can oversee and engage in is data mining, or the extraction of data and information from sizeable data sets collected and warehoused. Data mining helps to identify patterns in aggregate data, gain insights, and ultimately discover and generate knowledge applicable to nursing science. Nursing administrators must become astute informaticists—knowledge workers who harness the information and knowledge at their fingertips to facilitate the practice of their clinicians, improve patient care, and advance the science of nursing. Clinical information systems (CIS) have traditionally been designed for use by one unit or department within an institution. However, because clinicians working in other areas of the organization need access to this information, these data and information are generally used by more than one area. The new initiatives arising with the development of the electronic health record place institutions in the position of striving to manage their CIS through the electronic health record. Currently, there are many CISs, including nursing, laboratory, pharmacy, monitoring, and order entry, plus additional ancillary systems to meet the individual institutions' needs. Chapter 13 provides an overview of administrative information systems and helps the reader to understand powerful data aggregation and data mining tools afforded by these systems.

Chapter 14, related to improving the human–technology interface, discusses the need to improve quality and safety outcomes significantly in this country. Through the use of IT, the designs for human–technology interfaces can be radically improved so that the technology better fits both human and task requirements. A number of useful tools are currently available for the analysis, design, and evaluation phases of development life cycles and should be used routinely by informatics professionals to ensure that technology better fits both task and user requirements. In this chapter, the author stresses that the focus on interface improvement using these tools has had a huge impact on patient safety in one area of health care: anesthesiology. With increased attention from informatics professionals and engineers, the same kinds of improvements should be possible in other areas. This human–technology interface is a crucial area if the theories, architectures, and tools provided by the building block sciences are to be implemented.

Each organization must determine who can access and use their information systems, and provide robust tools for securing information in a networked environment. It is also imperative that nurses understand copyright and fair use rules as they apply to both written and electronic information. Chapter 15 introduces these important safeguards for protecting information. As new technologies designed to enhance patient care are adopted, barriers to implementation and resistance by practitioners to change are frequently encountered. Chapter 16 provides insights into clinical workflow analysis and provides advice on improving efficiency and effectiveness to achieve meaningful use of caring technologies.

Pause to reflect on the Foundation of Knowledge Model (Figure III-1) and its relationship to both personal and organizational knowledge management. Consider that organizational decision making must be driven by appropriate information and knowledge developed in the organization and applied with wisdom. Equally important to adopting technology within an organization is the consideration of the knowledge base and knowledge capabilities of the individuals within that organization. Administrators must use the system development life cycle wisely, and carefully consider organizational workflow as they adopt NI technology for meaningful use.

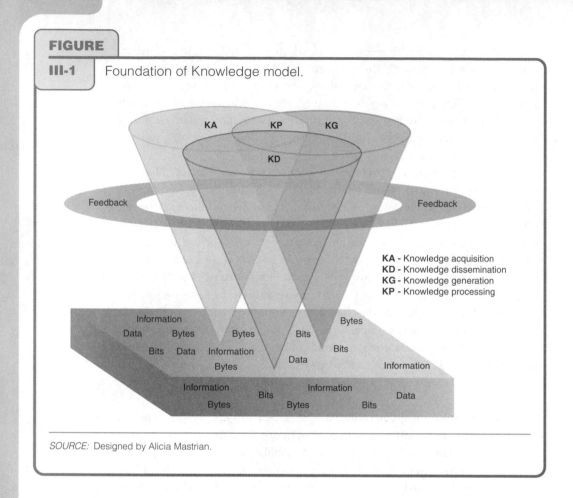

FIGURE III-1 Foundation of Knowledge model.

KA - Knowledge acquisition
KD - Knowledge dissemination
KG - Knowledge generation
KP - Knowledge processing

SOURCE: Designed by Alicia Mastrian.

The reader of this section is challenged to ask the following questions: (1) How can I apply the knowledge gained from my practice setting to benefit my patients and enhance my practice; (2) How can I help my colleagues and patients understand and use the current technology that is available; and (3) How can I use my wisdom to create the theories, tools, and knowledge of the future?

CHAPTER 12

Systems Development Life Cycle: NI and Organizational Decision Making

Dee McGonigle and Kathleen Mastrian

Objectives

1. Describe the system development life cycle (SDLC).
2. Explore select approaches to SDLC.
3. Assess interoperability and its importance in addressing and meeting the challenges of implementing the HITECH Act in health care.
4. Reflect on the past to move forward into the future to determine how new systems will be developed, integrated and interoperable in health care.

www

Key Terms **www**

Chief information officer
Computer-aided software engineering
Dynamic system development method
End-users
Free/open source software
Health management information system
Hospital information system
Information technology
Integration
Interoperability
Iteration
Milestones
MoSCoW
Object-oriented systems development
Open source software
Prototype
Rapid application development
Rapid prototyping
Repository
Systems development life cycle
TELOS strategy
Waterfall model

INTRODUCTION

The following case scenario demonstrates the need to have all of the stakeholders involved from the beginning to the end of the SDLC. Creating the right team to manage the development is a key. Various methodologies have been developed to guide the process. This chapter reviews the following approaches to SDLC: waterfall, **rapid prototyping** or **rapid application development** (RAD), **object-oriented system development** (OOSD), and DSDM. When reading about each approach, think about the case scenario and how important it is to understand the specific situational needs and the various methodologies for bringing a system to life. As in this case, it is generally necessary or beneficial to use a hybrid approach that blends two or more models for a robust development process.

As the case demonstrates, the process of developing systems or SDLC is an ongoing development with a life cycle. The first step in developing a system is to understand the problem or business needs; followed by understanding the solution or how to address those needs; developing a plan; implementing the plan; evaluating the implementation; and finally, maintenance, review, and destruction. If the system needs major upgrading outside of the scope of the maintenance phase, needs to be replaced because of technologic advances, or if the business needs change, a new project is launched, the old system is destroyed, and the life cycle begins anew.

SDLC is a way to deliver efficient and effective information systems that fit with the strategic business plan of an organization. The business plan stems from the mission of the organization. In the world of health care, this includes the needs assessment for the entire organization, which should include outreach linkages (as seen in the case scenario) and partnerships and merged or shared functions. The organization's participating physicians and other ancillary professionals and their offices are included in thorough needs assessments. When developing a strategic plan, the design must take into account the existence of the organization within the larger health care delivery system and also assess those factors outside of the organization itself including technologic, legislative, and environmental issues that impact the organization. The plan must identify the needs of the organization as a whole and solutions to meet the needs or a way to address the issues.

SDLC can occur within an organization, be outsourced, or be a blending of the two. By outsourcing, the team hires an outside organization to carry out all or some of the development. Developing systems that truly meet business needs is not an easy task and is quite complex. Therefore, it is common to run over budget and miss **milestones**. When reading this chapter, reflect on the case scenario and in general the challenges teams face when developing systems.

CASE SCENARIO

Envision two large healthcare facilities that merge resources to better serve their community. This merger is called the Wellness Alliance and its mission is to establish and manage community health programming that addresses the health needs of their rural, underserved populations. They would like to establish pilot clinical sites in five rural areas to promote access and provide health care to these underserved consumers. Each clinical site will have a full-time program manager and three part-time employees (a secretary, a nurse, and a doctor). Each program manager will report to the Wellness Program Coordinator, a newly created position within the Well-ness Alliance.

Because you are a community health nurse with extensive experience, you have been appointed as the Wellness Program Coordinator. Your directive is to establish these clinical sites within 3 months and report back in 6 months as to the following: (1) community health programs offered, (2) level of community involvement in outreach health programs and clinical site-based programming, (3) consumer visits made to the clinical site, and (4) personnel performance.

You are excited and challenged, but soon reality sets in; you know that you have five different sites with five different program managers. Therefore, there must be some way to gather this information from each of them in a similar manner so that it is meaningful and useful to you as you develop your reports and evaluate the strengths and weaknesses of the pilot project. You know that you need a system that will handle all of the pilot project's information needs.

Your first stop is the **chief information officer** of the health system, a nurse informaticist. You know her from the **health management information system** mini seminar that she led. After explaining your needs, you also share with her that this system must be in place in 3 months when the sites are up and running. When she begins to ask questions, you realize that you do not know the answers. All you know is that you must be able to report on what community health programs were offered, track the level of community involvement in outreach health programs and clinical site-based programming, monitor consumer visits made to the clinical site, and monitor the performance of site personnel. You do know that you want accessible, real-time tracking but as far as programming and clinical site-related activities, you do not have a precise description of the process and procedures that will be involved in implementing the pilot nor how they will gather and enter data.

The chief information officer requires that you and each program manager remain involved in the development process. She assigns an **information technology** (IT) analyst to work with you and your team in the development of a system that will meet your current needs. After the first meeting, your head is spinning because the IT analyst has challenged your team not only to work out the process for your immediate needs but also to envision what your needs will be in the future. At the next meeting, you tell the analyst that your team does not feel comfortable trying to map everything out at this point. He states that there are several ways to go about building the system and software by using the systems' developmental life cycle (SDLC). Noticing the blank look on everyone's faces, he explains, SDLC is a series of actions used to develop an information system. The SDLC is similar to the nursing process where the nurse must assess, diagnose, plan, implement, evaluate, and revise. If this does not meet the patient's need or if a new problem arises, the nurse either revises and updates the plan or starts anew. Therefore, you will plan, analyze, design, implement, operate, support, and secure the system. The SDLC is an iterative process, a conceptual model that is used in project management describing the phases involved in building or developing an information system from assessing feasibility or project initiation, design analysis, system specification, programming, testing, implementation, maintenance, and destruction, literally from beginning to end. Once again, he saw puzzled looks and quickly stated that even the destruction of the system is planned, how it will be retired, broken down, and replaced with a new system. Even during upgrades, destruction tactics can be invoked to secure the data and even decide if servers are to be disposed of or repurposed. The security people will tell you that this is their phase, where they make sure that any sensitive information is properly handled whether the data is to be securely and safely archived or destroyed.

After reviewing all of the possible methods and helping you to conduct your feasibility and business study, the analyst chose the **dynamic system development method** (DSDM). This SDLC model was chosen because it works well when the time span is short and the requirements are fluctuating and mainly unknown at the outset. He explains that this model works well on tight schedules and is a highly iterative and incremental approach stressing continuous user input and involvement. As a highly iterative process, this means that the team will revisit and loop through the same development activities numerous times; this repetitive examination provides ever-increasing levels of detail, thus improving accuracy. The analyst explains that you will use a mockup of the **hospital information system** (HIS) and design for what is known and then create your own mini system that will interface with the HIS. Because time is short, the analysis, design, and development phases will occur simultaneously while formulating and revising your specific requirements through the iterative process so that they can be integrated into the system.

The functional model **iteration** phase will be completed in 2 weeks based on what you have given to the analyst. He explains further that, at that time, the **prototype** will be reviewed by the team. He tells you to expect at least two or more iterations of the prototype based on your input. You should end with software that provides some key capabilities. Design and testing will occur in the design and build iteration phase until the system is ready for implementation, the final phase. This DSDM should work well because any previous phase can be revisited and reworked through its iterative process.

One month into the SDLC process, the IT analyst tells the team that he will be leaving his position at Wellness Alliance.   He introduces his replacement. She is new to Wellness Alliance and is eager to work with the team. The initial IT analyst will be there 1 more week to help the new analyst with the transition. When he explains that you are working through DSDM, she looks a bit panicky and states that she has never used that approach. She says that she has used the waterfall, prototyping, iterative enhancement, spiral, and object oriented methodologies but never the DSDM. From what she heard, DSDM is new and often runs amok because of the lack of understanding as to how to implement it appropriately. After 1 week, she believes that this was not the best choice. As the leader of this SDLC, she is growing concerned about having a product ready for when the clinical sites open. She might combine another method to create a hybrid approach with which she would be more comfortable; she is thinking out loud and has everyone very nervous.

She reviews the equipment that has arrived for the sites and is excited that the Mac computers were ordered from Apple. They will be powerful and versatile enough for your needs. Two months after the opening of the clinical sites, you as the wellness program coordinator are still tweaking the system with the help of the IT analyst. It is hard to believe how quickly the team was able to get a robust system in place. As you think back on the process it seems so long ago that you reviewed the HIS for deficiencies and screen shots. You re-examined your requirements and watched them come to life through five prototype iterations and constant security updates. You trained your personnel on its use, tested its performance, and made final adjustments before implementation. Your own standalone system that met your needs was installed and fully operational on the Friday before you opened the clinic doors on Monday, 1 day ahead of schedule. You are continuing to evaluate and modify the system, but that is how the SDLC works: it is never finished, but rather constantly evolving.

WATERFALL MODEL

The **waterfall model** is one of the oldest methods and literally depicts a waterfall effect; the output from each previous phase flows into or becomes the initial input for the next phase. This model is a sequential development process because there is one pass through each component activity from conception or feasibility through implementation in a linear order. The deliverables for each phase result from the inputs and any additional information that is gathered. There is minimal or no iterative development where one takes advantage of what was learned during the development of earlier deliverables. Many projects are broken down into six phases (Figure 12-1), especially small- to medium-size projects.

FIGURE 12-1

Waterfall phases.

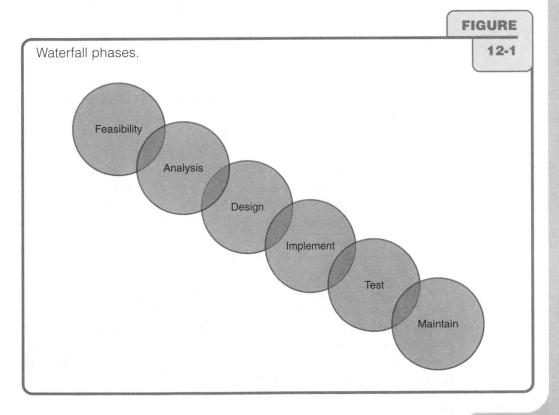

Feasibility

As the term implies, the feasibility study is used to determine if the project should be initiated and supported. This study should generate a project plan and estimated budget for the SDLC phases. Often, the **TELOS strategy** is followed: *t*echnologic and systems, *e*conomic, *l*egal, *o*perational, and *s*chedule feasibility. Technologic and systems feasibility addresses the issues of technologic capabilities including the expertise and infrastructure to complete the project. Economic feasibility is the cost–benefit analysis, weighing the benefits versus the costs to determine if the project is fiscally possible to do and worth undertaking. Formal assessments should include return on investment. Legal feasibility assesses the legal ramifications of the project including current contractual obligations, legislation, regulatory bodies, and liabilities that could affect the project. Operational feasibility determines how effective the project will be in meeting the needs and expectations of the organization and actually achieving the goals of the project or addressing and solving the business problem. Schedule feasibility assesses the viability of the timeframe, making sure it is a reasonable estimation of the time and resources necessary for the project to be developed in time to attain the benefits and meet constraints. TELOS helps to provide a clear picture of the feasibility of the project.

Analysis

During the analysis phase, the requirements for the system are teased out from a detailed study of the business needs of the organization. This is when work flows and business practices are examined. It may be necessary to consider options for changing the business process.

Design

The design phase focuses on high- and low-level design and interface and data design. At the high-level phase, the team establishes what programs are needed and ascertains how they are going to interact. At the low end phase, they explore how the individual programs are actually going to work. The interface design determines what the look and feel will be or what the interfaces will look like. During data design, the team critically thinks about and verifies what data are required or essential.

The analysis and design phases are vital in the development cycle and great care is taken during these phases to ensure that the software's overall configuration is defined properly. Mockups or prototypes of screen shots, reports, and processes may be generated to clarify the requirements and get the team or stakeholders on the same page, limiting the occurrence of glitches resulting in costly software development resolutions later in the project.

Implement

During this phase, the designs are brought to life through programming code. The right programming language, such as C++, Pascal, Java, and so forth, is chosen based on the application requirements.

Test

The testing is generally broken down into five layers: (1) the individual programming modules, (2) **integration**, (3) volume, (4) the system as a whole, and (5) beta testing. Typically, the programs are developed in a modular fashion and these individual modules are subjected to detailed testing. The separate modules are then synthesized and the interfaces between the modules are tested. The system is evaluated with respect to its platform and expected amount or volume of data. The system is then tested as a complete system by the team. Finally, to determine if the system performs appropriately for the user, it is beta tested. During beta testing, users put the new system through its paces to make sure that it does what they need it to do to perform their jobs.

Maintain

Once the system has been finalized from the testing phase, it must be maintained. This could include user support through actual software changes necessitated through use or time.

The waterfall approach is linear and progresses sequentially. The main lack of iterative development is seen as a major weakness according to Purcell (2007). No projects are static and typically changes occur during the SDLC. As requirements change there is no way formally to address them using the waterfall method after project requirements are developed. The waterfall model should be used for simple projects when the requirements are well-known and stable from the outset.

RAPID PROTOTYPING OR RAPID APPLICATION DEVELOPMENT

As technology advances and faster development is expected, RAD provides a fast way to add functionality through prototyping and user testing. It is easier for users to examine actual prototypes rather than documentation. There is a rapid requirements gathering phase using workshops and focus groups to build a prototype application using real data. This is then beta tested with users and their feedback is used to perfect or add functionality and capabilities to the system. According to Alexandrou (2010), "RAD (rapid application development) proposes that products can be developed faster and of higher quality" (para. 1). The RAD approach uses informal communication, repurposes components, and typically follows a fast-paced schedule. Object-oriented programming using such languages as C++ and Java promotes software repurposing and reuse.

The major advantage is the speed with which the system can be deployed; a working, usable system can be built within 3 months. The use of prototyping allows the developers to skip steps in the SDLC process in favor of getting a mockup in front of the user. At times, the system is deemed acceptable if it meets a predefined minimum set of requirements rather than all of the identified requirements. This rapid deployment also limits the project's exposure to change elements. The fast pace can also be its biggest disadvantage. Once one is locked into a tight development schedule, the process may be too fast for adequate testing to be in place and completed. The most dangerous lack of testing is in the realm of security.

The RAD approach is chosen because it builds systems quickly through user-driven prototyping and adherence to quick, strict delivery milestones. This approach continues to be refined and honed and other contemporary manifestations of RAD continue to emerge in the agile software development realm.

OBJECT-ORIENTED SYSTEMS DEVELOPMENT

The OOSD model "combines the logic of the **systems development life cycle** with the power of object-oriented modeling and programming" (Stair & Reynolds, 2008, p. 501). Object-oriented modeling makes an effort to represent real world objects; modeling the real world entities or things (e.g., hospital, patient, account, nurse) into abstract computer software objects. Once the system is object oriented, all of the interactions or exchanges take place between or among the objects. The objects are derived from classes and "an object consists of both data and the actions that can be performed on the data" (Stair & Reynolds, p. 501). Class hierarchy allows objects to inherit characteristics or attributes from parent classes and this fosters object reuse resulting in less coding. The object-oriented programming languages, such as C++ and Java, promote software repurposing and reuse. Therefore, the class hierarchy must be clearly and appropriately designed to reap the benefits of this SDLC approach, which uses object-oriented programming to support the interactions of objects.

For example, in the case scenario, a system could be developed for the Wellness Alliance to manage the community health programming for the clinic system being set up for outreach. There could be a class of programs and well-baby care could be an object in the class of programs; programs is a relationship between Wellness Alliance and well-baby care. The program class has attributes, such as clinic site, location address, or attendees or patients. The relationship itself may be considered an object having attributes, such as pediatric programs. The class hierarchy from which all of the system objects are created with resultant object interactions must be clearly defined.

The OOSD model is a highly iterative approach. The process begins by investigating where object-oriented solutions can address business problems or needs, determining user requirements, designing the system, programming or modifying object modeling (class hierarchy and objects), implementing, user testing, modifying, and implementing the system, and ends with the new system being reviewed regularly at established intervals and modifications being made as needed throughout its life.

DYNAMIC SYSTEM DEVELOPMENT METHOD

DSDM is a highly iterative and incremental approach with a high level of user input and involvement. The iterative process requires repetitive examination that enhances detail and improves accuracy. The DSDM has three phases: (1) preproject; (2) project life cycle (feasibility and business studies, functional model iteration, design and build iteration, and implementation); and (3) postproject.

In the preproject phase, buy-in or commitment is established and funding is secured. This helps to identify the stakeholders (administration and **end-users**) and gain support for the project.

In the project life cycle phase, the project's life cycle begins. There are five steps during this phase: (1) feasibility, (2) business studies, (3) functional model iteration, (4) design and build iteration, and (5) implementation.

In steps one and two, the feasibility and business studies are completed. The team ascertains if this project meets the required business needs while identifying the potential risks during the feasibility study. In step one, the deliverables are a feasibility report, project plan, and a risk log. Once the project is deemed feasible step two, the business study, is begun. The business study extends the feasibility report by examining the processes, stakeholders, and their needs. It is important to align the stakeholders with the project and secure their buy-in because it is necessary to have user input and involvement throughout the entire DSDM process. Therefore, bringing them in at the beginning of the project is imperative.

Using the **MoSCoW** approach, the team works with the stakeholders to develop a prioritized requirements list and a development plan. The MoSCoW approach stands for *M*ust have, *S*hould have, *C*ould have, and *W*ould have. The "must have" requirements are needed to meet the business needs and are critical to the success of the project. "Should have" requirements are those that would be great to have if possible, but the success of the project does not depend on them being addressed. The "could have" requirements are those that would be nice to have met, and the "would have" are those requirements that can be put off until later; these may be undertaken during future developmental iterations. Timeboxing is generally used to develop the project plan. In timeboxing, the project is divided into sections with each having its own fixed budget and dates or milestones for deliverables. The MoSCoW approach is then used to prioritize the requirements within each section; the requirements are the only variables because the schedule and budget are set. If a project is running out of time or money, the team can easily omit the requirements that have been identified as the lowest priority to meet their schedule and budget obligations. This does not mean that the final deliverable, the actual system, would be flawed or incomplete. Instead, it meets the business needs. According to Haughey (2010), the 80/20 rule or Pareto principle can be applied to nearly everything. Using the Pareto principle, 80% of the project comes from 20% of the system requirements; therefore, the 20% of requirements must be the crucial requirements or those with the highest priority. One also must consider the pancake principle: the first pancake is not as good as the rest, and one should know that the first development is not going to be perfect. This is why it is extremely important to clearly identify the "must have" and "should have" requirements.

In the third step, functional model iteration, the deliverables are a functional model and prototype ready for user testing. Once the requirements are identified the next step is to translate them into a functional model with a functioning prototype that can be evaluated by users. This could take several iterations to develop the wanted functionality and incorporate the users' input. At this stage, the team should examine the quality of the product and revise the list requirements and risk log. The requirements are adjusted, the ones that have been realized are deleted, and the remaining requirements are prioritized. The risk log is revised based on the risk analysis completed during and after prototype development.

The design and build iteration step focuses on integrating functional components and identifying the nonfunctional requirements that need to be in the tested system. Testing is crucial; the team will develop a system that the end-users can safely use on a daily basis. The team will garner user feedback and generate user documentation. These efforts provide this step's deliverable, a tested system with documentation for the next and final phase of the development process.

In the final step, implementation, deliverables are the system (ready to use), documentation, and trained users. The requirements list should be satisfied along with the users' needs. Training users and implementing the approved system is the first part of this phase, and the final part consists of a full review. It is important to review the impact of the system on the business processes and determine if it addressed the goals or requirements established at the beginning of the project. This final review determines if the project is completed or if further development is necessary. If further development is needed, preceding phases are revisited. If it is complete and satisfies the users, then it moves into postproject (maintenance and ongoing development).

The final phase is labeled "postproject." The team verifies that the system is functioning properly. Once verified, the maintenance schedule is begun. Because the DSDM is iterative, this postproject phase is seen as ongoing development and any of the deliverables can be refined. This is what makes the DSDM such an iterative development process.

DSDM is one of an increasing number of agile methodologies, such as Scrum and Extreme Programming. These new approaches address the organizational, managerial, and interpersonal communication issues that bog down SDLC projects. Empowering teams and user involvement enhance the iterative and programming strengths provided in these SDLC models.

COMPUTER-AIDED SOFTWARE ENGINEERING TOOLS

When reviewing SDLC, the **computer-aided software engineering** (CASE) tools must be described. The "CASE tools automate many of the tasks required in a systems development effort and encourage adherence to the SDLC, thus instilling a high degree of rigor and standardization to the entire systems development process" (Stair & Reynolds, 2008, p. 500). These tools help to reduce cost and development time while enriching the quality of the product. The CASE tools contain a **repository** with information about the system: models, data definitions, and references linking models together. They are valuable in their ability to make sure the models follow diagramming rules and are consistent and complete. They can be referred to as upper CASE tools or lower CASE tools. The upper CASE tools support the analysis and design phases, whereas the lower CASE tools support implementation. The tools can also be general or specific in nature with the specific tools being designed for a particular methodology. Two examples of CASE tools are Visible Analyst and Rational Rose. According to Andoh-Baidoo, Kunene, and Walker (n.d.), Visible Analyst "supports structured and object-oriented design (UML)," whereas Rational Rose "supports solely object-oriented design (UML)" (p. 372). They can both "build and reverse database schemas for SQL and Oracle" and "support code generation for pre.NET versions of Visual Basic" (p. 372). Visible Analyst can also support shell code generation for pre.NET versions of C and COBOL, whereas Rational Rose can support complete code for C++ and Java. In addition, Andoh-Baidoo et al. found that Rational Rose "Provides good integration with Java, and incorporates common packages into class diagrams and decompositions through classes" (p. 372). The CASE tools have many advantages including decreasing development time and producing more flexible systems. On the down side, they can be difficult to tailor or customize and use with existing systems.

OPEN SOURCE SOFTWARE AND FREE/OPEN SOURCE SOFTWARE

Another area that must be discussed with SDLC is **open source software** (OSS). An examination of job descriptions or advertisements for candidates shows that many IS and IT professionals need a thorough understanding of SDLC and OSS development tools (e.g., PHP, MySQL, and HTML). This is because, with OSS, any programmer can implement, modify, apply, reconstruct, and restructure the rich libraries of source codes available from proven, well-tested products. Vauldes (2008) offers "Examples of FOSS successes are the Internet, Google, Web 2.0, the GNU/Linux operating system, courseware such as Moodle, and the Veterans Affairs VistA hospital system" (p. 7).

To transform health care it is necessary for clinicians to use information systems that can share patient data (Goulde & Brown, 2006). This all sounds terrific and many people wonder why it has not as yet happened, but the challenges are many. How does one establish the networks necessary to share data between and among all healthcare facilities easily and securely? "Healthcare IT is beginning to adopt open source software to address these challenges" (Goulde & Brown, p. 4). Early attempts at OSS ventures in the healthcare realm failed because of a lack of support or buy-in for sustained effort, technologic lags, authority and credibility, and other such issues. "Spurred by a greater sense of urgency to adopt IT, health industry leaders are showing renewed interest in open source solutions" (Goulde & Brown, p. 5). Health care is realizing the benefits of OSS. Goulde and Brown stated that "other benefits of open source software—low cost, flexibility, opportunities to innovate—are important but independence from vendors is the most relevant for health care" (p. 10).

INTEROPERABILITY

Interoperability, the ability to share information across organizations, will remain paramount under the HITECH Act (see Chapter 10). The ability to share patient data is extremely important, both within an organization and across organizational boundaries. According to HIMSS (2010), few healthcare systems take advantage of the full potential of the current state of the art in computer science and health informatics. The consequences of this situation include a drain on financial resources from the economy, the inability to truly mitigate the occurrence of medical errors, and a lack of national preparedness to respond to natural and man-made epidemics and disasters. HIMSS has created the Integration and Interoperability Steering Committee to guide the industry on allocating resources to develop and implement standards and technology needed to achieve interoperability (para. 2).

As we enter into SDLCs, we must be aware of the impact on our own healthcare organization and the impact on the healthcare delivery system as a whole. In an ideal world, we would all work together to create systems that are integrated within our own organization while having the interoperability to cross organizational boundaries and unite the healthcare delivery system to realize the common goal of improving the quality of care provided to consumers.

SUMMARY

At times during the SDLC, new information affects the outputs from earlier phases and the development effort may be re-examined or halted until these modifications can be reconciled with the current design and scope of the project. There are times that teams are overwhelmed with new ideas from the iterative SDLC process that result in new capabilities or features that exceed the initial scope of the project. Astute team leaders preserve these ideas or initiatives so they can be considered at a later time. The team should develop a list of recommendations to improve the current software when the project is complete. This iterative and dynamic exchange makes the SDLC robust.

As technology and research continue to advance, new SDLC models are pioneered and introduced to enhance techniques. The interpretation and implementation of any model selected reflects the knowledge and skill of the team applying the model. The success of the project is often directly related to the quality of the organizational decision making throughout the project; how well the plan was followed and documented. United efforts to create systems that are integrated and interoperable will define the future of health care.

THOUGHT-PROVOKING Questions

www

1. How would you describe cognitive informatics? Reflect on a plan of care that you have developed for a patient. How could cognitive informatics be used to create tools to help with this important work?

2. Think of a clinical setting you are familiar with and envision artificial intelligence tools. Are there any current tools in use? What tools would enhance practice in this setting and why?

3. Reflect on the SDLC in relation to the quality of the organizational decision making throughout the project. What are some of the major stumbling blocks faced by healthcare organizations?

For a full suite of assignments and additional learning activities, use the access code located in the front of your book to visit this exclusive website: **http://go.jblearning.com/mcgonigle**. If you do not have an access code, you can obtain one at the site.

References

Alexandrou, M. (2010). *Rapid application development (RAD) methodology.* Retrieved from http://www .mariosalexandrou.com/methodologies/rapid-application-development.asp

Andoh-Baidoo, F., Kunene, K., & Walker, R. (n.d.). *An evaluation of CASE tools as pedagogical aids in software development courses.* Retrieved from http://www.swdsi.org/swdsi 2009/Papers/9K10.pdf

Brown, P. (2010). *Free software is a matter of liberty, not price.* Retrieved from http://www.fsf.org/ about/

Goulde, M., & Brown, E. (2006). *Open source software: A primer for health care leaders.* Retrieved from http://www.chcf.org/~/media/Files/PDF/O/OpenSourcePrimer.pdf

Haughey, D. (2010). *Pareto analysis step by step.* Retrieved from http://www.projectsmart.co .uk/pareto -analysis-step-by-step.html

HIMSS. (2010). *Integration and interoperability.* Retrieved from http://www.himss.org/ASP/topics_ integration.asp

Lee, M. (2009). *FSF announces new executive director.* Retrieved from http://www.fsf.org/news/new-executive-director.html

Purcell, J. (2007). *Comparison of software development lifecycle methodologies.* Retrieved from http:// www2.giac.org/resources/whitepaper/application/217.pdf

Stair, R., & Reynolds, G. (2008). *Principles of information systems* (8th ed.). Boston, MA: Thomson Course Technology.

Vauldes, I. (2008). *Free and open source software in healthcare 1.0: American Medical Informatics Association. Open Source Working Group White Paper.* Retrieved from Https://Www.Amia.Org/ Files/Final-Os-Wg%20white%20paper_11_19_08.Pdf

CHAPTER 13

Administrative Information Systems

Original contribution by Marianela Zytkowski and Susan Paschke, updated for the Second Edition by Dee McGonigle and Kathleen Mastrian

1. Explore agency-based health information systems.
2. Evaluate how administrators use core business systems in their practice.
3. Assess the function and information output from selected information systems used in healthcare organizations.

WWW

Key Terms

WWW

Acuity system
Admission, discharge, and
    transfer system
American National Standards
    Institute (ANSI)
Attribute
Care plan
Case management
    information system
Clinical documentation
    system
Clinical information system
Collaboration
Column
Communication system
Computerized physician
    order entry system
Core business system
Data dictionary
Data file
Data mart
Data mining
Data warehouse
Database
Database management
    system
Decision support

Continues

INTRODUCTION

To compete in the ever-changing healthcare arena, organizations require quick and immediate access to a variety of types of information, data, and bodies of knowledge for daily clinical, operational, financial, and human resource activities. Information is continuously shared between units and departments within healthcare organizations and is also required or requested from other healthcare organizations, regulatory and government agencies, educational and philanthropic institutions, and consumers.

Healthcare organizations integrate a variety of clinical and administrative types of **information systems**. These systems collect, process, and distribute patient-centered data to aid in managing and providing care. Together they create a comprehensive **record** of the patient's medical history and support organizational processes. Each of these systems is unique in the way it functions and provides information to clinicians and administrators. An understanding of how each of these types of systems works within healthcare organizations is fundamental in the study of informatics.

TYPES OF HEALTHCARE ORGANIZATION INFORMATION SYSTEMS

Case Management Information Systems

Case management information systems identify resources, patterns, and variances in care to prevent costly complications related to chronic conditions and to enhance the overall outcomes for patients with chronic illness. These systems span past episodes of treatment and search for trends among the records. Once a trend is identified, case management systems provide **decision support** promoting preventive care. **Care plans** are a common tool found in case management systems. A care plan is a set of care guidelines that outline the course of treatment and the recommended interventions that should be implemented to achieve optimal results. By using a **standardized plan of care**, these systems present clinicians with treatment protocols to maximize patient outcomes and support best practices. Case management information systems are especially beneficial for patient populations with a high cost of care and complex health needs, such as the elderly or patients with chronic disease conditions. One example of case management systems at work is in treating patients with AIDS. The case management system applies a care plan to treat the patient to manage care better from outpatient to inpatient visits where opportunistic infections, such as *Pneumocystis carinii* pneumonia, are common complications (DiJerome, 1992). Avoiding these types of complications requires identifying the right resources for care and implementing preventive treatments across all medical visits. Ultimately, this preventive care decreases the costs of care for these patients and supports a better quality of life. These systems increase the value of individual care while controlling the costs and risks associated with long-term health care. Case management systems assimilate massive amounts of information obtained over a patient's lifetime by reaching far beyond the walls of the hospital and track care from one medical visit to the next (Simpson & Falk, 1996). Information collected by case management systems is processed in a way that helps to reduce risks, ensure quality, and decrease costs.

Communication Systems

Communication systems promote interaction among healthcare providers and between providers and patients. Communication systems have historically been separate from other types of health information systems and from one another. Health-care professionals overwhelmingly recognize the value of these systems so they are now more commonly integrated into the design of other types of systems as a newly developing standard within the industry. Examples of communication systems include call light systems, wireless telephones, pagers, e-mail, and instant messaging, which have traditionally been forms of communication targeted at clinicians. However, communication systems are more frequently beginning to target patients and their families. Some patients are now able to access their electronic chart from home via Internet connections. They can update their own medical record to inform their physician of changes to their health or personal practices that impact their physical condition. Inpatients in hospital settings also receive communication directly to their room. Patients and their families review individualized messages with scheduled tests and procedures for the day and confirmation of menu choices for their meals. These types of systems may also communicate educational messages, such as smoking cessation advice.

As health care begins to introduce more of this technology into practice, the value of having communication tools integrated with other types of systems is recognized. Integrating communication systems with clinical applications provides a real-time approach that facilitates care among the entire healthcare team, patients, and their families. These systems enhance the flow of communication within an organization and promote an exchange of information to care better for patients. The next generation of communication systems will be integrated with other types of healthcare systems and are guaranteed to integrate with one another. The Research Brief discusses the economic impact of communication inefficiencies in United States hospitals.

Research Brief

Researchers attempted to quantify the costs of poor communication, termed "communication inefficiencies," in hospitals. This qualitative study was conducted in seven acute-care hospitals of varying sizes via structured interviews with key informants at each facility. The interview questions focused on four broad categories: (1) communication bottlenecks, (2) negative outcomes as a result of bottlenecks, (3) subjective perceptions of the potential effectiveness of communication improvements on the negative outcomes, and (4) ideas for specific communication improvements. The researchers independently coded the interview data and then compared results to extract themes. All of the interviewees indicated that communication was an issue. Inefficiencies revolved around time spent tracking people down to communicate with them, with various estimates provided: 3 hours per nursing shift wasted tracking people down, 20% of productive time wasted on communication bottlenecks, and a reported average of five to six telephone calls to locate a physician. Several pointed to costly medical errors that were the direct result of communication issues. Communication lapses also result in inefficient use of clinician resources and increases in patient length of stay.

The researchers developed a conceptual model of communication quality with four primary dimensions: (1) efficiency of resource use, (2) effectiveness of resource use, (3) quality of work life, and (4) service quality. They conclude that the total cost of communication inefficiencies in United States hospitals is over $12 billion annually and estimate that a 500-bed hospital could lose up to $4 million annually. They urge the adoption of information technologies to redesign work-flow processes and promote better communication.

SOURCE: Agarwal, R., Sands, D., Schneider, J., & Smaltz, D. (2010). Quantifying the economic impact of communication inefficiencies in U.S. hospitals. *Journal of Healthcare Management, 55*(4), 265–281.

Core Business Systems

Core business systems enhance administrative tasks within healthcare organizations. Unlike **clinical information systems** (CISs), whose aim is to provide direct patient care, these systems support the management of health care within an organization. Core business systems provide the framework for reimbursement, support of best practices, quality control, and resource allocation. There are four common core business systems: (1) **admission, discharge, and transfer (ADT) systems**; (2) financial systems; (3) acuity systems; and (4) scheduling systems.

ADT systems provide the backbone structure for the other types of clinical and business systems (Hassett & Thede, 2003). Admitting, billing, and bed management departments most commonly use ADT systems. These systems contain key information on which all other systems interface. A few examples of information that ADT systems provide include the patient name; medical record number; visit or account number; and demographic information, such as age, gender, home address, and contact information. ADT systems are considered the central source for collecting this type of patient information and communicating it to other types of healthcare information systems.

Financial systems manage the expenses and revenue for providing health care. The finance, auditing, and accounting departments within an organization most commonly use financial systems. These systems determine the direction for maintenance and growth for a given facility. Financial systems often interface to share information with materials management, staffing, and billing systems to balance the financial impact of these resources within an organization. These systems report fiscal outcomes to track them against the organizational goals of an institution. Financial systems are one of the major decision-making factors as healthcare institutions prepare their fiscal budgets. These systems often play a pivotal role in determining the strategic direction for an organization.

Acuity systems monitor the range of patient types within a healthcare organization using specific indicators. Acuity systems track these indicators based on the current patient population within a facility. By monitoring the patient acuity, these systems provide feedback about how intensive the care requirement is for an individual patient or group of patients. Identifying and classifying a patient's acuity can promote better organizational management of expenses and resources necessary to provide care. Acuity systems help to predict the ability and capacity of an organization to care for its current population. These types of systems also forecast future trends to allow an organization to successfully strategize on how to meet upcoming market demands.

Scheduling systems coordinate staff, services, equipment, and allocation of patient beds. These systems frequently integrate with the other types of core business systems. By closely monitoring staff and physical resources, these systems provide data to the financial systems. For example, resource-scheduling systems provide information about operating room use or availability of intensive care unit beds and regular nursing unit beds. These systems also serve as a great asset to the financial systems when they are used to track medical equipment within a facility. Procedures and care are planned when the tools and resources are available. Scheduling systems help to track resources within a facility while managing the frequency and distribution of those resources.

Order Entry Systems

Order entry systems are one of the most important systems in use today. These systems automate the way that orders have traditionally been initiated for patients. Clinicians place orders within these systems instead of placing them with traditional handwritten transcription onto paper. Order entry systems provide major safeguards by ensuring that physician orders are legible and complete, thereby providing a level of patient safety that was historically missing with paper-based orders. **Computerized physician order entry systems** provide decision support and automated alert functionality that was unavailable with paper-based orders. The Institute of Medicine estimates that medical errors cost the nation approximately $37.6 billion each year; about $17 billion of those costs are associated with preventable errors. In addition, this report recommends eliminating reliance on handwriting for ordering medications and other treatment needs (Agency for Healthcare Research and Quality, 2000). Because of this global concern for patient safety as a result of incorrect and misinterpreted orders, healthcare organizations are incorporating these types of systems as a standard tool for practice. Order entry systems allow for clear and legible orders promoting patient safety and streamlining care. Although much of the health **information technology** literature suggests that physicians are resistant to adopting health information technology, a recent study by Elder, Wiltshire, Rooks, BeLue, and Gary (2010) found that physicians who use information technology were more satisfied overall with their careers. Chapter 22 provides more information about the use of computerized physician order entry systems in clinical care.

Patient Care Support Systems

Most specialty disciplines within health care have an associated **patient care information system**. These patient-centered systems focus on collecting data and disseminating information related to direct care. Several of these systems have become mainstream types of systems used in health care. The four systems most commonly found include (1) **clinical documentation systems**, (2) **pharmacy information systems**, (3) **laboratory information systems**, and (4) **radiology information systems** (RIS).

Clinical documentation systems, also known as "clinical information systems," are the most commonly used type of **patient care support system** within healthcare organizations. CISs are designed to collect patient data in real time. They enhance care by providing data at the clinician's fingertips and enabling decision making where it needs to occur, at the bedside. For that reason, these systems often are easily accessible at the point of care for caregivers interacting with the patient. CIS systems are **patient centered**, meaning they contain the observations, interventions, and outcomes noted by the care team. Team members enter information, such as the plan of care, hemodynamic data, laboratory results, clinical notes, allergies, and medications. All members of the treatment team use clinical documentation systems; pharmacists, allied health workers, nurses, physicians, support staff, and many others access the clinical record for the patient using these systems. Frequently these types of systems are also referred to as the "electronic patient record" or the "**electronic health record**." Chapter 17 provides a comprehensive overview of CISs and the electronic health record.

Pharmacy information systems also have become a mainstream patient care support system. These systems typically allow pharmacists to order, manage, and dispense medications for a facility. They also commonly incorporate information regarding allergies and height and weight for effective medication management. Pharmacy information systems streamline the order entry, dispensing, verification, and authorization process for medication administration. These systems often interface with clinical documentation and order entry systems so that clinicians can order and document the administration of medications and prescriptions to patients while having the benefits of decision support alerting and interaction checking.

Laboratory information systems were perhaps some of the first systems ever used in health care. Because of this strong history within medicine, laboratory systems have been models for the design and implementation of other types of patient care support systems. Laboratory information systems report on blood, body fluid, and tissue samples along with biologic specimens collected at the bedside and received in a central laboratory. These systems provide clinicians with reference ranges for tests indicating high, low, or normal values to make care decisions. Often, the laboratory system provides result information directing clinicians toward the next course of action within a treatment regime.

The final type of patient care support system commonly found within health care is the RIS in radiology departments. These systems schedule, result, and store information as it relates to diagnostic radiology procedures. One common feature found in most radiology systems is a **picture archiving and communication system** (PACS). These systems may also be stand-alone systems, separate from the main radiology system, or they can be integrated with RIS and CIS. These systems collect, store, and distribute medical images, such as computed tomography scans, magnetic resonance imaging, and X-rays. PACS replace traditional hard copy films with digital media that is easy to store, retrieve, and present to clinicians. The benefit of RIS and PACS is their ability to assist in diagnosing and storing vital patient care support data. Beird (2000) identified the main benefits of PACS as streamlined workflow, enhanced productivity, and better patient care. Imaging studies can be available in minutes as opposed to 2–6 hours for images in a film-based system. The digital workstations provide enhanced imaging capabilities and on-screen measuring tools to improve diagnostic accuracy. Finally, the archive system stores images in a **database** that is readily accessible and can be easily retrieved and compared to subsequent testing or shared instantly with consultants.

The mobility of patients geographically and within one healthcare delivery system challenges information systems because data must be captured wherever and whenever the patient receives care. In the past, **managed care information systems** began to address these issues. Ciotti and Zodda (1996) stated that the managed care information systems "can nimbly cross organizational boundaries, includes an enterprise-wide **master patient index** (MPI), and offers access across provider, geographic, and departmental lines" (para. 10). This means that data can be obtained at any and all of the patient areas. Patient tracking mechanisms continue to be honed while the financial impact of health care also has been changing systems. Information systems currently in use make it possible for nurses and physicians to make clinical decisions while being mindful of their financial ramifications. There will continue to be vast improvements in information systems and systems that support health information exchange.

Many organizations are aggregating data in a **data warehouse** (DW) for the purpose of mining the data to discover new relationships and to build organizational knowledge. Mekhjian, Vasila, and Jones (2008) provide insights into how their healthcare system integrated data from 30 different silos containing physician information into a single comprehensive database. None of the disparate information systems was able to communicate with any of the others resulting in poor communications, billing errors, and issues with continuity of care. By developing a single comprehensive database, they were able to facilitate communications among physicians, particularly consulting physicians from outside the system, and maintain compliance with privacy regulations.

The most basic element of a database system is the data. Data refers to raw facts that can consist of unorganized text, graphics, sound, or video. Information is data that has been processed—it has meaning; information is organized in a way that people find meaningful and useful. Even useful information can be lost if one is mired in unorganized information. Computers can come to the rescue by helping to create order out of chaos. Computer science and information science are designed to help cut down the amount of information to a more manageable size and organize it so that one can cope with it more efficiently through the use of databases and database programs technology. Learning about basic databases and database management programs is paramount so that one can apply data and information management principles in health care.

Databases are structured or organized collections of data that are typically the main component of an information system. Databases and database management software allow the user to input, sort, arrange structure, organize, and store data and turn it into useful information. One can set up a personal database to organize recipes, music, names and addresses, notes, bills, and other data. In health care, the databases and information systems make key information available to healthcare providers and ancillary personnel to promote the provision of quality patient care. Box 13-1 provides a detailed description of a database.

BOX 13-1

Overview of Database Construction

Databases are comprised of **fields** or **columns** and records or **rows**. Within each record, one of the fields is identified as the **primary key** or **key field**. This primary key contains a code, name, number, or other information that acts as a unique identifier for that record. In your healthcare system, for example, your patient is assigned a patient number or ID that is unique for that patient. As you compile related records, you create **data files** or **tables**. A data file is a collection of related records. Therefore, databases consist of one or more related data files or tables.

The term "**entity**" represents a table and each field within the table becomes an attribute of that entity. The database developer must critically think about the attributes for each specific entity. For example, the entity "disease" might have the attributes of chronic disease, acute disease, or communicable disease. The name of the entity, disease, implies that the entity is about diseases. The fields or attributes are chronic, acute, or communicable. The **entity relationship diagram** specifies the relationship among the entities in the database. Sometimes the implied relationships are apparent based on the entities' definitions; however, all relationships should be specified as to how they relate to one another. There are typically three relationships: (1) one to one, (2) one to many, and (3) many to many. A one-to-one relationship exists between the entities of the table about a patient and the table about the patient's birth. The one-to-many relationship could exist when one entity is repeatedly used by another entity. The one-to-many relationship could then be a table query for age that could be used numerous times for one patient entity. The many-to-many relationship reflects entities that are all used repeatedly by other entities. This is easily explained by the entities of patient and nurse. The patient could have several nurses caring for them and the nurse could have many patients assigned to him or her (see Figure 13-1). When describing and discussing databases, depending on the context, the terms "entity" and "attribute" or "table" and "field" are used.

The relational model is a database model that describes data in which all data elements are placed in relation in two-dimensional tables; the relations or tables are analogous to files. A **relational database management system** (RDMS) is a system that

Continues

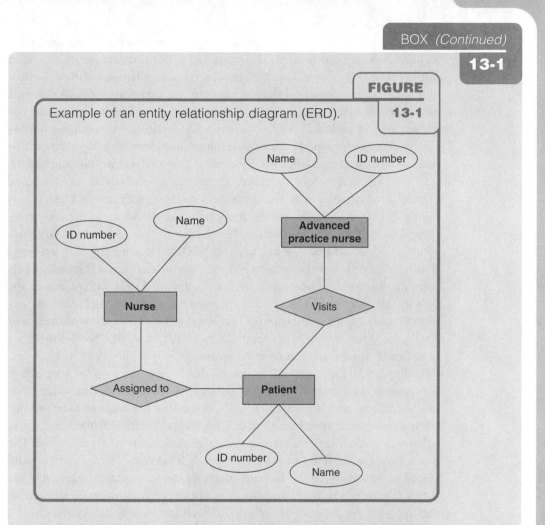

FIGURE
13-1

Example of an entity relationship diagram (ERD).

manages data using the relational model. A relational database could link a patient's table to a treatment table (e.g., by a common field, such as the patient ID number). To keep track of the tables that comprise a database, the **database management system** uses software called a "**data dictionary**." The data dictionary contains a listing of the tables and their details including field names, validation settings, and data types. The data type refers to the type of information, such as a name, a date, or a time. The database management system is an important program because before it was available, many health systems and businesses had dozens of database files with incompatible formats. Because patient data come from a variety of sources, these separated, isolated data files required duplicate entry of the same information, thereby increasing the risk of data entry error. The design of the relational databases eliminates data duplication. Some examples of popular database management system software include Microsoft's Access or Visual FoxPro, Corel's Paradox, Oracle's Oracle Database 10g, and IBM's DB2.

On a large scale, a DW is an extremely large database or **repository** that stores all of an organization's or institution's data and makes this data available for **data mining**. The DW can combine an institution's many different databases to provide management personnel flexible access to the data. On the smaller scale, a **data mart** represents a large database where the data used by one of the units or a division of a healthcare system is stored and maintained. For example, a university hospital system might store clinical information from its many affiliate hospitals in a DW, and each separate hospital might have a data mart housing its data.

There are many ways to access and retrieve information in databases. Searching information in databases can be done through the use of a **query**, as is used in Microsoft's Access database. A query asks questions of the database to retrieve specific data and information. Please refer to Box 13-2 for a detailed description of **Structured Query Language** (SQL). Data mining software sorts thorough data to discover patterns and ascertain or establish relationships. This software discovers or uncovers previously unidentified relationships among the data in a database by conducting an exploratory analysis looking for hidden patterns in data. Using this software, the user searches for previously undiscovered or undiagnosed patterns by analyzing the data stored in a DW. "**Drill-down**" is a term that means the user can view DW information by drilling down to lower levels of the database to focus on information that is pertinent to his or her needs at the moment. As users move through databases within the healthcare system, they can move from enterprise-wide DWs to data marts. For example, an infection-control nurse might notice a pattern of methicillin-resistant *Staphylococcus aureus* infections in the local data mart (a single hospital within a larger system). The nurse may want to find out if the outbreak is local (data mart) or more widespread in the system (DW). The nurse might also query the database to determine if there are certain patient **attributes** (e.g., age or medical diagnosis) that are associated with the incidence of infection. These data mining capabilities are also quite useful for those who wish to conduct clinical research studies. For example, one might query a database to tease out attributes (patient characteristics) associated with asthma-related hospitalizations.

There are five typical clinical applications for databases: (1) hospitals, (2) clinical research, (3) clinical trials, (4) ambulatory care, and (5) public health. Some healthcare systems are connecting their hospitals together because they have chosen a single CIS to capture data system wide. In this case, healthcare organizations are modeling businesses where multiple application programs share a pool of related data. Think about how potent databases can be in managing organizations and providing insights into new relationships that may ultimately transform the way work is done.

BOX

13-2

SQL

SQL was originally called SEQUEL or Structured English Query Language. SQL, still pronounced "sequel," stands for Structured Query Language, a database querying language, not a programming language. It is a standard language for accessing and manipulating databases. SQL is "used with relational databases, it allows users to define the structure and organization of stored data, verify and maintain data integrity, control access to the data, and define relationships among the stored data items" (U.C. San Diego, 2010, para. 8). Therefore, it simplifies the process of retrieving information from a database in a functional or usable form while facilitating the reorganization of data within the databases.

The Relational Database Management System (RDMS) is the foundation or basis for SQL. A RDMS stores data in "database objects called tables" (W3Schools.com, 2010, para. 6). A table is a collection of related data that consists of columns and rows; columns are also referred to as fields and rows are also referred to as records or **tuples**. Databases can have many tables and each table is identified by a name (see the Database Example: School of Nursing Faculty).

SQL statements handle most of the actions users need to perform on a database. SQL is an ISO (**International Organization for Standardization**) standard and ANSI (**American National Standards Institute**) standard but many different versions of the SQL language exist (Indiana University, 2010). To remain compliant with the ISO and ANSI standards, SQL must handle or support the major commands of SELECT, UPDATE, DELETE, INSERT and WHERE in a similar manner (W3Schools.com, 2010). The SELECT command allows you to extract data from a database. UPDATE would update the data, DELETE would delete the data and INSERT would insert new data. WHERE is used to specify selection criteria, thereby restricting the results of the SQL query. Thus, SQL allows you to create databases and manipulate them by storing, retrieving, updating, and deleting data.

The database example below reflects the faculty listing for a School of Nursing. The table that contains the data is identified by the name Faculty. The faculty members are each categorized by the following fields (columns): Last Name, First Name, Department Affiliation, Office Phone Number, Office Location, and UserID. Each individual faculty member's information is a record (tuple or row).

Database Example: School of Nursing Faculty

Table named "Faculty"

Continues

BOX *(Continued)*

13-2

P_ID	Last Name	First Name	Department Affiliation	Office Phone Number	Office Location	UserID
1	Eggleers	Renee	Informatics	444-111-1104	104A	Eggleersr100
2	Feistyz	Judi	Gerontology	444-111-2202	202B	Feistyzj562
3	Martinez	Bethann	Neurology	444-111-3336	336C	Martinezb789
4	Smythe	Ralph	Informatics	444-111-1110	110 A	Smyther355

Using the following SQL command, SELECT, all of the records in the "Faculty" table would be selected.

SELECT * FROM Faculty

This command would SELECT all (*) of the records FROM the table known as FACULTY. The asterisk (*) is used to select all of the columns.

Lee (2009) states that "Developers face a new set of challenges and opportunities managing data for cloud computing" (para. 1). Data mining in the clouds is emerging and evolving. This new frontier is becoming a potent way to extract the power of cloud computing and combine it with SQL. The world as we know it is changing since clouds are leading us to develop revolutionary data mining technologies.

DEPARTMENT COLLABORATION AND EXCHANGE OF KNOWLEDGE AND INFORMATION

The implementation of systems within health care is the responsibility of many people and departments. All systems require a partnership of **collaboration** and knowledge sharing to implement and maintain successful standards of care. Collaboration is the sharing of ideas and experiences for the purposes of mutual understanding and learning. **Knowledge exchange** is the product of collaboration when sharing an understanding of information promotes learning from past experiences to make better future decisions.

Depending on the type of project, collaboration occurs at many different levels within an organization. At an administrative level, collaboration among key **stakeholders** is critical to the success of any project. Stakeholders have the most responsibility for completing the project. They have the greatest influence in the overall design of the system, and ultimately, stakeholders are the ones who are most impacted by a system implementation. Together with the organizational executive team, stakeholders collaborate on the overall budget and time frame for a system implementation.

Collaboration also occurs among the various departments impacted by the system. These groups are frequently comprised of representatives from information technology, clinical specialty areas, support services, and software vendors. Once a team is assembled, it defines the objectives and goals of the system. The members work strategically to align their goals with the goals of the organization where the system is to be used. The focus for these groups is on planning, resource management, transitioning, and ongoing support of the system. This collaboration determines how the project is managed, the deliverables for the project, who is accountable for the project, the time frame for the project, opportunities for process improvement using the system, and how resources are allocated to support the system.

From collaboration comes the exchange of information and ideas through knowledge sharing. Specialists exchange knowledge within their respective areas of expertise to ensure that the system works for an entire organization. From one another, they learn requirements that make the system successful. This exchange of ideas is what makes healthcare information systems so valuable. A multidisciplinary approach ensures that systems work in the complex environment of healthcare organizations that have diverse and complex patient populations.

SUMMARY

The integration of technology within healthcare organizations has limitless possibilities. As new types of systems emerge, clinicians will become smarter and more adept at implementing these tools into daily practice. Success will be achieved when health care incorporates technology systems in a way that they are not viewed as separate tools to support healthcare practices, but rather as necessary instruments to provide health care. Patients, too, will become savvier at using healthcare information systems as a means of communication and managing their personal and preventive care. In the future, these two mindsets will become expectations for health care and not simply a high-tech benefit as they are often viewed today. When it comes to healthcare information technology, the possibilities are endless. Ultimately, it is not the type of systems that are important but rather the method in which they are put into practice. In an ideal world there will be robust and transparent information technologies that support clinical and administrative functions promoting safe, quality, and cost-effective care.

THOUGHT-PROVOKING Questions

1. What type of technology exists today that could be converted into new types of information systems to be used in health care?

2. How could collaboration and knowledge sharing at a single organization be used to help individuals preparing for information technology at a different facility?

3. Discuss the administrative information systems and their applications.

For a full suite of assignments and additional learning activities, use the access code located in the front of your book to visit this exclusive website: http://go.jblearning.com/mcgonigle. If you do not have an access code, you can obtain one at the site.

References

Agarwal, R., Sands, D., Schneider, J., & Smaltz, D. (2010). Quantifying the economic impact of communication inefficiencies in U.S. hospitals. *Journal of Healthcare Management, 55*(4), 265–281; discussion 281–282. Retrieved from ABI/INFORM Global. (Document ID: 2108239361).

Agency for Healthcare Research and Quality. (2000). *Medical errors: The scope of the problem. An epidemic of errors.* Retrieved from http://www.ahrq.gov/qual/errback.htm

Beird, L. (2000). How to satisfy both clinical and information technology goals in designing a successful picture archiving and communication system. *Journal of Digital Imaging: Supplement, 13,* 10–2. Retrieved from ProQuest Nursing & Allied Health Source. (Document ID: 1951921891).

Ciotti, V., & Zodda, F. (1996). Selecting managed care information systems. *Journal of the Healthcare Financial Management Association, 50*(6), 35–36. Retrieved from http://findarticles.com/p/articles/mi_m3257/is_n6_v50/ai_18515376

DiJerome, L. (1992). The nursing case management computerized system: Meeting the challenge of health care delivery through technology. *Computers in Nursing, 10*(6), 250–258.

Elder, K., Wiltshire, J., Rooks, R., BeLue, R., & Gary, L. (Summer 2010). Health information technology and physician career satisfaction. *Perspectives in Health Information Management,* 1–18. Retrieved from ProQuest Nursing & Allied Health Source. (Document ID: 2118694921).

Hassett, M., & Thede, L. (2003). Information in practice: Clinical information systems. In B. Cunningham (Ed.), *Informatics and nursing opportunities and challenges* (2nd ed., rev., pp. 222–239). Philadelphia: Lippincott Williams & Wilkins.

Indiana University. (2010). University Information Technology Services Knowledge Base: What is SQL? Retrieved from http://kb.iu.edu/data/ahux.html

Lee, J. (2009). SQL for cloud computing: Microsoft SQL data services. Retrieved from http://www.devx.com/MSDN/Article/40704

Mekhjian, H., Vasila, M., & Jones, K. (2008). Combine and conquer: Computing from a single database. *Physician Executive, 34*(5), 30–32, 34–35. Retrieved from ABI/INFORM Global. (Document ID: 1651800501).

Simpson, R. L., & Falk, C. (1996). Technology and case management. In J. Hodgson (Ed.), *Information management in nursing and healthcare* (pp. 144–152). Springhouse, PA: Springhouse Corporation.

U.C. San Diego. (2010). Data warehouse terms. Retrieved from http://blink.ucsd.edu/technology/help-desk/queries/warehouse/terms.html#s.

W3Schools.com. (2010). Introduction to SQL. Retrieved from http://www.w3schools.com/SQL/sql_intro.asp

CHAPTER 14

Improving the Human–Technology Interface

Judith A. Effken

INTRODUCTION

Several years ago I stayed in a new hotel on the outskirts of London. When I entered my room, I encountered three wall-mounted light switches in a row, but with no indication of which lights they operated. In fact, the mapping of switches to lights was so peculiar that I was more often than not surprised by the light that came on when I pressed a particular switch. One might conclude that I have a serious problem, but I prefer to attribute my difficulty to poor design.

When these kinds of technology design issues surface in health care, they are more than just an annoyance. Poorly designed technology can lead to errors, lower productivity, or even the removal of the system (Alexander & Staggers, 2009). Unfortunately, as more and more kinds of increasingly complex health information technology applications are integrated, the problem becomes even worse (Johnson, 2006). However, nurses are very creative and, if at all possible, will design **workarounds** that allow them to circumvent troublesome technology. However, workarounds are only a band-aid; they are not a long-term solution.

In his classic book, *The Psychology of Everyday Things*, Norman (1988) argued that life would be a lot simpler if people who built the things others encounter (like light switches) paid more attention to how they would be used. At least one everyday thing meets Norman's criteria for good design: the scythe. Even people who have never encountered one will pick up a scythe in the manner needed to use it because the design makes only one way feasible. The scythe's design fits perfectly with its intended use and a human user. Would it not be great if all technology were so well fit to human use? In fact, this is not such a far-fetched idea. Scientists and engineers are making excellent strides in understanding human–technology interface problems and proposing solutions.

By the end of this chapter the reader will be able to (1) define what is meant by the "human–technology interface"; (2) describe problems with human–technology interfaces currently available in health care; and (3) describe models, strategies, and exemplars for improving interfaces during the analysis, design, and evaluation phases of the development life cycle.

THE HUMAN–TECHNOLOGY INTERFACE

What is the human–technology interface? Broadly speaking, any time a human uses technology, there is some type of hardware or software that enables and supports the interaction. It is this hardware and software that defines the interface. The array of light switches described previously was actually an interface (although not a great one) between the lighting technology in the room and the human user.

In today's healthcare settings, one encounters a wide variety of human–technology interfaces. Those who work in hospitals may use bar-coded identification cards to log their arrival time into a human resources management system. Using the same cards, they might log into their patients' electronic medical record (EMR), access their drugs from a drug administration system, and even administer their drugs using bar-coding technology. Other examples of human–technology interfaces one might encounter include a defibrillator, a patient-controlled analgesia (PCA) pump, any number of physiologic monitoring systems, electronic thermometers, and telephones and pagers.

The human interfaces for each of these technologies are different, and can even differ among different brands or versions of the same device. For example, to enter data into an EMR one might use a keyboard, a light pen, a touch screen, or voice. Healthcare technologies may present information via computer screen, printer, or a personal data assistant. Patient data might be displayed in the form of text, pictures (e.g., the results of a brain scan), or even sound (an echocardiogram); and the information may be arrayed or presented differently, based on roles and preferences. Some human–technology interfaces mimic face-to-face human encounters. For example, faculty increasingly uses videoconferencing technology to communicate with students. Similarly, telehealth allows nurses to use telecommunication and videoconferencing software to communicate more effectively and more frequently with patients at home by using the technology to monitor patients' vital signs, supervise their wound care, or demonstrate a procedure. Telehealth technology has fostered other virtual interfaces, such as system-wide intensive care units in which intensivists and specially trained nurses monitor critically ill patients in intensive care units, some of whom may be in rural locations. Sometimes telehealth interfaces allow patients to interact with a virtual clinician (actually a computer program) that asks questions, provides social support, and tailors education to identify patient needs based on the answers to screening questions. These human–technology interfaces have been remarkably successful; sometimes patients even prefer them to live clinicians.

Human–technology interfaces may present information using text, numbers, pictures, icons, or sound. Auditory, visual, or even tactile alarms may alert one to important information. One may interact with (or control) the technology using keyboards, digital pens, voice activation, or even touch.

A small, but growing number of clinical and educational interfaces rely heavily on tactile input. For example, many students learn to access an intravenous site using virtual technology. Other, more sophisticated virtual reality applications help physicians learn to do endoscopies or practice complex surgical procedures in a safe environment. Still others allow drug researchers to design new medications by combining virtual molecules (here, the tactile response is quite different for molecules that can be joined from those that cannot). In each of these training environments, accurately depicting tactile sensations is critical. For example, feeling the kind and amount of pressure required to penetrate the desired tissues, but not others, is essential to a realistic and effective learning experience.

The growing use of large databases for research has led to the design of novel human–technology interfaces that help researchers visualize and understand patterns in the data that generate new knowledge or lead to new questions. Many of these interfaces now incorporate multidimensional visualizations, in addition to scatter plots, histograms, or cluster representations (Vincent, Hastings-Tolsma, & Effken, 2010). Some designers, like Quinn (the founder of the Design Rhythmics Sonification Research Laboratory at the University of New Hampshire) and Meeker (2000), use variations in sound to help researchers hear the patterns in large data sets. In Quinn's (2000) "climate symphony," different musical instruments, tones, pitches, and phrases are mapped onto variables, such as the amounts and relative concentrations of minerals to help researchers detect patterns in ice core data covering over 110,000 years. Climate patterns take centuries to emerge and can be difficult to detect. The music allows the entire 110,000 years to be condensed into just a few minutes, making detection of patterns and changes much easier.

The human–technology interface is ubiquitous in health care and takes many forms. A look the quality of these interfaces follows. Be warned: it is not always a pretty picture.

THE HUMAN–TECHNOLOGY INTERFACE PROBLEM

In *The Human Factor*, Vicente (2004) cited the many safety problems in health care identified by the Institute of Medicine's (1999) report and how the technology (defined broadly) used often does not fit well with human characteristics. As a case in point, Vicente described his own studies of nurses' PCA pump errors. Nurses made the errors, in large part, because of the complexity of the user interface, which required up to 27 steps to program the device. Vicente and his colleagues developed a PCA in which programming required no more than 12 steps. Nurses who used it in laboratory experiments made fewer errors, programmed drug delivery faster, and reported lower cognitive workloads compared to the commercial device. Further evidence that human–technology interfaces do not work as well as they might is evident in the following events.

Doyle (2005) reported that when a bar-coding medication system interfered with their workflow, nurses devised workarounds, such as removing the armband from the patient and attaching it to the bed, because the bar-code reader failed to interpret bar codes when the bracelet curved tightly around a small arm. Koppel et al. (2005) reported that a widely used computer-based provider order entry (CPOE) system meant to decrease medication errors actually facilitated 22 types of errors because the information needed to order medications was fragmented across as many as 20 screens, available medication dosages differed from those the physicians expected, and allergy alerts were triggered only after an order was written.

Han et al. (2005) reported increased mortality among children admitted to Children's Hospital in Pittsburgh after CPOE implementation. Three reasons were cited for this unexpected outcome: (1) CPOE changed the workflow in the emergency room. Before CPOE, orders were written for critical time-sensitive treatment based on radio communication with the incoming transport team before the child arrived. After CPOE implementation, orders could not be written until the patient arrived and was registered in the system (a policy that was later changed). (2) Entering an order required as many as 10 clicks and took as long as 2 minutes; moreover, computer screens sometimes froze or response time was slow. (3) When the team changed its workflow to accommodate CPOE, face-to-face contact among team members diminished. Despite the problems with study methods identified by some of the informatics community, there certainly were serious human–technology interface problems.

In 2005, a *Washington Post* article reported that Cedars-Sinai Medical Center in Los Angeles had shut down a $34 million system after 3 months because of the medical staff's rebellion. Reasons for the rebellion included the additional time it took to complete the structured information forms; failure of the system to recognize misspellings (as nurses had previously done); and intrusive and interruptive automated alerts (Connolly, 2005). Even though physicians actually responded appropriately to the alerts, modifying or cancelling 35% of the orders that triggered them, designers had not found the right balance of helpful-to-interruptive alerts. The system simply did not fit the clinicians' workflow.

Such unintended consequences (Ash, Berg, & Coiera, 2004) or unpredictable outcomes (Aarts, Doorewaard, & Berg, 2004) of healthcare information systems may be attributed, in part, to a flawed implementation process; but there were clearly also **human–technology interaction** issues. That is, the technology was not well matched to the users and the context of care. In the pediatric case, a system developed for medical–surgical units was implemented in a critical care unit.

Human–technology interface problems are the major cause of up to 87% of all patient monitoring incidents (Walsh & Beatty, 2002). It is not always that the technology itself is faulty. In fact, the technology may perform flawlessly, but the interface design may lead the human user to make errors (Vicente, 2004).

IMPROVING THE HUMAN–TECHNOLOGY INTERFACE

A lot can be learned from the related fields of cognitive engineering, **human factors**, and **ergonomics** about how to make interfaces more compatible with their human users and the context of care. Each of these areas of study is multidisciplinary and integrates knowledge from multiple disciplines (e.g., computer science, engineering, cognitive engineering, psychology, and sociology). Over the years, the following three axioms have evolved for developing effective **human–computer interactions** (Staggers, 2003): (1) users must be an early and continuous focus during interface design; (2) the design process should be iterative, allowing for evaluation and correction of identified problems; and (3) formal evaluation should take place using rigorous experimental or qualitative methods.

Axiom 1: Users Must Be an Early and Continuous Focus During Interface Design

Rubin (1994) uses the term "user-centered design" to describe the process of designing products (e.g., human–technology interfaces) so that users can carry out the tasks needed to achieve their goals with "minimal effort and maximal efficiency" (p. 10). Thus, in user-centered design, the end user is emphasized.

Vicente (2004) argued that technology should fit human requirements at five levels of analysis (physical, psychologic, team, organizational, and political). Physical characteristics of the technology (e.g., size, shape, or location) should conform to the user's size, grasp, and available space). Information should be presented in ways that are consistent with known human psychologic capabilities (e.g., the number of items that can be remembered is seven plus or minus two). In addition, systems should conform to the communication, workflow, and authority structures of work teams; to organizational factors, such as culture and staffing levels; and even to political factors (e.g., budget constraints, laws, or regulations).

A number of analysis tools and techniques have been developed to help designers better understand the task and user environment for which they are designing. Discussed next are **task analysis**, **cognitive task analysis**, and **cognitive work analysis** (CWA).

Task analysis examines how a task must be accomplished. Generally, analysts describe the task in terms of inputs needed for the task; outputs (what is achieved by the task); and any constraints on actors' choices on carrying out the task. Analysts then lay out the sequence of temporally ordered actions that must be carried out to complete the task in flow charts (Vicente, 1999). Task analysis is very useful in defining what human workers must do and what functions might be distributed between the worker and technology.

Cognitive task analysis usually starts by identifying, through interviews or questionnaires, the particular task and its typicality and frequency. Analysts then may review the written materials that describe the job or are used for training and determine, through structured interviews or by observing experts perform the task, what knowledge is involved and how that knowledge might be represented.

CWA was developed specifically for the analysis of complex, high technology work domains, such as nuclear power plants, intensive care units, or emergency departments where workers need considerable flexibility in responding to external demands (Burns & Hajdukiewicz, 2004; Vicente, 1999). A complete CWA includes five types of analysis: (1) work domain, (2) control tasks, (3) strategies, (4) social–organizational, and (5) worker competencies. The work domain analysis describes the functions of the system and what information users need to accomplish task goals. The control task analysis investigates the control structures through which the user interacts with or controls the system. The analysis also identifies which variables and relations among variables discovered in the work domain analysis are relevant for particular situations so that context-sensitive interfaces can present the right information (e.g., prompts or alerts) at the right time. The strategies analysis looks at how work is actually done by users to facilitate the design of appropriate human–computer dialogues. The social–organizational analysis identifies the responsibilities of various users (e.g., doctors, nurses, clerks, or therapists) so that the system can support collaboration, communication, and a viable organizational structure. Finally, the worker competencies analysis identifies design constraints related to the users themselves (Effken, 2002). Specialized tools are available for the first three types of analysis (Vicente, 1999). Analysts typically borrow tools (e.g., ethnography) from the social sciences for the two remaining types. Hajdukiewicz, Vicente, Doyle, Milgram, and Burns (2001) used CWA to model an operating room environment. Effken (2002) and Effken, Loeb, Johnson,

Johnson, and Reyna (2001) used CWA to analyze the information needs for an oxygenation management display for an ICU. Other examples of the application of CWA in health care are described by Burns and Hajdukiewicz (2004) in their chapter on medical systems (pp. 201–238).

Axiom 2: The Design Process Should Be Iterative, Allowing for Evaluation and Correction of Identified Problems

Today there are available both principles and techniques for developing human–technology interfaces that people can use with minimal stress and maximal efficiency. An excellent place to start is with Norman's (1988, pp. 188–189) principles:

1. Use both knowledge in the world and knowledge in the head. In other words, pay attention not only to the environment or to the user, but to both, and to how they relate. By using both, the problem actually may be simplified.
2. Simplify the structure of tasks. For example, reduce the number of steps or even computer screens needed to accomplish the goal.
3. Make things visible: bridge the gulfs of execution and evaluation. Users need to be able to see how to use the technology to accomplish a goal (e.g., what buttons does one press and in which order to program this PCA); if they do, then designers have bridged the **gulf of execution**. They also need to be able to see the effects of their actions on the technology (e.g., if a nurse practitioner prescribes a drug to treat a certain condition, the actual patient response may not be perfectly clear). This bridges the **gulf of evaluation**.
4. Get the mappings right. Here, the term "mapping" is used to describe how environmental facts (e.g., the order of light switches or variables in a physiologic monitoring display) are accurately depicted by the information presentation.
5. Exploit the power of constraints, both natural and artificial. Because of where the eyes are located in the head, humans have to turn their heads to see what is happening behind them; however, that is not true of all animals. As the location of one's eyes constrains what one can see, so also do physical elements, social factors, and even organizational policy constrain the way tasks are accomplished. By taking these constraints into account when designing technology, it can be made easier for humans use.
6. Design for error. Mistakes happen. Technology should eliminate predictable errors and be sufficiently flexible to allow humans to identify and recover from unpredictable errors.
7. When all else fails, standardize. To get a feel for this principle, think how difficult it is to change from a Macintosh to a Windows environment or from the Windows operating system to Vista.

Kirlik and Maruyama (2004) described a real-world human–technology interface that follows Norman's principles. The authors observed how a busy expert short-order cook strategically managed to grill many hamburgers at the same time, but each to the customer's desired level of doneness. The cook put those burgers that were to be well-done on the back and far right portion of the grill, those to be medium well-done in the center of the grill, and those to be rare at the front of the grill, but farther to the left. The cook moved all burgers to the left as grilling proceeded and turned them over during their travel across the grill. Everything the cook needed to know was available in this simple interface. As a human–technology interface, the grill layout was elegant. The interface used knowledge housed both in the environment and in the expert cook's head; and things were clearly visible, both in the position of the burgers and the way they were moved. The process was clearly and effectively standardized, and with built-in constraints. What might it take to create such an intuitive human–technology interface in health care?

Several useful books have been written about effective interface design (e.g., Burns & Hajdukiewicz, 2004; Cooper, 1995; Mandel, 1997). In addition, there is a growing body of research exploring new ways to present clinical data that might facilitate clinicians' problem identification and accurate treatment. Often designers use graphical objects to show how variables relate. The first to do so were likely Cole and Stewart (1993), who used changes in the lengths of the sides and area of a four-sided object to show the relationship of respiratory rate to tidal volume. Other researchers have demonstrated that histograms and polygon displays are better than numeric displays for detecting changes in patients' physiologic variables (Gurushanthaiah, Weinger, & Englund, 1995). When Horn, Popow, and Unterasinger (2001) presented physiologic data via a single circular object with 12 sectors (where each sector represented a different variable), nurses reported that it was easy to recognize abnormal conditions, but difficult to comprehend the patient's overall status. This kind of graphical object approach has been most widely used in anesthesiology, where a number of researchers have shown improved clinician **situational awareness** or problem detection time by mapping physiologic variables onto display objects that have meaningful shapes, such as using a bellows-like object to represent ventilation (Agutter et al., 2003; Blike, Surgenor, Whallen, & Jensen, 2000; Michels, Gravenstein, & Westenskow, 1997; Zhang et al., 2002).

Effken (2006) compared a prototype display that represented physiologic data in a structured pictorial format with two bar graph displays. The first bar graph display and the prototype both presented data in the order that experts were observed to use them. The second bar graph display presented the data in the way that nurses collected them. In an experiment in which resident physicians and novice nurses used simulated drugs to treat observed oxygenation management problems using each display, residents' performance was improved with the displays ordered as experts used them, but nurses' performance was not improved. Nurses performed better when the variables were ordered as they were used to collecting them, demonstrating the importance of understanding user roles and the tasks they need to accomplish.

Data need not only be represented visually. Gaver (1993) proposed that because ordinary sounds map onto familiar events, they could be used as icons to facilitate easier technology navigation and use and also to provide continuous background information about how a system is functioning. In health care, auditory displays have been used to provide clinicians with information about patients' vital signs (e.g., in pulse oximetry), such as by altering volume or tone when there is a significant change (Sanderson, 2006).

Admittedly, auditory displays are probably more useful for quieter areas of the hospital, such as the operating room. Perhaps that is why researchers have most frequently applied the approach in anesthesiology. For example, Loeb and Fitch (2002) reported that anesthesiologists detected critical events more quickly when auditory information about heart rate, blood pressure, and respiratory parameters was added to a visual display. Auditory tones also have been combined as "earcons" to represent relationships among data elements, such as the relationship of systolic to diastolic blood pressure (Watson & Gill, 2004).

Axiom 3: Formal Evaluation Should Take Place Using Rigorous Experimental or Qualitative Methods

Perhaps one of the highest accolades that any interface can achieve is that it is transparent. An interface becomes transparent when it is so easy to use that users no longer think about it, but only about the task at hand. For example, a transparent clinical interface would enable clinicians to focus on patient decisions rather than on how to access or combine patient data from multiple sources. In Figure 14-1, instead of the nurse interacting with the computer, the nurse and patient interact through the technology interface. The more transparent the interface, the easier should be the interaction.

Usability is a term that denotes the ease with which people can use an interface to achieve a particular goal. Usability of a new human–technology interface needs to be evaluated early and often throughout its development. Typical usability indicators include ease of use, ease of learning, satisfaction with using, efficiency of use, error tolerance, and fit of the system to the task (Staggers, 2003). Some of the more commonly used approaches to usability evaluation are discussed next.

FIGURE

14-1

Nurse–patient interaction framework in which the technology supports the interaction.

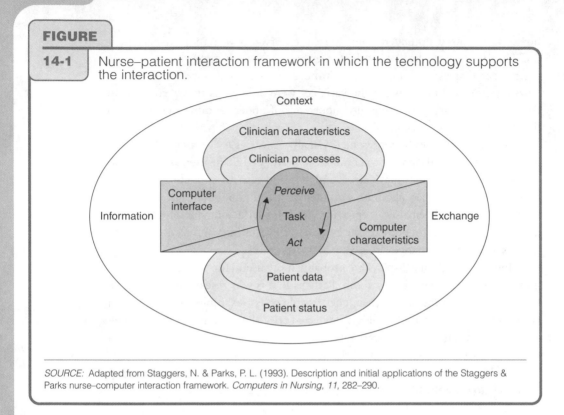

SOURCE: Adapted from Staggers, N. & Parks, P. L. (1993). Description and initial applications of the Staggers & Parks nurse–computer interaction framework. *Computers in Nursing, 11,* 282–290.

Surveys of Potential or Actual Users

Chernecky, Macklin, and Waller (2006) assessed cancer patients' preferences for website design. Participants were asked their preferences for a number of design characteristics, such as display color, menu buttons, text, photo size, icon metaphor, and layout, by selecting on a computer screen their preferences for each item from two or three options.

Focus Group

Typically used at the very start of the design process, focus groups can help the designer better understand users' responses to potential interface designs and to content that might be included in the interface.

Cognitive Walkthrough

In a **cognitive walkthrough**, evaluators assess a paper mock-up, working prototype, or completed interface by observing the steps users are likely to take to use the interface to accomplish typical tasks. The analysis helps designers determine how understandable and easy to learn the interface is likely to be for these users and the typical tasks (Wharton, Rieman, Lewis, & Polson, 1994).

Heuristic Evaluation

A **heuristic evaluation** has become the most popular of what are called "discount usability evaluation" methods. The objective of a heuristic evaluation is to detect problems early in the design process when they can be most easily and economically corrected. The methods are termed discount because they typically are easy to do; involve fewer than 10 experts (often expert in relevant fields such as human computer technology or cognitive engineering); and are therefore much less expensive than other methods. They are called heuristic because evaluators assess the degree to which the design complies with recognized usability rules of thumb or principles (the heuristics), such as those proposed by Nielsen (1994) and available on his website (http://www.useit.com/papers/heuristic/heuristic_list.html). For example, McDaniel and colleagues (2002) conducted a usability test of an interactive computer-based program to encourage smoking cessation by low-income women. As part of the initial evaluation, healthcare professionals familiar with intended users reviewed the design and layout of the program. The usability test revealed several problems with the decision rules used to tailor content to users that were corrected before implementation.

Formal Usability Test

Formal usability tests typically use either experimental or observational studies of actual users using the interface to accomplish real-world tasks. A number of researchers use these methods. For example, Staggers, Kobus, and Brown (2007) conducted a usability study of a prototype electronic medication administration record. Participants were asked to add, modify, or discontinue medications using the system. The time they needed to complete the task, their accuracy in the task, and their satisfaction with the prototype were assessed (the latter through a questionnaire). Although satisfaction was high, the evaluation also revealed design flaws that could be corrected before implementation.

Field Study

In a **field study**, end users evaluate a prototype in the actual work setting just before its general release. For example, Thompson, Lozano, and Christakis (2007) evaluated the use of touch screen computer kiosks containing child health-promoting information in several low-income, urban community settings using an online questionnaire that could be completed after the kiosk was used. Most users found the kiosk easy to use and the information it provided easy to understand. Researchers also gained a better understanding of the characteristics of the likely users (e.g., 26% had never used the Internet and 48% had less than a high school education), and the information most often accessed (television and media use, and smoke exposure).

Dykes and her colleagues (2006) used a field test to investigate the feasibility of using digital pen and paper technology to record vital signs as a way to bridge an organization from a paper to an electronic health record. In general, satisfaction with the tool increased with use, and the devices conformed well to nurses' workflow. However, 8% of the vital sign entries were recorded inaccurately because of inaccurate handwriting recognition; entries outside the recording box; or inaccurate data entry (data entered were not valid values). The number of modifications needed in the tool and the time that would be required to make them ruled out using the digital pen and paper as a bridging technology.

Ideally, every healthcare setting would have a usability laboratory of their own to test new software and technology in their own setting before actual implementation. However, this can be expensive, especially for small organizations. Kushnirik and Borycki (2006) developed a low-cost rapid usability engineering method in which was created a "portable" usability laboratory comprised of videocameras and other technology that one can take out of the laboratory into hospitals and other locations to test the technology on site using as close to a "real world" environment as possible. This is a much more cost-effective and efficient solution and makes it possible to test all technologies before implementation.

A FRAMEWORK FOR EVALUATION

Ammenwerth, Iller, and Mahler (2006) proposed a Fit between Individuals, Tasks, and Technology (FITT) model that suggests that each of these factors be considered in designing and evaluating human-technology interfaces. It is not enough to consider only the user and technology characteristics; the tasks that the technology supports must also be considered. The FITT model builds on DeLone and McLean's (1992) Information Success Model; Davis' (1993) Technology Acceptance Model; and Goodhue and Thompson's (1995) Task Technology Fit Model. A strength of the FITT model is that it encourages the evaluator to examine the fit between each two of the components: user and technology, task and technology, and user and task.

Johnson and Turley (2006) compared how doctors and nurses describe patient information and found that doctors emphasized diagnosis, treatment, and management, whereas the nurses emphasized functional issues. Although both physicians and nurses share some patient information, how they thought about patients differed. For that reason, an EMR needs to present information (even the same information) to the two groups in different ways.

Hyun, Johnson, Stetson, and Bakken (2009) used a combination of two models (Technology Acceptance Model and Task Technology Fit Model) to design and evaluate an electronic documentation system for nurses. To facilitate the design, they used a combination of methods, including brainstorming of experts, to identify design requirements. To evaluate how well the prototype design fit both task and user, they had nurses carry out specific tasks using the prototype in a laboratory setting, and then complete a questionnaire on ease of use, usefulness, and fit of the technology with their documentation tasks. Because they engaged nurses at each step of the design process, the result was a more useful and usable system.

FUTURE OF THE HUMAN–TECHNOLOGY INTERFACE

Increased attention to improving the human–technology interface through human factor approaches has already led to significant improvement in one area of health care: anesthesiology. Anesthesia machines that used to have hoses that would fit into any delivery port now have hoses that can only be plugged into the proper port. Anesthesiologists have also been actively working with engineers to improve the computer interface through which they monitor their patients' status and are among the leaders in investigating the use of audio techniques as an alternative way to help anesthesiologists stay situationally aware. As a result, anesthesia-related deaths dropped from 2 in 20,000 to 1 in 200,000 in under 10 years (Vicente, 2004). It is hoped that continued emphasis on the human factor (Vicente, 2004) and user-centered design (Rubin, 1994) by informatics professionals and human–computer interactions experts will be equally successful in other parts of the healthcare system. The increased amount of informatics research in this area is encouraging, but there is a long way to go.

A systematic review of clinical technology design evaluation studies (Alexander & Staggers, 2009) found 50 nursing studies. Of those, nearly half (24) evaluated effectiveness, fewer (16) evaluated satisfaction, and still fewer (10) evaluated efficiency. The evaluations were not systematic. That is, there was no attempt to evaluate the same system in different environments or with different users. Most evaluations were done in a laboratory, rather than in the setting where the system would be used. The authors argued for a broader range of studies that use an expanded set of outcome measures. For example, instead of looking at user satisfaction, evaluators should dig deeper into the design factors that led to the satisfaction or dissatisfaction. In addition, performance measures, such as diagnostic accuracy, errors, and correct treatment, should be used. There is a long way to go.

SUMMARY

There are at least three messages the reader should take away from this discussion. First, if there is to be significant improvement in quality and safety outcomes in this country through the use of information technology, the designs for human–technology interfaces must be radically improved so that the technology better fits human and task requirements. However, that improvement is possible only if clinicians identify and report problems, rather than simply creating workarounds. That means that each clinician has a responsibility to participate in the design process and to report designs that do not work.

Second, a number of useful tools are currently available for the analysis, design, and evaluation phases of development life cycles and should be used routinely by informatics professionals to ensure that technology better fits both task and user requirements. Finally, focusing on interface improvement using these tools has had a huge impact on patient safety in the area of anesthesiology. With increased attention from informatics professionals and engineers, the same kind of improvement should be possible in other areas. In the ideal world one can envision that every human–technology interface will be designed to enhance users' workflow, will be as easy to use as ATM machines, and will be fully tested before its implementation in a setting that mirrors the setting where it will be used.

THOUGHT-PROVOKING Questions

WWW

1. You are a member of a team that has been asked to evaluate a prototype personal data assistant–based application for calculating drug dosages. Based on what you know about usability testing, what kind of test (or tests) might you do and why?
2. Is there a human–technology interface that you have encountered that you think needs improving? If you were to design a replacement, what of the analysis techniques that you read about would you choose? Why?

For a full suite of assignments and additional learning activities, use the access code located in the front of your book to visit this exclusive website: http://go.jblearning.com/mcgonigle. If you do not have an access code, you can obtain one at the site.

References

Aarts, J., Doorewaard, H., & Berg, M. (2004). Understanding implementation: The case of a computerized physician order entry system in a large Dutch university medical center. *JAMA, 11*, 207–216.

Agutter, J., Drews, F., Syroid, N., Westneskow, D., Albert, R., Strayer, D.Burmedez, J. & Weinger, M. (2003). Evaluation of graphic cardiovascular display in a high-fidelity simulator. *Anesthesia and Analgesia, 97*, 1403–1413.

Alexander, G., & Staggers, N. (2009). A systematic review of the designs of clinical technology findings and recommendations for future research. *Advances in Nursing Science, 32*(3), 252–279.

Ammenwerth, E., Iller, C., & Mahler, C. (2006). IT-adoption and the interaction of task, technology and individuals: A fit framework and a case study. *BMC Medical Informatics and Decision Making, 6*, 3.

Ash, J. S., Berg, M., & Coiera, E. (2004). Some unintended consequences of information technology in health care: The nature of patient care information system-related errors. *Journal of the American Medical Informatics Association, 11*, 104–112.

Blike, G. T., Surgenor, S. D., Whallen, K., & Jensen, J. (2000). Specific elements of a new hemodynamics display improves the performance of anesthesiologists. *Journal of Clinical Monitoring & Computing, 16*, 485–491.

Burns, C. M., & Hajdukiewicz, J. R. (2004). *Ecological interface design.* Boca Raton, FL: CRC Press.

Chernecky, C., Macklin, D., & Waller, J. (2006). Internet design preferences of patients with cancer. *Oncology Nursing Forum, 33*, 787–792.

Cole, W. G., & Stewart, J. G. (1993). Metaphor graphics to support integrated decision making with respiratory data. *International Journal of Clinical Monitoring and Computing, 10*, 91–100.

Connolly, C. (2005, March 21). Cedars-Sinai doctors cling to pen and paper. *Washington Post*, p. A01.

Cooper, A. (1995). *About face: Essentials of window interface design.* New York, NY: Hungry Minds, Inc.

Davis, F. D. (1993). User acceptance of information technology: System characteristics, user perceptions and behavioral impacts. *International Journal of Man-Machine Studies, 38*, 475–487.

DeLone, W. H., & McLean, E. (1992). Information systems success: The question for the dependent variable. *Information Systems Research, 3*(1), 60–95.

Doyle, M. (2005). *Impact of the Bar Code Medication Administration (BCMA) system on medication administration errors.* Unpublished doctoral dissertation, University of Arizona, Tucson, AZ.

Dykes, P. C., Benoit, A., Chang, F., Gallagher, J., Li, Q.,Spurr, C., McGrath, E., Kilroy, S., & Prater, M. (2006). The feasibility of digital pen and paper technology for vital sign data capture in acute care settings. In *AMIA 2006 Symposium Proceedings* (pp. 229–233). Washington, DC: American Medical Informatics Association.

Effken, J. A. (2002). Different lenses, improved outcomes: A new approach to the analysis and design of healthcare information systems. *International Journal of Medical Informatics, 65*, 59–74.

Effken, J. A. (2006). Improving clinical decision making through ecological interfaces. *Ecological Psychology, 18*(4), 283–318.

Effken, J., Loeb, R., Johnson, K., Johnson, S., & Reyna, V. (2001). Using cognitive work analysis to design clinical displays. In V. L. Patel, R. Rogers, & R. Haux (Eds.). *Proceedings of MedInfo-2001* (pp. 27–31). London: IOS Press.

Gaver, W. W. (1993). What in the world do we hear? An ecological approach to auditory event perception. *Ecological Psychology, 5*, 1–30.

Goodhue, D. L., & Thompson, R. L. (1995). Task-technology fit and individual performance. *MIS Quarterly, 19*(2), 213–236.

Gurushanthaiah, K. I., Weinger, M. B., & Englund, C. E. (1995). Visual display format affects the ability of anesthesiologists to detect acute physiologic changes: A laboratory study employing a clinical display simulator. *Anesthesiology, 83*, 1184–1193.

Hajdukiewicz, J. R., Vicente, K. J., Doyle, D. J., Milgram, P., & Burns, C. M. (2001). Modeling a medical environment: An ontology for integrated medical informatics design. *International Journal of Medical Informatics, 62,* 79–99.

Han, Y. Y., Carcillo, J. A., Venkataraman, S. T., Clark, R. S. B., Watson, R. S., Nguyen, T. Bayir, H. & Orr, R. (2005). Unexpected increased mortality after implementation of a commercially sold computerized physician order entry system. *Pediatrics, 116,* 1506–1512.

Horn, W., Popow, C., & Unterasinger, L. (2001). Support for fast comprehension of ICU data: Visualization using metaphor graphics. *Methods in Informatics Medicine, 40,* 421–424.

Hyun, S., Johnson, S. B., Stetson, P. D., & Bakken, S. (2009). Development and evaluation of nursing user interface screens using multiple methods. *Journal of Biomedical Informatics, 42*(6), 1004–1012.

Institute of Medicine. (1999). *To err is human: Building a safer health system.* Washington, DC: Institute of Medicine.

Johnson, C. W. (2006). Why did that happen? Exploring the proliferation of barely usable software in healthcare systems. *Quality & Safety in Healthcare, 15*(Suppl. 1), 176–181.

Johnson, C. M., & Turley, J. P. (2006). The significance of cognitive modeling in building healthcare interfaces. *International Journal of Medical Informatics, 75*(2), 163–172.

Kirlik, A., & Maruyama, S. (2004). Human–technology interaction and music perception and performance: Toward the robust design of sociotechnical systems. *Proceedings of the IEEE, 92*(4), 616–631.

Koppel, R., Metlay, J. P., Cohen, A., Abaluck, B., Localio, A. R., Kimmel, S. E., & Stron, B. (2005). Role of computerized physician order entry systems in facilitating medication errors. *JAMA, 293*(10), 1197–1203.

Kushniruk, A. W., & Borycki, E. M. (2006). Low-cost rapid usability engineering: Designing and customizing usable healthcare information systems. *Healthcare Quarterly (Toronto, Ont.), 9*(40), 98–100, 102.

Loeb, R. G., & Fitch, W. T. (2002). A laboratory evaluation of an auditory display designed to enhance intraoperative monitoring. *Anesthesia and Analgesia, 94,* 362–368.

Mandel, T. (1997). *The elements of user interface design.* New York, NY: John Wiley & Sons.

McDaniel, A., Hutchinson, S., Casper, G. R., Ford, R. T., Stratton, R., & Rembush, M. (2002). Usability testing and outcomes of an interactive computer program to promote smoking cessation in low income women. In *Proceedings AMIA 2002* (pp. 509–513). Washington, DC: American Medical Informatics Association.

Michels, P., Gravenstein, D., & Westenskow, D. R. (1997). An integrated graphic data display improves detection and identification of critical events during anesthesia. *Journal of Clinical Monitoring & Computing, 13,* 249–259.

Nielsen, J. (1994). Heuristic evaluation. In J. Nielsen & R. L. Mack (Eds.), *Usability inspection methods* (pp. 25–62). New York, NY: John Wiley & Sons.

Norman, D. A. (1988). *The psychology of everyday things.* New York, NY: Basic Books.

Quinn, M. (2000). *The climate symphony: Rhythmic techniques applied to the sonification of ice core data.* Retrieved from http://www.bcca. org/ief/dquin00c.htm

Quinn, M., & Meeker, L. (2000). *Research set to music: The climate symphony and other sonifications of ice core, radar, DNA, seismic and solar wind data.* Retrieved from http://www.drsrl.com/climate_paper.html

Rubin, J. (1994). *Handbook of usability testing: How to plan, design, and conduct effective tests.* New York, NY: Wiley & Sons.

Sanderson, P. (2006). The multimodal world of medical monitoring displays. *Applied Ergonomics, 37,* 501–512.

Staggers, N. (2003). Human factors: Imperative concepts for information systems in critical care. *AACN Clinical Issues, 14*(3), 310–319.

Staggers, N., Kobus, D., & Brown, C. (2007). Nurses' evaluations of a novel design for an electronic medication administration record. *CIN: Computers, Informatics, Nursing, 25*(2), 67–75.

Staggers, N., & Parks, P. L. (1993). Description and initial applications of the Staggers & Parks nurse–computer interaction framework. *Computers in Nursing, 11*, 282–290.

Thompson, D. A., Lozano, P., & Christakis, D. A. (2007). Parent use of touchscreen computer kiosks for child health promotion in community settings. *Pediatrics, 119*(3), 427–434.

Vicente, K. (2004). *The human factor.* New York, NY: Routledge.

Vicente, K. J. (1999). *Cognitive work analysis: Toward safe, productive, and healthy computer-based work.* Mahwah, NJ: Lawrence Erlbaum Associates.

Vincent, D., Hastings-Tolsma, M., & Effken, J. (2010). Data visualization and large nursing datasets. *Online Journal of Nursing Informatics (OJNI), 14*(2). Available at http://ojni.org/14_2/Vincent.pdf

Walsh, T., & Beatty, P. C. W. (2002). Human factor error and patient monitoring. *Physiological Measurement, 23*, R111–R132.

Watson, G., & Gill, T. (2004). Earcon for intermittent information in monitoring environments. In Proceedings of the 2004 Conference of the Computer-Human Interaction Special Interest Group of the Human Factors and Ergonomics Society of Australia (OzCHI2004), Wollonggong, New South Wales, November 22-24, 1994.

Wharton, C., Rieman, J., Lewis, C., & Polson, P. (1994). The cognitive walkthrough: A practitioner's guide. In J. Nielsen & R. L. Mack (Eds.), *Usability inspection methods* (pp. 105–139). New York, NY: John Wiley & Sons, Inc.

Zhang, Y., Drews, F. A., Westenskow, D. R., Foresti, S., Agutter, J., Burmedez, J.C., Bilke, G. & Loeb, R. (2002). Effects of integrated graphical displays on situation awareness in anaesthesiology. *Cognition, Technology & Work, 4*, 82–90.

CHAPTER 15

Information Copyright and Fair Use and Network Security

Lisa Reeves Bertin

Objectives

1. Explore information fair use and copyright restrictions.
2. Describe processes for securing information in a computer network.
3. Identify various methods of user authentication and relate authentication to security of a network.
4. Explain methods to anticipate and prevent typical threats to network security.

www

Key Terms

www

Acceptable use
Antivirus software
Authentication
Biometrics
Confidentiality
Copyright
Fair use
Firewall
Flash drive
Hacker
Integrity
Intrusion detection devices
Intrusion detection system
Jump drive
Malicious code
Malicious insider
Mask
Network
Network accessibility
Network availability
Network security
Password
Proxy server
Radio frequency identity chip
Secure information
Security breach
Shoulder surfing
Social engineering
Spyware

Continues

INTRODUCTION

In addition to complying with federal HIPAA guidelines regarding the privacy of patient information, healthcare systems also need to be vigilant in the way that they **secure information** and manage **network security**. Mowry and Oakes (n.d.) discuss the vulnerability of electronic health records to data breaches. They suggest that as many as 77 persons could view a patient's record during a hospital stay. It is critical for information technology (IT) policies and procedures to ensure appropriate access by clinicians and to protect private information from inappropriate access. However, **authentication** procedures can be cumbersome and time consuming, thus reducing clinician performance efficiency.

Physicians spend on average seven minutes per patient encounter, of which they spend nearly two minutes on managing logins and application navigation. Likewise, an average major healthcare provider has more than 150 applications—most requiring different user names and **passwords**—making it difficult for caregivers to navigate and receive contextual

Key Terms Continued

Thumb drive
Trojan horse
Virus
Worm

information. Healthcare organizations must strike the right balance, in terms of simplifying access to core clinical data sets while maximizing the time providers can interact with patients without jeopardizing data **integrity** and security (para. 7).

This chapter explores **copyright** and **fair use** of information and processes for securing information in a health system computer **network**.

FAIR USE OF INFORMATION AND SHARING

Copyright laws in the world of technology are notoriously misunderstood. The same copyright laws that cover physical books, artwork, and other creative material are still applicable in the digital world. Have you ever given a friend a CD that contains a computer game or some other type of software that you paid for and registered? Have you ever downloaded a song from the Internet without paying? Have you ever copied a section of online content from a reference site and used that content as if it was your own? Have you ever copied a picture from the Internet without asking permission from the photographer who took the picture? Have you copied and pasted information about a disease or drug from a website and then printed out the information to give to a patient or family member? These are all examples of the type of copyright infringements enabled by technology that occur almost without thought.

The value of creative material, whether it is written content, a song, a painting, or some other type of creative work is not in the physical medium on which it is stored. The value is in the intangible areas of creativity, skills, and labor that went into creating that item. The person who created the material should be properly credited and possibly reimbursed for the use of the material. How would a musician be reimbursed for their music if everyone just downloaded their songs illegally from the Internet? Imagine creating a game to teach type 1 diabetics how to manage their diet and other nurses copied and distributed it without permission.

Almost all software, music CDs, and movie DVDs come with restrictions of how and why copies can be made. The license included with the software clarifies exactly what restrictions are applicable. Be aware that the most common type of software license is a "shrink wrap" license, meaning as soon as one removes the shrink wrap from the CD or DVD case one has agreed to the license restriction. Most computer software developers allow for a backup copy of the software without restriction. If the hard drive fails on one's computer, the software can usually be reinstalled through the backup copy. Some software companies even allow one to transfer software to a new user. In this case, the software typically must be uninstalled from the computer before the new owner is free to install the software on his or her computer. Most of these restrictions depend on the honesty of the user in reading and following the licensing agreement. As a result of widespread abuses, the music and film industries commonly use hardware security features that block users from making a working copy of a music CD or movie DVD.

The bottom line is to recognize that copyright laws also apply to the digital world and that copyright violations can lead to prosecution. Advances in technology have made the sharing of information easy and extremely fast. A scanner can convert any document to digital form instantly, and that document can then be shared with people anywhere in the world. The person who created that document has a right to approve of the sharing of the work. Carefully read the fine print of any software purchased and be sure to clarify any questions regarding how that software can be copied. Avoid downloading music illegally from the Internet and do not use information from the Internet without permission to do so or citing the reference appropriately. Healthcare organizations that allow access to the Internet from a network computer should ensure that users are well aware of and compliant with copyright and fair use principles.

SECURING NETWORK INFORMATION

Typically, a healthcare organization has computers linked together to facilitate communication and operations within and outside the facility. This is commonly referred to as a "network." The linking of computers together and to the outside creates the possibility of a breach of network security and exposes the information to unauthorized use.

The three main areas of secure network information are (1) **confidentiality**, (2) availability, and (3) integrity. As discussed in the chapters dealing with ethics and legislative aspects (Chapters 5 and 10, respectively), an organization must follow a well-defined policy to ensure that private health information remains appropriately confidential. The confidentiality policy should clearly define what data are confidential and how the data should be handled. Employees also need to understand the procedures for releasing confidential information outside the organization or to others within the organization and what procedures to follow if confidential information is accidentally or intentionally released without authorization. In addition, the policy should contain consideration for elements as basic as the placement of monitors so that information cannot be read by passersby. **Shoulder surfing**, or watching over someone's back as that person is working, is still a major way that confidentiality is compromised.

Availability refers to network information being accessible when needed. This area of the policy tends to be much more technical in nature. An accessibility policy covers issues associated with protecting the key hardware elements of the computer network and the procedures to follow with a major electric outage or Internet outage. Food and drinks spilled onto keyboards of computer units, dropping or jarring hardware, and electrical surges or static charges are all examples of ways that the hardware elements of a computer network may be damaged. In the case of an electrical outage or a weather-related disaster, the network administrator must have clear plans for data backup, storage, and retrieval. There must also be clear procedures and alternative methods of ensuring that care delivery is largely uninterrupted.

Another way organizations protect the availability of their networks is to institute an **acceptable use** policy. Elements covered in such policy could include what types of activities are acceptable on the corporate network. For example, are employees permitted to download music at work? Restricting downloads is a very common way for organizations to avoid **viruses** and other **malicious code** from entering their networks. The policy should also clearly define what activities are not acceptable and the consequences for violations.

The last area of information security is integrity. Employees need to have confidence that the information they are reading is true. To accomplish this, organizations need clear policies to clarify how data are actually inputted, who has the authorization to change such data, and to track how and when data are changed. All three of these areas use authorization and authentication to enforce the corporate policies. Access to networks can easily be grouped into areas of authorization (e.g., users can be grouped by job title). For example, anyone with the job title of floor supervisor may be authorized to change the hours worked by an employee, but an employee with the title of patient care assistant may not make such changes.

AUTHENTICATION OF USERS

Authentication of employees is also used by organizations in their security policies. The most common ways to authenticate are by something the user knows, something the user has, or something the user is (Figure 15-1). Something a user knows is a password. Most organizations today enforce a strong password policy, because free software available on the Internet can break a password from the dictionary very quickly. Strong password policies include using combinations of letters, numbers, and special characters, such as plus signs and ampersands. Policies typically include the enforcement of changing passwords every 30 or 60 days. Passwords should never be written down in an obvious place, such as a sticky note attached to the monitor or under the keyboard. The second area of authentication is something the user has, such as an identification (ID) card. ID cards can be magnetic, similar to a credit card, or have a **radio frequency identity chip** embedded into the card. The last area of authentication is **biometrics**. Devices that recognize thumb prints, retina patterns, or facial patterns are available. Depending on the level of security needed, organizations commonly use a combination of these types of authentication.

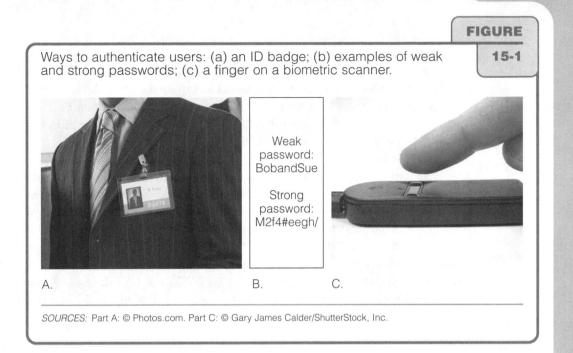

FIGURE 15-1

Ways to authenticate users: (a) an ID badge; (b) examples of weak and strong passwords; (c) a finger on a biometric scanner.

Weak password: BobandSue

Strong password: M2f4#eegh/

A.   B.   C.

SOURCES: Part A: © Photos.com. Part C: © Gary James Calder/ShutterStock, Inc.

THREATS TO SECURITY

The largest benefit of a computer network is the ability to share information. However, organizations need to protect that information and ensure that only authorized individuals have access to the network and the data appropriate to their role. A 2003 nationwide survey by the Computing Technology Industry Association found that human error was the most likely cause of problems with **security breaches**. The survey indicated that only 8% were caused by purely technical errors, with more than 63% being caused by some type of human error (Gross, 2003). According to Degaspari (2010), "Given the volume of electronic patient data involved, it's perhaps not surprising that breaches are occurring. According to the Department of Health and Human Services' Office of Civil Rights (OCR), 146 data breaches affecting 500 or more individuals occurred between December 22, 2009 and July 28, 2010. The types of breaches encompass theft, loss, hacking, and improper disposal; and include both electronic data and paper records" (para. 4). How, then, should organizations approach security knowing that human beings are the most likely cause of a security breach?

The first line of defense is strictly physical. The power of a locked door, an operating system that locks down after 5 minutes of inactivity, and regular security training programs are extremely effective. Proper workspace security discipline is a critical aspect. Employees need to be properly trained to be aware of computer monitor visibility, shoulder surfing, and policy regarding the removal of computer hardware. A major issue facing organizations is removable storage devices (Figure 15-2). CD/DVD burners, **jump drives**, **flash drives**, or **thumb drives** (which use USB port access) are all potential security risks. These devices can be slipped into a pocket and thus are easily removed from the organization. One way to address this physical security risk is to limit the authorization to write files to a device. Organizations are also turning off the CD/DVD burners and USB ports on company desktops.

The most common threats a corporate network faces are **hackers**; malicious code (**spyware**, viruses, **worms**, **Trojan horses**); and the **malicious insider**. Acceptable use policies help to address these problems. It is common practice for employees to be restricted from downloading files from the Internet. Downloaded files, including e-mail attachments, are the most common way viruses and other malicious code enters a computer network. Network security policies typically prohibit employees from using personal CDs/DVDs and USB drives, and thus prevent the transfer of malicious code from a personal computer to the network.

FIGURE

15-2   A removable storage device.

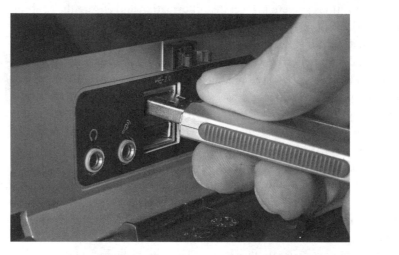

SOURCE: © Alex Kotlov/ShutterStock, Inc.

Spyware is normally controlled by limiting functions of the browser used to surf the Internet. For example, the browser privacy options can control how cookies are used. A cookie is a very small file written to the hard drive of a computer whose user is surfing the Internet. The file simply contains information about the user. For example, many shopping sites write cookies to the user's hard drive containing the user's name and preferences. When that user returns to the site, the site will greet her by name and list products in which she is possibly interested. Weather websites send cookies to users' hard drives with their zip code so that when each user returns to that site, the local weather forecast is immediately displayed. On the negative side, cookies can also follow the user's travels on the Internet. Marketing companies use spying cookies to track popular websites that could provide return on advertising expenditures. Spying cookies related to marketing typically do not track keystrokes to steal user IDs and passwords. They simply exist to track what websites are popular, and thus are used to develop advertising and marketing strategies. Spyware that does steal user IDs and passwords contains malicious code that is normally hidden in a seemingly innocent file download. This threat to security explains why healthcare organizations typically do not allow employees to download files. The rule of thumb to protect the network and one's own computer system is to download only files from a reputable site that provides complete contact information. Organizations may also use such devices as **firewalls** (covered in the next section) and **intrusion detection devices** to protect from hackers.

Another huge threat to corporate security is **social engineering**, or the manipulation of a relationship based on one's position in an organization. For example, someone attempting to access a network might pretend to be an employee from the corporate IT office who then simply asks for an employee's digital ID and password. The outsider can then gain access to the corporate network. Once this access has been obtained, all corporate information is at risk. A second example of social engineering is a hacker impersonating a federal government agent. After talking an employee into revealing network information, the hacker has an open door to enter the corporate network.

The number one security threat to a corporate network is the malicious insider. This can be a disgruntled employee or a recently fired employee whose rights of access to the corporate network have not yet been removed. In the case of the latter, network access should be suspended immediately on notice of termination. To avoid issues created by malicious insiders, healthcare organizations need some type of policy to monitor employee activity to ensure that employees are only carrying out duties that are part of their normal job. Separation of privileges is a common security tool; no one employee should be able to complete a task that could cause a critical event without the knowledge of another employee. For example, the employee who processes the checks and prints them should not be the same person who signs them. Another example is that the employee who alters pay rates and hours worked must submit a weekly report to a supervisor before the changes take effect. There is also software available to track and monitor employee activity. This software can log what files an employee accesses, if changes were made to files, and if the files were copied. Depending on the number of employees, organizations may also employ a full-time electronic auditor who does nothing but monitor activity logs.

SECURITY TOOLS

There is a wide range of tools available to an organization to protect the organizational network and information. These tools can be either a software solution, such as **antivirus software**, or a hardware tool, such as a **proxy server**. These tools are only effective if used along with employee awareness training. For example, e-mail scanning is a commonly used software tool. All incoming e-mail messages are scanned to ensure they do not contain a virus or some other malicious code. This software can only find viruses that are currently known, so it is important that the virus software be set to search automatically for and download updates. Organizations can further protect themselves by training employees to never open an e-mail attachment unless they are expecting the attachment and they know the sender. Even IT managers have fallen victim to email viruses and sent "affected" emails to everyone in their address book. Help protect an organization from new viruses that may not yet be included in their scanning software by never opening an email attachment unless the sender is known and the attachment is expected. E-mail scanning software and antivirus software should never be turned off and updates should be installed at least weekly, but ideally, daily. Software is also available to scan instant messages and to delete automatically spam e-mail. There are many antivirus and adware software packages available ranging from free to over $25 per month. The main factors to consider when purchasing antivirus software are its effectiveness or the number of viruses it has missed, the ease of installation and use, the effectiveness of the updates, and the help and user support available. There are numerous websites that compare and contrast the most recent antivirus software packages available. Be aware, however, that some of these sites are also selling antivirus software, and thus may be presenting biased information.

Firewalls are another common tool used by organizations to protect their corporate networks when they are attached to the Internet. A firewall can be either hardware or software or a combination of both. A firewall examines all incoming messages or traffic to the network. The firewall can be set up to allow only messages from known senders into the corporate network. Firewalls can also be set up to look at outgoing information from the corporate network. If the message contains some type of corporate secret, the firewall prevents the message from leaving. Firewalls are electronic security guards at the gate of the corporate network. Box 15-1 contains links to short videos explaining Internet security and firewalls.

Proxy servers also protect the organizational network. Proxy servers prevent users from directly accessing the Internet. They must first request passage from the proxy server. The server looks at the request and makes sure the request is from a legitimate user and that the destination of the request is permissible. For example, organizations can block requests to view a website with the word "sex" in the title or the actual uniform resource locator of a known pornography site. The proxy server can also lend the requesting user a **mask** to use while he or she is surfing on the World Wide Web. In this way, the corporation is protecting the identity of its employees. The proxy server keeps track of which employees are using which masks and directs the traffic appropriately.

With hacking becoming more common, healthcare organizations must have some type of protection to avoid this invasion. **Intrusion detection systems** (both hardware and software) allow an organization to monitor who is using the network and what files that user has accessed. Detection systems can be set up to monitor a single computer or an entire network. Corporations must diligently monitor for unauthorized access of their networks. Any time someone uses a secured network, a digital footprint is left of all of their travels, and their use can be easily tracked by electronic auditing software. The Research Brief provides an overview of the HIMSS 2010 Security Survey results that report on progress made by institutions in securing private information.

BOX 15-1

Check out YouTube for the following videos on the Internet and firewalls:

"Warriors on the Net, (Full Version)"
http://www.youtube.com/watch?v=RhvKm0RdUY0

"What is a firewall?"
http://www.youtube.com/watch?v=0_EVfWpL6L4

"Firewalls—An Introduction"
http://www.youtube.com/watch?v=kIAu7mvjBUU&feature=related

Research Brief

Overview of HIMSS 2010 Security Survey

In the 3rd Annual Security Survey, 272 persons who had some responsibility for information security in their organization participated. Roles and titles varied among respondents, such as CIO, senior IT executive, Chief Security Officer or Chief Technology Officer, but all reported responsibility for privacy and information security. Key survey results from the Executive Summary are reproduced here:

Maturity of Environment: Respondents characterized their environment at a middle rate of maturity, with an average score of 4.43 on a scale of one to seven, where one is not at all mature and seven is a high level of maturity.

Security Budget: Approximately half percent of respondents reported that their organization spends three percent or less of their organization's IT budget on information security. However, while this was consistent with what was reported last year, many respondents indicated that their budget actually increased in the past year, primarily as a result of federal initiatives. There is little difference in response in this area by organization type.

Formal Security Position: Slightly more than half (53 percent) of respondents reported they have either a CSO/CISO or full-time staff in place to handle their organizations' security function. Those working for a hospital were more likely to report that they had a CSO/CSIO in place compared to individuals working for medical practices. Also, while 17 percent of respondents working for medical practices indicated that they handled their security function exclusively using external resources. None of the respondents from the hospitals reported that they used external resources exclusively.

Risk Analysis: Slightly more than half of respondents (59 percent) that reported that their organization conducts a formal risk analysis indicated that this type of analysis is conducted annually. Susceptibility to internal threats and external threats are nearly universally included in the risk analysis.

Patient Data Access: Surveyed organizations most widely use user-based and rolebased controls to secure electronic patient information. More than half of respondents from hospital organizations reported that they used two or more types of controls to manage data access, compared to 40 percent of respondents from medical practices. Approximately half of respondents reported that their organization allows patients/surrogates to access electronic patient information.

Management of Security Environment: Nearly all respondents reported that their organization actively works to determine the cause/origin of security breaches and two thirds reported having a plan in place for responding to threats or incidents related to a security breach. Respondents working for the hospital organizations in this sample were more likely to report that they worked to determine the cause/origin of security breaches than were their counterparts at medical practices.

Security in a Networked Environment: Approximately 85 percent of respondents reported that their organization shares patient data in an electronic format. Data is most frequently shared with third party providers, state government, third party providers and other facilities within the corporate organization. While respondents from hospitals are somewhat more likely to report (83 percent) that they will share data in the future than are those from medical practices (77 percent), the likelihood of data sharing in the future is high among both groups.

Future Use of Security Technologies: Mobile device encryption, e-mail encryption and single sign on and were most frequently identified by respondents as technologies that were not presently installed at their organization but were planned for future installation. Respondents from hospitals that were not presently using these technologies are more likely to report installing them in the future, compared to respondents in medical practices.

Patient Identity: Half of respondents indicated that they validate patient identity by both requiring a government/facility-issued ID and checking the ID against information in the master patient index. A similar percent reported that they have a formal process for reconciling duplicate records in their master patient index.

Continues

Research Brief Continued

Medical Identity Theft: One-third of respondents reported that their organization has had at least one known case of medical identity theft at their organization. Those working for a medical practice were much less likely to report that an instance of medical identity theft occurred at their organization (17 percent), when compared to those working for a hospital organization (38 percent).

In summary, undertaking a formal risk analysis and then using the outcomes to change use of controls and make modifications within policies and procedures is required to qualify for Stage One meaningful use incentives. At present, one-quarter of the sample population would not qualify for meaningful use. In addition, establishing a robust security environment is crucial as hospitals and medical practices increasingly share information outside of their organizations (pp. 4–5).

Permission for use of the data is granted in the publication. Individuals are encouraged to cite this report and any accompanying graphics in printed matter, publications, or any other medium, as long as the information is attributed to the 3nd Annual HIMSS Security Survey, sponsored by Intel.

OFF-SITE USE OF PORTABLE DEVICES

Off-site uses of portable devices, such as laptops, personal data assistants (PDA), home computing systems, smart phones, and portable data storage devices, can help to streamline the delivery of health care. For example, home health nurses may need to access electronic protected health information (EPHI) via a wireless laptop connection during a home visit, or a physician might use a PDA to get specific patient information related to a prescription refill in response to a patient request. These mobile devices are invaluable to healthcare efficiency and responsiveness to patient need in such cases. At the very least, agencies should require data encryption when EPHI is being transmitted over unsecured networks or transported on a mobile device as a way of protecting sensitive information. "Hotspots" provided by companies, such as McDonald's, and airports are not secured networks. Virtual private networks must be used to ensure that all data transmitted on unsecured networks is encrypted. The user must log into the virtual private networks actually to reach the organization's network.

Only data essential for the job should be contained on the mobile device, and other nonclinical information, such as Social Security numbers, should never be carried outside the secure network. Some institutions make use of thin clients, which are basic interface portals that do not keep secure information stored on them. Essentially, users must log in to the network to get the data they need. Use of thin clients may be problematic in patient care situations where the user cannot access the network easily. For example, some rural areas of the country still do not have wireless coverage. In these instances, private health information may need to be stored in a clinician's laptop or PDA. This is comparable to home health nurses carrying paper charts in their cars to make home visits, and the responsibilities accompanying such use of private information outside the institution's walls.

What happens if one of these devices is lost or stolen? The agency is ultimately responsible for the integrity of the data contained on these devices and is required by HIPAA regulations (Department of Health and Human Services, 2006) to have policies in place covering such items as appropriate remote use, removal of devices from their usual physical location, and how these devices are to be protected from loss or theft. Simple rules, such as covering laptops left in a car and locking car doors during transport of mobile devices containing EPHI, can help to deter theft. If a device is lost or stolen, the agency must have clear procedures in place to help ensure that sensitive data are not released or used inappropriately. Software packages that provide for physical tracking of the static and mobile computer inventory including laptops and PDAs are being used more widely and help in the recovery of lost or stolen devices. In addition, some software that allows for remote data deletion in the event of theft or loss of a mobile device can be invaluable to the agency in preventing the release of EPHI.

If a member of an agency is caught accessing EPHI inappropriately or steals a mobile device, the sanctions should be swift and public. Sanctions may range from a warning or suspension with retraining to termination or prosecution depending on the severity of the security breach. The sanctions must send a clear message to all that protecting EPHI is serious business.

The Department of Health and Human Services (2006) identifies potential risks and proposes risk management strategies for accessing, storing, and transmitting EPHI. Visit the following website for detailed tabular information (pp. 4–6) on potential risks and risk management strategies: http://www.cms.hhs.gov/Security Standard/Downloads/SecurityGuidanceforRemoteUseFinal122806.pdf.

SUMMARY

Technology changes so quickly that even the most diligent user will likely encounter a situation that could constitute a threat to their network. Organizations must provide their users with the proper training to avoid known threats but more importantly to be able to discern a possible new threat. Consider that 10 years ago wireless networks were the exception to the rule, where today access to wireless networks is almost taken for granted. How will computer networks be accessed 10 years from now? The most important concept to remember from this chapter is that the only completely safe network is one that is turned off. **Network accessibility** and **network availability** are necessary evils that pose security risks. The information must be available to be accessed yet secured from hackers, unauthorized users, and any other potential security breaches. In an ideal world, everyone would understand the potential threats to fair use and network security and diligently monitor for unauthorized access of their networks, data, and information.

THOUGHT-PROVOKING Questions

WWW

1. Jean, a diabetes nurse educator, recently read an article in an online journal that she accessed through her health agency's database subscription. The article provided a comprehensive checklist for managing diabetes in older adults, which she prints and distributes to her patients in a diabetes education class. Does this constitute fair use or is this a copyright violation?

2. Sue is a chronic obstructive pulmonary disorder clinic nurse enrolled in a master's education program. She is interested in writing a paper on the factors that are associated with poor compliance with medical regimens and associated repeat hospitalization of chronic obstructive pulmonary disorder patients. She downloads patient information from the clinic database to a thumb drive that she later accesses on her home computer. Sue understands rules about privacy of information and believes that because she is a nurse and needs this information for a graduate school assignment she is entitled to the information. Is Sue correct in her thinking?

For a full suite of assignments and additional learning activities, use the access code located in the front of your book to visit this exclusive website: http://go.jblearning.com/mcgonigle. If you do not have an access code, you can obtain one at the site.

WWW

References

3nd Annual HIMSS Security Survey, sponsored by Intel. Retrieved from http://www.himss.org/content/ files/2010_HIMSS_SecuritySurvey.pdf

Degaspari, J. (2010). Staying ahead of the curve on data security. *Healthcare Informatics 27*(10):32-36. Retrieved from http://www.healthcare-informatics.com/ME2/dirmod.asp?sid=9B6FFC446FF 74869 81EA3C0C3CCE4943&nm=Articles%2FNews&type=Publishing&mod=Publications%3A% 3AArticle&mid=8F3A7027421841978F18BE895F87F791&tier=4&id=35F1496AE0B144D3A9716 D5D9C2D03CF

Department of Health and Human Services. (2006). *HIPAA security guidance*. Retrieved from Security Guidance for Remote Use Website: http://www.cms.hhs.gov/SecurityStandard/Downloads/ Security GuidanceforRemoteUseFinal122806.pdf

Gross, G. (2003). *Human error causes most security breaches.* InfoWorld. Retrieved from http://www
  .infoworld.com/article/03/03/18/HNhumanerror_1.html

Mowry, M., & Oakes, R. (n.d.). *Not too tight, not too loose.* Healthcare Informatics, Healthcare IT
  Leadership, Vision & Strategy. Retrieved from http://www.healthcare-informatics.com/ME2/
  dirmod.asp?nm=&type=Publishing&mod=Publications%3A%3AArticle&mid=8F3A702742184
  1978F18BE895F87F791&tier=4&id=B7823E299AC64041AC3F253CE19DF298

CHAPTER 16

Nursing Informatics: Improving Workflow and Meaningful Use

Denise Hammel-Jones

If you want to truly understand something, try to change it. ~ Kurt Lewin

Objectives

1. Provide an overview of the purpose of conducting workflow analysis and design.
2. Deliver specific instructions on workflow analysis and redesign techniques.
3. Cite measures of efficiency and effectiveness that can be applied to redesign efforts.

Key Terms

American Recovery and Reinvestment Act
Barcode medication administration
Clinical transformation
Computerized provider order entry
Electronic medical records
Events
Health information exchanges
Health information technology
Information systems
Interactions
Meaningful use
Medical home/health information exchange
Metrics
Process analysis
Process owners
Quality
Six Sigma/Lean
Tasks
Workflow
Workflow analysis
Work process

INTRODUCTION

The healthcare environment has grown more complex and continues to evolve every day. The complexities that help clinicians to deliver better care and improved patient outcomes also take a toll on clinicians themselves. This toll is exemplified through hours spent learning new technology, loss in productivity as the user adjusts and adapts to new technology, and the "unintended workflow consequences" from the use of technology.

Despite the perceived negative downstream effects to end-users and patients as a result of technology, this very same technology can improve efficiency and yield a leaner healthcare environment. This chapter outlines the driving forces that create the need to redesign workflow, how to conduct workflow redesign, and how to measure the impact of workflow changes.

Research Brief

Mazur and Chen (2009), in a study designed to identify workflow issues related to a medication delivery system, emphasize that the "underestimation of the impact of basic workflow analysis on operational failures appears to dominate the healthcare industry, ultimately subjecting patients to significant risks" (p. 57). They used the Toyota Production Systems model to first identify where workflow issues occurred in medication administration and then to develop a robust workflow model that would minimize errors. In their data collection and analysis, they discovered three issues that contributed to medication errors, productivity pressures, nurses and technicians felt stress related to efficiency requirements; group behavior that indirectly supported noncompliance with standard procedures to increase efficiency and group behaviors that condoned under reporting of medication errors; and compliance/autonomy where professionals did not comply with specified procedures. As a result Mazur and Chen specified two workflow design rules that must be implemented in an un-autonomous culture to improve medication administration workflow:

- Highly specify all medication delivery workflow procedures as to content, sequence, timing, outcome and resources used.
- Make every connection (communication) unambiguous and feedback capable to confirm all requests and receive responses (p. 62–63).

Source: Mazur, L. & Chen, S. (2009). An empirical study for medication delivery improvement based on healthcare professionals' perceptions of medication delivery system. *Health Care Management Science, 12*(1), 56–66. Retrieved from ABI/INFORM Global. (Document ID: 1636187001).

WORKFLOW ANALYSIS PURPOSE

An astounding 98,000 Americans are injured each year as a result of medication errors (Institute of Medicine [IOM], 1999). Not only is there an impact on patients from these errors but there is also a significant financial impact to healthcare organizations. The IOM report suggests many actions to improve care delivery and minimize error, but one of the most important tools to use is electronic records and **information systems** to provide point-of-care decision support and automation.

Technology provides a mechanism to improve care delivery and create a safer patient environment provided it is implemented appropriately and considers the surrounding workflow. In an important article by Campbell, Guappone, Sittig, Dykstra, and Ash (2009), the authors suggest that technology implemented without consideration of workflow can provide greater patient safety concerns than no technology at all. This article represents the second installment of research surrounding **computerized provider order entry** (CPOE) and focuses more specifically on workflow considerations. Ash, Stavri, and Kuperman (2003) refer to these workflow implications as the unintended consequences of CPOE implementation, and they are just some of the effects of poorly implemented technology. This landmark publication and other sources, such as the Healthcare Information Management Systems Society (2010) ME-PI Toolkit, address workflow redesign and why it is so critical to successful technology implementations.

Technology is recognized to have a potentially positive effect on patient outcomes, but even with the promise of improving how care is delivered technology has been slow to adopt. The cost of technology solutions, such as CPOE, **barcode medication administration**, and **electronic medical records**, remains staggeringly high. The cost of technology coupled with lengthy timelines has made this endeavor out of reach for many healthcare organizations. Technology timelines for complex clinical technologies are lengthy and upgrades or enhancements to the technology are necessary either mid-implementation or shortly after a launch leaving little time to focus efforts on the optimization of the technology within the current workflow. Furthermore, the existence of technology does not in itself guarantee that it is being used in a manner that promotes better outcomes for patients.

Given sluggish adoption of technology, in 2009 the United States government for the first time recognized the importance **health information technology** has on patient care outcomes. Through the **American Recovery and Reinvestment Act** (ARRA) healthcare organizations can qualify for financial incentives based on the level of **meaningful use** achieved. To qualify for the incentives, the data to support the 25 meaningful use measures must be gathered and reported on electronically, necessitating the use of technology in all patient care areas. Additionally, a fundamental aspect of meaningful use is the assurance that a significant number of healthcare providers have adopted technology. Meaningful use measures will push healthcare organizations to re-examine the use of clinical technologies within their organization and approach implementation in a new way.

Not only is there a potential for patient safety and **quality** issues from technology implementations that do not address workflow, but a financial impact to the organization is also possible. All organizations regardless of industry must operate efficiently to maintain profits and continue to provide services to their customers. For hospitals that normally have significantly smaller profit margins than other organizations the need to maintain efficient and effective care is essential for survival. With hospital profit margins diminishing, never has there been a more crucial time to examine the cost of errors, poorly designed workflow, and the financial burden this presents to an organization. Moreover, what are the costs to an organization for failing to address the integration of technology? This is an area where there are little supporting data to substantiate the claim that technology without workflow considerations can impact the bottom line.

Today, many healthcare organizations are experiencing the effects of poorly implemented clinical technology solutions, manifested in the form of redundant documentation, non–value-add steps, and additional time spent at the computer rather than in direct care delivery. A recent study by the University of Maryland indicated that nursing is spending the equivalent of one full-time equivalent (FTE) per year at a computer instead of on direct patient care. Technology ought not to be implemented for the sake of automation unless there are gains in patient outcomes and proper workflow. In fact, the cost to organizations for duplicate and redundant documentation by nursing can range from $6,500 to $13,000 per nurse, per year (Clancy, Delaney, Morrison, & Gunn, 2006).

Examining the workflow surrounding the use of technology enables better use of the technology and more efficient work. It also promotes safer patient care delivery. The focus on workflow and technology has gained increasing importance and recognition; however, there remains a dearth of literature to address the importance of this area. As more organizations work to achieve a level of technology adoption that enables them to receive ARRA financial incentives more attention will likely be given to the area of workflow design, leading to a greater body of research and evidence.

WORKFLOW AND TECHNOLOGY

Workflow is a term used to describe the action or execution of a series of **tasks** in a prescribed sequence. Another definition of workflow is a progression of steps (tasks, **events**, and **interactions**) that comprise a **work process;** involve two or more persons; and create or add value to the organization's activities. In a sequential workflow, each step is dependent on the occurrence of the previous step; in a parallel workflow, two or more steps can occur concurrently. The term "workflow" is sometimes used interchangeably with process or process flows, particularly when used in the context of implementations. Observation and documentation of workflow to understand better what is happening in the current environment and how it can be altered is referred to as "process" or "**workflow analysis**." A typical output of workflow analysis is a visual depiction of the process, which is called a "process map." The process map ranges from simplistic to fairly complex and provides an excellent tool to identify specific steps. The process map also can provide a vehicle for communication and a tool on which to build educational materials and policies and procedures.

One school of thought suggests that technology should be designed to meet the needs of clinical workflow. This model implies that system analysts have a high degree of control over screen layout and data capture. It also implies that technology is malleable enough to allow for the flexibility to adapt to a variety of workflow scenarios. Lessons learned from over three decades of clinical technology implementations suggest that clinical technologies still have a long path on the road to maturity to allow this to be possible. The second and most prevalent thought process is that workflow should be adapted to the use of technology. This is by far the most commonly used model given the progress of clinical technology.

A concept that has gained popularity within recent years relative to workflow redesign is clinical transformation. **Clinical transformation** by definition is the complete alteration of the clinical environment and therefore should be used cautiously to describe redesign efforts. Earl, Sampler, and Short (1995) define transformation as "a radical change approach that produces a more responsive organization that is more capable of performing in unstable and changing environments that organizations continue to be faced with" (p. 31). Many workflow redesign efforts are focused on relatively small changes and not the widespread change that accompanies transformational activities. Moreover, clinical transformation implies that the manner in which work is carried out and the outcomes achieved are completely different than the prior state, which is not always true in the case of simply implementing technology. Technology can be used to launch or in conjunction with a clinical transformation initiative; however, the implementation of technology alone is not justifiably transformational. Before undertaking transformative initiatives:

Leadership must take the lead and create a case for transformation
Establish a vision for the end-point
Allow those with specific expertise to provide the details
Think about the most optimal experience for the patient and clinician
Do not replicate the current state
Focus on those initiatives that offer greatest value to organization
Understand that small gains have no real impact on transformation

OPTIMIZATION

Most of what is discussed in this chapter is related to workflow analysis in conjunction with implementation of technology; however, it should be noted that not all workflow analysis and redesign occurs before the implementation of technology. Some analysis and redesign efforts may occur weeks, months, or even years after the implementation. When workflow analysis occurs post-implementation it is often referred to as "optimization." Optimization is the process of moving conditions past their current state and into more efficient and effective methods of performing tasks. The Merriam-Webster Online Dictionary (2010) considers optimization the act, process, or methodology of making something (as a design, system, or decision) as fully perfect, functional, or effective as possible. Some organizations routinely engage in optimization efforts after an implementation and other organizations may undertake this activity in response to clinician concerns or marked change in operational performance.

Furthermore, workflow analysis can be conducted as a stand-alone effort, or as part of an operational improvement event. When process is addressed alone this is process improvement. Nursing informatics should always be included in these activities to represent the needs of clinicians and to serve as liaison for technologic solutions to process problems. Additionally, informaticists will likely become operationally focused and will need to transform their role accordingly to address workflow in an overall capacity and respective to technology. Hospitals operate with smaller profit margins than other industries and these profits will continue to diminish forcing organizations to function smarter not harder, and to accomplish this using technology.

If optimization efforts are undertaken the need to revisit workflow design should not be considered a flaw in the implementation approach. Even a well-designed future state workflow during a technology implementation must be re-examined post-implementation to ensure that what was projected about the future state remains valid and to incorporate any additional workflow elements into the process redesign.

Exploring the topic of workflow analysis with regard to clinical technology implementation will yield considerably fewer literature results than other topical areas of implementation. More research is needed in the area of financial implication of workflow inefficiencies and impact on patient care. Time studies require an investment of resources and may be subject to patient privacy issues and the challenges of capturing time measurements on processes that are not exactly replicable. Another confounding factor affecting the quality and quantity of workflow research is the lack of standardized terminology for this area. A comprehensive literature search was conducted and published through the Agency for Healthcare Quality and Research in 2008 as an evidence-based handbook for nurses. This literature search yielded findings indicating that a lack of publications and standardized terminology in the area of workflow have made this a difficult topic to support through research findings.

What all organizations ultimately strive for is efficient and effective delivery of patient care. The terminology of efficient and effective is widely known in quality areas or **Six Sigma** and **Lean** departments but not necessarily known or used in informatics. Effective delivery of care or workflow suggests that the process or end product is in the most desirable state. An efficient delivery of care or workflow means that little waste, or unnecessary motion, transportation, over-processing, or defects were incurred. Health systems, such as Virginia Mason University Medical Center, have experienced significant quality and cost gains from the widespread implementation of Lean throughout their organization.

Case Study

In my experience consulting, I have seen several examples of organizations that incorporate the printing of paper reports, which replicate information that has been entered and is available with the electronic patient record. These reports are often reviewed, signed, and acted on instead of the electronic information. Despite the knowledge that the information contained in these reports was outdated the moment the report was printed and the very nature of using the report for workflow is an inefficient practice, this method of clinical workflow is prevalent in many hospitals across the United States. There is an underlying fear that drives the decision to mold a paper-based workflow around clinical technology. There is also a lack of the appropriate amount of integration that would otherwise allow this information to be available in an electronic form.

WORKFLOW ANALYSIS AND INFORMATICS PRACTICE

The American Nurses Association (ANA, 2008) defines nine functional areas of practice for the informatics nurse specialist. The functional area of analysis identifies the specific functional qualities related to workflow analysis. Particularly, the *Nursing Informatics: Scope and Standard of Practice* indicates that the informatics nurse specialist should develop techniques necessary to assess and improve the human–computer interaction. It is important to note that workflow analysis is not only relevant to analysis but is part of every functional area in which the informatics nurse specialist engages. The functional area of consultants, researchers, and other areas needs to understand workflow and how lack of efficient workflow impacts patient care.

A critical aspect of the informatics role is workflow design. Nursing informatics is uniquely positioned to engage in the analysis and redesign of processes and tasks surrounding the use of technology. The ANA cites workflow redesign as one of the fundamental skills sets that make up the discipline of this specialty. Moreover, workflow analysis should be part of every technology implementation and the role of the informaticist within this team is to direct others in the execution of this task or to perform the task directly.

Unfortunately, many nurses find themselves in an informatics capacity without sufficient preparation for a **process analysis** role. One area of practice that is particularly susceptible to inadequate preparation is the ability to facilitate process analysis. Workflow analysis requires careful attention to detail, the ability to moderate group discussion, organizing concepts, and generating solutions. These skills can be acquired through a formal academic informatics program or through courses that teach the discipline Six Sigma or Lean by example. Regardless of where these skills are acquired, it is important to understand that they will continue to remain a vital aspect of the informatics role.

Some organizations have believed strongly enough in the need for workflow analysis that departments have been created to address this very need. Whether the department carries the name of clinical excellence, organizational effectiveness, or Six Sigma/Lean it is nevertheless critical to recognize the value this group can offer technology implementations and clinicians overall. As one examines how workflow analysis is conducted it is important to note that although the nursing informaticist is an essential member of the team to participate in or enable workflow analysis, a team dedicated to this effort is necessary for its success.

BUILDING THE DESIGN TEAM

The workflow redesign team is an interdisciplinary team consisting of "**process owners.**" Process owners are those who directly engage in the workflow to be analyzed and redesigned. They are individuals who can speak about the intricacy of process, including process variations from the norm. When constructing the team include individuals who are able to contribute information about the exact current state workflow and offer suggestions for future state improvement. Individuals on the workflow redesign team should also have the authority to make decisions about how the process should be redesigned. This authority is sometimes issued by managers or could come from participation of the managers directly. This careful blend of decision makers and "process owners" can be difficult to assemble but is critical for forming the team and enabling success. Often, individuals at the manager level want to participate exclusively in the redesign process. Although having management participate provides the advantage of having decision makers and management level buy-in, these individuals may also make erroneous assumptions about how the process should be versus how the process truly occurs. Conversely, including only process owners who do not possess the authority to make decisions can slow the work of the team down while decisions are made outside the group sessions.

Team focus needs to occur at the outset of assembling the team. Decisions on what workflow will be examined is a decision that the team should make early on in the effort to avoid confusion or spending unnecessary time on workflow that does not ultimately matter to the outcome. In the early stages of workflow redesign the team defines the beginning and end of a process and a few high-level steps of the process. Avoid focusing on process steps in great detail in the beginning because the conversation can get sidetracked, and do not spend time focusing on details and not moving along at a good pace. Six Sigma expert George Eckes uses the phrase "stay as high as you can as long as you can," which is a good catch phrase to remember to keep the team focused and at a high level. The pace at which any implementation team progresses ultimately impacts the overall timeline of a project. Therefore, focus and speed are skills the informatics expert should develop and use throughout every initiative, particularly when addressing workflow redesign.

The workflow redesign team develops a detailed process map after agreement is reached on the current state process beginning and end points and a high-level map depicting major process steps is finalized. Because workflow crosses many different care providers it may be useful to construct the process map using a swim-lane technique (Figure 16-1). A swim-lane technique uses such categories as functional workgroups and roles to depict visually groups of work and who performs the work. The swim-lane map shows how workflow and data transitions to clinicians and can demonstrate areas of potential process and information breakdowns.

It may take several sessions of analysis to complete a process map as details are uncovered and workarounds discussed. There is a tendency for individuals who participate in process redesign sessions to describe workflow as they believe it to be occurring rather than how it is in reality. It is the role of the informatics expert

FIGURE
16-1

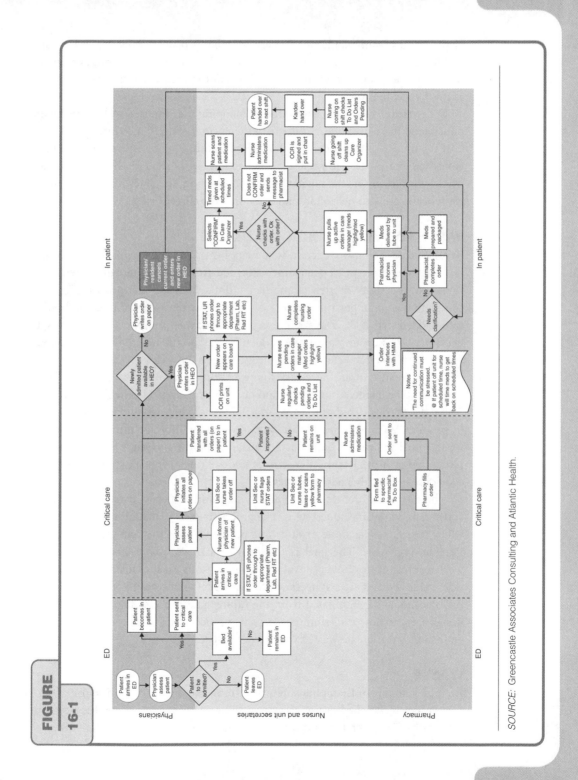

SOURCE: Greencastle Associates Consulting and Atlantic Health.

or the process team facilitator to determine what is really happening and to capture it accurately. Regardless of whether a swim-lane or simplistic process map design is used the key is to capture enough detail to portray the process accurately as it is happening today.

Other techniques aside from process mapping may be used to help the team understand the workflow as it exists in the current state. The future state workflow planning will only be as good as the reliability of the current state can provide; therefore, partake in whatever other actions are needed to understand better what is happening in the current state. Observation, interviews, and process or waste-walks are also helpful in understanding the current state.

VALUE ADD VERSUS NON–VALUE ADD

Beyond analysis of tasks, current state mapping provides the opportunity for the process redesign team to determine value add from non–value add activities. A value-added activity or step is one that ultimately brings the process closer to completion or changes the product or service for the better. An example of a value-added step is placing a name tag on a specimen sample. The name tag is necessary for laboratory personnel to identify the specimen and therefore is an essential or value-added step in the process. Some steps in a process do not necessarily add value but are necessary for regulatory or compliance reasons. These steps are still considered necessary and need to be included in the future process. A step that is considered non–value added does not alter the outcome of a process or product. Such activities as handling, moving, and holding are not considered value-added and should be evaluated during workflow analysis. Manipulating papers, moving through computer screens, and walking or transporting items are all considered non–value add activities.

The five "whys" represent one technique to drive toward determining value-add versus non–value added steps. The process redesign facilitator asks the group why a specific task is done or done in a particular way through a series of questions asking "why." The goal is to uncover tasks that came about because of workarounds or for other unsubstantiated reasons. Tasks that are considered non–value add and are not necessary for the purpose of compliance or regulatory reasons should be eliminated from the future state process. The purpose in redesigning workflow is to eliminate steps in a process that do not add value to the end-state or that create waste by their very nature.

WASTE

An underpinning of Lean philosophy is the removal of waste activities from workflow. Waste is classified as unnecessary activities or an excess of products to perform tasks. The seven categories listed below are the mostly widely recognized:

1. Overproduction: pace is faster than necessary to support process
2. Waiting
3. Transport
4. Inappropriate processing: over processing
5. Unnecessary inventory: excess stock
6. Unnecessary motion: bending, lifting, moving, and so forth
7. Defects: reproduction

VARIATION

Variation in workflow is considered the enemy of all good processes and therefore should always be eliminated when possible. Variation occurs when workers perform the same function in different ways and usually occurs because of flaws in the way a process was originally designed, lack of knowledge about the process, or because a process cannot be executed as originally designed because of disruption or disturbances in the workflow. Examining the process as it currently exists today helps to identify variation. A brief word about variation that cannot be eliminated; processes that involve highly customized products or services are generally not conducive to standardization and the elimination of variation inherent to the process.

Some argue that delivery of care is subject to variation by its very nature and the individual needs of patients. There is little doubt that each patient's care should be tailored to meet their specific needs; however, there are common processes that can be standardized and improved on without jeopardizing care.

TRANSITIONING TO FUTURE STATE

After redesign efforts regardless of whether they occurred during or after an implementation or as a stand-alone process improvement event, steps must be taken to ensure that change takes hold and the new workflow continues after the support team has disbanded. Management support and involvement during the transition phase is essential because management is necessary to enforce new workflow procedures and further define and refine roles and responsibilities. Documentation of the future state workflow should have occurred during the redesign effort but does not completely conclude until after the redesign is complete and the workflow has become operational. Policy and procedures are addressed and rewritten to encompass the changes to workflow and role assignment. Helpdesk, system analyst, nursing education, and other support personnel need to be educated to the workflow specifics as part of the post-improvement effort. It is considered good practice to involve the operational staff in the future process discussions and planning to incorporate specifics of these areas and ensure the buy-in of the staff.

When workflow changes begin to fail and workarounds develop this is a signal that something is flawed about the way in which the new process was constructed and further evaluation is needed. The workflow redesign team is brought together to review and if necessary, redesign the process.

Future state is constructed with the best possible knowledge of how the process will ideally work. To move from the current state to the future state gap analysis is necessary. Gap analysis zeros in on the major areas most affected by the change, namely technology. What often happens in redesign efforts is an exact or near-exact replication of the current state using automation. The gap analysis discussion should generate ideas from the group about how best to use the technology to transform practice. It is prudent to consider having legal and risk representatives at the table when initiating future state discussions to know the parameters the group should work within; however, do not use existing parameters as the only boundaries.

Future state process maps become the basis of educational materials for end users, communication tools for the project team, and the foundation of new policies and procedures. Simplified process maps provide an excellent schematic for communication change.

INFORMATICS AS A CHANGE AGENT

Technology implementations alone represent a significant change for clinicians as does the workflow redesign that accompanies technology. Often the degree of change and its impact is underappreciated and unaccounted for by leadership and staff alike. A typical response to change is anger, frustration, and a refusal to accept the proposed change. All of these responses are expected and need to be accounted for so that early on a plan to address the emotional side of change is developed. Every workflow redesign effort should begin with a change management plan. Engagement of the end-user is a critical aspect of change management and therefore adoption. Without end-user involvement, change is resisted and efforts are subject to failure. Users are engaged and brought into the prospective change through question and answer forums, technology demonstrations, frequent communications regarding change, and as department-specific representatives in working meetings.

There are many change theories to explore but regardless of the change theory adopted by the informatics specialist communication, planning, and support are key factors of any change management strategy. Informaticists should become knowledgeable about at least one change theory and use this knowledge as the basis for change management planning as part of every effort. John Kotter, one of the most recognized change theorists, suggests the following conditions to deal with change in an organization (Kotter, 1996):

Education and communication
Participation and involvement
Facilitation and support
Negotiation and agreement
Manipulation and co-optation
Explicit and implicit coercion

In the HIMSS (2009) nursing informatics impact survey, nursing informaticists were identified as the most significant resource among a project team to impact adoption and change management. The nurse brings the ability to interact with various clinicians, knowledge of clinical practice, and the ability to empathize with the clinicians as they experience the impact of workflow change. These innate skills differentiate the nursing informaticist from other members of the implementation team and are highly desirable in the informatics community.

It must be kept in mind that regardless of the change management techniques used by the informatics specialist and the project team, adoption of technology and workflow may be slow to evolve. Change is often a slow process that requires continual positive reinforcement and involvement of supporting resources. Failure to achieve strong adoption results early on is not necessarily a failure of the methods used but may be caused by other factors not entirely within the control of the informaticist.

Perhaps a complete alteration in behavior is not possible but modifications to behaviors to support a desired outcome are possible. Similar to the individual who stops smoking, the desire for the cigarette remains but the behavior has been modified to no longer sustain smoking. To manage change in an organization, modify behavior to produce the intended outcome.

Change takes hold when there is strong leadership support. This support manifests itself as a visible presence to staff, clear and concise communications, an unwavering position, and an open door policy to field concerns about change. Too often, leadership gives verbal endorsement of change and then fails to follow-through with actions or withdraws their support when the going gets tough. Inevitably, if leadership wavers so too will staff.

MEASURING THE RESULTS

Metrics provide understanding about the performance of a process or function. Typically, within clinical technology projects one identifies and collects specific metrics about the performance of the technology or metrics that capture the level of participation or adoption. Equally important is the need for process performance metrics. Process metrics are collected at the initial stage of a project or problem identification. Current state metrics are then benchmarked against internal indicators. When there are no internal indicators to benchmark against, a suitable course of action is to benchmark against an external source, such as a similar business practice within a different industry. Consider examining the hotel room changeover strategy or the customer service approach of Disney or the Ritz Carlton to determine suitable metrics for a particular project or focus area.

The right workflow compliment provides the organization with the data they need to understand operational and clinical performance. This area is highlighted through the need for healthcare organizations to capture meaningful use measures. Good metrics should tell the story of accomplishment. The presence of technology alone does not guarantee an organization's ability to capture and report on these measures without also addressing the surrounding workflow. Metrics should focus on the variables of time, quality, and costs. Table 16-1 provides examples of metrics.

The ARRA highlights the need to collect information that represents the impact of technology on patient outcomes. Furthermore, data are necessary to demonstrate how a process is performing in its current state. Despite ARRA, the need to collect data to demonstrate improvement in workflow remains strong yet all too often is absent in implementations or redesign efforts. A team cannot demonstrate improvements on an existing process without collecting information about how the process is currently performing. Current state measures also help the process team validate that the correct area for improvement was identified. Once a process improvement effort is over and the new solution has been implemented, post-improvement measures should be gathered to demonstrate progress.

In some organizations, the informatics professional has a reporting structure to the Director of Operations or the Chief Operations Officer. In this relationship, the need to demonstrate operational measures is even stronger. Operational measures, such as turnaround times, throughput, and equipment or technology availability are some of the measures captured.

FUTURE DIRECTIONS

Workflow analysis is not an optional part of clinical implementations. It is a necessity for safe patient care fostered by technology. The ultimate goal of workflow analysis is not to "pave the cow path" but rather create a future state solution that maximizes the use of technology and eliminates non–value add activities.

TABLE 16-1

Turnaround times	Cycle times	Throughput
Change over time	Set-up time	System availability
Patient satisfaction	Employee satisfaction	

Although there are many tools to accomplish workflow redesign the best method is the one that compliments the organization and supports the work of clinicians. Redesigning how people do work evidentially creates change and therefore the nursing informaticist needs to apply change management principles for the new way of doing things to take hold.

Workflow analysis has been described in this chapter within the context of the most widely accepted tools that are fundamentally linked to the concepts of Six Sigma and Lean. Other methods of workflow analysis exist and may become commonly used to assess clinical workflow. An example of an alternate workflow analysis tool is the use of radiofrequency badges to detect movement within a defined clinical area. Clinician and patient movement are tracked using these devices and corresponding actions are documented painting the picture of workflow for a specific area (Vankipuram, 2010.)

Another example of workflow analysis is the use of modeling software. An application, such as ProModel, provides images of the clinical work area where clinician workflows can be plotted out and reconfigured best to suit the needs of a specific area. Simulation applications enable decision-makers to visualize realistic scenarios and draw conclusions about how to leverage resources, implement technology, and improve performance. ProModel, cited here, is one example of a simulation application; however, there are other vendors in this marketplace including Maya and Autodesk.

Health care must examine how other industries have analyzed and addressed workflow to streamline business practices and improve quality outputs, to glean best practices to incorporate into the clinical and business approach. An organization must step outside itself and recognize that not all aspects of patient care are unique and therefore many aspects can be subject to standardization. Many models of workflow redesign from manufacturing and the service sector can be extrapolated to health care. The healthcare industry is facing difficult economic times and can benefit from performance improvement strategies used in other industries.

Although workflow analysis principles are described within the context of acute and ambulatory care, the need to perform process analysis on a macro level

Research Brief

One reason for studying workflow processes is to improve efficiency and thus impact cost by using resources effectively. Marjamaa, Torkki, Hirvensalo, and Kirvelä (2009) used computer simulation technology to compare workflow models to improve operating room scheduling and efficiency. They compared the traditional model where anesthesia induction takes place in the room to alternative models: an operating room with a separate but connected induction room; a circulating induction team; a centralized multi-bed induction room; and four teams in four rooms for three surgeons. They considered labor costs, number of procedures performed, and under and over-utilized time. They determined that all of the alternative models were more efficient than the traditional model. The value of this study is two-fold in that it provides insight into how workflow processes can be studied using computer modeling, and it provides information related to planning and redesign of operating rooms.

Source: Marjamaa, R., Torkki, P., Hirvensalo, E., & Kirvelä, O. (2009). What is the best workflow for an operating room? A simulation study of five scenarios. *Health Care Management Science, 12*(2), 142-6. Retrieved from ABI/INFORM Global. (Document ID: 1673784291).

will expand as more organizations move forward with **health information exchanges** and **medical home** models. Health information exchanges require the nursing informaticist to visualize how patients move through the entire continuum of care and not just a select patient care area.

As technology initiatives become increasingly complex, nursing informaticists need greater preparation in the areas of process analysis and improvement techniques to meet growing technologic challenges and operational performance demands of fiscally impaired healthcare organizations.

SUMMARY

Workflow redesign is a critical aspect of technology implementation and when done well yields technology that is more likely to achieve the intended patient outcomes and safety benefits. Nursing informatics professionals are taking on a greater role with respect to workflow design and this aspect of practice will grow in light of meaningful use-driven objectives. Other initiatives that impact hospital performance will also drive informatics professionals to influence how technology is used in the context of workflow to improve on the bottom line. In an ideal world, nurse informaticists who are experts at workflow analysis will be core members of every technology implementation team.

THOUGHT-PROVOKING Questions

WWW

1. What do you perceive as the current obstacles to redesigning workflow within your clinical settings?
2. Thinking about your last implementation, were you able to challenge the policies and practices that comprise today's workflow or were you able to create a workflow solution that eliminated non–value add steps?
3. Is the workflow surrounding technology usage providing the organization with the data they need to make decisions and eventually meet meaningful use criteria?
4. How does current educational preparation need to change to address the skills necessary to perform workflow analysis and redesign clinical processes?

For a full suite of assignments and additional learning activities, use the access code located in the front of your book to visit this exclusive website: http://go.jblearning.com/mcgonigle. If you do not have an access code, you can obtain one at the site.

WWW

References

Agency for Healthcare Research and Quality. (2008). *Patient safety and quality: An evidence-based handbook for nurses.* Retrieved from http://www.ahrq.gov/qual/nurseshdbk/

American Nurses Association (2008). *Nursing informatics: Scope and standards of practice.* Silver Spring, MD: American Nurses Association.

Ash, J., Stavri, P., & Kuperman, G. (2003). The practice of informatics. Synthesis of research paper. A consensus statement on considerations for a successful CPOE implementation. *Journal of the American Medical Informatics Association (JAMIA), 10,* 229–234.

Campbell, E., Guappone, K., Sittig, D., Dykstra, R., & Ash, J. (2009). Computerized provider order entry adoption: Implications for clinical workflow. *Journal of General Internal Medicine, 24*(1), 21–26.

Clancy, T., Delaney, C., Morrison, B., & Gunn, J. (2006). The benefits of standardized nursing languages in complex adaptive systems such as hospitals. *Journal of Nursing Administration, 36*(9), 426-434. Earl, M., Sampler, J., & Short, J. (1995). Strategies for business process reengineering: Evidence from field studies . *Journal of Management Information Systems, 12*(1), 31–56.

Earl, M., Sampler, J., & Short, J. (1995). Strategies for Business Process Reengineering: Evidence from Field Studies. *Journal of Management Information Systems, 12*(1), 31–56.

Healthcare Information Management Systems Society. (2009). *Nursing informatics impact study.* Retrieved from http://himss.org/content/files/HIMSS2009NursingInformaticsImpactSurveyFull Results.pdf

Healthcare Information Management Systems Society. (2010). *ME-PI Toolkit: Process management, workflow & mapping: Tools, tips and case studies to support the understanding, optimizing and monitoring of processes.* Retrieved from http://www.himss.org/ASP/topics_FocusDynamic.asp?faid=322

Kotter, J. (1996). Leading change. *Harvard Business Press. 1st Edition.* pp. 33–147.

Merriam-Webster Online Dictionary. (2010). *Optimization.* Retrieved from http://www.merriam-webster.com/dictionary/optimization

Institute of Medicine. (1999). *To err is human: Building a better health system.* Washington, DC: National Academy Press.

Vankipuram, K. (2010). Toward automated workflow analysis and visulization in clinical environment. *Journal of Biomedical Informatics,* doi.10.1016/jbi.2010.05.015.

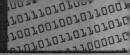

Nursing Informatics Practice Applications: Care Delivery

Nursing information systems must support nurses as they fulfill their roles delivering quality patient care. The system must be responsive to nurses' needs, allowing them to manage their data and information as needed and providing access to necessary references, literature sources, and other networked departments. Nurses have always practiced in a field where they have had to use their ingenuity, resourcefulness, creativity, initiative, and skills. To improve patient care and advance the science of nursing, clinicians as knowledge workers also need to apply these same abilities and skills to become astute users of available information systems.

In this section the reader learns about clinical practice tools, electronic health records, and clinical information systems; consumer information and education needs; population and community health tools; telehealth and telenursing; and informatics tools to enhance patient safety. Many of the chapters in this section were contributed by informatics experts from around the world. Although there may be some similarities in the information presented, it is important to preserve the perspective provided by these expert contributors.

Information systems, electronic documentation, and electronic health records are changing the way nurses and physicians practice. Nursing informatics systems are also changing how patients enter and receive data and information. Some institutions are permitting patient access to their own records electronically via the Internet. Confidentiality and privacy issues loom with the new electronic systems. HIPAA regulations (covered in Section III) and professional ethics principles (covered in Section I) must remain at the forefront when clinicians interact electronically with intimate patient data and information.

The material within this book is placed within the context of the Foundation of Knowledge model (Figure IV-1) to meet the needs of healthcare delivery systems, organizations, patients, and nurses. The reader should continue to assess where they are in the model. The Foundation of Knowledge model reflects that knowledge is powerful, and for that reason, nurses focus on information as a key resource. This section addresses the information systems that clinicians interact with in their healthcare environments affected by legislation, professional codes of ethics, consumerism, and reconceptualization of practice paradigms, such as in telenursing. All of the various nursing roles—practice, administration, education, research, and informaticians—involve the science of nursing.

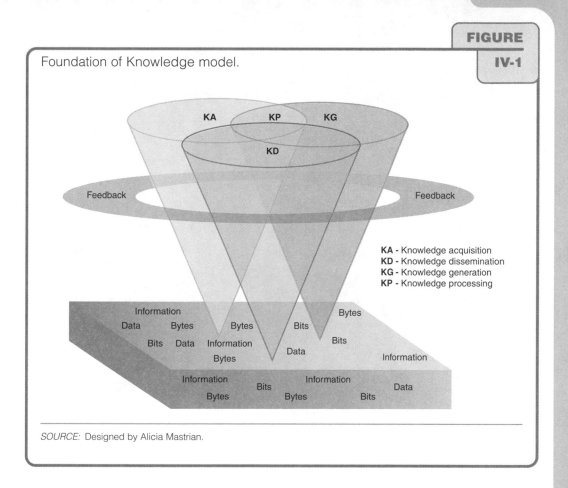

FIGURE
IV-1

Foundation of Knowledge model.

KA - Knowledge acquisition
KD - Knowledge dissemination
KG - Knowledge generation
KP - Knowledge processing

SOURCE: Designed by Alicia Mastrian.

CHAPTER 17

The Electronic Health Record and Clinical Informatics

Emily B. Barey

Objectives

1. Describe the common components of an electronic health record.
2. Assess the benefits of implementing an electronic health record.
3. Explore the ownership of an electronic health record.
4. Evaluate the flexibility of the electronic health record in meeting the needs of clinicians and patients.

www

Key Terms

www

Administrative processes
ARRA - HITECH
Connectivity
Decision support
Electronic communication
Electronic health record
Healthcare information
Interoperability
Meaningful use
Order entry management
Patient support
Population health management
Reporting
Results management

INTRODUCTION

The significance of **electronic health records** (EHRs) to nursing cannot be underestimated. Although EHRs on the surface suggest a simple automation of clinical documentation, in fact the implications are broad ranging from how care is delivered, the types of interactions nurses have with patients, in conjunction with the use of technology to the research surrounding EHRs that will inform nursing practice for tomorrow. A basic knowledge of EHRs and nursing informatics is now considered by many to be an entry level nursing competency.

The Technology Informatics Guiding Education Reform (TIGER, 2006) summit on evidence and informatics transforming nursing stated that, "the nation is working full-speed to realize the 10-year goal of Electronic Health Records for its citizens" (p. 1). Nurses must become active participants in this effort to capture **healthcare information**, generate knowledge, and enhance patient care. "This is a critical juncture for nurses, who comprise 55% of the healthcare workforce, number more than 3 million, and who must become more aware and involved at every level of the Informatics Revolution" (TIGER, p. 1). Although EHR standards are evolving and barriers to adoption remain, the collective work has a positive momentum that can only benefit clinician and patient alike.

This has been underscored with the passage of the Health Information Technology for Economic and Clinical Health Act of 2009 (HITECH). It is essential that this competency be developed to participate fully in the changing world of healthcare information technology. This chapter has four goals. The first is to describe the common components of an EHR. The second and third are to review the benefits of implementing an EHR and to provide an overview of successful ownership of an EHR, including nursing's role in promoting the safe adoption of the use of an EHR in day-to-day practice. The fourth goal is to discuss the flexibility of an EHR in meeting the needs of both clinicians and patients, including an introduction to **interoperability**.

SETTING THE STAGE

The United States healthcare system faces the enormous challenge to improve the quality of care and simultaneously control costs. EHRs have been proposed as one solution to achieve this goal (Institute of Medicine [IOM], 2001). In January 2004, President George W. Bush raised the profile of EHRs in his State of the Union address by outlining a plan to ensure that most Americans have an EHR by 2014. He stated that "by computerizing health records we can avoid dangerous medical mistakes, reduce costs, and improve care" (Bush, 2004). This proclamation generated an increased demand for understanding EHRs and how to promote their adoption, but relatively few healthcare organizations were motivated to pursue more rapid adoption of EHRs. The Healthcare Information and Management Systems Society (HIMSS) has been tracking EHR adoption since 2005 through its "Stage 7" Award and reports that most of the country's healthcare organizations are in Stage 0–3, reflecting only the basic components of laboratory, radiology, and pharmacy ancillaries installed; a clinical data repository including a controlled medical vocabulary; and simple nursing documentation and clinical **decision support** available (HIMSS, 2010b).

Since then, President Barack Obama passed the **American Recovery and Reinvestment Act** of 2009 (ARRA), including the **HITECH Act** to specifically incentivize health organizations and providers to become "meaningful users" of EHRs. These incentives will come in the form of increased reimbursement rates from the Centers for Medicaid and Medicare Services (CMS) and ultimately will result in a payment penalty to the healthcare organization if adoption of an EHR is not obtained by January 2015. The final rule was published by the Department of Health and Human Services (DHHS) in July 2010 for the first phase of implementation, and more details are expected to be completed for a second and third phase in 2011 and 2012, leading up to the 2015 deadline (DHHS, 2010).

COMPONENTS

Overview

Before the ARRA there were several definitions of EHRs, each with its own terminology and developed with a different audience in mind. The sources ranged from the federal government (Certification Commission for Healthcare Information Technology, 2007); the IOM (2003); the HIMSS (2007); and the National Institutes of Health (Robert Wood Johnson [RWJ], 2006). Under ARRA, there is now an explicit requirement for providers and hospitals to use a certified EHR that meets a set of standard functional definitions to be eligible for the increased reimbursement incentive. DHHS has granted two organizations the authority to accredit EHRs: The Drummond Group and the Certification Commission for Healthcare Information Technology. These bodies are authorized to test and certify EHR vendors against the standards and test procedures developed by the National Institute of Standards and Technology (NIST) and endorsed by the Office of the National Coordinator for Health Information Technology for EHRs.

The NIST test procedure includes 45 certification criteria ranging from the basic ability to record patient demographics, document vital signs, and maintain an up-to-date problem list to more complex functions, such as electronic exchange of clinical information and patient summary records (NIST, 2010). Box 17-1 provides a list of the 45 certification criteria outlined by NIST.

BOX 17-1

Criteria #	Certification Criteria
§170.302 (a)	Drug–drug, drug–allergy interaction checks
§170.302 (b)	Drug formulary checks
§170.302 (c)	Maintain up-to-date problem list
§170.302 (d)	Maintain active medication list
§170.302 (e)	Maintain active medication allergy list
§170.302 (f)(1)	Vital signs
§170.302 (f)(2)	Calculate body mass index
§170.302 (f)(3)	Plot and display growth charts
§170.302 (g)	Smoking status

Continues

BOX *(Continued)*

17-1

§170.302 (h)	Incorporate laboratory test results
§170.302 (i)	Generate patient lists
§170.302 (j)	Medication reconciliation
§170.302 (k)	Submission to immunization registries
§170.302 (l)	Public health surveillance
§170.302 (m)	Patient specific education resources
§170.302 (n)	Automated measure calculation
§170.302 (o)	Access control
§170.302 (p)	Emergency access
§170.302 (q)	Automatic log-off
§170.302 (r)	Audit log
§170.302 (s)	Integrity
§170.302 (t)	Authentication
§170.302 (u)	General encryption
§170.302 (v)	Encryption when exchanging electronic health information
§170.302 (w)	Accounting of disclosures (optional)
§170.304 (a)	Computerized provider order entry
§170.304 (b)	Electronic prescribing
§170.304 (c)	Record demographics
§170.304 (d)	Patient reminders
§170.304 (e)	Clinical decision support
§170.304 (f)	Electronic copy of health information
§170.304 (g)	Timely access
§170.304 (h)	Clinical summaries
§170.304 (i)	Exchange clinical information and patient summary record
§170.304 (j)	Calculate and submit clinical quality measures
§170.306 (a)	Computerized provider order entry
§170.306 (b)	Record demographics
§170.306 (c)	Clinical decision support
§170.306 (d)(1)	Electronic copy of health information
§170.306 (d)(2)	Electronic copy of health information
	Note: For discharge summary
§170.306 (e)	Electronic copy of discharge instructions
§170.306 (f)	Exchange clinical information and patient summary record
§170.306 (g)	Reportable lab results
§170.306 (h)	Advance directives
§170.306 (i)	Calculate and submit clinical quality measures

SOURCE: National Institute of Standards and Technology (NIST). (2010). *Meaningful use test measures: Approved test procedures.* Retrieved from http://healthcare.nist.gov/use_testing/finalized_requirements.html

Despite ARRA, the IOM definition also remains a valid reference point. The definition is useful because it has distilled all the possible features of an EHR into eight essential components with an emphasis on functions that promote patient safety, a universal denominator that everyone in health care can accept. The eight components include (1) health information and data, (2) **results management**, (3) **order entry management**, (4) decision support, (5) **electronic communication** and **connectivity**, (6) **patient support**, (7) **administrative processes**, and (8) **reporting** and **population health management** (IOM, 2003). Each is described in more detail here, and with the exception of EHR infrastructure functions, such as security and privacy management, controlled medical vocabularies, and interoperability standards, the 45 NIST standards easily map into the IOM categories.

Health Information and Data
Health information and data is the patient data required to make sound clinical decisions including demographics, medical and nursing diagnoses, medication lists, allergies, and test results (IOM, 2003).

Results Management
Results management is the ability to manage results of all types electronically, including laboratory and radiology procedure reports, both current and historical (IOM, 2003).

Order Entry Management
Order entry management is the ability of a clinician to enter medication and other care orders, including laboratory, microbiology, pathology, radiology, nursing, supply orders, ancillary services, and consultations directly into a computer (IOM, 2003).

Decision Support
Decision support is the computer reminders and alerts to improve the diagnosis and care of a patient including screening for correct drug selection and dosing, medication interactions with other medications, preventive health reminders in such areas as vaccinations, health risk screening and detection, and clinical guidelines for patient disease treatment (IOM, 2003).

Electronic Communication and Connectivity
Electronic communication and connectivity is the online communication among healthcare team members, their care partners, and patients including e-mail, Web messaging, and an integrated health record within and across settings, institutions, and telemedicine (IOM, 2003).

Patient Support

Patient support is the patient education and self-monitoring tools, including interactive computer-based patient education, home telemonitoring, and telehealth systems (IOM, 2003).

Administrative Processes

Administrative processes are the electronic scheduling, billing, and claims management systems including electronic scheduling for inpatient and outpatient visits and procedures, electronic insurance eligibility validation, claim authorization and prior approval, identification of possible research study participants, and drug recall support (IOM, 2003).

Reporting and Population Health Management

Reporting and population health management are the data collection tools to support public and private reporting requirements including data represented in a standardized terminology and machine-readable format (IOM, 2003).

NIST is not an exhaustive list of all possible features and functions of an EHR. Different vendor EHR systems combine different components in their offerings, and often a single set of EHR components does not meet the needs of all clinicians and patient populations. For example, a pediatric setting may demand functions for immunization management, growth tracking, and more robust order entry features to include weight-based dosing (Spooner & The Council on Clinical Information Technology, 2007). These types of features may not be provided by all EHR systems, and it is important to consider EHR certification as a minimum standard.

ADVANTAGES

There are mixed reviews of the advantages of an EHR. Much has been written about the potential promise of reduced cost, improved quality, and outcomes, but very little of it has been substantiated except anecdotally (Sidorov, 2006). Possible methods to estimate EHR benefits include using vendor-supplied data that has been retrieved from their customer systems, synthesizing and applying studies of overall EHR value, creating logical engineering models of EHR value, summarizing focused studies of elements of EHR value, and conducting and applying information from site visits (Thompson, Osheroff, Classen, & Sittig, 2007). However, the time and effort involved completing this work is further burdened by the fact that historically there was no standard by which to measure adoption or expected benefits (RWJ, 2006; Thompson et al.). With the advent of ARRA there are now 25 **meaningful use** objectives for eligible providers and 24 for eligible hospitals (CMS, 2010a). Chapter 16 provides an expanded discussion of meaningful use. In addition, the final rule also calls for providers to report on three required clinical quality measures and three additional quality measures of their choice from a list of 44 possible measures (CMS, 2010b). Eligible hospitals must report on 15 clinical quality measures. Although these objectives and measures will provide a universal benchmark moving forward for EHR benefits, for most healthcare organizations these outcomes alone will not provide sufficient return on investment for the capital investment made to implement an EHR, and additional benefits will continue to be sought.

The four most common benefits are (1) an increased delivery of guideline-based care, (2) an enhanced capacity to perform surveillance and monitoring for disease conditions, (3) a reduction in medication errors, and (4) a decreased use of care (Chaudhry et al., 2006). These findings were echoed by two similar literature reviews. The first focused on the use of informatics systems for chronic illness and found that the processes of care most positively impacted were guideline adherence; visit frequency (i.e., a decrease in emergency department visits); provider documentation; patient treatment adherence; and screening and testing (Dorr et al., 2007).

The second review was a cost–benefit analysis of health information technology completed by the Agency for Healthcare Research and Quality that studied the value of an EHR in the ambulatory care and pediatric settings, including its overall economic value. The Agency for Healthcare Research and Quality highlighted the common findings already described and also noted that most of the data available for review is from six leading healthcare organizations in the United States, underscoring the challenge of generalizing these results to the broader healthcare industry (Shekelle, Morton, & Keeler, 2006). As noted previously by the HIMSS Stage 7 Awards, the challenge to generalize results persists in 2010 and in the hospital arena and with less than 1% of United States hospitals or eight leading organizations providing most of the experience with a comprehensive EHR available (HIMSS, 2010d). Finally, all three literature reviews cited here indicated that there are a limited number of hypothesis-testing studies and even fewer that reported cost data.

The descriptive studies, however, do have value and should not be hastily dismissed. Although not as rigorous in their design, they do describe advantages to an EHR well and often also include useful implementation recommendations learned from practical experience. Among these types of reviews, EHR advantages include simple benefits, such as no longer having to interpret poor handwriting and handwritten orders, reduced turnaround time for laboratory results in an emergency department, and decreased time to administration of the first dose of antibiotics in an inpatient nursing unit (Husk & Waxman, 2004; Smith et al., 2004).

In the ambulatory care setting, evidence of improved management of cardiac-related risk factors in patients with diabetes and effective patient notification of medication recalls have been demonstrated (Jain et al., 2005; Reed & Bernard, 2005). Two other unique advantages that have great potential are the ability to use the EHR and decision support functions to identify patients who qualify for research studies or who qualify for prescription drug benefits offered by pharmaceutical companies at safety-net clinics and hospitals (Embi et al., 2005; Poprock, 2005).

The HIMSS Davies Award may be the best resource for combined quantitative and qualitative results of successful EHR implementation. The Davies Award recognizes healthcare organizations who have achieved both excellence in implementation and value from health information technology (HIMSS, 2010a). One recent winner demonstrated a significant avoidance of medication errors because of barcode scanning alerts, a $3 million decrease in medical records expenses as a result of going paperless, and a 5% reduction of duplicate laboratory orders by using computerized provider order entry alerting (HIMSS, 2010c). Another recent winner also noted a 13% decrease in adverse drug reactions through the use of computerized physician order entry, and a decrease in methicillin-resistant *Staphylococcus aureus* nosocomial infections from 9.8 per 10,000 discharges to 6.4 per 10,000 discharges in less than a year using the EHR flagging function that made clinicians immediately aware that contact precautions were required on methicillin-resistant *S. aureus*–positive patients (HIMSS, 2009). At both organizations there was also qualitative and quantitative evidence of high end user adoption and satisfaction with use of the EHR.

Without an EHR system, any of these benefits would be very difficult and costly to accomplish. Thus, despite limited standards and published studies, there is enough evidence to warrant pursuing widespread implementation of the EHR (Halamka, 2006) and certainly enough as discussed here to warrant further study of the use and benefit of EHRs.

OWNERSHIP

The implementation of an EHR has the potential to affect every member of a healthcare organization. The process of becoming a successful owner of an EHR has multiple steps and requires integrating the EHR into both the organization's day-to-day operations and long-term vision, and the clinician's day-to-day practice. All members of the healthcare organization, from the executive level to the clinician at the point of care, must feel a sense of ownership to make the implementation successful for themselves, their colleagues, and their patients. Successful ownership of an EHR may be defined in part by the level of clinician adoption of the tool, and this section reviews key steps and strategies for the selection, implementation and evaluation, and optimization of an EHR in pursuit of that goal.

Historically, many systems were developed locally by the information technology department of a healthcare organization. It was not unusual for software developers to be employed by the organization to write needed systems and interfaces between them. As commercial offerings were introduced and matured, it became less and less common to see homegrown or locally developed systems. As a result, the first step of ownership is typically a vendor selection process for a commercially available EHR. During this step, it is important to survey the organization's level of interest, identify possible barriers to participation, document desired functions of an EHR, and assess the willingness to fund the implementation (Holbrook, Keshavjee, Troyan, Pray, & Ford, 2003). Although clinicians should drive the project, the assessment should also include the needs and readiness of the executive leadership, information technology, and project management teams. It is essential that leadership understands that this type of project is as much about redesigning clinical work as it is about technically automating it, and that they agree to hold accountability for its success (Goddard, 2000). In addition, this preacquisition phase should also concentrate on understanding the current state of the health information technology industry to identify appropriate questions and the next steps in the selection process (American Organization of Nurse Executives, 2006). These first steps begin to identify any organizational risks toward a successful implementation and pave the way for initiating a change management process to educate the organization about the future state of delivering health care with an EHR system.

The second step of the selection process is to select a system based on the organization's current and predicted needs. It is common during this phase to see a demonstration of several vendors' EHR products. Based on the completed needs assessment, the organization should establish key evaluation criteria to compare the different vendors and products. The criteria should include both subjective and objective items that cover such topics as common clinical workflows, decision support, reporting, usability, technical build, and maintenance of the system. Providing the vendor with these guidelines will ensure the process meets the organization's needs; however, it is also essential to let the vendor demonstrate a proposed future state from its own perspective. This is critical to ensuring that its vision and the organization's vision are well aligned. It also helps spark additional dialogue about the possible future state of clinical work at the organization and the change required in obtaining it. The demonstrations provide not only the ability to compare and contrast the features and functions of different systems, but are also a good way to engage the organization's members in being a part of this strategic decision.

Implementation planning should occur concurrently with the selection process, particularly the assessment of the scope of the work, initial sequencing of the EHR components to be implemented, and resources required. However, it begins in earnest once a vendor and product have been selected. In addition to further refining the implementation plan, this is also the time to identify key metrics by which to measure the EHRs success. An organization may realize numerous benefits from implementing an EHR. The organization should choose metrics that match its overall strategy and goals in the coming years and may include expected improvements in financial, quality, and clinical outcomes. Common metrics include reducing the number of duplicate laboratory tests through duplicate orders alerting, reducing the number of adverse drug events through the use of barcode medication administration, meaningful use objectives and measures, and those EHR advantages mentioned previously. To be sure benefits are realized, it is important to avoid choosing so many that they become meaningless or unobtainable, to carefully and practically define those that are chosen, to measure before and after the implementation, and to assign accountability to a member of the organization to ensure the work is completed.

End user adoption of the EHR is also essential to realizing its benefits. Clinicians must be engaged to use the EHR successfully in their practice and daily workflows so that data may be captured to drive the decision support that underlies so many of the advantages and metrics described. To promote adoption, a change management plan must be developed in conjunction with the EHR implementation plan. The most effective change management plans offer end users several exposures to the system and relevant workflows in advance of its use, and continue through the go-live and post-live time periods. Successful pre-live strategies include end user involvement as subject matter experts to validate the EHR workflow design and content build, hosting end user usability testing sessions, shadowing end users in their current daily work in parallel with the new system, and formal training activities. The goal of these pre-live activities is not only to ensure that the EHR implementation will meet end user needs but also to assess the impact of the new EHR on current workflow and process. The larger the impact, the more change management is required above and beyond system training. For example, simulation laboratory experiences may be offered to more thoroughly dress rehearse a significant workflow change, executive leadership may need to convey their support and expectations of clinicians about a new way of working, and generally more anticipatory guidance is required to communicate to those impacted.

Training may be delivered in a variety of mediums, and often a combination of approaches works best including classroom time, electronic learning, independent exercises, and peer to peer at the elbow support. Training must be workflow based and reflect real clinical processes. Training must also be planned and budgeted for through the post-live period to ensure that competency with the system is assessed at go-live and any necessary retraining or reinforcements are made in the 30 to 60 days post-live. This not only promotes reliability and safe use of the system as it was designed, but also can have a positive impact on end user morale that they are being supported beyond the initial go-live period and have an opportunity to move from basic skills to advanced proficiency with the system.

Finally, the implementation plan should also account for the long-term optimization of the EHR. This step is commonly overlooked and often results in benefits falling short of expectations because the resources are not available to realize them permanently. It also often means the difference between end users of EHRs merely surviving the change as opposed to becoming savvy about how to adopt the EHR as another powerful clinical tool, such as the stethoscope. Optimization activities of the EHR should be considered a routine part of the organization's operations, should be resourced accordingly, and should emphasize the continued involvement of clinician users to identify ways that the EHR can enable meeting the overall mission of the organization. Many organizations start an implementation of an EHR with the goal of transforming their care delivery and operations. Different than simply automating a previously manual or fragmented process, transformation often includes improving the process to realize better patient care outcomes or added efficiency. Although some transformation is experienced with the initial use of the system, most of this work is done post-implementation and is reliant on widespread clinician adoption of the EHR. As such, it makes optimization a critical component to successful ownership of an EHR. Review Box 17-2 for the barriers and methods for successful acceptance.

FLEXIBILITY AND EXPANDABILITY

Health care is as unique as the patients themselves. It is delivered in a variety of settings, for a variety of reasons over the course of a patient's lifetime. In addition, patients rarely receive all their care from one healthcare organization and choice is a cornerstone of the American healthcare system. An EHR must be flexible and expandable to meet the needs of patients and caregivers in all these settings, despite the challenges.

At a very basic level, there is as yet no EHR system available that can provide all functions for all specialties to a degree that all clinicians would successfully adopt. A good example is oncology. Most systems do not yet provide the advanced ordering features required for complex treatment planning. An oncologist could use a general system, but he or she would not find as many benefits without additional features for chemotherapy ordering, lifetime cumulative dose tracking, or the ability to adjust a treatment day schedule and have the remaining days of the plan recalculate a new schedule.

BOX

17-2

Resistance to Implementation

Julie A. Kenney and Ida Androwich

For an implementation to be successful, a few things need to happen. The informatics nurse specialist (INS) will need to understand and use change management theory to ensure that the implementation of the new EHR system will be successful. It is a well-known fact that nurses can make or break a system implementation. A nursing staff that is involved early in the implementation process has been found to be a major determinant in a successful implementation. Assessing nursing attitudes and concerns early in the process can aid the INS in determining the best way to proceed with staff education and implementation rollout. Nurses may feel that the implementation that should be making their job easier may actually make it more challenging (Trossman, 2005). Nurses who feel that the system has been forced onto them will very likely be highly resistant to the change. This is why it is imperative that nurses be involved in the design, development, and implementation of the EHR. Nurses who have been involved in the implementation process will ensure that the product meets the needs of the staff, which will result in high end user satisfaction (McLane, 2005).

Another challenge facing those wishing to implement an EHR is that writing is nearly automatic for most but using a computer is not. This can be overcome by ensuring that data entry and system navigation make for a system that is user friendly (Walsh, 2004). Voice data entry is an easy way to enter data into the system and may be a way for those who are not comfortable with computers to still use the system effectively (Walsh). An additional way for staff to accept the new EHR is to ensure that they have had adequate training prior to the implementation as well as ensure continued support and education after the implementation. The implementation of a new EHR system requires the staff to make significant changes to how they work and how they handle patient information. The INS who is familiar with change management and the NI process should have an integral role in the redesign of workflow processes in order to ensure a smooth transition from a paper record to an electronic record. Many excellent EHR systems that have been installed fail due to poor implementation planning. It is imperative that nurses are employed in the information systems (IS) department (Trossman, 2005).

References

McLane, S. (2005). Designing an EMR planning process based on staff attitudes toward and opinions about computers in healthcare. *CIN: Computers, Informatics, Nursing, 23*(2), 85–92.

Trossman, S. (2005). Bold new world: Technology should ease nurses' jobs, not create a greater work load. *American Journal of Nursing, 105*(5), 75–77.

Walsh, S. (2004). The clinician's perspective on electronic health records and how they can affect patient care. *BMJ: British Medical Journal, 328*(7449), 1184–1187.

Further, most healthcare organizations do not yet have the capacity to implement and maintain systems in all care areas. As one physician stated, "implementing an EMR is a complex and difficult multidisciplinary effort that will stretch an organization's skills and capacity for change" (Chin, 2004, p. 47). These two conditions are improving every day at both vendor and healthcare organizations alike, and were recently fueled by ARRA incentives (see Box 17-3).

ARRA has also set the expectation that despite the number of settings in which a patient may receive care, there is a minimum set of data from those records that must flow or "interoperate" between each setting and the unique EHR systems used. Today, interoperability exists through what is called a continuity of care document. This data set includes patient demographics, medication, allergy, and problem lists among others and the continuity of care document formatting and exchange is required to be supported by EHR vendors and healthcare organizations seeking ARRA meaningful use incentives. Despite this positive step forward, financial and patient privacy hurdles still must also be overcome to achieve an expansive EHR. Most health care is delivered by small community practices and hospitals, many of which do not have the financial or technical resources to implement an EHR. DHHS recently loosened regulations so that physicians may now be able to receive healthcare information technology software, hardware, and implementation services from hospitals to alleviate the cost burden on individual providers and foster adoption of the EHR.

BOX
17-3

Cloudy EHRs

A paradigm shift from healthcare facility-owned machine-based computing to off-site, vendor-owned cloud computing, Web browser-based login accessible data, software and hardware, could link systems together and reduce costs. Hospitals with shrinking budgets and extreme IT needs, are exploring the successes in other industries such as Amazon's S3. As providers strive to implement potent EHRs, they are looking for the cloud-based models that offer the necessary functionality without having to assume the burden associated with all of the hardware, software, application, and storage issues. However, in the face of the HITECH Act and its associated penalties, how can we overcome the challenges to realize the benefits? There are advantages and disadvantages of cloud computing and while they explore this new paradigm, healthcare providers must relinquish control as they continue to strive to maintain security. The vendors, responsible for developing and maintaining this new environment, are also facing challenges brought on by the legislature and healthcare providers. As the vendors and healthcare providers work together to improve the implementation and adoption of the cloud-based EHR, the sky is the limit!

Finally, patient privacy is a pivotal issue to determine how far and how easy it will be to share data across healthcare organizations. In addition to the Health Insurance Portability and Accountability Act privacy rules, many states have regulations in place related to patient confidentiality. The recent experience of the state of Minnesota foreshadows what all states will soon be facing. In 2007, Governor Tim Pawlenty announced the creation of the Minnesota Health Information Exchange (State of Minnesota, 2007). Although the intentions of the exchange are to promote patient safety and increase healthcare efficiency across the state, it raised significant concerns about security and privacy. New questions arose about the definition of when and how patient consent is required to exchange data electronically, and older paper-based processes needed to be updated to support real-time electronic exchange (Minnesota Department of Health, 2007). For health exchanges such as these to reach their full potential, the public must be able to trust that their privacy will be protected, or else the healthcare industry risks that patients may not share a full medical history, or worse yet, may not seek care, effectively making the exchange useless.

THE FUTURE

Despite the challenges, the future of EHRs is an exciting one for patient and clinician alike. Benefits may be realized by stand-alone EHRs as described here, but the most significant transformation will come as interoperability is realized between systems. As the former national information technology coordinator in the DHHS, David Brailer, notes the potential of interoperability:

> For the first time, clinicians everywhere can have a longitudinal medical record with full information about each patient. Consumers will have better information about their health status since personal health records and similar access strategies can be feasible in an interoperable world. Consumers can move more easily between and among clinicians without fear of their information being lost. Payers can benefit from the economic efficiencies, fewer errors, and reduced duplication that arises from interoperability. Healthcare information exchange and interoperability (HIEI) also underlies meaningful public health reporting, bioterrorism surveillance, quality monitoring, and advances in clinical trials. In short, there is little that most people want from health care for which HIEI isn't a prerequisite (Brailer, 2005, p. W 5-20).

The future also holds tremendous potential for EHR features and functions that will not only include more sophisticated decision support and clinical reporting capacity, but also improved biomedical device integration, ease of use and intuitiveness, and access through more hardware platforms.

Implementations of EHRs will also become more commonplace in the near future with ARRA putting pressure on healthcare organizations to move more quickly toward adoption. More organizations adopting EHRs will facilitate broader dissemination of implementation best practices, with the hope of further shortening the time to taking advantage of advanced EHR features.

SUMMARY

It is an important time for health care and technology. EHRs have come to the forefront and will remain central to shaping the future of health care. In an ideal world, all nurses from entry level to executives will have a basic competency in nursing informatics to participate fully in shaping the future use of technology in the practice at a national level and wherever care is delivered. Such initiatives as TIGER are imperative for adoption and ultimately more visibility of nursing in the later phases of the ARRA meaningful use standards, which are still being defined.

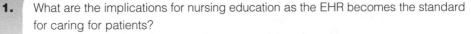

THOUGHT-PROVOKING Questions   WWW

1. What are the implications for nursing education as the EHR becomes the standard for caring for patients?
2. What are the ethical considerations related to interoperability and a shared EHR?

For a full suite of assignments and additional learning activities, use the access code located in the front of your book to visit this exclusive website: http://go.jblearning.com/mcgonigle. If you do not have an access code, you can obtain one at the site.

References

American Organization of Nurse Executives. (2006, September). *Defining the role of the nurse executive in technology acquisition and implementation.* Washington, DC: Author. Retrieved from http://www.aone.org/aone/pdf/Guiding%20Principles%20for%20Acquisition%20and%20Implementation%20of%20Information%20Technology.pdf

Brailer, D. J. (2005, January). *Interoperability: The key to the future healthcare system. Health Affairs— Web Exclusive, W 5-19–W 5-21.* Available from http://content.healthaffairs.org/cgi/reprint/hlthaff.w5.19v1

Bush, G. W. (2004). *State of the Union address.* Retrieved from http://www.whitehouse.gov/news/releases/2004/01/20040120-7.html

Centers for Medicare and Medicaid Services. (2010a). *EHR incentive programs: Meaningful use.* Retrieved from https://www.cms.gov/EHRIncentivePrograms/35_Meaningful_Use.asp

Centers for Medicare and Medicaid Services. (2010b). *Quality measures: Electronic specifications.* Retrieved from http://www.cms.gov/QualityMeasures/03_ElectronicSpecifications.asp#TopOfPage

Certification Commission for Healthcare Information Technology. (2007). *Certification commission announces new work group members.* Retrieved from http://www.cchit.org/about/news/releases/Certification-Commission-Announces-New-Work-Group-Members.asp

Chaudhry, B., Wang, J., Wu, S., Maglione, M., Mojica, W., Roth, E., Morton, S. & Shekelle, P. (2006). Systematic review: Impact of health information technology on quality, efficiency, and costs of medical care. *Annals of Internal Medicine, 144*(10), E-12–E-22.

Chin, H. L. (2004). The reality of EMR implementation: Lessons from the field. *The Permanente Journal, 8*(4), 43–48.

Department of Health and Human Services. (2007). *HIT certification: Background.* Retrieved from http://www.dhhs.gov/healthit/certification/background

Department of Health and Human Services. (2010). *Medicare and Medicaid programs: Electronic health record incentive program.* Retrieved from http://www.ofr.gov/OFRUpload/OFRData/2010-17202_PI.pdf

Dorr, D., Bonner, L. M., Cohen, A. N., Shoai, R. S., Perrin, R., Chaney, E. & Young, A. (2007). Informatics systems to promote improved care for chronic illness: A literature review. *Journal of the American Medical Informatics Association, 14*(2), 156–163.

Embi, P. J., Jain, A., Clark, J., Bizjack, S., Hornung, R., & Harris, C. M. (2005). Effect of a clinical trial alert system on physician participation in trial recruitment. *Archives of Internal Medicine, 165,* 2272–2277.

Goddard, B. L. (2000). Termination of a contract to implement an enterprise electronic medical record system. *Journal of American Medical Informatics Association, 7,* 564–568.

Halamka, J. D. (2006, May). Health information technology: Shall we wait for the evidence? [Letter to the editor]. *Annals of Internal Medicine, 144*(10), 775–776.

Healthcare Information and Management Systems Society (HIMSS). (2007). *Electronic health record.* Retrieved from http://www.himss.org/ASP/topics_ehr.asp

Healthcare Information and Management Systems Society (HIMSS). (2009). *HIMSS Davies Organizational Award Application: MultiCare.* Retrieved from http://www.himss.org/davies/docs/2009_RecipientApplications/MultiCareConnectHIMSSDaviesManuscript.pdf

Healthcare Information and Management Systems Society (HIMSS). (2010a). *HIMSS Davies Organizational Award Application: Sentara.* Forthcoming.

Healthcare Information and Management Systems Society (HIMSS). (2010b). *EMR Adoption Model.* Retrieved from http://www.himssanalytics.org/hc_providers/stage7Award.asp

Healthcare Information and Management Systems Society (HIMSS). (2010c). *Recipient list.* Retrieved from http://www.himssanalytics.org/hc_providers/stage7Hospitals.asp

Healthcare Information and Management Systems Society (HIMSS). (2010d). *Davies Award.* Retrieved from http://www.himss.org/davies/

Holbrook, A., Keshavjee, K., Troyan, S., Pray, M., & Ford, P. T. (2003). Applying methodology to electronic medical record selection. *International Journal of Medical Informatics, 71,* 43–50.

Husk, G., & Waxman, D. A. (2004). Using data from hospital information systems to improve emergency care. *Academic Emergency Medicine, 11*(11), 1237–1244.

Institute of Medicine. (2001). *Crossing the quality chasm: A new health system for the 21st century.* Washington, DC: National Academies Press.

Institute of Medicine. (2003). *Key capabilities of an electronic health record system: Letter report.* Washington, DC: National Academies Press.

Jain, A., Atreja, A., Harris, C. M., Lehmann, M., Burns, J., & Young, J. (2005). Responding to the rofecoxib withdrawal crisis: A new model for notifying patients at risk and their healthcare providers. *Annals of Internal Medicine, 142*(3), 182–186.

Minnesota Department of Health. (2007, June). *Minnesota Health Records Act—HF 1078 fact sheet.* Minneapolis, MN: Author. Retrieved from http://www.health.state.mn.us/e-health/mpsp/hrafact sheet2007.pdf

National Institutes of Health. (April, 2006). *Electronic health records overview.* McLean, Virginia: The MITRE Corporation.

National Institute of Standards and Technology. (2010). *Meaningful use test measures: Approved test procedures.* Retrieved from http://healthcare.nist.gov/use_testing/finalized_requirements.html

Poprock, B. (2005, September). *Using Epic's alternative medications reminder to reduce prescription costs and encourage assistance programs for indigent patients.* Presented at the Epic Systems Corporation user group meeting, Madison, WI.

Reed, H. L., & Bernard, E. (2005). Reductions in diabetic cardiovascular risk by community primary care providers. *International Journal of Circumpolar Health, 64*(1), 26–37.

Robert Wood Johnson Foundation. (2006). *Health information technology in the United States: The information base for progress.* Retrieved from http://www.rwjf.org/programareas/resources/product .jsp?id=15895&pid=1142&gsa=1

Shekelle, P. G., Morton, S. C., & Keeler, E. B. (2006). *Costs and benefits of health information technology. Evidence report/technology assessment, No. 132* [Prepared by the Southern California Evidence-based Practice Center under Contract No. 290-02-0003]. Agency for Healthcare Research and Quality Publication No. 06-E006. Rockville, MD: Agency for Healthcare Research and Quality.

Sidorov, J. (2006). It ain't necessarily so: The electronic health record and the unlikely prospect of reducing healthcare costs. *Health Affairs, 25*(4), 1079–1085.

Smith, T., Semerdjian, N., King, P., DeMartin, B., Levi, S., Reynolds, K., Ryan, J. & Dowd, J. (2004). *Nicolas E. Davies Award of Excellence: Transforming healthcare with a patient-centric electronic health record system.* Evanston, IL: Evanston Northwestern Healthcare. Retrieved from http://www.himss.org/content/files/davies2004_evanston.pdf

Spooner, S. A., & The Council on Clinical Information Technology. (2007). Special requirements of electronic health record systems in pediatrics. *Pediatrics, 119,* 631–637.

State of Minnesota, Office of the Governor. (2007). *New public-private partnership to improve patient care, safety and efficiency.* Retrieved from http://www.governor.state.mn.us/mediacenter/press releases/2007/PROD008303.html

Technology Informatics Guiding Education Reform. (2006). *Evidence and informatics transforming nursing.* Retrieved from http://www.amia.org/inside/releases/2006/tiger_press%20release_amia .pdf

Thompson, D. I., Osheroff, J., Classen, D., Sittig, D. F. (2007). A review of methods to estimate the benefits of electronic medical records in hospitals and the need for a national database. *Journal of Healthcare Information Management, 21*(1), 62–68.

CHAPTER 18

An Insider's View of the Utility of a Clinical Information System

Denise Tyler

1. Assess an insider's description of a clinical information system (CIS).
2. Explore knowledge dissemination and generation tools supported by the CIS.
3. Describe quality assurance and clinical outcomes measurement supported by the CIS.
4. Explore evidence-based practice and translational research tools provided by the CIS.

www

Key Terms www

Aggregate data
American Recovery and Reinvestment Act
Clinical analytics
Clinical guidelines
Clinical information system
Clinical outcomes
Clinical practice council
Coded terminology
Electronic health record
Evidence-based practice
Knowledge dissemination
Legacy systems
Performance improvement
Performance improvement analyst
Professional development
Quality assurance
Staff development
Translational research

INTRODUCTION

A **clinical information system** (CIS) is a technology-based system applied at the point of care and designed to support the acquisition and processing of information and to provide storage and processing capabilities. Sittig et al. (2002) provide a comprehensive definition of a CIS:

> A clinical information system is a collection of various information technology applications that provides a centralized repository of information related to patient care across distributed locations. This repository represents the patient's history of illnesses and interactions with providers by encoding knowledge capable of helping clinicians decide about the patient's condition, treatment options, and wellness activities. The repository also encodes the status of decisions, actions underway for those decisions and relevant information that could help in performing those actions. The database could also hold other information about the patient including genetic, environmental, and social contexts (Sittig et al., 2002, para. 3).

Early CISs were limited in scope and provided such information as laboratory results or medication administration and drug interaction information. The goal of many organizations is to expand the scope of the CIS to a comprehensive system that provides clinical decision support, an electronic patient record, and in some instances **professional development** training tools. Benefits of such a comprehensive system include providing easy access to patient data at the point of care; structured and legible information that can be searched easily and lends itself to data mining and analysis; and improved patient safety, especially the prevention of adverse drug reactions and the identification of health risk factors, such as falls. The implementation of such a comprehensive system, however, will cost the organization both dollars and losses in clinician productivity during development and implementation. Reports from organizations that have implemented such comprehensive systems point to the critical need for end users to be intimately involved in choosing and developing the CIS. Additional issues associated with implementation of a CIS include the need to interface with **legacy systems** (those already in place); privacy and security (covered elsewhere in this book); and clinician resistance to learning new technology (Biohealthmatics, 2006).

At Kaweah Delta, staff nurses, nurse managers, support staff, and **performance improvement analysts** were all intimately involved in the design of the system used by nursing. Ancillary staff was also very involved in the design of their systems. This has enabled a consistency in the charting done by different clinicians, while enabling their pathways to be designed according to their specific needs. As the system matures and more staff from different areas use the system both for charting and for accessing information, changes are put in place to enhance the system, and reports are created for **quality assurance** and reporting.

As the system evolved, views were created to incorporate an interdisciplinary display of patient education, care planning, and exchange of information for communication between providers and shift reports. These displays have greatly improved the way the information is accessed and shared. The displays and reports also allow for easier and timelier quality assurance of charting to provide better feedback for improvement. Reports are available online and are e-mailed daily to clinical analysts for the review of priority assessment data to ensure accurate and timely entry of information on each new admission. These reports also help nursing administrators prioritize educational needs of staff, and fine tune the computerized nursing documentation to enable staff to comply better with charting requirements.

Paying attention to the human–technology interface (see Chapter 14) elements of the system is essential. Adequate testing before implementation can prevent problems for users. Inadequate testing can result in a negative attitude and a lack of trust in the system. This testing involves not only the system itself but the hardware used by staff (computers, printers, and so forth). Getting input from both the clinicians who will be using the system and the staff who will be using the output information is critical to the success of system design and implementation. The INS is a key player in these project management processes. For a comprehensive overview of usability considerations and design collaboration strategies, see the Tiger Usability Report: http://www.tigersummit.com/uploads/Tiger_Usability_Report.pdf

One glitch that remains with many CISs is the quality of the printed document generated by the system. Because the systems are designed for virtual use, their display when printed can produce volumes of paper that is difficult to follow. This may be resolved one day as a result of improvements suggested by outside agencies, payers, and attorneys who may need printed reports. In the meantime, early testing of what the record will look like may not result in huge improvements, but it can at least decrease the surprise when confronted with the new printed record.

CLINICAL OUTCOMES AND QUALITY ASSURANCE SUPPORTED BY THE CIS

The ability to measure outcomes can be enhanced or impeded by the way an information system is designed and used. Although many practitioners can paint a very good picture of the patient by using a narrative (free text), using this mode of expression in a clinical system without the use of a coded entry makes it difficult to analyze the care given or the patient's response. Free text reporting also leads to inconsistencies of reporting from clinician to clinician and patient information that is fragmented or disorganized. This can limit the usefulness of patient data to other clinicians and interfere with the ability to run reports off of the data for quality assurance and measurement. The other issue with using free text is that not all clinicians are skilled at this form of communication, yielding inconsistent documentation.

Integrating standardized nursing terminologies into computerized nursing documentation systems enhances the ability to use the data for reporting and further research. Saba (2007) elaborates on the benefits of using the **aggregate data** available when nursing documentation is linked to a **coded terminology** for research from practice.

The ability to refine the CIS to create different reports and displays based on the need of the user is very helpful. For example, the **performance improvement** department may want to look at charting based on safety indicators or regulatory requirements, whereas the clinicians caring for a patient might need to see the most recent vital signs, intake and output, results, and specific charting elements that summarize or give a picture of what is happening with that patient.

McLaughlin and Halilovic (2006) describe the use of **clinical analytics** to promote medical care outcomes research. The use of a CIS with standardized codes for patient clinical issues helps to support the rigorous analysis of clinical data. Outcomes data as a result of these analyses may include length of stay, mortality, readmissions, and complications. Future goals include the ability to compare data and outcomes across various institutions as a means of developing **clinical guidelines** or best practices guidelines. With the implementation of a comprehensive CIS, similar analyses of nursing outcomes could also be performed and shared. Such a system could also aid nurse administrators in cross-unit comparisons and staffing decisions, especially when coupled with acuity systems data. In addition, clinical analytics can support required data reporting functions, especially those required by accreditation bodies. Box 18-1 describes clinical outcomes measures and reporting requirements.

BOX
18-1

Clinical Outcomes Measurement

Julie A. Kenney and Ida Androwich

Currently, all hospitals are required to gather data in regards to four core measures: (1) acute myocardial infarction, (2) heart failure, (3) pneumonia, and (4) surgical care improvement and surgical infection prevention. Each of these four core measures is composed of evidence-based care that should be received by patients who fall into these categories. These data are required to be published on the institution's or corporation's website and be available as a hard copy on site. The data are also published on the United States Department of Health and Human Services website Hospital Compare, which can be found at http://www.hospitalcompare.hhs.gov/Hospital/Search/SelectConditionsAndMeasures.asp. This website lists each hospital's compliance with the four core measure bundles. The public can compare hospitals based on these four clinical outcomes measures. Each hospital supplies the information quarterly (United States Department of Health and Human Services, 2007).

With the worldwide emphasis on measuring and evaluating the quality of health care, the American Nurses Association decided that nursing should begin a program that builds a database for nursing-sensitive quality indicators and use the collected data to educate practicing nurses on quality activities and educate the public about nursing (Gallagher & Rowell, 2003). This was the beginning of the national database of nursing quality indicators (NDNQI). Facilities were recruited to gather data and return it to NDNQI, which would then store the data to begin developing facility indicator profiling and the eventual data comparison of hospitals that share similar characteristics (Gallagher & Rowell). Each facility is given a unique number in order that no identifying information is released unintentionally. Each facility decides if it wants to publicize its participation in the NDNQI project (Gallagher & Rowell).

Continues

This project has resulted in numerous studies that have used the data within the database. One study is looking at the relationship between nursing staffing and patient outcomes. Currently, there is little quantifiable evidence to show nursing's impact on patient outcomes, especially when looking at nursing staff ratios to patient outcomes. The database provides the ability to differentiate areas of concern down to the unit level because of the type of data that is collected (Gallagher, 2001; Gallagher & Rowell, 2003).

The information is more useful when differentiated by nursing unit type than when grouped together as a whole. The separated information allows for a more accurate picture of unit level activity compared to the institution as a whole. If the information is viewed together, a weaker unit is balanced out by a stronger unit, which sways the way the picture is painted by the data. In addition, the erroneous conclusions drawn by lumping unit data together hamper the ability to provide administrative support to the unit that is struggling and provide positive reinforcement to the unit that is performing above average (Gallagher & Rowell, 2003). If an institution owns an electronic health record (EHR), a significant portion of these data can be pulled from the system, which saves the institution from employing a person to pull data manually from the paper chart. The following is the current list of data that are being collected by NDNQI (American Nurses Association, 2007):

- Patient falls
- Patient falls with injury, including level of injury
- Pressure ulcer rate
- Hospital-acquired pressure ulcer rate
- Registered nurse satisfaction
- Nursing hours per patient day
- Registered nurse hours per patient day
- Licensed practical/vocational nurse hours per patient day
- Unlicensed assistive personnel hours per patient day
- Staff mix
- Registered nurse
- Licensed practical/vocational nurses
- Unlicensed assistive personnel
- Percent agency staff
- Registered nurse education and certification
- Pediatric pain assessment, intervention, reassessment cycle
- Pediatric peripheral intravenous infiltration
- Psychiatric physical and sexual abuse

Additional data collected include the following:

- Patient population, adult or pediatric
- Hospital category (teaching, nonteaching, and so forth)
- Type of unit (critical care, step-down, medical, surgical, combined medical/ surgical, rehabilitation, and psychiatric)
- Number of staffed beds designated by the hospital

Continues

BOX *(Continued)*

18-1

New indicators undergoing development include the following:

- Restraints
- Practice environment scale
- Nursing turnover
- Nursing musculoskeletal injuries

The introduction of the EHR has changed the way data are collected. There is an abundance of data available for study, but because of the large number of systems and the lack of a universal medical language, transferring the data to the databases has proved difficult (Lu, Park, Ucharattana, Konicek, & Delaney, 2007). This is where nursing informatics plays a significant role. The nurse informatics specialist works with the program developers to ensure that EHR systems are using a universal language, which allows researchers to extract data from the EHR and import it into the database without having to translate the data into a different nomenclature. Developing and using a universal language aids in allowing different systems to move toward interoperability.

References

American Nurses Association. (2007). *Nursing sensitive indicators*. Retrieved from http://nursingworld.org/MainMenuCategories/ThePracticeofProfessionalNursing/PatientSafetyQuality/NDNQI/NDNQI_1/NursingSensitiveIndicators.aspx

Gallagher, R. M. (2001). Nursing quality indicators: Research proves nursing's impact on patient care. *Arkansas Nursing News, 18*(4), 23–25.

Gallagher, R. M., & Rowell, P. A. (2003). Claiming the future of nursing through nursing-sensitive quality indicators. *Nursing Administration Quarterly, 27*(4), 273–284.

Lu, D.-F., Park, H.-T., Ucharattana, P., Konicek, D., & Delaney, C. (2007). Nursing outcomes classification in the systematized nomenclature of medicine clinical terms: A cross-mapping validation. *CIN: Computers, Informatics, Nursing, 25*(3), 159–170.

United States Department of Health and Human Services. (2007). *Hospital compare Web site*. Retrieved from http://www.hospitalcompare.hhs.gov/Hospital/Search/SelectConditionsAndMeasures.asp

Quality assurance in the electronic world deals not only with quality indicators in regards to the care provided, but it also applies to the way the information is captured, displayed, and reported. To ensure that the system design and linking are done so that the discrete data elements are easy to identify whether the data is reviewed online or used for research measurement is now important.

Reviewing the way staff are charting using the system is still necessary but should be less time consuming than it was in the paper era because of the ability to access the information from anywhere in real time and in the reporting functions based on the needs of the user.

EVIDENCE-BASED PRACTICE AND THE CIS

Evidence-based practice (EBP) can be thought of as the integration of clinical expertise and best practices based on systematic research to enhance decision making and improve patient care. EBP does not take away from the critical-thinking skills used by expert nurses; it enhances their informed decision making. According to Simpson (2004), "Evidence-based nursing is the process by which nurses make clinical decisions using the best available research evidence, their clinical expertise, and patient preferences. Three areas of research competence are: interpreting and using research, evaluating practice, and conducting research" (p. 10).

EBP should be embedded in computerized documentation of a CIS, providing both prompts for interventions and different questions based on the charted assessment. These prompts can be done by required fields that display only when the criterion is met, by pop-up boxes, or even by printed reminders. How the prompts are delivered is best determined by the workflow during that process, but system capabilities and organizational policies must also be considered.

References supporting EBP should be available for review at the click of a mouse or by a few keystrokes. This ease of access to more detailed information establishes a trust among clinicians in the prompts built into the documentation system and increases the user's understanding of the information provided. As clinical knowledge is acquired, it can be applied to situations where the CIS prompting is not present to improve clinical decision making. The CIS prompting capabilities can also reinforce the practice of looking for evidence to support nursing interventions rather than relying on how things have been done historically. This enhances processing and understanding of the information, and allows the nurse to apply the information to other areas, increasing the knowledge obtained about why certain conditions or responses result in prompts for additional questions or actions.

For example, a healthcare agency accrediting body, the Joint Commission, has added core measures for quality as part of its reporting and inspection process. When parts of the nursing process, such as problem identification and care planning, are embedded in the documentation, they may become such an integral part of the workflow that staff at the bedside no longer consciously separates them out as unique actions. This reflects well on the system design but can make it difficult for care providers to explain to regulatory agencies, such as the Joint Commission, what they are doing. Preparing staff involved in bedside care to communicate effectively what they are doing can be a challenge. Some institutions rely on standardized clinical practice guidelines that can be modified for application to individual patients. In this way, there is a clear illustration for the application of the nursing process to clinical care.

To incorporate EBP into the practice of clinical nursing, the information needs to be embedded in the computerized documentation system so that it is part of the workflow. The most typical way of embedding this timely information is through clinical practice guidelines. The resulting interventions and **clinical outcomes** need to be measurable and reportable for further research. The supporting documentation for the EBP needs to be easily retrievable and meaningful. Links, reminders, and prompts can all be used as vehicles for transmission of this information. The format needs to allow for rapid scanning, with the ability to expand the amount of information when more detail is required or desired. Balancing a consistency in formatting with creativity can be difficult but worth the effort to stimulate an atmosphere for learning.

EBP is supported by **translational research**, which is a "dynamic and fluid exchange of scientific and clinical knowledge" (Clements & Crane, 2006, p. 42). This is an exciting movement that has enormous potential for the sharing and use of EBP. By creating a fluid sharing of research and application between research experts (those who know) and clinical experts (those who do) at the bedside, more meaningful research and improved clinical outcomes should result. The use of translational research to support EBP may help to close the gap between what is known (research) and what is done (practice).

THE CIS AS A STAFF DEVELOPMENT TOOL

Joy Hilty, a registered nurse from Kaweah Delta, came up with a creative way to provide **staff development** or education without taking staff away from the bedside to a classroom setting. She created pop-up boxes on the opening charting screens for all staff who chart on the computer. These pop-ups vary in color and content and include a short piece of clinical information, along with a question. Staff can earn "vacations" from these pop-ups for up to 14 days by e-mailing the correct answer to the question. This media has provided information, stimulation, and a definite benefit: the vacation from the pop-up boxes. The pop-up box education format has encouraged staff to share the answers, thus creating interaction, **knowledge dissemination**, and reinforcement of the education provided.

This same logic can be used to reinforce new standards of care based on current evidence. By adding interaction to embedded practices, the information is reinforced. As this information is repeatedly used and reinforced, an awareness of the way the information can be used to improve patient care is developed. When the information is applied to other similar situations, knowledge has been achieved.

Embedding EBP into nursing documentation can also increase the compliance with Joint Commission core measures, such as providing information on influenza and pneumovac vaccinations to at-risk patients. In the author's experience at Kaweah Delta, educating staff via classes, flyers, and storyboards was not successful in improving compliance with the documentation of immunization status or offering education on these vaccinations to at-risk patients. Embedding the prompts, information, and related questions in the nursing documentation with a link to the protocol and educational material has improved the compliance to 96% for pneumococcal vaccinations and to 95% for the influenza vaccination (Hettinger, 2007).

Creating an environment that encourages and expects professional development and learning needs to be a consistent expectation across all levels of an organization. The volume of information available makes it extremely difficult to find information that is current, valid, and applicable to the problem or question at hand. Relying on memory or past knowledge may not be the best way of providing care based on current evidence. Further, maintaining knowledge on best practices based on current research is almost impossible because of the sheer volume of information. To provide the medical community with a way to manage this volume of information, several companies have developed strategies for reviewing research and have developed software applications where this information can be easily retrieved. These knowledge vendors are now working with clinical systems to embed this knowledge and provide links to timely and continuously updated information.

By embedding a standard language (see Chapter 7) into the computerized documentation, the data can be used for instruction and for facilitating the sharing of information for research. This sharing of information improves the ability to track the effects of nursing interventions. Many institutions have implemented **clinical practice councils** that use information generated by the CIS to design clinical education programs. Councils may also update policies or procedures or clinical practice guidelines according to changes based on the analysis of institutional strengths, weaknesses, and goals.

CURRENT STATE

In this scenario, the supervisor reports using an automated bed board to review the current open beds and staffing. Requests for new admissions are communicated using the bed board to the bed coordinator or supervisor, who evaluates them and pushes the alert to the nursing unit who he or she has determined is the best place based on level of care required, patient acuity, and staffing. The unit responds electronically, which generates an alert to the professional making the assignment and the unit (including the emergency department) requesting the bed.

Staff input their charting, including problem identification and planning, into the computer system. Telemetry wave forms can be accessed real time using a transparent link from the patient's **electronic health record** (EHR). In a similar manner, electrocardiograms and radiographic images can also be easily accessed without leaving the EHR. This enables providers to review the chart from any location. A nurse can call the supervisor or clinical specialist with a concern.

Real Life Example

A nurse called the supervisor with a concern about a change that she noted in cardiac rhythm and corresponding symptoms (even though the monitors are in a different area). The supervisor contacted the cardiologist to ask him if he thought a consult was needed. He remotely reviewed the new and old electrocardiogram, laboratory work, and the nurses' charting of the patients symptoms along with the real-time cardiac rhythm and determined that a consult was in the patient's best interest. The attending physician agreed, and the cardiologist was able to order additional laboratory work, which was completed and available when he arrived on the unit to see the patient.

What This Means to the Nursing Informatics Professional

As more information is stored electronically, nurse informaticists must translate the technology so that the input and retrieval are developed in a manner that is easy for clinicians to learn and use. Usability is described in the TIGER Usability Report (n.d) as how easy it is for users to learn, remember, and use a product. A highly usable product should decrease errors and improve information entry and retrieval. Nurse informaticists must be able to work with staff and expert users to design systems that meet the needs of the staff using the systems. The work is not done after the system is installed; the system must continue to be developed and improved, because as staff uses the system they will be able to suggest changes to improve the system. This results in a system that is mature and meets the needs of the users.

MEANINGFUL USE

In 2004, President Bush mandated that all Americans be using EHRs by 2014. Shortly after taking office in 2009, President Obama continued this vision by signing the **American Recovery and Reinvestment Act** (ARRA), which earmarked $19 billion to develop an electronic health information technology infrastructure that will improve the efficiency and access of health care to all Americans (see Chapter 10). These executive directives clarified the need for healthcare providers, and nurses in particular, to be able to function in an age of automated healthcare tools.

As more facilities become automated, the ability to find paper policies, clinical resources, and patient information is becoming more and more limited. Combined with the number of patients and families with computers in their homes, the situation is beyond the need for basic computer skills and to the point of requiring computer literacy and information literacy to function.

According to the Healthcare Information and Management Systems Society, in 2009, 67% of hospitals installed some parts of the electronic record, requiring only one or two applications to meet the basic ARRA EHR criteria. Staff nurses at many facilities use the computerized kardex, or rand card, to share information during report. They use bar-coding technology to give medications more safely. Alerts notify them of new orders; of specimens that need to be collected; and of potential nursing problems (nursing diagnoses).

Hospitals that are already automated are reviewing the ARRA criteria and then comparing the criteria to what they already have in place. This information is then used to prioritize what (if any) applications need to be implemented. This may require minor or major modifications to their current timeline for implementations. After developing a plan for what to implement and when, a gap analysis needs to be done comparing the current resources to the resources required for the new timeline.

SUMMARY

The CIS is a technology-based system applied at the point of care and designed to support the acquisition and processing of information and providing storage and processing capabilities. Early CISs were limited in scope. Today, the goal of many organizations is to expand the scope of the CIS to a comprehensive system that provides clinical decision support, an electronic patient record, and in some instances professional development training tools. Benefits of such a comprehensive system could provide easy access to patient data at the point of care; structured and legible information that can be searched easily and lends itself to data mining and analysis; and improved patient safety, especially the prevention of adverse drug reactions and the identification of health risk factors, such as falls. Quality assurance is a positive outcome from CISs and the clinical analytics promote medical care outcomes research. The incorporation of EBP and the integration of clinical expertise and best practices based on systematic research to enhance decision making and improve patient care will further enhance the system. The use of translational research to support EBP may help to close the gap between what is known (research) and what is done (practice). As a staff development medium, embedding the prompts, information, and related questions in the nursing documentation with a link to the protocol and educational material has improved compliance. CISs are becoming more robust and are assuming increasing roles in the healthcare delivery system.

In an ideal world, all clinical documentation will be shared through a national database, in a standard language to enable evaluation of nursing care, increase the body of evidence, and improve patient outcomes. With minimal effort, the information will be translated into new research that can be analyzed, and linked to new evidence that will be intuitively applied to the CIS. Alerts will be meaningful, and will be patient and provider specific. The steps required of the clinician to find current, reliable information will be almost transparent, and the information will be presented in a personalized manner based on user preferences stored in the CIS.

THOUGHT-PROVOKING Questions

 WWW

1. You have been asked to prioritize the requirements of a clinical documentation system. It has already been determined that ease, usability, and dependability are priorities. What else would you include in the system requirements?
2. You have been asked to design a test scenario for a new CIS. What are some of the details you would test? Who would you involve?
3. You are asked about a diagnosis with which you are unfamiliar. Where would you start looking for information? How would you determine the validity of the information?

For a full suite of assignments and additional learning activities, use the access code located in the front of your book to visit this exclusive website: **http://go.jblearning.com/mcgonigle**. If you do not have an access code, you can obtain one at the site.

WWW

References

Biohealthmatics. (2006). *Clinical information system.* Retrieved from http://www.biohealthmatics.com/technologies/his/cis.aspx

Clements, P. T., & Crane, P. A. (2006). Building bridges: The importance of translational forensic nursing research. *Journal of Forensic Nursing, 2*(1), 42–44.

Hettinger, M. (2007, March). Core measure reporting: Performance improvement. Kaweah Delta Health Care District publication. Visalia, California.

McLaughlin, T., & Halilovic, M. (2006). Clinical analytics, rigorous coding bring objectivity to quality assertions. *Medical Staff Update Online, 30*(6). Retrieved from http://med.stanford.edu/shs/update/archives/JUNE2006/analytics.htm

Saba, V. K. (2007). Clinical care classification (CCC) system manual: A guide to nursing documentation (2nd ed.). New York, NY: Springer.

Simpson, R. L. (2004). Evidence-based nursing offers certainty in the uncertain world of health care. *Nursing Management, 35*(10), 10–12.

Sittig, D., Hazlehurst, B., Palen, T., Hsu, J., Jimison, H., & Hornbrook, M. (2002). A clinical information system research landscape. *The Permanente Journal, 6*(2). Retrieved from http://xnet.kp.org/permanentejournal/spring02/landscape.html

Technology Informatics Guiding Education Reform (TIGER). (n.d.). Designing usable clinical information systems: Recommendations from the TIGER usability and clinical applications design collaborative team. Retrieved from http://www.tigersummit.com/uploads/Tiger_Usability_Report.pdf

CHAPTER 19

Telenursing and Remote Access Telehealth

Original contribution by Audrey Kinsella and Kathleen Albright with contributions by Sheldon Prial and Schuyler F. Hoss, updated for the Second Edition by Dee McGonigle and Kathleen Mastrian

Objectives

1. Explore the use of telehealth technology in nursing practice.
2. Identify the socioeconomic factors likely to increase the use of telehealth interventions.
3. Describe clinical and nonclinical uses of telehealth.
4. Specify and describe the most common telehealth tools used in nursing practice.
5. Explore telehealth pathways and protocols.
6. Identify legal, ethical, and regulatory issues of home telehealth practice.
7. Describe the role of the telenurse.
8. Apply the Foundation of Knowledge model to home telehealth.

WWW

Key Terms

WWW

Call centers
Central stations
Chronic disease
Home health care
Home telehealth care
Medication management
    devices
Patient informed consent
Peripheral biometric
    (medical) devices
Personal emergency
    response system
Portals
Real-time telehealth
Sensor and activity
    monitoring systems
Store-and-forward telehealth
    transmission
Telehealth
Telehealth care
Telemedicine
Telemonitoring
Telenursing
Telepathology
Telephony
Teleradiology
Web servers

INTRODUCTION

Telehealth is a relatively new term in the medical and nursing vocabulary, and refers to a wide range of health services that are delivered by telecommunications-ready tools, such as the telephone, videophone, and computer. The most basic of telecommunications technology, the telephone, has been used by health professionals for many years, sometimes by nurses to counsel a patient or by doctors to change a patient's plan of care. Because of these widespread uses, people are already somewhat familiar with the value of the direct, expedient contact that telecommunications-ready tools provide for healthcare professionals. The growing field of telehealth, particularly in nursing practice, will allow clinicians to improve care delivery services even more.

HISTORY OF TELEHEALTH

The late President John F. Kennedy gave NASA a goal of landing an American on the moon. A surprise benefit of the space program was the demonstration of effective remote monitoring of the astronauts, and thus modern telehealth was born. Although most of the advances in telehealth have taken place in the last 20 to 30 years, Craig and Patterson (2005) describe much earlier examples, such as the use of bonfires to alert neighboring villages of the arrival of bubonic plague during the Middle Ages. Postal services and telegraphs were used to transmit health information in the mid-19th century, and 1910 marks the first transmission of stethoscope sounds over a telephone. Radio communications were used to provide medical support for crews on ships; the Seaman's Church Institute of New York (1920) and the International Radio Medical Center (1938) are two examples of organizations founded to provide health support at a distance. These services were later expanded to cover air travel (Craig & Patterson). The National Institutes of Mental Health supported a program in the mid-1950s that connected seven state hospitals in four different states via a closed-circuit telephone system (Venable, 2005). As technology evolved, its use in health care continued to grow. The first reported use of television to monitor patients in a clinical facility occurred in the 1950s, which then led to the development of interactive closed-circuit applications in the mid-1960s. These early TV applications to health care occurred within the facility but still had the benefit of extending the reach of the caregivers because they did not need to be in the same room to monitor their patients effectively (Prial and Hoss, 2009).

In the 1970s, uses of more advanced forms of telehealth in the medical field, referred to as **telemedicine**, included **teleradiology** and **telepathology**—radiologic and pathologic images transmitted to specialists who were located at some distance (Allan, 2006). As additional specialties, such as dermatology and ophthalmology, entered the telemedicine arena, telehealth use enabled even more physicians to access information about their patients regardless of distances between themselves and the patients and conventional healthcare settings.

Success in telehealth was achieved after decades spent refining the technology, which resulted in clearer imaging, more speedy transmissions, and accurate replication of data from remote locations to a central hub. Technical advances in imaging, for example, have increased the usage of telehealth in wound care and increased specialists' satisfaction with quality of patient data received from remote sites (Kinsella, 2002b). The end results of telehealth interactions today have helped to ensure that professionals, whether working off site or directly with patients, can replicate usual clinical interactions in all specialties regardless of the distance involved in the contact.

This capacity to supervise patients away from an office is predicted to continue to grow rapidly and "worldwide telemedicine markets at $7 billion in 2009 are expected to reach $24 billion by 2016" (Aarkstore Enterprise, 2010, para. 30). The ability to provide better healthcare access is the number one benefit of using telehealth. By reducing the need for face-to-face interaction with the patient, the nurse, physician, or even the technician can be much more productive. When information is collected in the home, it becomes much more convenient for the patient and the quality and timeliness of the information is improved dramatically. Home **telemonitoring** should be viewed as an enhancement to care, because it allows more direct, physical intervention to occur only when it is actually needed. Care is not directed by prescheduled appointment or subjective perceptions of condition; it can instead be determined by objective measures of physical status. With telehealth, it can also be delivered at the most appropriate site of care, reducing reliance on emergency departments and inpatient facilities (Prial and Hoss, 2009).

NURSING ASPECTS OF TELEHEALTH

Understanding telehealth and the potential use of telehealth technology in nursing practice is necessary in today's changing healthcare arena. As this chapter describes, nurses using telehealth have much greater access to their patients' conditions and needs and are able to respond in a more timely way than is possible using only face-to-face visits. Patients' responses to new medications, for example, can be tracked within hours rather than the several days that elapse between face-to-face visits. The telecommunications-ready tools that can be used to achieve these results are described, and cases that have demonstrated successful outcomes are highlighted.

Today, the use of many telehealth tools by nurses is new. Telehealth interventions or contacts are performed off site and often require less time spent on task because of the efficiencies offered by the technology applications. Their use, however, must never be associated with less care. It is important to note that nursing activity in telehealth still follows the same best practice standards as those espoused in conventional care. One should, look at the use of telehealth tools as a means for nurses to do their work better.

The following case study indicates the capability of a **home health care** nurse's working with telehealth tools to detect and respond to a patient's condition more expediently so that needed care could be accessed.

Case Study:
Early Detection of a Change in Condition

Mrs. C., an independent, 96-year-old woman, has a history of rehospitalization because of atrial fibrillation resulting from congestive heart failure (CHF) and hypertension.

After her most recent hospitalization, Mrs. C. was treated and released into home care at an agency in Washington. A home telemonitoring system that tracks and transmits patients' vital signs was placed in her home. The primary goal of placing this patient on the telemonitor was to provide daily monitoring of the patient's condition, thereby avoiding unnecessary rehospitalizations.

One morning, Mrs. C's telenurse detected an alarmingly low oxygen saturation level in the patient's transmitted data. As a result, the nurse telephoned Mrs. C. and asked her to retake her oxygen reading. The reading was confirmed and the telenurse contacted the patient's physician, who requested immediate transportation of the patient to the hospital emergency room. Medics were called and the patient was taken to the hospital, where she was diagnosed with a pulmonary embolism.

The prompt response resulted from early detection and timely intervention enabled by the home telehealth equipment and a home health nurse's oversight. One notable fact in this case is that although the primary goal of monitoring patients is to avoid unnecessary hospitalization, in this case the hospitalization was necessary for the patient as a result of her elevated blood pressure and compromised oxygen saturation levels. The patient was still asymptomatic at the time of detection. However, the telehealth intervention and subsequent hospitalization allowed for the embolism to be treated before any serious damage occurred.

Under the traditional home care model, this patient may only have been seen by a nurse two to three times a week. The clinician does not have knowledge of the patient's condition in between visits; however, having vital patient data tracked and transmitted daily allowed for rapid response that resulted in a positive outcome, perhaps a life-saving intervention for this patient.

DRIVING FORCES FOR TELEHEALTH

A significant increase is expected in the use of information technology tools in nursing venues in the coming decades. This use is affected by a number of factors in all of western society. The following factors are drivers of the growing trend toward telehealth and technology use and will influence nursing practice significantly in the next decades: demographics; nursing and healthcare worker shortages; **chronic diseases** and conditions; the new, educated consumers; and excessive costs of healthcare services that are increasing in need and kind.

Demographics

One hears it every day: the baby boomers are getting older and people are living longer. In 2000, 13% of the American population was over 65, and the numbers are growing significantly. According to the U.S. Bureau of the Census (1993), 2,500 Americans turn 65 years old every day. Consequently, by 2040, 21% of the United States Population (one in five Americans) will be 65 years old or older and there will be almost four times as many people over 85 as there are today, as documented by the Institute of Aging (1996). Also on the rise is the number of aged Americans living with at least one chronic disease or condition (Hoffman, Rice, & Sung, 1996), a factor alerting clinicians to the much greater demand for planned professional care in the near future.

Nursing and Healthcare Worker Shortages

The crisis in the well-known nursing shortage is twofold: there is a greater need for nurses by more persons, particularly those living lifetimes with sometimes multiple comorbidities; and there is a significant decrease in the number of young persons entering the nursing profession. In 2004, there were 2.9 million registered nurses (RNs) in the United States, with well over 41% of them aged 50 years old or older (U.S. Department of Health and Human Services, 2004). Nationwide, the demand for nurses is clearly exceeding supply. A report from the Health Resources and Services Administration (U.S. Department of Health and Human Services, 2002) on the shortage of RNs notes that the shortage is expected to rise from 6% today to 12% by 2010, and more than triple in size to 20% as soon as 2015.

The very serious shortage of healthcare workers in the United States must be addressed with some foresight. Although there is currently more focus on training lay people, such as aides and other paraprofessionals, in certain nursing tasks, this venture certainly cannot replicate the clinical expertise of trained nurses skilled in nursing routines. One must begin to look seriously at using effective adjuncts to skilled care, telehealth being one of these important adjuncts. Some have already begun to do so. For one, a recent study by the Pennsylvania Homecare Association and Penn State University (2004) looked at how telehealth can be used to address workforce issues in the home healthcare industry and determined that telehealth use may enhance nurses' job satisfaction and help to retain nurses in their current positions.

Chronic Diseases and Conditions

Chronic conditions are the leading cause of illness, disability, and death in the United States today. The aging population living with chronic diseases and conditions is expected to increase dramatically in the United States in the next decades. Many age groups are also affected by chronic diseases, not just the elderly.

Currently, more than 100 million Americans are living with one or more chronic diseases or conditions. The costs of their direct medical care are excessive; as much as $539 billion a year, according to the Institute of Aging's 1996 report, *Chronic Care in America: A 21st Century Challenge*. As noted in a more recent report, from the Centers for Disease Control and Prevention (2005), medical care costs of people with chronic diseases account for more than 75% of the United States' $1.4 trillion medical care expenditures. Furthermore, by the year 2030, 148 million Americans will join these ranks, at least one third of them limited in their ability to go to school or to live independently. Securing appropriate, adequate, and affordable care services for these populations should be a national concern.

Educated Consumers

The wave of today's aging baby boomers is driving some of the usual health service practices toward a very different course. Many of these individuals are more educated than their parents and more comfortable with the use of technology. They want to become more informed and involved with their care plans. These empowered consumers will be financially motivated with the introduction of consumer-directed healthcare plans that reward healthier lifestyles and better disease management of chronic conditions. All of these circumstances will further drive the use and the innovation of new technologies to meet consumer need. However, as Kinsella (2002a) has pointed out, this new consumer-driven trend of which the boomers are a part will not only be affected by technologic innovation but will affect how healthcare services are delivered. New plans for this new generation of consumers are very much leaning toward meeting their demands for when-needed, as-needed care, or care services delivered on their own terms and timing.

Economics

When one connects the drivers of today's healthcare market—the demographics, nursing shortages, and increased number of persons living with chronic conditions and their extensive use of healthcare services—with excessive costs of this health care, the need for solutions is vital. The American healthcare system spends $1.4 trillion per year on conventional medical care. Much more will be spent annually in the coming decades. One must ask: taking all of the driving factors of today's healthcare market into account, what needs to be done to address healthcare issues in the United States and meet the burgeoning numbers and needs of patients?

A solution is to develop a new clinical model for American health care that includes technology. Most particularly, telehealth technology should be included to fill the gap resulting from an overabundance of patients and a scarcity of healthcare providers. This concept is indicated in Figure 19-1.

Consider the use of technology that can fill current gaps in the healthcare system. Tools of telehealth can, for example, help render needed services without re-

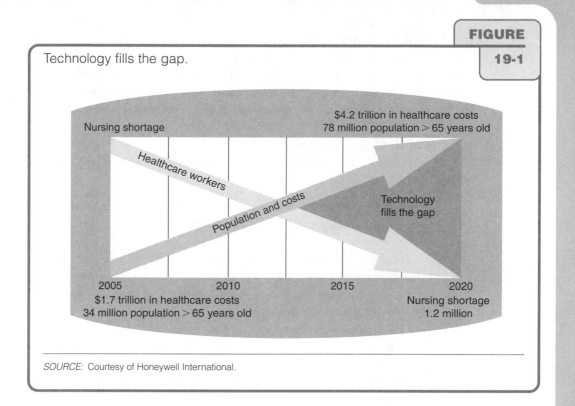

FIGURE 19-1

Technology fills the gap.

Nursing shortage

$4.2 trillion in healthcare costs
78 million population > 65 years old

Healthcare workers

Population and costs

Technology fills the gap

2005
$1.7 trillion in healthcare costs
34 million population > 65 years old

2010

2015

2020
Nursing shortage
1.2 million

SOURCE: Courtesy of Honeywell International.

quiring in-person professional care at all contacts. The remote or virtual visit made by skilled clinicians is only one approach to using a range of health technologies available today. More needs to be learned about what telehealth is, how it works, and what aspects have been successful so that clinicians can plan to incorporate its use into routine clinical care.

TELEHEALTH CARE

Let us start with a basic definition of **telehealth care**. Keep in mind, however, that telehealth is an emerging field, and definitions are subject to change and improvement as technology evolves. The American Telemedicine Association (2010) provides the following definition:

> Telemedicine is the use of medical information exchanged from one site to another via electronic communications to improve patients' health status. Closely associated with telemedicine is the term "telehealth," which is often used to encompass a broader definition of remote health care that does not always involve clinical services. Videoconferencing, transmission of still images, e-health including patient **portals**, remote monitoring of vital signs, continuing medical education and nursing **call centers** are all considered part of telemedicine and telehealth. (para. 1).

Indeed, "telehealth" is generally used as an umbrella term to describe all of the possible variations of healthcare services that use telecommunications. Telehealth can refer to clinical and nonclinical uses of health-related contacts. Delivery of patient education, such as menu planning for diabetic patients or the transmission of medication reminders, is an example of health-promoting aspects of telehealth.

Clinical Uses of Telehealth

A few clinical uses for telehealth technologies and some sample clinical applications include the following:

1. Transmitting images for assessment or diagnosis. One example is transmission of digital images, such as images of wounds for assessment and treatment consults.
2. Transmitting clinical data for assessment, diagnosis, or disease management. One example is remote patient monitoring and transmitting patients' objective or subjective clinical data, such as monitoring of vital signs and answers to disease management questions.
3. Providing disease prevention and promotion of good health. One example is telephonic case management and patient education provided through asthma and weight management programs conducted in schools.
4. Using telephonic health advice in emergent cases. One example is performing teletriage in call centers.
5. Using real-time video. One example is exchanging health services or education live via videoconference.

Telehealth Transmission Formats and Their Clinical Applications

Nurses must become familiar with the many and varied clinical and nonclinical transmission formats and applications of telehealth technologies so that they can make informed choices about the tools that are available for their use, as needed. Among these applications are store-and-forward telehealth, **real-time telehealth**, remote monitoring, and **telephony**.

Store-and-Forward Telehealth

In a **store-and-forward telehealth transmission**, digital images, video, audio, and clinical data are captured and stored on the client computer or device; then, at a convenient time, the data are transmitted securely (forwarded) to a specialist or clinician at another location where they are studied by the relevant specialist or clinician. If indicated, the opinion of the specialist or clinician is then transmitted back. Based on the requirements of the participating healthcare entities, this round-trip interaction could take from minutes to 48 hours. In many store-and-forward specialties, such as teleradiology, an immediate response is not critical. Dermatology, radiology, and pathology are common specialties that are conducive to store-and-forward technologies. Transmission of wound care images for assessment by specialty care nurses or other specialists has become a frequently used and important form of home telehealth nursing practice.

Real-Time (or interactive) Telehealth

In real-time telehealth, a telecommunications link between the involved parties allows a real-time or live interaction to take place. Videoconferencing equipment is one of the most common forms of technologies used in synchronous telehealth. There are also peripheral devices that can be attached to computers or to the videoconferencing equipment that can aid in an interactive examination. Use of computers for real-time two-way audio and video streaming between centers over ever-improving and cheaper communication channels is becoming common. These developments have contributed to lowering of costs in telehealth.

Examples of real-time clinical telehealth applications include the following:

- Telemental health, which uses videoconferencing technology to connect a psychiatric nurse with a mental health client.
- Telerehabilitation, which uses videocameras and other technologies to assess patients' progress in home rehabilitation.
- Telehomecare, which uses video technologies to observe, assess, and teach patients living in rural areas.
- Teleconsultations, which use a variety of technologies to enable collaborative exchanges or consultations between individuals or among groups that are involved with a case. These teleconsults may be transmitted live using videoconferencing technology. They may, for instance, involve teaching a certain technique to a less-experienced clinician or they may provide several clinicians with an opportunity for discussing an appropriate approach to a difficult case.
- Telehospice or telepalliative care, which can use real-time or remote monitoring to provide psychologic support to patients and caregivers. Telehealth devices can also play a role in symptom management, in effect helping end-of-life patients to achieve an optimum quality of life.

Remote Monitoring (Telemonitoring or Remote Patient Monitoring)

In remote monitoring, devices are used to capture and transmit biometric data. For example, a tele-electroencephalogram device monitors the electrical activity of a patient's brain and then transmits that data to an assigned specialist. This interaction could be done in either real time or as a stored and then forwarded transmission. Examples of telemonitoring include the following:

- Monitoring patient parameters during home-based nocturnal dialysis
- Cardiac and multiparameter monitoring of remote intensive care units
- Home telehealth, in which examples can include daily home telemonitoring of vital signs by patients and transmitting data that enables off-site nurses to track their patients regularly and precisely and address noticeable changes through education and information suggestions about diet or exercise
- Disease management

Telephony

Telephone monitoring (telephony) is the most basic type of telehealth. It can be described as scheduled remote care delivery or monitoring in which scheduled patient encounters via the telephone occur between a healthcare provider and a patient or caregiver (Quality Insights of Pennsylvania, 2005). More details about interaction using telephony are discussed later.

Nonclinical Uses of Telehealth Technologies

There are also many nonclinical uses of telehealth technologies. Currently, these include distance education including continuing medical and nursing education, grand rounds, and patient education; administrative uses including meetings among telehealth networks, supervision, and presentations; and research using the Internet and other online sources for information and health data management.

All of these telecommunications-assisted activities overcome obstacles of distance and provide access to needed health-related information. Clearly, with telehealth, the range of patient care possibilities broadens significantly.

TELENURSING

Where do nurses using telehealth, as in **telenursing**, play a role in today's healthcare delivery arena? Telenursing refers to the use of telecommunications and information technology for providing nursing services in health care to enhance care whenever a physical distance exists between patient and nurse or between any numbers of nurses (Skiba, 1998). As a clinical field, telenursing is part of telehealth and has many points of contacts with other medical and nonmedical applications, such as telediagnosis, teleconsultation, and telemonitoring. In their study, St George et al. (2009) concluded that "In terms of the kinds of calls received, the dispositions reached after triage and clinical safety, we could detect no differences between nurses working from home and those working in the call centre" (p. 123). Telenurses do not, in effect, work outside of the broader clinical team effort, no matter where they are located. They are indeed an integral part of the healthcare delivery team.

Applications of Telenursing in Home Care

The most developing area of telenursing today is in **home telehealth care**. An accepted definition of home telehealth care provided by Kinsella (2004) is as follows: "Home telehealth care is clinician-driven remote care delivery and education services that are delivered to the home via telecommunications-ready tools" (p. 36).

As home telehealth care evolved, the definition has expanded to include a broader arena of delivery. In fact, some have defined the home as anywhere outside of an acute inpatient setting, and so includes nursing homes, assisted living facilities, and other living situations beyond the single family home or apartment. Wherever the home setting may be people want to be cared for there. Today's burgeoning senior population, in particular, has become quite vocal about this preference. According to regular surveys by the American Association for Retired Persons (AARP, 1996), more than 90% of seniors want to remain independent at home and age in a familiar place. Care at home is clearly a key concern and preference.

Fortuitously, the reach of nurses using telecommunications-ready tools in the home is now remarkably extended. Not only are the settings for home care extended beyond what was usual (the family home) in the last four decades of home health's formal existence, but the types of services delivered to the home are more advanced than ever before. The home care industry's newest challenge is to work with sicker patients, many of whom have been discharged from hospitals to home earlier than in the past.

This challenge to extend the range of conventional home care is why telehealth can be and needs to be provided to a wide range of patients, including those who:

- Are immobilized
- Live in remote or difficult-to-reach places
- Have chronic ailments, such as chronic obstructive pulmonary disease, diabetes, and congestive heart disease
- Have debilitating diseases, such as neural degenerative diseases (Parkinson disease, Alzheimer disease, amyotrophic lateral sclerosis)

All of these patients may stay at home and be visited and assisted regularly by a nurse via videoconferencing, Internet, videophone, or other telecommunications means. These telecommunications-ready tools enable home telenurses to follow through advanced levels of care, as needed.

Still other varied applications of home telehealth care are the care of patients in immediate postsurgical situations, those needing care of wounds and ostomies, and handicapped individuals needing physical therapy interventions or telerehabilitation. In addition to this extended range of patients who can be served with telehealth, many more patients can be seen when telehealth is used. For example, in conventional home health care, depending on the distances of travel involved, one nurse is able to visit up to seven patients per day. Using telenursing, however, one nurse can remotely visit or televisit 12–16 patients in the same amount of time using interactive telehealth. Over the last decade, efficiencies of telenursing have become well documented, as have the resulting improved patient care outcomes that can be expected by frequent telecontact.

Another outpatient application of telenursing is telephony-based call centers, which may be operated by managed care organizations, hospitals, and other health organizations. Some call centers also include telemonitoring services, which allow the patient to stay at home and use different telehealthcare devices to transmit biometric and other medical information back to the call center. Monitoring can be intermittent or continuous. This use of the teletechnology allows clinicians to evaluate patients' status and use the data to make decisions to manage patients' health conditions better.

Many features of call centers' services are comparable to conventional hands-on care in the home. For instance, call centers are typically staffed by RNs who act as case managers or perform patient triage. These professionals can provide information and counseling to patients as part of a disease management program and as a means to educate them on their disease process. In effect, their goal is to offer appropriate access to care (from nurses at the call centers) and help patients to prevent avoidable emergency room visits and rehospitalizations. An example of this assistance includes a nurse calling (i.e., not waiting for a patient to contact the call center) a recently discharged diabetic patient on a regularly scheduled basis to evaluate progress at home, activity tolerance, medication compliance, foot care, and diet management. This empowering of patients towards self-management is a very significant and needed part of telenursing.

Home care telenursing can also involve other activities, such as providing customized patient education in dietary or exercise needs, nursing teleconsultations, review of results of medical tests and examinations, and assistance to physicians in the implementation of medical treatment protocols. The work can be wide ranging; for example, there are some home-based telecardiology programs that involve the patient, the family, the physician, and a specialized cardiac monitoring center. A multidisciplinary approach is used along with best practice–defined protocols to manage the patient; improve the patient's quality of life; and reduce healthcare costs, most particularly reduced hospitalization costs. Nurses play a key role in this network of care.

By reviewing all of these examples of telenursing practice, one can see that nurses using telenursing can broaden their involvement in the targeted care of each of their patients. It is predicted that home care will soon become a hub of all patient activity; the home will be where care that is begun in hospitals and other settings will be managed over the very long term and in the most cost-effective healthcare setting. Home care telenurses can well expect to play a vital and dynamic role in the changing delivery systems that are likely to be in place in the coming decades.

TELEHEALTH PATIENT POPULATIONS

(FROM PRIAL AND HOSS, 2009)

Any patient who has a condition that must be monitored is a candidate for home telemonitoring. Patients with chronic illnesses have particularly benefited from ongoing monitoring to prevent acute episodes. Patients who are homebound or who have limited access to transportation are also appropriate for monitoring.

Chronic Disease Patients

Given demographics and advances in medical practice, there has been unprecedented growth in patients with chronic diseases. Those patients are at significant risk of having an acute episode when subtle but significant changes in their medical condition occur. The ability to identify these changes in a timely fashion allows for changes in medication, lifestyle, or treatment to occur. Identification of a 3-lb weight gain over 5 days in a CHF patient allows for interventions that prevent an emergency room visit and subsequent hospitalization. The most common categories of chronic patients that are currently monitored include those with CHF, chronic obstructive pulmonary disease (COPD), diabetes, or those who require long-term wound care.

These patients, particularly those with higher acuity levels, are at significant risk of having a medical crisis that necessitates emergency or unplanned acute interventions. There are many other categories of chronic patients who are less susceptible to a health crisis, but would greatly benefit from home telemonitoring to improve care and reduce costs.

At-Risk Populations

Telemonitoring can be used effectively on patients who are at risk for an episode of acute illness. Patients who have a predisposition to disease are at risk of medical problems associated with employment, lifestyle, or location, or those patients who have displayed early signs of potential serious health problems could be placed on preventive monitoring. Monitoring is used to ensure that interventions are timely and acute incidents avoided. Such technology could be part of a healthcare early warning system and could support preventive models of care.

Isolated Patients

Home telemonitoring is effective for patients who cannot physically access healthcare services. The homebound elderly have been among the first to benefit from this technology in conjunction with the home health services they receive. With increasing limits on the ability of patients to receive services in the home because of staffing shortages and coverage limitations, telemonitoring technology takes on greater importance in managing homebound patients.

Patients in remote geographic areas have been long-time users of telemedicine interventions, such as robodocs. According to Strauss (2010), "The Remote Presence Robot (RP-7) from InTouch Health is a mobile telemedicine unit that connects physicians and specialists with patients and other doctors who are too distant to consult with them in person" (para. 2). With few rural healthcare facilities being built and access problems becoming more difficult, the use of technology in the home will increase. Even in suburban and rural areas, access is becoming more problematic, requiring greater use of home telemonitoring interventions. A lack of primary care and emergency resources in many urban core areas has many health systems looking at managing certain patients through telemonitoring options and better staging patient access. Telemedicine also is effective for patients in such institutions as prisons, for whom it is logistically difficult to have them travel to traditional care sites.

Hospitalized Patients

Home telemonitoring has proved effective in managing the flow of patients into and out of hospitals and other inpatient facilities. Patients are monitored to determine when they are admitted, how long they are expected to stay, and to prevent unfunded readmissions. Patients undergoing semi-elective procedures can be better staged with scheduling options when they are monitored in the home before admission. If there is an observed deterioration in a condition, a procedure can be accelerated or planned interventions changed. Monitoring can also be used effectively in length of stay reduction strategies. Physicians and surgeons are more confident to discharge early when they know that vital signs will be monitored and any decline in condition noted in a timely fashion. Use of monitoring effectively allows for an extension of step-down models of care into the patient's home. These length of stay management strategies have been particularly useful in situations where there is a lack of available hospital beds. Unplanned readmissions are a serious patient care and financial management issue for hospitals. The use of monitoring in the home has consistently reduced unplanned and unfunded readmissions by being able to obtain reliable information on the patient and intervene appropriately to keep the patient at home.

Emergency Response Situations

Telemedicine will likely be a major component of effective patient management in a major disaster, large-scale nuclear or biochemical attack, or in the case of an outbreak of highly infectious disease. In such a situation, traditional healthcare delivery systems may be overwhelmed and patients will need to be more effectively triaged and managed by remote providers. Telemedicine applications allow for a dramatic extension of patient management and triaging options and allow off-site providers to be involved in care. If an infectious or communicable disease is involved, patient isolation could be accomplished in the home using telemedicine technology.

Concerned Patients and Families

Perhaps the largest potential market for home telemonitoring is patients and families who want to have reliable and objective information that allows for their involvement in healthcare decision making. At one extreme is a young person who wants to monitor physiologic data as part of a personal wellness or fitness program. At the other extreme are families that want information on the status of a terminally ill loved one in another city. In between there is a wide range of opportunities for individuals and families to obtain information that promotes realistic and meaningful dialogue with healthcare professionals.

Assisted Living and Subacute Patients

In assisted living facilities or subacute care centers, a kiosk can be used to obtain vital signs for large groups of people. Vital sign reports can then be forwarded on a regularly established schedule to physicians and others involved in the patient's care. This allows for better individual care management and lends itself to developing intervention strategies and education options to benefit the entire population of a facility. Some facilities have even used access to telemonitoring systems as an inducement to attract potential residents.

Employers and Wellness Programs

Health care is a vital concern for employers. They have a direct financial interest in lowering costs and are financial beneficiaries of long-term illness preventive strategies. If they can monitor their workers (offering telehealth options as a wellness program), they will see many benefits for themselves, such as reduced absenteeism and increased productivity. Effective monitoring programs can ultimately lower healthcare costs and associated insurance premiums. Some companies are now exploring the creation of financial incentives for employees who achieve healthcare objectives, such as appropriate weight, reduced blood pressure, and levels of exercise. Monitoring could very well be used as a means of tracking performance in this regard.

TOOLS OF HOME TELEHEALTH

There is a wide and growing range of telecommunications-ready tools readily available for nurses' and patients' use in the home. These tools are examined in more detail next.

Central Stations, Web Servers, and Portals

Central stations, **Web servers**, and portals are various terms presently used for multifunctional telehealthcare platforms and application servers. The terms indicate clinical management software programs that receive and display patients' vital signs and other information transmitted from a medical device, including blood pressure and glucose information. This transmission is most commonly accomplished over plain old telephone system lines (POTS); however, network access and wireless communication is gaining popularity as technology advances and access improves.

Central stations and Web servers are key components to telehealth that can be as minimal as a single screen display or may be more comprehensive software applications that provide various functions including triaging the data according to medical alerts, which allows clinicians quickly to identify patients requiring immediate attention. Other features found in these packages allow clinicians to build personal medical records for patients and provide trended patient data and analysis reports supporting improved patient outcomes using telehealth. In addition, some of the software packages provide remote programming capabilities that allow the clinician to remotely program the medical device in the patient's home. This application can change monitoring report times for patients, individualize alert parameters, set up reminders, and send educational content to a patient.

Peripheral Biometric (Medical) Devices

Peripheral biometric (medical) devices can consist of fully integrated systems, such as a vital signs monitor, or they may be stand-alone telecommunications-ready devices, such as blood pressure cuffs and blood glucose meters. Many plug directly into the household telephone jack to send data to a central server location.

There is an ever-increasing number of peripheral devices coming to market. Some examples of other peripheral devices seen in home telehealth today include pulse oximeters; prothrombin time, international normalized ratio meters; spirometers; peak flow meters; electrocardiogram monitors; and card readers and writers that use smart card technology and enable multiple users to use one device.

Telephones

Telephones are already the most familiar household communications tool used in telehealth care. A telephone device can also be augmented for easier use by patients, as needed, with a lighted dial pad, an auto-dial system, or a louder ringer.

Videocameras and Videophones

Videocameras and videophones are easily available consumer items that can be used in telehealth for show-and-tell demonstrations by nurses for patients or to capture wound healing progress, among other applications. Typically, these products can operate as a standard telephone or as a video picture telephone, using standard telephone lines to transmit information or interactions. It should be noted that the image quality over a POTS is limited by the bandwidth of POTS technology. It favors assessment rather than diagnostic quality images. These imaging capabilities will improve as integrated services digital network lines become more widely available in the home environment. Typically, medical centers and hospitals have access to larger bandwidth capabilities for image transmission and viewing, thus ensuring high-quality diagnostic images and point-to-point consultations in hospital- or medical center-based settings.

Personal Emergency Response Systems

Personal emergency response systems are well-known signaling devices worn as a pendant or otherwise made easily accessible to patients to ensure their safety and to access emergency care when needed, usually in case of a fall. A preset telephone number is alerted by the patient's pushing a button on the pendant and predesignated emergency help is dispatched. Many newer sensor options for tracking patients at home are being incorporated into multifunctioning personal emergency response systems devices, such as alerting a central call center to water flooding or smoke in a patient's home. See the next section for details on these sensors and monitors.

Sensor and Activity-Monitoring Systems

Sensor and activity-monitoring systems can track activities of daily living of seniors and other at-risk individuals in their place of residence. The sensors and monitoring systems can provide insight into behavior changes that might signal changes or deterioration of health status. These technologies consist of wireless motion sensors that are strategically placed around the residence and can detect motion on a 24-hour basis.

One authority on these new technologies, David J. Stern, describes their operation further (Stern, 2007), noting that data from these sensors are wirelessly sent to a receiver and base station that periodically transmits the information to a centralized server through standard telephone lines. Sophisticated algorithms analyze the data, compiling each individual's normal patterns of behavior including bathroom usage, sleep disturbance, meal preparation, medication interaction, and general levels of activity including fall detection. Deviations from these norms can be important warning signs of emerging health problems and can enable caregivers to intervene early.

In addition to widely used fire, security, and home gas detectors, there are other sensors that can monitor appliances to detect whether a household appliance is turned on or off and can sometimes switch the appliance on and off for the resident. Typical applications for affixing programmable sensors can include lamps, television sets, irons, and kitchen stoves. Such sensors might be very valuable for ensuring the safety of elderly, forgetful persons who live alone. One excellent example of today's sensor use for assistance with the elderly are sensors placed in or on stovetops to alert the user when he or she is standing too close to the equipment or when the kettle has over boiled. Benefits realized from these technologies include enabling people to live independently with an improved quality of life. They can also provide peace of mind for other family members living at a distance.

Medication Management Devices

Medication management devices address a well-recognized major problem in health care: medication management and compliance. According to the American Heart Association (2007), 49% of Americans use prescription drugs. In fact, 32 million people are taking three or more medications daily, with even more medications typically being taken by those 65 years of age or older.

What has become a national problem in health care today is the failure of patients to take medications as prescribed. Failing to do so can have devastating consequences, particularly for those patients living with chronic illnesses. Here are some of the facts about medication management and compliance in the United States, based on data from the National Pharmaceutical Council (2003):

- The cost of hospital admissions is an estimated $8.5 billion annually just for patients who do not take their medications as prescribed.
- About 23% of all nursing home admissions are caused by failure to take medications as prescribed.
- About 10% of all hospital admissions are related to improper self-administration of medication.
- People who miss medication doses need three times as many doctor visits as others and face increased medical costs.

To address some of these very pressing problems, there are a host of telecommunications-ready medication devices available and many new ones in development. Some are as simple as a watch that reminds a person to take medications, others are pill organizers with audible reminders, and some actually can be programmed to dispense prefilled containers with medications and alert a patient or caregiver of a missed dose. Furthermore, there are medication tools that send data from the device back to a central server so that patient's medication compliance can be tracked. These telecommunications-ready devices can organize, manage, dispense, or remind, and they can play an increasingly important role in helping people live independently and manage their disease processes through medication compliance. For more information on these devices, see Chapter 22.

Special Needs Telecommunications-Ready Devices

Special needs telecommunications ready-devices can include preprogrammed, multifunctional infusion pumps for providing a range of infusion needs, including medications for pain management and other infusion delivery needs, such as hydration and nutrition, peak flow meters, electrocardiogram monitors, and so on. Many such tools are in development to meet the more demanding and challenging needs of today's at-home patients. The common goal among all of these tools is that of increasing communications between the nurse and patient and providing the opportunity to increase nurses' knowledge of their patients' status in a timely manner.

HOME TELEHEALTH SOFTWARE

(FROM PRIAL AND HOSS, 2009)

As important as the gathering of data is the organizing of information to support decision making by clinical professionals. The telehealth software supporting home telehealth programs has become much more sophisticated, allowing for greater numbers of patients to be better managed by a single clinician. Areas of significant improvement in software include trending, triage, communications protocols, access, and sharing.

Trending

One of the advantages of home telemonitoring is the creation of a digital health record that allows information to be recorded over time. If a patient takes his or her weight and blood pressure daily, most software graphically displays this data over time so that subtle trends can be observed. This type of trend data is much more useful in identifying emerging or developing conditions than snapshot data that is collected every 6–8 weeks at a physician's office. Trend information can also be developed for groups of patients or populations, allowing for population-based analyses of interventions. It is possible to gather trend information on COPD patients, patients of a particular physician, or all patients receiving a certain medication.

Triage

Most home telemonitoring systems set an acceptable range of values for an individual patient when he or she is enrolled in the monitoring program. For example, if oxygen saturation, blood pressure, or weight values go above or below predetermined amounts, then the software alerts the appropriate party. More sophisticated software looks at readings from multiple pieces of equipment on a single patient and can give higher priority to patients at risk of an acute episode. This helps clinicians better organize their work and arrange for appropriate interventions.

Communications

Advanced telemonitoring software has sophisticated electronic notification protocols. It is often predetermined when information will be communicated and to whom it is sent. Sophisticated protocols can be developed related to both routine and alert information organizing communications with physicians, nurses, and caregivers. Some systems also have the capacity to communicate back to the patient or seek additional information under predetermined circumstances.

Data Access and Information Sharing

Many telemonitoring systems house information in Web-based formats. This allows for easy access to the data from any location that has access to the Internet. Multiple parties can simultaneously share and view data. Information can also be conveniently transmitted to other clinicians and is updated almost immediately when new values are received. Web-based records are fully HIPAA compliant when appropriate protections and controls are in place.

HOME TELEHEALTH PRACTICE AND PROTOCOLS

The tools of telehealth described previously are devices that enable remote care delivery, enhance patient care, and improve outcomes. They should be incorporated into nursing practice because nurses would typically use, for example, a blood pressure cuff. It is important to note that the data received from these tools is useless without some type of clinical oversight. The tools do not replace the nurse; rather, they give the nurse the ability to make more informed clinical decisions based on reliable data and a comprehensive picture of the patient's status. In home care they also direct the clinical resources to patients based on need. It becomes a patient-centered approach to care that delivers improved patient outcomes and clinical efficiencies.

Home telehealth is indeed a practice. It is a change in the current clinical model of practice for home care. Use of the telehealth tools is integrated into the practice to improve patient outcomes. Like any tool, however, the effectiveness is directly proportional to its application and use. Home telehealth programs differ depending on the type of technology used and the foci of the telehealth programs. However, every program should have telehealth use criteria established. The guidelines discussed here are broad-based, generic clinical guidelines for the deployment of home telehealth developed by the Home Telehealth Special Interest Group of the American Telemedicine Association (ATA, 2002).

The first guideline focuses on ensuring that the home is suitable for home telehealth delivery, and the second example focuses on ensuring that patients sign an informed consent form before receiving telehealth services. During the initial face-to-face visit, an assessment should be conducted to determine access to utilities and safety concerns appropriate for the installation of the equipment. Informed written consent must be obtained from the client or designee before beginning the use of telehealth consultations. The consent should be part of the plan of care and stored in the clinical record. These and similar guidelines issued by other health organizations including the American Nurses Association (2001) and the Community Health Accreditation Program (whose guidelines are not publicly available to nonmembers) can apply to both interactive home telehealth and telemonitored activity. Patient criteria should have inclusion and exclusion guidelines established, detailing who is eligible and appropriate for each type of technology. Other criteria include establishing policies and procedures that address patient enrollment, education, and equipment setup; patient and caregiver and home assessment; **patient informed consent**; and privacy and confidentiality rights. In addition, a clinical plan of care that is specific to patient needs should be developed. Telehealth pathways and protocols ensure more focused work with patients and allow for targeted interventions. A sample pathway to use for a patient who is being remotely monitored is provided in Figure 19-2. Home health agencies may use such samples as templates from which to design their own in-house, customized guidelines for home telenursing practice.

In addition, in Figure 19-3, a sample protocol is provided for telemonitoring patients living with hypertension. As with use of the pathway in Figure 19-2, nursing agencies may use this sample as a template for better managing these chronic disease patients and use it as a template to design other in-house protocols for telemanaging patients living with other chronic diseases. These protocols provide a focused start for nurses to learn and use home telehealth correctly and consistently.

Clearly, by using the protocol for patients who regularly use telehealth equipment for tracking their status, nurses receive a good deal more targeted information than is possible by scheduled, in-person visits. As a result, the use of telehealth tools, together with clinical oversight and practice, allows for more efficient and

FIGURE

19-2   Sample clinical pathway.

Hypertension
Daily Home Monitoring Pathway

Client Name: _____ SOC: _____

POC/Visit Frequency: **2w1, 1w8 with daily home monitoring until end of episode.**

                            2 PRN visits to assess cardiovascular status based upon data received from daily home monitoring.

                            *Visits may be reduced throughout the episode based upon client assessment, daily home monitoring and the achievement of goals.

GOALS OF DAILY HOME MONITORING & INTERMITTENT SKILLED SERVICES

1) Increase client knowledge regarding the disease process, treatment and management of hypertension utilizing the clinical data received from daily home monitoring.
2) Client will comply with treatment regimen and lifestyle changes to promote the optimum level of functioning at the time of discharge.
3) Improve clinical outcomes through the review of daily and trended data, allowing for early detection and intervention.
4) Maintain BP within parameters to avoid rehospitalization/ED visits allowing the client to remain at home with focus on self-management.

WEEK ONE: 2w1

Visit One: _____

☐ Admission SOC/OASIS
☐ Assess client/caregiver/home for daily home monitoring
☐ Initiate client/caregiver teaching as indicated
☐ Skilled interventions as ordered
☐ Evaluate appropriate parameters
☐ Add daily home monitoring to 485
☐ Installation of monitor and transmission of baseline vital signs

Visit Two: _____

☐ Installation and inservice of home monitor
☐ Client assessment
☐ Continue client/caregiver teaching as indicated
☐ Skilled interventions as ordered
☐ Discharge planning
☐ Assess appropriateness of parameters
☐ Other: _____

WEEK TWO: Nine: 1w8 and prn SNV based upon data from daily home monitoring

Skilled Nursing Visits:

☐ Client assessment
☐ Client/caregiver teaching as indicated
☐ Skilled interventions as ordered
☐ Confer with central station clinician as required
☐ Discharge planning
☐ Oversight and coordination of home care services and disciplines
☐ Assess need for continuing daily monitoring after discharge from home healthcare services
☐ Other: _____

Daily Home Monitoring:

☐ Daily review of clinical data
☐ Contact client to obtain additional subjective data if needed
☐ Reinforce client teaching
☐ Provide early detection and intervention as needed
☐ Confer with CM to review client status
☐ Weekly review of trends to evaluate client status and identify subtle changes in condition
☐ Fax trend reports to physician per protocol
☐ Assess need for continuing monitor after discharge from home care

Date	Initials	Signature
_____	_____	_____
_____	_____	_____
_____	_____	_____

Continues

SOURCE: Courtesy of Honeywell International.

FIGURE

19-2

Sample clinical pathway—*continued*.

Client/Caregiver Teaching Client/Caregiver Demonstrates/Verbalizes:	Goal Met	Not Met	N/A	Variance
1. Goal, purpose and importance of daily home monitoring related to disease process and management of hypertension. (↓ ED visits/hospitalizations)				
2. Demonstrates correct use of Honeywell HomMed monitor and identified peripherals.				
3. Early warning signs and symptoms of hypertension and when to call 911, MD, or the agency.				
4. Measures to avoid long-term complications of hypertension.				
5. Factors affecting hypertension and preventive measures/lifestyle changes to promote or improve health.				
6. Importance of MD follow-up visits.				
7. Medications: Indications, dosage, timing, route, desired, and adverse effects.				
8. Compliance with medication regimen.				
9. Importance of diet modifications and restrictions including sodium, cholesterol, calories, and fluid balance.				
10. Compliance with diet and fluid regimen.				
11. Importance of rest, exercise, energy conservation, and pacing activities following MD guidelines.				
12. Importance of lab testing and relation of results to the continuing treatment plan.				
13. Importance of daily maintenance or improvement of VS within individually set parameters.				
14. Health-promoting behaviors at or before discharge.				

VARIANCE CODES

V1: Client physically/cognitively unable	V13: Assistive aids unavailable _____
V2: Client refuses/noncompliant	V14: Assistive aid other_____
V3: Client hospitalized	V15: Environment unsafe_____
V4: Client terminated services	V16: Environment other_____
V5: Client transferred	V17: New diagnosis/Comorbidity
V6: Client moved	V18: Exacerbation of disease
V7: Client expired	V19: Client no longer meets criteria for HHC
V8: Client other_____	V20: Other:_____
V9: Caregiver none/absent	V21: Other:_____
V10: Caregiver refuses	V22: Other:_____
V11: Caregiver not capable	V23: Other:_____
V12: Caregiver other_____	V24: Other:_____

FIGURE

19-3   Protocol for CHF.

Telemonitoring Disease Management Protocol
Chronic Heart Failure

Overview: To increase the efficiency of healthcare resouce utilization and to improve patient health status, care coordination will be enhanced with the daily collection of patient specific objective and subjective data via the HomeMed Monitor.

GOALS:

1) Improve clinical outcomes through daily collection and review of patient's objective and subjective data allowing for early detection and intervention.
2) Increase patient knowledge regarding the disease process, treatment, and management of the disease utilizing the clinical data received from daily home monitoring.
3) Improve patient compliance with treatment regimen and lifestyle changes for promotion of health and optimal daily life functioning.
4) Promote patient independence and enhance behavior modification through daily vital sign awareness and follow-up.
5) Increase patient satisfaction through avoided rehospitalizations/ED visits/inappropriate clinic utilization and promotion of self-management in home.

CARE MANAGEMENT OVERVIEW: PATIENT IDENTIFICATION AND EDUCATION

Home Monitoring Patient Identification/ Installation

☐ Admit patient into monitoring program
☐ Provide phone notification to patient to introduce daily home monitoring
☐ Explain benefits of home monitoring, discuss location of monitor, and identify scheduled daily monitoring time(s)
☐ Evaluate appropriateness of home monitor based on diagnosis/secondary diagnoses, family dynamics, and home situation
☐ Customize monitor with programmed subjective questions and/or peripheral medical devices for individual patient need(s)
☐ Install and instruct patient on use of HomeMed monitor and transmit baseline vital signs
☐ Provide written monitor instructions
☐ Verify vital sign transmission, set patient-specific vital sign parameters (alert limits), and activiate "CHF alert" within central station

Patient/Caregiver/Family Education

☐ Provide basic disease process educational information: *What is Congestive Heart Failure?*
☐ Give diet, sodium, and fluid recommendations based on patient condition
☐ Provide medication education: Indications, dosage, timing, route, adverse effects
☐ Stress importance of maintaining MD appointments
☐ Educate patient about basic vital sign awareness, appropriate ranges, and when follow-up occurs based on vital sign values
☐ Teach patient recognition of common signs and symptoms
☐ Explain when, how, and whom to notify when symptoms occur
☐ Explain goals and benefits of daily home monitoring
☐ Instruct patient on answering disease-specific questions and the purpose of subjective questions

CARE MANAGEMENT OVERVIEW: DAILY MONITORING

Daily Review and Response of Clinical Data

☐ Patient objective and subjective data monitored daily by a skilled clinician
☐ Review of color-coded, triaged (stratified), and trended clinical data to determine follow-up
☐ Contact patient for further assessment if vital signs dictate
☐ Provide education, positive reinforcement, and follow-up to patient during phone contact to enhance behavior modification
☐ Facilitate visit to clinic, home, hospital, or other based on data gathered from home monitor

Ongoing Review and Response of Clinical Data

☐ Evaluate patient status and identify subtle changes in condition via weekly trend review
☐ Reinforce patient teaching, medication compliance, etc.
☐ Provide early detection and intervention as needed
☐ Work collaboratively with healthcare personnel to maximize efficiency
☐ Review vital sign parameters (alert limits) based upon patient condition
☐ Evaluate clinical progress and response to teaching via periodic documentation review

SOURCE: Courtesy of Honeywell International.

effective clinical management by allowing the patient's needs to drive the care. As home telehealth protocols are used more extensively, the improved clinical and operational efficiencies may ultimately impact the home care agency's bottom lines.

One must understand this clinically driven, as-needed approach to care services more fully so that it is not misunderstood as providing less care. In the following case study, a proactive, patient-centered approach enabled a home healthcare agency to identify early exacerbations in a patient's condition and take appropriate action.

Case Study:
Home Telemonitoring of Multiple Illnesses

WWW

The focus patient is a 71-year-old male who suffers with stage 4 cardiomyopathy/ pulmonary hypertension, atrial fibrillation, COPD, and type 2 diabetes mellitus. He has been an active patient with a home healthcare agency in Michigan since November 28, 2000, with an admitting diagnosis of CHF.

Initially, the patient was seen three times a week by an RN for CHF assessment and management. The patient's history included frequent hospitalizations for exacerbation of CHF and uncontrolled atrial fibrillation. He encountered a total of four hospitalizations in the year before placement of a telemonitoring system in his home, after about 6 months of receiving conventional home care.

Ever since he was placed on a telemonitoring system for daily tracking more than 8 months ago, he has not been rehospitalized. The telemonitoring interactions with his nurse have made him very conscientious of the role that his medications, diet, and fluid restrictions play in his overall health status.

In addition, the telemonitor has proved its benefits to local physicians. The patient's family physician, cardiologist, and pulmonologist all were able to care better for their patient with the tabular and graphical trends that were elicited from the daily vital signs monitor. This information aided in the titration and addition of the various medications needed to control the patient's CHF and atrial fibrillation. The physicians were able to ascertain the response to the medication adjustments and other treatment modalities, such as oxygen titration. At the start of care, the patient's weight was 196 pounds and is now at a stable 187 pounds, with the symptoms more controlled than they have ever been.

The patient's nurses, meanwhile, have peace of mind knowing they can keep an eye on their patient daily while making additional visits as needed, with the documentation to justify the additional nursing visit. This tool can also be incorporated into the nurses' care plan, enabling a higher standard of care to the patient.

At present, the patient is being case managed by nursing staff visits of once per month. He now enjoys a newfound peace of mind and security and an improved state of health, something this patient has not experienced in over a year.

Research Brief

Nurses' Scope of Practice in a Call Center

Butler, Danby, Emmison, and Thorpe (2009) examined nursing scope of practice issues for nurses who staff a child health hotline. They used a qualitative research approach to examine call transcripts and found that nurses used three main strategies to avoid providing medical advice and information: (1) informing callers that they were nurses and thus specifying boundaries of expertise; (2) prompting parents to recognize their own personal authority to make decisions regarding their child's health (termed "privileging parental authority"); and (3) reframing medical questions and medical information seeking as child development issues to keep within the boundaries of nursing expertise. Butler et al. emphasize the need for specific institutional guidelines and policies, and training to ensure that call-center nurses are not practicing telehealth beyond the scope of their practice license.

Butler, C., Danby, S., Emmison, M., & Thorpe, K. (2009). Managing medical advice seeking in calls to Child Health Line. *Sociology of Health & Illness*, 31(6), 817–834. Retrieved from Health Module. (Document ID: 1884062501).

LEGAL, ETHICAL, AND REGULATORY ISSUES

Telehealth is affected by certain legal, ethical, and regulatory issues of which nurses should be aware. In the United States, interstate practice of telenursing, for example, requires attending nurses to be licensed to practice in all of the states in which they provide telehealth services. This is particularly important when nurses work for health systems that are located near state borders and draw patients from both states.

Legal issues, such as scope of practice, accountability for practice, and the potential for and definition of malpractice are still largely unresolved concerns that are difficult to address, according to attorney and medical doctor Barry Cepelewicz (2003). Nurses must be vigilant about keeping extensive documentation of their visits on and off site. Charges of negligence, for instance, can be countered by nurses' providing documented evidence of visits and interventions made to their patients, particularly when the nurses were located off site. See Research Brief on nurses' scope of practice in a call center.

Patient confidentiality and the privacy and safety of clinical data must be given special consideration. Informed consent releases to receive telehealth services is a critical first step. Demiris, Doorenbos, and Towle (2009) suggest that informed consent be treated as a process and not a onetime event. They argue that because telehealth is a completely new experience, patients and families should have the opportunity to revise consent after they fully understand its implications, especially the intrusiveness of home monitoring. In addition, they suggest that informed consent be obtained from all persons living in the household because there are potential privacy considerations for all who live in the home. When the patient is presented with the informed consent form, the nurse must ensure the patient that physiologic data, such as blood pressure readings that will be transmitted over telephone lines or other public communication means, will be kept confidential and protected. In addition, for safety considerations, pointed efforts must be continually undertaken by the nurses' agencies to upgrade information systems to ensure that a high level of data security is provided at all times. Telehealth providers must adhere to all data privacy and confidentiality guidelines and be vigilant to ensure that all involved parties, including the technical staff assistants, have appropriate training in privacy and confidentiality issues.

A DAY IN THE LIFE OF A HOME TELENURSE

Within the range of available telehealth tools, telenurses must choose tools that are appropriate to the patients' needs and capabilities. A very important consideration is whether the patient can perform what is expected. Take, for instance, an automated weight scale to be used daily to track an elderly CHF patient's weight status. Simple procedures for patients using these devices are typically unplugging the telephone from the household telephone jack, plugging in the scale to the telephone jack, stepping on the scale, pushing a send button, and replugging the telephone. Weight readings received at a central nursing station are accurate and timed on the patient's stored record.

Certainly the procedure is automated and low touch. However, there is also ample room for patient–nurse contact, most particularly if a weight gain is noted by the patient's nurse. The following is an example of usual telephone contact procedures made by one telenurse, Mary Bondmass, who responds to her CHF patients' 2-pound weight gain in the past 24 hours with what she calls "teaching opportunities" (quoted in Kinsella, 1998).

> Typically, Bondmass reports, she asks patients who showed a weight increase: "What did you have for dinner last night?" Then, "Tell me what you've been eating this week." Hmm, Chinese take-out again.
>
> She might then say, "Sounds like a lot of salt," which would then lead into the "teaching opportunity" about salt intake and fluid retention that the patient should have heard at least once before. Mary, the nurse, might say: "Look at your ankles," which may be swollen with retained fluids; or, if she noted a shortness of breath, indicating fluid in the lungs, she would point that out. Patients would then get an immediate, practical lesson in cause, effect, and correctable actions for managing and preventing fluid retention (p. 47).

This case well illustrates one nurse's contention (Bernier, 2001) about the value of home telehealth: she notes that with home telehealth, nurses are working "at a distance but not in the dark" (p. 640). Nurses can see how patients are managing from the data sent and identify the interventions that might be needed to correct problems.

Many telenurses have their patients' weight information and alerts of gains automatically transferred to their pagers and use the telephone to call the patient and reinforce details for, say, CHF patients' newly learned dietary routines. At that time, the nurses may also request an order from a physician for a diuretic for the patient, doing so in a timelier manner than would likely be the case with less frequent patient–nurse in-person contact. In fact, with relatively long periods (days) between in-person visits, many patients seek help at emergency rooms for troubled breathing and pain, symptoms that might well be identified and corrected more speedily through telehealth interventions.

THE PATIENT'S ROLE IN TELEHEALTH

The range and sophistication of home telehealth tools is expanding regularly, and a concern by nurses when choosing appropriate tools for their patients is to ask, will my patient use this device? Elderly patients may find the monitoring technology that may speak to them in their homes and videocameras to assist in wound care tracking a daunting introduction to home health care. To assuage the possible discomfort, these and other such tools have undergone much iteration so that they are easier to use and the capability to be turned on and off ensured. When patients are scheduled for a televisit, these devices can be turned on and used. This use by patients is a key, of course, so that the necessary information about them will be gathered and transmitted, and so that their needs can be acted on by telenurses. Demiris et al. (2009) emphasized considerations for usability issues when using telehealth applications with elders who may have sensory, cognitive, and motor disabilities. They suggest rigorous usability testing to maximize the quality of the user experience and special attention to design details for Web-based interfaces, such as font choices and color schemes to improve readability. Similarly, Kaplan and Litweka (2008) emphasized the need for ethical design principles:

- How provider or patient-centric is the technology?
- Does the shift to remote services promote rationality and efficiency at the expense of values traditionally at the heart of caregiving?
- How does the design affect home life and family dynamics?
- To what extent should technology usage involve attempts to manipulate users into different behaviors?
- How might the replacement of human contact by new technologies be ameliorated?
- To what extent is the deployment of technology an end in itself, aimed not toward the improvement of health or well-being, but to create market needs?
- How do we identify the boundaries between genuine solutions and futility in light of technologies that may shift them? (p. 404)

The importance of ensuring patient satisfaction with home health service delivery was predicted to be a megatrend in 2007 (Remington, 2007). Data gathered from the Hospital Consumer Assessment of Health Providers and System survey tool will measure consumer satisfaction, which in turn will enable patient satisfaction to become a performance measurement for every provider across the healthcare delivery system. For this reason, nurses must pay attention to the many examples of studies in home telehealth indicating a great deal of patient satisfaction with telehealth, particularly those that note a preference for telehealth, not conventional care. One example reports on patients' indicating that the telehealth monitor helped them change the way they performed self-care (Chetney, 2006). Other studies also note that patients seen with telehealth have a better understanding of their own disease process and note the ease with which patients are able to manage self-care and so enjoy an improved quality of life (Sanderson, 2007). By patients' achieving a good understanding of and performing self-care by the end of their home health admission periods, an important goal of home telehealth has been attained.

However, when one moves beyond issues of technical ease of use and looks more closely at patients' preferences for privacy or at their desires to use the telehealth devices according to their own schedules, one moves head-on toward the growing trend of consumer-directed health care. This is the new reality in health care. In part, the baby boom generation, many of whom are educated and comfortable with technology, are driving this trend toward as-needed, when-wanted care. Challenges of scheduling and possibly even reengineering telehealthcare services may be a concern (or an opportunity) for tomorrow's home telehealthcare nurses. That is because clinicians are only now beginning to learn how to care differently for this new generation of patients, with telehealth care on their own terms. Kaplan et al. (2008) emphasized that we must consider cultural and community meanings associated with technology when we suggest telehealth as a care delivery model.

TELEHEALTH RESEARCH

Telehealth research focuses primarily on clinical outcomes, such as effectiveness of telehealth compared to usual care, cost effectiveness of telehealth intervention, and patient and family satisfaction. For example, Dansky, Vasey, and Bowles (2008) studied the effects of telehomecare on several clinical outcomes in patients with heart failure. They found that patients with telehomecare had fewer hospitalizations and costly emergency room visits during the study period, and a greater reduction in heart failure symptoms than the control group. They suggest that the frequent monitoring of symptoms afforded by telehealth allowed for more frequent encounters than home visits, providing more timely intervention when clinical status changed, and more frequent teaching and support by nurses. Similarly, Jia, Chuang, Wu, Wang, and Chumbler (2009) studied the long-term effects of telehealth on preventable hospital use and found a statistically significant reduction in hospital use for the first 18 months of follow-up, but that the effects diminished over the 4-year study period. There were no differences found between telehealth and standard care groups in a study of rates of infection, rejection, and hospitalization in a group of transplant recipients, leading the researchers to conclude that telehealth is as effective as usual care for posttransplant follow-up (Leimig, Gower, Thompson, & Winsett 2008). Telehealth was shown to be effective in providing support and problem-solving assistance for family caregivers of victims of polytrauma (Bendizen et al. 2008) and persons with spinal cord injuries (Elliott, Brossart, Berry, & Fine 2008). In a qualitative study of patient and physician perspectives on treating rural depression, Swinton, Robinson, and Bischoff (2009) concluded, "Although an acceptable solution, both patients and PCPs expressed reservations about using telehealth for the treatment of depression because they felt that technology mediated communication would not lend itself to establishing and maintaining the type of provider-patient relationship that would allow treatment to be effective" (p. 178). However, given the access issues associated with rural communities, telehealth provided an opportunity for intervention in cases where traditional care was challenging. Telehealth was also shown to be an effective alternative to usual care in conducting hearing screenings for rural elementary schools, extending the reach and controlling costs of conducting hearing screenings (Lancaster, Krumm, Ribera, & Klich 2008). Julie Polisena et al. (2009) conducted a meta-analysis of 22 studies that compared telehealth to usual care in patients with chronic diseases and included a cost-effectiveness analysis. They concluded that in general telehealth can be cost-saving for the health system and insurance providers, but caution that because the overall methodologic quality of the studies was low, the societal impact of telehealth is uncertain.

It is clear that research in telehealth interventions demonstrates that telehealth is at least as effective as usual care in managing chronic conditions in the home, and in many cases is more cost-effective than home visits. Demiris et al. (2009) suggest that more studies are needed to focus on the patient–provider relationship changes, especially the loss of human touch associated with telehealth interventions. They also caution that researchers who are studying telehealth in remote populations must consider long-term sustainability of telehealth support beyond the study period to ensure that the "research does not exacerbate existing disparities" in access to technologies (p. 132). To follow progress in telehealth research, bookmark the sites provided in Box 19-1.

BOX 19-1

Telehealth Research and Information Centers

- Center for Telehealth and E-Health Law: http://www.telehealthlawcenter.org/
- Global Telehealth Resource Center at Global Health Council: http://www.globalhealth.org/sources/view.php3?id=188
- Telehealth Research Institute at University of Hawaii: http://www.tri.jabsom.hawaii.edu/cms/
- Telehealth Resource Centers: http://telehealthresourcecenter.org/
- Telemedicine Information Exchange: http://telemed.org/news/
- UTMB Center for Center for Telehealth Research and Policy at University of Texas Medical Branch: http://telehealth.utmb.edu/
- Virginia Telehealth Network: http://ehealthvirginia.org/

THE FOUNDATION OF KNOWLEDGE MODEL AND HOME TELEHEALTH

There is much to learn about usual home telehealthcare service delivery, particularly to the elderly and chronically ill, and for this important purpose using the Foundation of Knowledge model is key to learning how to use telehealthcare tools with typical patients (elderly, needing pointed care) and operate effectively as telenurses. To understand the mechanics and effectiveness of home telehealth delivery within the Foundation of Knowledge model, one must begin with a typical home telehealth case from which one can learn the telenurse's role in this model.

Case Study:
The Role of a Home Telehealth Nurse

Mrs. A is an 84-year-old woman recently discharged from the hospital with a diagnosis that includes an exacerbation of CHF. She also has diabetes and hypertension. Mrs. A was discharged from the hospital on multiple medications and lives alone.

Home care services were initiated with skilled nursing care visits, some home health aide support, and orders to include daily telemonitoring of her vital signs. The telehealth device will remotely monitor her blood pressure, heart rate, oxygen saturation, and weight. In addition, the patient will answer customized questions about her disease on a daily basis. This information will then be transmitted daily to the home care agency where the telenurse can determine appropriate clinical actions based on the data trends and preset baseline alerts that indicate when set parameters have been exceeded.

Knowledge Acquisition

In the previous case study, knowledge acquisition involves the telenurse's receiving the information from the telehealth devices via a variety of communication modes. For example, the telenurse receives the patient's vital signs taken in the home and the patient's responses to customized questions. All of this information is transmitted to a remote server or site (a central station or website) that is easily accessible to the telenurse.

Knowledge Processing

As a result of the telenurse's knowledge acquisition, the next step to be followed is knowledge processing (i.e., understanding a set of information and ways it can be useful to a specific task). In the case study, the telenurse assesses the patient's vital signs along with subjective data received from the patient as a result of customized questions that she is asked. For example, she might be asked if she feels more short of breath today compared to a normal day. The telenurse then combines this information with the overall patient history and diagnosis to get an up-to-date view of the patient's status and asks where this information fits into the clinical picture being presented for this patient.

As an example, the telenurse notes: postacute heart failure patient shows trended data with weight gain of 5 lb over 2 days, elevated blood pressure, decreased oxygen saturation, and answers yes to questions about increased shortness of breath and increased fatigue. After processing all of the current information, the telenurse is able to target the appropriate next steps involving knowledge generation and knowledge dissemination.

Knowledge Generation

By using her own nursing skills and clinical knowledge of the disease process, the telenurse considers all of the data as they apply to Mrs. A and decides the best course of action to take and acts on the data. The telenurse may, in addition, ask a variety of questions to ensure that a complete and accurate decision about next steps for the patient is made. These questions may include the following:

- Do I need to gather additional data?
- Do I need to call the patient?
- Do I need to call the physician and inquire about a change in the current plan of care?

Knowledge Dissemination

Finally, the telenurse determines how the knowledge will be used and disseminated. Various questions that were posed in the knowledge generation stage are acted on, including the following:

- Calling the doctor
- Obtaining a change in medication order
- Calling the patient and instructing her in medication change
- Reviewing activities that could have led to the changes (e.g., eating salty foods)
- Educating the patient on disease process, symptom management, and self-management techniques
- Continuing to monitor the patient on an ongoing basis

SUMMARY

Telehealth is a rapidly developing mode of health service delivery in which nurses can expect to play a significant role. The most promising area of concentration for nurses is in home telehealth care, an area that is expected to provide extensive care to the burgeoning numbers of American elderly persons living with challenging chronic diseases and conditions. Many telecommunications-ready tools to assist nurses in delivering this care are available, and their effectiveness in maintaining or improving patients' health outcomes is well documented. Today's nurses are providing telehealth services to typical home care patients (elderly, needing regular and targeted care) and operating effectively as telenurses. The practice of telehealth will provide opportunities for telenurses to become key players in care management across the healthcare continuum.

PARTING THOUGHTS FOR THE FUTURE AND A VIEW TOWARD WHAT THE FUTURE HOLDS

Consumers will drive the way health care is delivered in the future. Consider that tomorrow's healthcare facility might have no walls. The evolving role of the Internet, personal health records, and telehealth all will support a more integrated healthcare model. This convergence of trends and solutions will continue to expand with new business practice models, such as retail clinics and concierge care.

The care continuum will need to be supported by a clinical and caregiver structure that will use data collected to make better and more informed healthcare decisions. Health parameter data could be used by the end user for personal direct care decision making, or it may be used by a member of the healthcare community to determine appropriate healthcare interventions.

Technology of today will be different from technology of tomorrow as access to broadband communications systems, acceptance of technology, and mobility and data transfer evolve. As a result of emerging needs, many companies will enter the market and offer a wide range of information technology tools from embedded and worn sensors to remote monitoring devices. There will continue to be different user interfaces to receive customized health services, such as the television, cell phones, and perhaps someday the iPod.

Clearly, by making key information readily accessible, there will be solutions across all areas (home health, hospitals, and a range of other settings) that facilitate collaboration in care delivery and health information. Products that integrate into consumers' and patients' everyday lives to improve the quality of life will continue to emerge. Telehealth and telenursing will play an important role in improving quality of life and care for the patients served.

Foremost, one must be open to change and be willing to embrace ever-evolving practice models. Tools should always be used to improve care delivery models to make more targeted contact with and about patients. In an ideal world, there would be seamless integration of clinical data systems and robust data exchange to provide quality care for patients no matter their location.

THOUGHT-PROVOKING Questions

1. Will the increased use of these telehealth technology tools be viewed as dehumanizing patient care, or will they be viewed as a means to promote more contact with healthcare providers and new ways for people to stay connected (as in online disease support groups), thereby creating better long-term disease management and patient satisfaction?

2. What types of resistance to new technologies might be evident among patients, caregivers, and nurses? What evidence and strategies might help to diminish these resistances?

3. As telehealth technology advances toward seamless data access regardless of distance or health system, how can patient privacy rights and the confidentiality of personal medical data be protected?

4. Consider a recent patient care scenario and describe how it could have been managed at a distance.
  • What training would be needed?
  • What equipment would be used?
  • How would the patient and his or her family respond to home telemonitoring?

For a full suite of assignments and additional learning activities, use the access code located in the front of your book to visit this exclusive website: **http://go.jblearning.com/mcgonigle**. If you do not have an access code, you can obtain one at the site.

References

Aarkstore Enterprise. (2010). *Telemedicine market shares, strategies, and forecasts, worldwide, 2010 to 2016.* Retrieved from http://www.articlebuster.com/2010/03/telemedicine-market-shares-strategies-and -forecasts-worldwide-2010-to-2016-aarkstore-enterprise/

Allan, R. (2006, June 29). *A brief history of telemedicine. Electronic design.* Retrieved from http://www .elecdesign.com/Articles/Index.cfm?AD=1&ArticleID=12859

American Association for Retired Persons (AARP). (1996). *Understanding senior housing into the next century: Survey of consumer preferences, concerns, and needs.* Washington, DC: AARP.

American Heart Association. (2007). *Statistics you need to know: Statistics on medication.* Retrieved from http://www.americanheart.org/presenter.jhtml?identifier=107

American Nurses Association (ANA). (2001). *Developing telehealth protocols: A blueprint for success.* Washington, DC: ANA.

American Telemedicine Association (ATA). (2002). *Home telehealth clinical guidelines.* Retrieved from http://www.americantelemed.org/icot/hometelehealthguidelines.htm

American Telemedicine Association (ATA). (2010). *Telemedicine defined.* Retrieved from http://www .americantelemed.org/i4a/pages/index.cfm?pageid=3333

Bendixen, R., Levy, C., Lutz, B., Horn, K., Chronister, K., & Mann, W. (2008). A telerehabilitation model for victims of polytrauma. *Rehabilitation Nursing, 33*(5), 215–220. Retrieved from Pro-Quest Nursing & Allied Health Source. (Document ID: 1550211771).

Bernier, L. (2001). Assessing respiratory status from a distance. *Home Health Care Nurse, 19*, 632–640.

Centers for Disease Control and Prevention. (2005). *Chronic disease overview.* Retrieved from http:// www.cdc.gov/nccdphp/overview

Cepelewicz, B. (2003). Legal issues in telemedicine. In A. Kinsella (Ed.), *Home healthcare: Wired and ready for telemedicine, the nurses' and nursing students' edition* (pp. AI–IX). Kensington, MD: Information for Tomorrow.

Chetney, R. (2006, July/August). What do patients really think about telehealth? In-depth interviews with patients and their caregivers. *The Remington Report, 26*, 28–29.

Craig, J., & Patterson, V. (2005). Introduction to the practice of telemedicine. *Journal of Telemedicine and Telecare, 11*(1), 3–9. Retrieved from ProQuest Psychology Journals database (Document ID: 805776671).

Dansky, K., Vasey, J., & Bowles, K. (2008). Impact of telehealth on clinical outcomes in patients with heart failure. *Clinical Nursing Research, 17*(3), 182. Retrieved from Health Module. (Document ID: 1521037211).

Demiris, G., Doorenbos, A., & Towle, C. (2009). Ethical considerations regarding the use of technology for older adults: The case of telehealth. *Research in Gerontological Nursing, 2*(2), 128–136. Retrieved from ProQuest Nursing & Allied Health Source. (Document ID: 1757456631).

Elliott, T., Brossart, D., Berry, J., & Fine, P. (2008). Problem-solving training via videoconferencing for family caregivers of persons with spinal cord injuries: A randomized controlled trial. *Behaviour Research and Therapy, 46*(11), 1220. Retrieved from Psychology Module. (Document ID: 1588 750351).

Health Data Management. (2007, September 4). *Report: Home monitoring growing fast.* Retrieved from http://www.healthdatamanagement.com/news/15703-1.html

Hoffman, C., Rice, D., & Sung, H-Y. (1996). Persons with chronic conditions: Their prevalence and costs. *JAMA, 276*, 1473–1479.

Institute of Aging, University of California at San Francisco. (1996). *Chronic care in America: A 21st century challenge.* Princeton, NJ: Robert Wood Johnson Foundation.

Jia, H., Chuang, H., Wu, S., Wang, X., & Chumbler, N. (2009). Long-term effect of home telehealth services on preventable hospitalization use. *Journal of Rehabilitation Research and Development, 46*(5), 557–566. Retrieved from Health Module. (Document ID: 1884235751).

Kaplan, B., & Litweka, S. (2008). Ethical challenges of telemedicine and telehealth. *Cambridge Quarterly of Healthcare Ethics, 17*(4), 401-16. Retrieved from Health Module. (Document ID: 1540615491).

Kinsella, A. (1998). *Home healthcare: Wired and ready for telemedicine, the second generation.* Sunriver, OR: Information for Tomorrow.

Kinsella, A. (2002a). Predicting home healthcare needs: A next step in patient monitoring. *Home Health Care Nurse, 20*, 725–729.

Kinsella, A. (2002b). Wound care and telehealth. *Telehealth Practice Report 3*, 9.

Kinsella, A. (2004). Obesity and new applications for home telehealth care. *Home Health Care Technology Report 1*(3), 36–45.

Lancaster, P., Krumm, M., Ribera, J., & Klich, R. (2008). Remote hearing screenings via telehealth in a rural elementary school. *American Journal of Audiology, 17*(2), 114–122. Retrieved from ProQuest Nursing & Allied Health Source. (Document ID: 1623340331).

Leimig, R., Gower, G., Thompson, D., & Winsett, R. (2008). Infection, rejection, and hospitalizations in transplant recipients using telehealth. *Progress in Transplantation, 18*(2), 97–102. Retrieved from ProQuest Nursing & Allied Health Source. (Document ID: 1537443161).

National Pharmaceutical Council. (2003). *Infos and facts about [medication] non-compliance.* Retrieved from http://www.m-pill.com/index.php?browse=compliance

Pennsylvania Homecare Association and Pennsylvania State University. (2004). *2003–2004 telehealth project evaluation year two: The impact of telehealth on nursing workload and retention.* Unpublished report.

Polisena, J., Coyle, D., Coyle, K., & McGill, S. (2009). Home telehealth for chronic disease management: A systematic review and an analysis of economic evaluations. *International Journal of Technology Assessment in Health Care, 25*(3), 339–49. Retrieved from ProQuest Nursing & Allied Health Source. (Document ID: 1797842261).

Prial, S., & Hoss, S. (2009). Overview of home telehealth. In D. McGonigle & K. Mastrian (Eds.), *Nursing Informatics and the Foundation of Knowledge* (pp. 265–281). Sudbury, MA: Jones and Bartlett.

Quality Insights of Pennsylvania. (2005). *Home telehealth reference 2005.* Unpublished report.

Remington, L. (2007, January/February). Healthcare MegaTRENDS, predictions and forecasts. *The Remington Report 15,* 5–10.

Sanderson, S. (2007, July/August). Cardiopulmonary disease management: A patient-focused approach to home health care. *The Remington Report, 15,* 46–47.

Skiba, D. J. (1998). Health-oriented telecommunications in nursing informatics. In M. J. Ball et al. (Eds.), *Where caring and technology meet* (pp. 40–53). New York, NY: Springer.

St George, I., Baker, J., Karabatsos, G., Brimble, R., Wilson, A. & Cullen, M. (2009). How safe is telenursing from home? *Collegian, Journal of the Royal College of Nursing Australia, 16*(3), 119–123. Retrieved from http://www.mckesson.com.au/index.php?option=com_docman&task=doc_download&gid=115

Stern, D. J. (2007, January/February). Intuitive system monitors resident behavior patterns. *Assisted Living Consult, 3*(1), 21–25.

Strauss, A. (2010). *Robot doctors bring specialty care to rural areas.* Retrieved from http://generalmedicine.suite101.com/article.cfm/robot-doctors-bring-specialty-care-to-rural-areas

Swinton, J., Robinson, W., & Bischoff, R. (2009). Telehealth and rural depression: physician and patient perspectives. *Families, Systems & Health, 27*(2), 172. Retrieved from Health Module. (Document ID: 1793129471).

U.S. Department of Commerce, Bureau of the Census. (1993). *Sixty-five plus in America.* Washington, DC: GPO.

U.S. Department of Health and Human Services. Health Resources Services Administration [HRSA]. Bureau of Health Professions. (2002). *Projected supply, demand, and shortages of registered nurses: 2000–2020.* Retrieved from http://www.ahca.org/research/rnsupply_demand.pdf

U.S. Department of Health and Human Services. Health Resources Services Administration [HRSA]. Bureau of Health Professions. (2004). *The registered nurse population: Findings from the 2004 National Sample Survey of RNs.* Retrieved from http://www.bhpr.hrsa.gov/healthworkforce/rnsurvey04

Venable, S. (2005). A call to action: Georgia must adopt a new standard of care, licensure, reimbursement, and privacy laws for telemedicine. *Emory Law Journal, 54*(2), 1183–1217. Retrieved from Law Module database (Document ID: 875322011).

CHAPTER 20

Supporting Consumer Information and Education Needs

Kathleen Mastrian and Dee McGonigle

Objectives

1. Define health literacy and e-health.
2. Explore various technology-based approaches to consumer health education.
3. Identify barriers to use of technology and issues associated with health-related consumer information.
4. Imagine future approaches to technology-supported consumer health information.

www

Key Terms

www

Blog
Digital divide
Domain name
e-brochure
e-health
eHealth Initiative
Empowerment
Grey gap
Health literacy
HONcode
Interactive technologies
Know-do gap
Static medium
Trust-e
Voice recognition
Web quest
Weblog

INTRODUCTION

Imagine that you have decided to take up running as your preferred form of exercise in a quest to get in shape. You start slowly by running a half mile and walking a half mile. You gradually build up your endurance and find yourself running nearly every day for longer distances and longer periods of time. You first notice a nagging pain in the right hip that over a few weeks gradually spreads to the center of your right buttocks and then down your right leg. You try rest and heat, but nothing seems to help. You visit your doctor, and she suggests that you have developed piriformis syndrome and prescribes a series of stretching exercises, ice to the involved area, and rest. You are intrigued by the diagnosis and on your return home you log on to the Internet and begin a search for information about piriformis syndrome. When you type the words into your favorite search engine, you get 60,500 results for your query. Your use of the Internet to seek health information mirrors the behavior of many consumers who increasingly rely on the Internet for health-related information. The challenge for consumers and healthcare professionals alike is the proliferation of information on the Internet and the need to learn how to recognize when information is accurate and meaningful to the situation at hand.

This chapter explores consumer information and education needs and how technology may help to meet those needs, and at the same time create ever-increasing demands for health-related information. It begins with a discussion of **health literacy**, **e-health**, and health education and information needs, and explores various approaches by healthcare providers to using technology to promote health literacy. Also examined is the use of games, **Web quests**, and simulations as means of increasing health literacy among the school-age population. Issues associated with the credibility of Web-based information and barriers to access and use are discussed. Finally, future trends related to technology-supported consumer information are explored.

CONSUMER DEMAND FOR INFORMATION

This is the Knowledge Age Era; many people want to be in the know. People demand news and information and they want immediate results and unlimited access. This is increasingly true with health information. More and more people, in a trend known as consumer **empowerment**, are interested in taking control of their health and are not satisfied being dependent on a healthcare provider to supply them with information. The Pew Internet and American Life Project survey report of 2011 (Fox, 2011) indicates that 8 in 10 (comparable to a previous survey of 2006) Americans who are online have searched for health information. The most frequent health topic searches (66%) are related to a specific disease or medical problem that the searcher or a member of the family is experiencing. Other frequent topics of health-related searches reported in a 2006 survey (Fox, 2006) are medical treatments or procedures (51%), nutrition and diet (49%), exercise or fitness (44%), and drug information (37%). The 2011 survey (n= 3,001) reports that consumers also searched for information on food (29%) and drug safety (24%). The 2006 Pew Internet survey tracked 8 million searches for health information by American adults in a single day and suggests that most begin their searches with a search engine. The impacts of the searches were reported as both positive and negative. The impacts ranged from affecting decisions about their care (58%), changes in the approaches to overall health maintenance (55%), providing material for asking questions of healthcare providers (54%), to feeling overwhelmed (25%) or confused (18%) by materials they found online about their health (Fox, 2006).

It is important to note that this survey is limited to those who are online and does not reflect the health information needs or demands of those who are not online. The **digital divide** is the term used to describe the gap between those who have and those who do not have access to online information. Fox (2007b) reports that the current estimate of connectivity among Americans is 71%. She also identifies a **grey gap** in that only 32% of persons over the age of 65 have ever gone online or lived in a connected household. Similarly, in another report from the Pew Internet group, Fox (2007a) describes connectivity disparities among various races and ethnicities, including Latinos, non-Hispanic whites, and non-Hispanic blacks, and analyzes the influences of English-speaking ability and level of education on connectivity. Nurses and healthcare providers need to be aware of the various components of the digital divide to ensure that patients and clients are receiving the health information they need in a format that they are interested in and can comprehend.

Missen and Cook (2007) discuss the potential impact that technology-based health information dissemination can have on the **know-do gap** in developing countries. The know-do gap reflects the fact that solutions to global health problems exist but are not implemented in a timely fashion because of the lack of access to important health information. The Internet connections in developing countries are widely scattered and may not be efficient or sufficient for viewing healthcare information. Missen and Cook describe the use of a freestanding hard drive that has been loaded with hundreds of CDs of health-related information in a webpage format that responds to a search command. This is a great example of providing technologies that work with the constraints of the situation. Another example of addressing the digital divide is the growing number of health-related websites that support a Spanish language format.

HEALTH LITERACY AND HEALTH INITIATIVES

The goal of health literacy for all is one that is widely embraced in many sectors of health care, a major goal of Healthy People 2010, and is being continued in the health communication and health information technology objective of Healthy People 2020 (Office of Disease Prevention & Health Promotion and U.S. Department of Health and Human Services, 2009). Clinicians who have been practicing for some time recognize that informed patients have better outcomes and pay more attention to their overall health and changes in their health than those who are poorly informed. Some of the earliest formally developed patient education programs that included postoperative teaching, diabetes education, cardiac rehabilitation, and diet education were implemented in response to research that suggested the positive impact of patient education on health outcomes and satisfaction with care. Glassman (2008) recently updated the National Network Libraries of Medicine webpage on health literacy (http://nnlm.gov/outreach/consumer/hlthlit.html). She concludes from the research on the economic impact of health literacy that those with low health literacy have less ability to manage a chronic illness properly and tend to use more healthcare services than those who are more literate. In addition, she uses results of health research to demonstrate the impact of low health literacy and the incidence of disease.

Glassman (2008) updated the National Network of Libraries of Medicine health literacy site that states, "Health literacy is defined in Healthy People 2010 as: 'The degree to which individuals have the capacity to obtain, process, and understand basic health information and services needed to make appropriate health decisions'" (para. 2). For example, healthcare providers depend on a patient's ability to understand and follow directions associated with preparation for surgery or taking medications. It is also assumed, sometimes erroneously, that people will correctly interpret symptoms of a serious illness and act appropriately. The ability to locate and evaluate health information for credibility and quality, to analyze the various risks and benefits of treatments, and to calculate dosages and interpret test results are among the tasks Glassman identifies as essential for health literacy. Other important and less easily learned health literacy skills are the ability to negotiate complex healthcare environments and understanding the economics of payment for services. Parker, Ratzan, and Lurie (2003) estimate that at least one third of all Americans have health literacy problems and lament that in a time-is-money economic climate, healthcare practitioners are not always reimbursed for patient education activities.

The **eHealth Initiative** was developed to address the growing need for managing health information and to promote technology as a means of improving health information exchange, health literacy, and healthcare delivery. The eHealth Initiative website provides more information (http://www.ehealthinitiative.org/default.mspx). Although the scope of the eHealth Initiative goes beyond health literacy, a major goal continues to be empowering consumers to understand their health needs better and to take action appropriate to those needs. Poor interoperability among healthcare systems and failure completely to embrace national data standards for health care continue to be identified as barriers to the eHealth Initiative. Further, concerns about privacy and security of information and the failure to invest appropriately in technology have slowed the development of this important initiative. Several states developed viable health information networks as part of the eHealth Initiative: the Utah Health Information Network (http://www.uhin.com/) and the Vermont Cooperative Consumer Health Information Project (http://library.uvm.edu/dana/vthealth/) are examples of attempts to implement e-health initiatives.

HEALTHCARE ORGANIZATION APPROACHES TO EDUCATION

Healthcare organizations (HCOs) use a wide variety of approaches and tools to promote patient education and health literacy. Although the old standby for disseminating information is the paper-based flyer, some HCOs are recognizing that today's consumers are more attracted to a dynamic rather than **static medium**. In addition, the cost of designing and of printing pamphlets and flyers becomes prohibitive when one considers the rapidity of change of information; the brochure may be outdated almost as soon as it is printed. One approach is to have patient education information stored electronically so that changes can be made as needed or information can be better tailored to the specific patient situation and then printed out and reviewed with the patient. Another old standby approach that is still widely used is the group education class. These classes initially were developed in response to helping people manage chronic health problems (e.g., diabetes) and were typically scheduled while people were hospitalized. Now, many HCOs also sponsor health promotion education classes as a way of marketing their facilities and showcasing some of their expert practitioners.

The movement from static to dynamic presentations began in many HCOs as DVDs and videotapes that were shown in groups or broadcast on demand over dedicated channels via television in a patient's room. HCOs are now also taking advantage of the fact that patients and families are captive audiences in waiting rooms and promote education via pamphlet distribution, health promotion programs broadcast on television, and health information kiosks. The kiosks are typically a computer station and often contain a variety of self-assessment tools (especially those related to risks for diabetes, heart disease, or cancer) and searchable pages of information about specific health conditions. The self-assessment tools represent yet another step forward in technologic support for education because in addition

Research Brief

Case studies of educational videos used on six hospital websites were the focus of this qualitative study by Huang (2009). He used both within-case and cross-case analyses to describe rationales for developing and using eHealth videos. He identified six main reasons for implementing eHealth videos:

1. The proliferation of high-speed Internet access has made online video a well-accepted culture in the United States.
2. Many online visitors, especially young people, like to watch videos more than reading lengthy articles.
3. Videos can attract online visitors' attention, thus attracting online traffic and further attracting visitors to the hosting hospital.
4. A video, when well produced, is worth more than a thousand words.
5. Videos can relate not only to online visitors' minds but also, more importantly, to their hearts to build trust and drive their decision-making.
6. Videos empower and inform the visitors outside of the hospital visit time and such self-driven homework is beneficial to both the visitor and the hospital (p. 67–68).

Source: Huang, E. (2009). Six cases of e-health videos on hospital Web sites. *E - Service Journal, 6*(3), 56–72. Retrieved from ABI/INFORM Global. (Document ID: 1945312291).

to being dynamic, the kiosk is also interactive. On the assessment page, the user is asked to respond to a series of questions and then the health risk is calculated by the computer program. One caution, however, is that just because the information is made available does not mean that people will participate or that they will understand what they have experienced. The level of health literacy, the digital divide, and the grey gap, still exist in these situations.

Many HCOs have invested time and money in developing interactive websites and believe that Web presence is a critical marketing strategy. Sternberg (2002) suggests that many websites begin as an **e-brochure** and progress through various stages to reach a true e-care status. Most offer physician search capabilities, e-newsletters, and call-center tie-ins. As with all patient education materials, there must be a sincere commitment to keeping information current and easily accessible. Web designers must pay particular attention to the aesthetics of the site, the ease of use, and the literacy level of those in the intended audience.

A usability study conducted by Lauterbach (2010) provides some insights into how to measure usability. The researcher compared the usability of the symptom checker functions of two popular websites by asking volunteers to navigate each using four different case scenarios. Users navigated the site to find the symptom checker and then entered the symptoms and evaluated site feedback. Users rated the ease of understanding for each site and completed a short comprehension quiz. Data were collected on descriptions of user site preferences, user satisfaction with the sites, results of the comprehension quiz, and efficiency, which was measured by tracking the number of webpage changes the user performed while navigating the site.

PROMOTING HEALTH LITERACY IN SCHOOL-AGED CHILDREN

Promoting health literacy in school-aged children presents special challenges to health educators. There is wide agreement that childhood obesity is a serious and growing issue and is related not only to poor choice of foods, but also to the sedentary lifestyles promoted by video games and television. In addition, the time devoted to health and physical education programs in schools has given way to the core subjects, such as math and science.

The Children's Nutrition Research Center has responded to these challenges by supporting the development of nutrition education programs as interactive computer games, video games, and cartoons referred to as "edutainment" (Flores, 2006). These e-health programs are developed specifically to appeal to the generational (highly connected and computer literate) and cultural needs of this group. Flores describes the Family Web project that uses comic strips to impart nutrition information; and Squires Quest, where the students earn points by choosing fruits and vegetables to fight the snakes and moles who are trying to destroy the healthy foods in the Kingdom of SALot. These are great examples of health education programs that are designed to appeal to this connected generation of learners and their intuitive ability to use **interactive technologies.**

Donovan (2005) describes an interdisciplinary Web quest designed to appeal to older school-aged children. The quest is interdisciplinary in that it requires reading comprehension, critical thinking, presentation, and writing so that core skills and health literacy skills are learned in a single assignment. Students are directed to the Web to search for information on the pros and cons of low-carbohydrate diets and obesity prevention. Students learn along the way as they search for information, collect and interpret it, and then develop a presentation and final paper.

The Cancer Game (Oda & Kristula, n.d.) was developed by a young man taking a college class on Macromedia software who had previously experienced a bone-marrow transplant. Subsequently, he and a professor collaborated and expanded the project to its present form. The game is designed as an arcade-style video game for cancer patients to relieve stress by visualizing the fighting of cancer cells. Although cancer victims of any age can access and play the game, it has a special appeal to children and adolescents. Similarly, Ben's Game (www.makea wish.org/ben) is a video game designed to help relieve the stress of cancer treatment for children (Anderson & Klemm, 2008). There are also games for other conditions, such as diabetes (Glymetrix, 2009).

SUPPORTING USE OF THE INTERNET FOR HEALTH EDUCATION

Nurses and other healthcare providers need to embrace the Internet as a source of health information for patient education and health literacy. Patients are increasingly turning there for instant information about their health maladies. Health-related **blogs** (short for **weblog**, an online journal) and electronic patient and parent support groups are also proliferating at an astounding rate. Clinicians need to be prepared to arm patients with skills to identify credible websites. They also need to participate in the development of well-designed, easy-to-use health education tools. Finally, they need to convince payers of the necessity of health education and the powerful impact education has on promoting and maintaining health. Box 20-1 provides more information about health education.

The Health on the Net (HON) Foundation (2005) survey describes the certifications and accreditation symbols that identify trusted health sites. The **HONcode** and **Trust-e** were identified as the two most common symbols that power users look for. The survey also indicates that Internet users look at the **domain name** and frequently gravitate toward university sites (.edu), government sites (.gov), and HCO sites (.org). Half of the survey respondents were in favor of the use of a domain name called .health to identify quality health information websites. In contrast, Pew/Internet (2006) indicates that nearly 75% of online searchers do not check the date or the source of information they are accessing on the Web and 3% of online health seekers report knowing someone who was harmed by following health information found on the Web.

The U.S. National Library of Medicine and the National Institutes of Health sponsor MedlinePlus, a website that has a tutorial for learning how to evaluate health information and an electronic guide to Web surfing that is available in both English and Spanish. The site is found at http://nccam.nih.gov/health/web resources. This guide explains the major things one should evaluate when accessing health-related resources on the Web (National Center for Complementary and Alternative Medicine, 2008). Suggest that patients visit this site to become better at identifying whether or not a website is credible before they adopt the recommendations provided. The clinician is very important in patient education. Refer to Boxes 20-1 and 20-2 to review effective education methods used in teaching patients and their families.

BOX

20-1

Considerations for Patient Education

Julie A. Kenney and Ida Androwich

Nurses need to take many things into account when teaching patients. Nurses need to assess a patient's willingness to learn, their reading ability, how they learn best, and how much they already know about the subject. Nurses also need to take cultural differences and language differences into account when teaching a patient. If the nurse chooses to use an electronic method to educate the patient, digital natives (patients who have grown up with technology) need to be taught differently than digital immigrants (those who have been forced to learn technology) (Educational Strategies, 2006). Digital natives are typically born after 1982 and may also be referred to as "Generation Y." This generation prefers to learn using technology. The younger group learns quite well if information is presented in a format they are accustomed to, such as an interactive video game to introduce them to a topic. This group is also comfortable using information that they can access via their iPods and MP3 players (Maag, 2006). Those born before 1982 have learning styles that range from preferring to learn in a classroom setting to reading a book about the topic to learning using a hands-on, interactive approach (Educational Strategies).

References

Educational strategies in generational designs. (2006). *Progress in Transplantation*, *16*(1), 8–9.

Maag, M. (2006). Pod casting and MP3 players: Emerging education technologies. *CIN: Computers, Informatics, Nursing*, *24*(1), 9–13.

Patient education websites

American Academy of Family Physicians: http://www.familydoctor.org
American Cancer Society: http://www.cancer.org
American Heart Association: http://www.americanheart.org
Centers for Disease Control and Prevention: http://www.cdc.gov
Krames (products to purchase): http://www.krames.com
Merck (products to purchase and free information for patients):
    http://www.merckservices.com/portal/site/merckservices/&tcode=K09FA
Thomson—Educational products for nurses (requires a subscription):
    http://www.micromedex.com/products/nurses and
    http://www.micromedex.com/products/carenotes/cn_brochure.pdf

Some providers have developed a list of credible websites that is shared with patients or family members. Recommendations might include the U.S. Department of Health and Human Services sponsored healthfinder site (http://www.healthfinder.gov), a website dedicated to helping consumers find

BOX
20-2

A Clinician's View on Patient Education

Denise D. Tyler

Knowledge dissemination in nursing practice includes sharing information with patients and families so that they understand their healthcare needs well enough to participate in developing the plan of care, make informed decisions about their health, and ultimately comply with the plan of care, both during hospitalization and as outpatients.

There are several effective methods for educating patients and their families. Providing one-on-one and classroom instruction are traditional and valuable forms of education. One-on-one education is interactive and can be adjusted anytime during the process based on the needs of the individual patient or family, and can be supplemented by written material, videos, and Web-based learning applications. Classroom education can be beneficial because patients and families with similar needs or problems can network, thus enhancing the individual experience. However, the ability to interact with each member of the group and to tailor the educational experience based on individual needs may be limited by the size and dissimilarities of the group. Individual follow-up should be available when possible.

Paper-based education that is created, printed, and distributed by individual institutions or providers can be very effective because they can be distributed at any time and reviewed when the patient feels like learning. Many agencies, such as the Centers for Disease Control and Prevention, have education for patients available on their websites. These can be reviewed online, or they can be printed by healthcare providers or patients. Organizations can also develop and distribute information and instructions specific to their policies and procedures. Printed educational material can also be purchased from companies who employ experts in the subject matter and instructional design.

One of the newer sources of patient education information is the Internet. Many hospitals and healthcare organizations provide proprietary information, such as directions, information on procedures, and instructions on what to expect during hospitalization, in this manner. Other health organizations, such as the National Institutes of Health, provide detailed information on their websites. Clinicians should be cautious when recommending websites to patients and families, because not all sites are reliable or valid.

Many companies who provide clinical information systems also include patient education materials linked to the clinical system via an intranet. Thus, standardized instructions that are specific to a procedure or disease process can be printed from this computer-based application. Discharge instructions that are interdisciplinary and patient specific can often be modified via drop-down lists or selectable items that can be deleted or changed by the clinician. This ability to modify before printing provides more consistent and individualized instruction. The computer-based genera-

Continues

BOX *(Continued)*

20-2

tion of instruction is preferable to free text and verbal instruction modification because it also allows the information to be linked to a coded nursing language and thus easily used for measurement and quality assurance reporting. Relevant triggers may be embedded in the clinical information systems. For example, when a patient answers "yes" to smoking, smoking cessation information should automatically print, or a trigger should remind the nurse to explore this with the patient and then provide the patient with preprinted information on smoking cessation.

Integration of standardized discharge instructions and patient education into the clinical system is another way to improve the compliance and documentation of education along with streamlining the workflow of clinicians. Printing the information to give to the patient should be seamless to the clinician who is charting. The format should be logical and easy to read. The more transparent the process, the more efficient the system and the easier it is to use for the clinician. What I envision for the future is a system that "remembers" the style of learning preferred by patients and their families, prompts the provider to print handouts, and programs the bedside computer/video education system based on their previous selections and surveys. This interactive patient and family education will be integrated into the clinical system and the patient's personal health record.

credible information on the Internet. Other excellent sources of reliable information are the National Institutes of Health (http://www.nih.gov), the Centers for Disease Control and Prevention (http://www.cdc.gov), Medline Plus (www.medlineplus.gov), NIHSeniorHealth (www.nihseniorhealth.gov), and the National Health Information Center (http://www.health.gov/nhic).

FUTURE DIRECTIONS

Predicting future directions for technology-based health education is somewhat difficult, because one may not be able completely to envision the technology of the future. One can predict, however, that some current technologies will be used increasingly to support health literacy. For example, audio and video podcasts may become more commonplace in health education and be provided as free downloads from the websites of HCOs.

Abreu, Tamura, Sipp, Keamy, and Eavey (2008) described the processes used to create patient and family surgical education video podcasts. They began by digitally recording actual pediatric otologic surgeries, and then edited the videos, developed a script, and finally recorded the audio. They report that the educational podcasts were developed in 8–10 hours (excluding the surgical recording time). These podcasts are used to supplement the traditional face-to-face patient and family education sessions for pediatric otologic surgeries.

Voice recognition software used to navigate the Web may reduce the frustration and confusion associated with attempting to spell complex medical terms. However, the confusion and frustration may increase if the patient or client is unable to pronounce the terms. Voice interactivity should help to reduce the digital access disparity associated with those who have limited keyboard or mouse skills. For those with visual impairments, some websites may provide both audio and text information and support increased text size for ease of reading (Anderson & Klemm, 2008).

Many websites associated with government and national organizations are also providing multiple language access to health information and decision-support tools. The multilanguage access broadens the population for which education can be provided and the decision-support programs allow users to access results that are tailored to their age, risk factors, or disease state (Anderson & Klemm, 2008).

Those who are frequent e-mail users may be interested in being able to communicate with physicians and other healthcare personnel via e-mail rather than the telephone. This idea may meet some resistance by physicians who perceive the e-mail correspondence as bothersome and time consuming. However, it is possible that work efficiency might also increase if patients and their needs are screened via e-mail before an office visit. For example, as a result of an e-mail correspondence in lieu of an initial office visit, medications could be changed or diagnostic tests could be performed before the office visit. In addition, patients could be directed to an interactive screening form housed on a website where they would answer a series of questions that would help them make a decision about whether they should call for an appointment, head for the emergency room, or self-manage the issue. If self-management is the outcome of the screening tool, then the patient or caregiver could be directed to a credible website for more information. The idea is not to interfere with or replace the face-to-face visit, but to supplement the physician–patient relationship and perhaps streamline the efficiency of healthcare delivery. McCray (2005) also suggests that physicians may be resistant to providing e-mail consultations and recommending health-related websites because of the potential for malpractice liability. Reimbursement mechanisms for electronic health care are also inadequate or nonexistent making providers even more resistant to this interaction.

Piette (2007) describes the use of interactive behavior change technology to improve the effectiveness of diabetes management. The goal of the interactive behavior change technology is to improve communication between patients and healthcare providers and provide educational interventions to promote better disease management between visits. The combination of electronic medication reminders, meters that track glycemic control longitudinally, and personal digital assistant–based calculators all supported the behavioral interventions necessary to better manage the diabetes. As a conclusion to their study, Watson, Bell, Kvedar, and Grant (2008) caution that even though patients are part of the digital divide (lacking access or skill in electronic communications and Internet use) one cannot assume that they will be resistant to using other forms of technology to support health. They compared Internet users to non-Internet users and found that both groups were willing to learn to use new technology to manage Type-2 diabetes, including wireless communication devices for information sharing with physicians.

Healthcare practitioners may soon embrace the use of "information prescriptions" (D'Alessandro, 2010) that direct patients and families to credible websites, including government and HCO websites, and wikis and blogs that may help them understand their health issues or share information with and seek support from others who have similar issues. "Information prescriptions are prescriptions of focused, evidence-based information given to a patient at the right time to manage a health problem" (p. 81).

SUMMARY

It is clear that the consumer empowerment movement will continue to drive the need for access to quality health education and support programs. In an ideal world, practitioners are willing to design educational materials that are user friendly, culturally competent, interesting, dynamic, and interactive, and that meet the skills, education needs, and interests of the user.

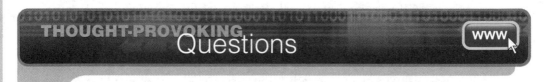

THOUGHT-PROVOKING Questions

WWW

1. How do you envision technology enhancing patient or consumer education in your setting?
2. Formulate a plan evidencing a potent patient education episode on methicillin-resistant Staphylococcus aureus. Provide a rationale for each approach and describe a tool you would use to educate the patient and his or her family.

For a full suite of assignments and additional learning activities, use the access code located in the front of your book to visit this exclusive website: http://go.jblearning.com/mcgonigle. If you do not have an access code, you can obtain one at the site.

WWW

References

Abreu, D., Tamura, T., Sipp, J., Keamy, D., & Eavey, R. (2008). Podcasting: Contemporary patient education. *Ear, Nose & Throat Journal, 87*(4), 208, 210–211. Retrieved from ProQuest Nursing & Allied Health Source. (Document ID: 1468588971).

Anderson, A., & Klemm, P. (2008). The Internet: Friend or foe when providing patient education? *Clinical Journal of Oncology Nursing, 12*(1), 55–63. Retrieved from ProQuest Nursing & Allied Health Source. (Document ID: 1430141231).

D'Alessandro, D. (2010). Challenges and options for patient education in the office setting. *Pediatric Annals, 39*(2), 78–83. Retrieved from Health Module. (Document ID: 1972816891).

Donovan, O. (2005). The carbohydrate quandary: Achieving health literacy through an interdisciplinary WebQuest. *The Journal of School Health, 75*(9), 359–362. Retrieved from Health Module database (Document ID: 924409661).

Flores, A. (2006). Using computer games and other media to decrease child obesity. *Agricultural Research, 54*(3), 8–9. Retrieved from Research Library Core database (Document ID: 1005199991).

Fox, S. (2006, October 29). *Online health search 2006.* Retrieved from http://pewinternet.org/pdfs/PIP_Online_Health_2006.pdf

Fox, S. (2007a, March 14). *Latinos online.* Retrieved from http://pewinternet.org/pdfs/Latinos_Online_March_14_2007.pdf

Fox, S. (2007b, June 22). *Broadband, cell phones, and the continuing reality of the grey cap.* Retrieved from http://pewinternet.org/PPF/r/101/presentation_display.asp

Fox, S. (2011, Feb. 1). *Health Topics.* Retrieved from http://www.pewinternet.org/Reports/2011/HealthTopics.aspx

Glassman, P. (2008). *Health literacy.* Retrieved from http://nnlm.gov/outreach/consumer/hlthlit.html

Glymetrix Diabetes Game. (2009). Retrieved from http://www.diabetesgame.com/

Health on the Net (HON) Foundation. (2005). *Analysis of 9th HON survey of health and medical Internet users.* Retrieved from http://www.hon.ch/Survey/Survey2005/res.html

Lauterbach, C. (2010). Exploring the usability of e-health websites. *Usability News, Vol. 12,* Issue 2. Retrieved from http://www.surl.org/usabilitynews/122/ehealth.asp

McCray, A. (2005). Promoting health literacy. *Journal of the American Medical Informatics Association, 12*(2), 152–163. Retrieved from ProQuest Nursing & Allied Health Source database (Document ID: 810410751).

Missen, C., & Cook, T. (2007). *Appropriate information-communications technologies for developing countries.* Retrieved from http://www.who.int/bulletin/volumes/85/4/07-041475/en/index.html

National Center for Complementary and Alternative Medicine (NCCAM)/National Institutes of Health. (2008). *10 things to know about evaluating medical resources on the Web.* Retrieved from http://nccam.nih.gov/health/webresources

Oda, Y., & Kristula, D. (n.d.) *The cancer game: A side-scrolling, arcade-style, cancer-fighting video game.* Retrieved from http://www.cancergame.org/

Office of Disease Prevention & Health Promotion and U.S. Department of Health and Human Services. (2009). *Proposed healthy people 2020 objectives.* Retrieved from http://www.healthypeople.gov/hp2020/Objectives/TopicAreas.aspx

Parker, R., Ratzan, C., & Lurie, N. (2003). Health literacy: A policy challenge for advancing high-quality health care. *Health Affairs, 22*(4), 147. Retrieved from ABI/INFORM Global database (Document ID: 376436551).

Pew/Internet. (2006). *The future of the Internet II.* Retrieved from http://news.bbc.co.uk/1/shared/bsp/hi/pdfs/22_09_2006pewsummary.pdf

Piette, J. (2007). Interactive behavior change technology to support diabetes self-management: Where do we stand? *Diabetes Care, 30*(10), 2425–2432. Retrieved from Health Module database (Doc ument ID: 1360494771).

Sternberg, D. (2002). Building on your quick wins. *Marketing Health Services, 22*(3), 41–43. Retrieved from ABI/INFORM Global database (Document ID: 155769441).

Watson, A., Bell, A., Kvedar, J., & Grant, R. (2008). Reevaluating the digital divide: Current lack of Internet use is not a barrier to adoption of novel health information technology. *Diabetes Care, 31*(3), 433–435. Retrieved from Health Module.

CHAPTER 21

Using Informatics to Promote Community/Population Health

Margaret Ross Kraft and Ida Androwich

Objectives

1. Provide an overview of community and population health informatics.
2. Describe informatics tools for promoting community and population health.
3. Define the roles of federal, state, and local public health agencies in the development of public health informatics.

www

INTRODUCTION

In late fall of 2002, severe acute respiratory syndrome (SARS) appeared in China. By March of 2003, SARS become recognized as a global threat. According to World Health Organization data more than 8,000 persons from 29 countries became infected with this previously unknown virus and more than 700 persons died. By 2004, the last SARS cases were caused by laboratory-acquired infections. Because of computerized global data collection, the potentially negative impact of a widespread global epidemic was averted. Many **surveillance** systems, loosely termed "syndromic surveillance systems," use data that are not diagnostic of a disease but that might indicate the early stages of an outbreak. Outbreak detection is the overriding purpose of **syndromic surveillance** for terrorism preparedness. Enhanced case-finding and monitoring the course and population characteristics of a recognized outbreak also are potential benefits of syndromic surveillance. New data have been used by **public health** to enhance surveillance, such as patients' chief complaints in emergency departments, ambulance log sheets, prescriptions filled, retail drug and product purchases, school or work absenteeism, and medical signs and symptoms in persons seen in various clinical settings. With faster, more specific and affordable diagnostic methods and

Key Terms **www**

Behavioral Risk
    Factor Surveillance
    System (BRFSS)
Bioterrorism
Centers for Disease Control
    and Prevention (CDC)
Community risk assessment
    (CRA)
Epidemiology
National Center for Public
    Health Informatics
    (NCPHI)
National health information
    network (NHIN)
National Health and Nutrition
    Examination Survey
    (NHANES)
Public Health
Public Health Informatics
Public health interventions
Regional health information
    organization (RHIO)
Risk Assessment
Suicide Prevention Community Assessment Tool
Surveillance
Surveillance data systems
Syndromic surveillance
Youth Risk Behavior
    Surveillance System
    (YRBSS)

decision-support tools timely recognition of reportable diseases with the potential to create a substantial outbreak is now possible. Tools for pattern recognition can be used to screen data for patterns needing further public health investigation. During the 2003 epidemic, the **Centers for Disease Control and Prevention (CDC)** worked to develop surveillance criteria to identify persons with SARS in the United States and the surveillance case definition changed throughout the epidemic, to reflect increased understanding of SARS (CDC, 2007).

Information acquired by the collection and processing of population health data becomes the basis for knowledge in the field of public health. There is an ever increasing need for timely information about the health of communities, states, and countries. Knowledge about disease trends and other threats to community health can improve program planning, decision-making, and care delivery. Patients seen from the perspective of major health threats within their communities can benefit from opportunities for early intervention. This chapter will focus on the application of informatics methods to public health surveillance. The availability of clinical information for public health has been fundamentally changed because of the electronic health record (EHR) and health information technology (IT), which now give public health "an unprecedented opportunity to leverage the information, technologies and standards to support critical public health functions such as alerting and surveillance" (Garrett, 2010).

CORE PUBLIC HEALTH FUNCTIONS

The core public health functions are "The assessment and monitoring of the health of communities and populations at risk to identify health problems and priorities; The formulation of public policies designed to solve identified local and national health problems and priorities; To assure that all populations have access to appropriate and cost-effective care, including health promotion and disease prevention services, and evaluation of the effectiveness of that care" (Medterms Medical Dictionary, 2007). "Public health is a field that encompasses an amalgam of science, action, research, policy, advocacy and government" (Yasnoff, Overhage, Humphreys, & LaVenture, 2001, p. 536).

Historically, Dr. John Snow can be designated the "father" of **public health informatics** (PHI). In 1854, he plotted information about cholera deaths and was able to determine that the deaths were clustered around the same water pump in London. He convinced authorities that cholera deaths were associated with that water pump; when the pump handle was removed, cholera disappeared. It was Dr. Snow's focus on the cholera population rather than on a single patient that led to his discovery of the source of the cholera outbreak (Vachon, 2005).

Florence Nightingale should also be recognized as an early public health informaticist. Her recommendations about medical reform and the need for improved sanitary conditions were based on data about morbidity and mortality that she compiled from her experiences in the Crimea and England. Her efforts led to a total reorganization of how and what healthcare statistics should be collected (Dossey, 2000).

Just as information has been recognized as an asset in the business world, health care is now recognized as information intensive requiring timely, accurate information from many different sources. Health information systems address the collection, storage, analysis, interpretation, and communication of health data and information. Many health disciplines, such as medicine and nursing, have developed their own concepts of informatics integrating computer, information, and cognitive science with the science of the professional domain. That trend has reached the field of public and community health and PHI represents "a systematic application of information and computer science and technology to public health (PH) practice, research and learning" (Yasnoff, O'Carroll, Koo, Linkings, & Kilbourne, 2000, p. 67). This area of informatics differs from others because it is focused on the promotion of health and disease prevention in populations and communities. PHI efficiently and effectively organizes and manages data, information, and knowledge generated and used by public health professionals to fulfill the core functions of public health: assessment, policy, and assurance (Agency for Toxic Substances and Disease Registry, 2003). Public health changes the social conditions and systems that affect everyone within a given community. It is because of public health that people understand the importance of clean water, the danger of second-hand smoke, and the fact that seat belts really do save lives (PHI, 2007).

The scope of PHI practice includes knowledge from a variety of additional disciplines including management, organization theory, psychology, political science, and law and fields related to public health, such as **epidemiology,** microbiology, toxicology, and statistics (O'Carroll, Yasnoff, Ward, Ripp, & Martin, 2003, p. 5). PHI focuses on applications of IT that "promote the health of populations rather than individuals, focus on disease prevention rather than treatment, focus on preventive intervention at all vulnerable points" (O'Carrroll et al., 2004, p. 3-4). PHI addresses the data, information, and knowledge that public health professionals generate and use to meet the core functions of public health (Public Health Data Standards Consortium [PHDSC], 2007b). Yasnoff et al. (2000) defined four principles that define and guide the activities of PHI: (1) applications promote the health of populations, (2) applications focus on disease and injury prevention, (3) applications should explore prevention at "all vulnerable points in the causal changes," and (4) PHI must reflect the "governmental context in which public health is practiced" (p. 69).

The Institute of Medicine defines the role of public health as "fulfilling society's interest in assuring conditions in which people can be healthy" (Khoury, 1997, p. 176). Functions of public health include prevention of epidemics and the spread of disease, protection against environmental hazards, promotion of health, disaster response and recovery, and providing access to health care (PHDSC, 2007a).

The initiative of integrating the healthcare enterprise to improve how health-care information can be shared more easily and used more effectively has created the domain of Quality, Research and Public Health (QRPH). Domain participants address the repurposing of clinical, demographic, and financial data collected in the process of providing clinical care to the monitoring of disease patterns; incidence, prevalence, and situational awareness of such patterns; and to the identification of new patterns of disease not previously known or anticipated. Such data can be incorporated within existing public health population analyses and programs for direct outreach and condition management through registries and locally determined appropriate treatment programs or protocols (QRPH, 2010).

COMMUNITY HEALTH RISK ASSESSMENT (TOOLS FOR ACQUIRING KNOWLEDGE)

As the public has become more aware of harmful elements in the environment, **risk assessment** tools have been developed. Such tools allow assessment of pesticide use, exposure to harmful chemicals, contaminants in food and water, and toxic pollutants in the air to determine if potential hazards need to be addressed. A risk assessment may also be called a "threat and risk assessment." A "threat" is a harmful act, such as the deployment of a virus or illegal network penetration. A "risk" is the expectation that a threat may succeed and the potential damage that can occur" (PCMag, 2007). "Risk factor assessments complement vital statistics data systems and morbidity data systems by providing information on factors earlier in the causal chain leading to illness, injury or death" (O'Carroll, Powell-Griner, Holtzman & Williamson, 2003, p. 316).

"Health risk assessments are used to estimate whether current of future exposures will pose health risks to a broad populations" (California Environmental Protection, 1998, p. 4) and are used to weigh the benefits and costs of various program alternatives for reducing exposure to potential hazards. They may impact public policy and regulatory decisions. Health risk assessment is a constantly developing process based in sound science and professional judgments. There are usually four basic steps ascribed to risk assessment: (1) hazard identification, (2) exposure assessment, (3) dose–response assessment, and (4) risk characterization. Hazard identification seeks to determine the types of health problems that could be caused by exposure to a potentially hazardous material. All research studies related to the potentially hazardous material are reviewed to identify potential health problems. Exposure assessment is done to determine the length, amount, and pattern of exposure to the potentially hazardous material. Dose–response is an estimation of how much exposure to the potential hazard would cause varying degrees of health effects. Risk characterization is an assessment of the risk of the hazardous material causing illness in the population (California Environmental Protection). The question the risk assessment has to answer is, "how much risk is acceptable?"

Risk factor systems are used throughout the country and may be local, regional, or national in scope. Specific risk assessment tools exist for specific health issues, such as the **Suicide Prevention Community Assessment Tool,** which addresses general community information, prevention networks, and the demographics of the target population and community assets and risk factors. Other risk assessment tools include the **Youth Risk Behavior Surveillance System,** the **Behavioral Risk Factor Surveillance System,** and the **National Health and Nutrition Examination Survey.** Pennsylvania's Office of Mental Retardation began an assessment initiative in 1998 to collect information on the movement of this specific population from state-operated facilities into community settings. The goal of this assessment process was to ensure that this population had access to necessary health care and that their needs were being met.

Determining the presence of risk factors in community is a key part of a **community risk assessment (CRA).** Communities may be concerned about what in the environment affects or may affect the community's health, the level of environmental risk, and other factors that should be included in public health planning. Ball (2003) defines value as "a function of cost, service, and outcome" (p. 41). The value of a CRA is in providing information crucial to planning, building consensus of how to mobilize community resources, and allowing for comparison of risks with those of other communities. The goal of a CRA is risk reduction and improved health. A CRA may identify unmet needs and opportunities for action that may help set new priorities for local public health units. A CRA may also be used to monitor the impact of prevention programs.

PROCESSING KNOWLEDGE AND INFORMATION TO SUPPORT EPIDEMIOLOGY AND MONITORING DISEASE OUTBREAKS

There is a need to define the role of federal, state, and local public health agencies in the development of PHI and IT applications. The availability of IT today challenges all stakeholders in the health of the public to adopt new systems that provide adequate disease surveillance and challenges people to improve outmoded processes. Preparedness in public health means more timely detection of potential health threats, situational awareness, surveillance, outbreak management, countermeasures, response, and communications. Surveillance uses health-related data that signal a sufficient probability of a case or an outbreak that warrants further public health response. Although historically syndromic surveillance has been used to target investigations of potential infectious cases, its use to detect possible outbreaks associated with **bioterrorism** is increasingly being explored by public health officials (CDC, 2007). Early detection of possible outbreaks can be achieved through timely and complete receipt, review, and investigation of disease case reports; by improving the ability to recognize patterns in data that may be indicative of a possible outbreak early in its course; and through receipt of new types of data that can signify an outbreak earlier in its course. New types of data might include identification of absences from work or school; increased purchases of health-care products, including specific types of over-the-counter medications; presenting symptoms to health-care providers; and laboratory test orders (CDC, 2007). A comprehensive surveillance effort supports timely investigation and identifies data needs for managing the public health response to an outbreak or terrorist event.

To appropriately process public health data, PHI has a need for a standardized vocabulary and coding structure. This is especially important as national public health data are collected so that data variables can be understood across systems and between agencies. A standardized vocabulary must address local language use versus universal language usage for public health.

In the early 1990s, the CDC launched a plan for an integrated surveillance system that moved from stand-alone systems to networked data exchange build with specific standards. Early initiatives were the National Electronic Telecommunications System for Surveillance and the Wide-ranging Online Data for Epidemiologic Research. Six current initiatives reflect this early vision:

1. PulseNet USA: A surveillance network for food-borne infections.
2. National Electronic Disease Surveillance System: Facilitates reporting on approximately 100 diseases with data feeding directly from clinical laboratories allowing for early detection.
3. Epidemic Information Exchange: A secure communication system for practitioners to access and share preliminary health surveillance information.
4. Health Alert Network: A state and nationwide alert system.
5. Biosense: Provides improved real-time biosurveillance and situational awareness in support of early detection.
6. Public Health Information Network: Promotes standards and software solutions for the rapid flow of public health information.

Certainly, the events of September, 2001, have accelerated the need for informatics in public health practice. Today response requirements include fast detection, science, communication, integration, and action (Kukafka, 2006). In 2005, the CDC created a **National Center for Public Health Informatics** to provide leadership in the field. This center aims to protect and improve health through PHI (McNabb, Koo, Pinner, & Seligman, 2006).

Information is vital to public health programming. The data processed into public health information can be from administrative, financial, and facility sources. Included may be encounter, screening, registry, clinical, and laboratory data and surveillance data. It has been recommended that the functions of population health beyond surveillance need to be integrated into the EHR and the personal health record. Such an initiative might allow for population-level alerts to be sent to clinicians through these electronic record systems. Systems now being developed allow for automated syndromic surveillance of emergency department records and media surveillance, which allow for early detection of potential pandemic occurrences. Systems such as this were tested during the 2009 H1N1 flu outbreak. The public health enhanced electronic medical record can provide immediate detection and reporting of "notifiable" conditions. The incorporation of geographic information systems allows public health data to be mapped to specific locations that may indicate an immediate need for intervention (Grannis & Vreeman, 2010).

Data on vital statistics from state and local governments are also used for public health purposes. It should be noted that databases created with public funds are "public" databases that are available for authorized public representatives for public purposes (Freedman & Weed, 2003).

Widespread implementation of EHRs now offers the concept of a "public health enabled record," which can automatically send patient information alerts from the point of care to public health departments when reportable symptoms, conditions, or diseases are encountered. A public health–enabled EHR can be bidirectional, allowing public health information and recommendations for treatment to be accessible at the point of care. One public health EHR prototype addresses the information flow related to newborn screenings (Orlova et al., 2005).

APPLYING KNOWLEDGE TO HEALTH DISASTER PLANNING AND PREPARATION

The availability of data and speed of data exchange can have a significant impact on critical public health functions, such as disease monitoring and syndromic surveillance. Currently, surveillance data are limited and historical in nature. Special data collections are needed to address specific public health issues and investigations and emergencies are addressed and managed with paper. The future of PHI will offer real-time surveillance data available electronically and investigations and emergences will be managed with the tools of informatics (Yasnoff, 2004). "**Surveillance data systems** such as infectious disease trackers that collect data on adverse health effects are invaluable tools for public health officials to tap for planning, evaluation, or implementation of **public health interventions**"(Agency for Toxic Substances and Disease Registry, 2003). "Syndromic surveillance for early outbreak detection is an investigational approach where health department staff, assisted by automated data acquisition and generation of statistical signals, monitor disease indicators continually (real-time) or at least daily (near real-time) to detect outbreaks of diseases earlier and more completely than might otherwise be possible with traditional public health methods" (Buehler, Hopkins, Overhage, Sosin, & Tong, 2004, para. 7). Traditionally, there has been no common infrastructure to respond to pandemics, but the development of health IT is creating opportunities that go far beyond national boundaries to impact global public health initiatives.

In New York City, a primary care information project funded by the CDC has developed a multifaceted initiative, the Center for Excellence in Public Health Informatics, to address issues of measurement of meaningful use, disease and outbreak surveillance, and decision support alerts at the point of care (Buck, Wu, Souliakis, & Kukalka, 2010).

INFORMATICS TOOLS TO SUPPORT COMMUNICATION AND DISSEMINATION

The revolution in IT has made the capture and analysis of health data and the distribution of healthcare information more achievable and less costly. Since the early 1960s, the CDC has used IT in its practice and PHI emerged as a specialty in the 1990s. PHI has become more important with improvements in IT; changes in the care delivery system; and the challenges related to emerging infections, resistance antibiotics, and the threat of chemical and biologic terrorism. Two-way communication between public health agencies, community, and clinical laboratories can identify clusters of reportable and unusual diseases. As a result, health departments can consult on case diagnosis and management, alerts, surveillance summaries, and clinical and public health recommendations. Ongoing healthcare provider outreach, education, and 24-hour access to public health professionals leads to the discovery of urgent health threats. The automated transfer of specified data from a laboratory database to a public health data repository improves the timeliness and completeness of reporting notifiable conditions.

Public health information systems represent a partnership of federal, state, and local public health professionals. Such systems allow the capture of large amounts of data, rapid exchange of information, and strengthened links between these three system levels. Dissemination of prevention guidelines and communication among public health officials, clinicians, and patients has become a major benefit of PHI. IT solutions can be used to provide accurate and timely information that guides public health actions. In addition, the Internet has become a universal communications pathway and allows individuals and population groups to be more involved and responsible for management of their own health status.

Few public health professionals have received formal informatics training and may not be aware of the potential impact of IT on their practice. A working group formed at the University of Washington Center for PHI has published a draft of PHI competencies needed (Karras, 2007). These competencies include the following (Center for Public Health Informatics, 2007):

- Supporting development of strategic direction for PHI within the enterprise.
- Participating in development of knowledge management tools for the enterprise.
- Using standards

- Ensuring that the knowledge, information, and data needs of project or program users and stakeholders are met.
- Managing information system development, procurement, and implementation.
- Managing IT operations related to project or program (for public health agencies with internal IT operations)
- Monitoring IT operations managed by external organizations.
- Communicating with cross-disciplinary leaders and team members.
- Participating in applied public health informatics research.
- Developing public health information systems that are interoperable with other relevant information systems.
- Supporting use of informatics to integrate clinical health, environmental risk, and population health.
- Implementing solutions that ensure confidentiality, security, and integrity, while maximizing availability of information for public health.
- Conducting education and training in PHI.

USING FEEDBACK TO IMPROVE RESPONSES AND PROMOTE READINESS

Improvement of community health status and population health depends on effective public and healthcare infrastructures. In addition to information from public health agencies, there is now interest in the capture of information from hospitals, pharmacies, poison control centers, laboratories, and environmental agencies. Timely collection of such data allows early detection and analysis, which can increase the rapidity of response with more effective interventions. Yasnoff et al. (2000) identify the "grand challenges" still facing PHI as the development of national public health information systems, a closer integration of clinical care with public health, and concerns of confidentiality and privacy.

Population health data must be considered an important part of the infrastructure of all **regional health information exchanges,** which are the building blocks for a **national health information network.** Organizations and agencies interested in promoting and protecting the public's health must commit to collaboration and seamless data sharing (PHDSC, 2007b). The public health data include information about surveillance, environmental health, and preparedness systems and has client information, such as immunization registries and laboratory results reporting and analysis. It can provide information about outbreaks, patterns of drug-resistant organisms, and other trends that can help improve the accuracy of diagnostic and treatment decisions (LaVenture, 2005). A regional health information exchange and national health information network can also support public health goals through broader opportunities for participation in surveillance and prevention activities, improved case management and care coordination, and increased accuracy and timeliness of information for disease reporting (LaVenture).

SUMMARY

Public health informatics strives to ensure that health data systems meet the data needs of all organizations interested in population health as national and international standards are developed for healthcare data collection. This includes standardization of environmental, sociocultural, economic, and other data that are relevant to public health (PHDSC, 2007b). Table 21-1 provides the names, addresses, and URLs for important organizations dedicated to public health data and informatics. Table 21-2 lists abbreviations commonly used in PHI.

TABLE 21-1
Important PHI Sites

Name	Address	Website
American Public Health Association	APHA 800 I Street, NW Washington, DC 20001	www.apha.org
Center for Public Health Informatics	CPHI University of Washington 1100 NE 45th Street, Ste 405 Seattle, WA 98105	www.cphi.washington.edu
Centers for Disease Control and Prevention	Centers for Disease Control and Prevention 1600 Clifton Road Atlanta, GA 30333	www.cdc.gov
National Center for Public Health Informatics	The National Center for Public Health Informatics (NCPHI) 1600 Clifton Road, N.E. Mailstop E-78 Atlanta, GA 30333	www.cdc.gov/ncphi
Public Health Data Standards Consortium	Public Health Data Standards Consortium c/o Johns Hopkins Bloomberg School of Public Health 624 N. Broadway, Room 325 Baltimore, MD 21205	www.phdsc.org
Public Health Institute	Public Health Institute 555 12th Street, 10th Floor Oakland, CA 94607	www.phi.org

TABLE 21-2
Abbreviations Used in PHI

BRFSS	Behavioral Risk Factor Surveillance System
CEPA	California Environmental Protection Agency
CDC	Center for Disease Control
CPHI	Center for Public Health Informatics
CRA	Community Risk Assessment
EPI-X	Epidemic Information Exchange
HAN	Health Alert Network
IT	Information Technology
IOM	Institute of Medicine
NCPHI	National Center for Public Health Informatics
NETSS	National Electronic Technology System for Surveillance
NHANES	National Health and Nutrition Examination Survey
NHIN	National Health Information Network
NEDSS	National Electronic Disease Surveillance System
PHRAP	Pennsylvania's Health Risk Assessment Process
PH	Public Health
PHDSC	Public Health Data Standards Consortium
PHI	Public Health Informatics
PHIN	Public Health Information Network
QRPH	Quality, Research, Public Health
RHIO	Regional Health Information Exchanges
SPRC	Suicide Prevention Community Assessment Tool
WONDER	Wide-ranging Online Data for Epidemiologic Research
YRBSS	Youth Risk Behavior Surveillance System

The future of practice in public health depends on how efficiently and effectively public health data are captured, analyzed, and disseminated for regional, national, and global health planning and management. In an ideal world one would see seamless data collection and sharing and a commitment to global health planning.

THOUGHT-PROVOKING Questions

WWW

1. Imagine that you are a public health informatics specialist and that you and your colleagues are concerned about a new strain of influenza. What public health data are used to determine the need for a mass inoculation?

2. What data will be collected to determine the success of such a program?

For a full suite of assignments and additional learning activities, use the access code located in the front of your book to visit this exclusive website: http://go.jblearning.com/mcgonigle. If you do not have an access code, you can obtain one at the site.

WWW

References

Agency for Toxic Substances and Disease Registry (2003). *ATSDR Glossary of Terms*. Retrieved from http://www.atsdr.cdc.gov/glossary.html.

Ball, M. (2003). Better health through informatics: Managing information to deliver value. In P. O'Carroll, W.L. Yasnoff, M.E. Ward, L. Ripp, & E. Martin (Eds.). *Public health informatics and information systems* (pp. 39–51). New York, NY: Springer-Verlag.

Buck, M., Wu, W., Souliakis, N., & Kukalka, R. (2010). *Achieving excellence in public health informatics: The New York City experience*. Washington, DC: AMIA.

Buehler, J. W., Hopkins, R. S., Overhage, J. M., Sosin, D. M., & Tong, V. (2004) *Framework for evaluating public health surveillance systems for early detection of outbreaks*. Retrieved from cdc.gov/mmwr/preview/mmwrhtml/rr5305a1.

California Environmental Protection (CEPA) (1998). *A guide to health risk assessment*. Retrieved from www.oehha.ca.gov.

Center for Disease Control (CDC) (2007). Retrieved from www.cdc.gov.

Center for Public Health Informatics (CPHI) (2007). *Draft competencies V7 for the public health informatician*. Seattle, WA: University of Washington.

Dossey, B. M. (2000). *Florence Nightingale: Mystic, visionary, healer*. Springhouse, PA: Springhouse Corporation.

Freedman, M.A. & Weed, J. A. (2003). National vital statistics system. In P. O'Carroll, W. Yasnoff, M. Ward, L. Ripp, & E. Martin (Eds.). *Public health informatics and information systems* (pp. 269–285). New York, NY: Springer-Verlag.

Garrett, N. (2010). *Leveraging the EHR for public health alerting.* CDC Clinician Outreach & Communication Activity (COCA) Conference Call, June 22, 2010.

Grannis, S. & Vreeman, D. (2010). *A vision of the journey ahead: Using public health notifiable condition mapping to illustrate the need to maintain value sets.* Washington, DC: AMIA.

Institute of Medicine Committee for the Study of the Future of Public Health. Division of Health Care Services. (1988). *The future of public health.* Washington, DC: Author.

Karras, B. (2007). *Competencies for the public health informatician.* Seattle, WA: University of Washington.

Khoury, M. J. (1997). Genetic epidemiology and the future of disease prevention and public health. *Epidemiology Reviews, 19*(1), 175–180.

Kukafka, R. (2006). Public health informatics. Medical Informatics Course for Health Professionals. Woods Hole, MA.

LaVenture, M. (2005, May). *Role of population/public health in regional health information exchanges.* PHDSC/eHealth Initiative Annual Conference. Washington, DC.

McNabb, S., Koo, D., Pinner, R., & Seligman, J. (2006) *Informatics and public health at CDC.* Retrieved from http://www.cdc.gov/mmwr/preview/mmwrhtml/su5502a10.

Medterms Medical Dictionary. (2007). Retrieved from www.medterms.com.

O'Carroll, P. (2003). Introduction to PH informatics. In P. O'Carroll, W. Yasnoff, M. Ward, L. Ripp, & E. Martin (Eds.). *Public health informatics and information systems* (pp. 3–15). New York, NY: Springer-Verlag.

O'Carroll, P.L., Powell-Griner, E., Holtzman, D., & Williamson, G. D. (2003). Risk factor information systems. In P. O'Carroll, W. Yasnoff, M. Ward, L. Ripp, & E. Martin (Eds.). *Public health informatics and information systems* (pp. 316–334). New York, NY: Springer-Verlag.

O'Carroll, P., Yasnoff, W., Ward, M., Ripp, L., & Martin, E. (Eds.). (2003). *Public health informatics and information systems.* New York, NY: Springer-Verlag.

Orlova, A., Dunnagan, M., Finitzo, T., Higgins, M., Watkings, T., Tien, A., & Beales, S. (2005). *An electronic health record-public health (EHR-PH) system prototype for interoperability in 21st century healthcare systems* (pp. 575–579). AMIA, Annual Symposium Proceedings.

PCMag.com Encyclopedia (2007). Retrieved from www.pcmag.com/encyclopedia.

Pennsylvania's Health Risk Assessment Process (PHRAP). Author.

Public Health Institute (2007). Retrieved from www.phi.org.

Public Health Data Standards Consortium (PHDSC) (2007a). *Tutorial Module 1: What is public health.* Retrieved from www.phdsc.org/knowresources/tutorials/module1.

Public Health Data Standards Consortium (PHDSC) (2007b). *Tutorial Module 8: Viewing public health data and data standards in a larger context.* Retrieved from www.phdsc.org/knowresources/tutorials/module1.

QRPH (2010). Retrieved from www.interoperabilityshowcase.org/.../HIMSS09_interop_QRPH.

Richards, J. (2003). Core competencies in PHI. In P. O'Carroll & W. Yasnoff (2004). *Current Issues in Public Health Informatics.* Amsterdam, The Netherlands. MEDINFO.

Rothman, K.J. & Greenland S. (1998). *Modern epidemiology.* (pp. 435). Philadelphia, PA: Lippincott Williams & Wilkins.

Suicide Prevention Resource Center. *Suicide prevention community assessment tool.* Retrieved from www.sprc.org.

Vachon, D. (2005). Dr John Snow blames water pollution for cholera epidemic. *Old News 16*(8), 8-10. Retrieved from www.ph.ucla/epi/snow.

Yasnoff, W., O'Carroll, P., Koo, D., Linkings, R., & Kilbourne, E. (2000). Public health informatics: Improving and transforming public health in the information age. *Journal of Public Health Management Practice 6*(6): 67–75.

Yasnoff, W., Overhage M., Humphreys B., LaVenture M. (2001). A national agenda for public health informatics. *Journal of the American Medical Informatics Association 8*(6): 535–545.

Yasnoff, W., and Humphreys, B., et al. (2004). A consensus action agenda for achieving the National Health Information Infrastructure. *Journal of the American Medical Informatics Association 11*(4): 332–338.

CHAPTER 22

Informatics Tools to Promote Patient Safety

Kathleen Mastrian and Dee McGonigle

Objectives

1. Explore the characteristics of a safety culture.
2. Examine strategies for developing a safety culture.
3. Recognize how human factors contribute to errors.
4. Appreciate the impact of informatics technology on patient safety.

WWW

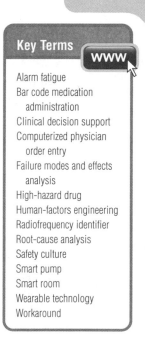

Key Terms WWW

Alarm fatigue
Bar code medication
    administration
Clinical decision support
Computerized physician
    order entry
Failure modes and effects
    analysis
High-hazard drug
Human-factors engineering
Radiofrequency identifier
Root-cause analysis
Safety culture
Smart pump
Smart room
Wearable technology
Workaround

INTRODUCTION

Nursing professionals have an ethical duty to ensure patient safety. Increasing demands on professionals in complex and fast-paced healthcare environments, however, may lead them to cut corners or develop **workarounds** that deviate from accepted and expected practice protocols. These deviations are not carried out deliberately to put patients at risk but are more often practiced in the interest of saving time or because the organizational culture is such that risky behaviors are commonplace. Occasionally, these inappropriate actions or omissions of appropriate actions result in harm or significant risk of harm to patients. Consider the following case scenario:

> A 19-year-old obese woman who had recently undergone C-section delivery of a baby presented in the emergency department (ED) with dyspnea. Believing the patient had developed a pulmonary embolism, the physician prescribed an IV heparin bolus dose of 5,000 units followed by a heparin infusion at 1,000 units/hour. After administering the bolus dose, a nurse started the heparin infusion but misprogrammed the pump to run at 1,000 mL/hour, not 1,000 units/hour (20 mL/hour). By the time the error was discovered, the patient had received more than 17,000 units (5,000 unit loading dose and about 12,000 units from the infusion) in less than an hour since arrival in the ED. A smart pump with dosing limits for heparin had been used.

Thus, the programming error should have been recognized before the infusion was started. However, the nurse had elected to bypass the dose-checking technology and had used the pump in its standard mode. It was quite fortunate that the patient did not experience adverse bleeding as her aPTT values were as prolonged as 240 seconds when initially measured and 148 seconds two hours later (Institute for Safe Medication Practices, 2007, para. 2).

The **smart pump** used in this scenario was equipped with dose calculation software that compares the programmed infusion rate to a drug database to check for dosing within safe limits. This technology is particularly important when high-alert or **high-hazard drugs** are being administered. In this case, however, the available dose checking technology had been turned off and the pump was operated in standard mode. A subsequent analysis of the error event revealed that many nurses in the institution were bypassing the safety technology afforded by the smart pump to save time. This chapter focuses on some of the recommended organizational strategies used to promote a culture of safety and some of the specific informatics technologies designed to reduce errors and promote patient safety.

WHAT IS A CULTURE OF SAFETY?

The 1999 Institute of Medicine report, *To Err is Human*, is widely credited for launching the current focus on patient safety in health care. This report was followed in 2001 by the Institute of Medicine *Quality Chasm* report bringing to national attention healthcare quality and safety. This national attention resulted in a $50 million grant by Congress to the Agency for Healthcare Research and Quality (AHRQ) to launch initiatives focused on safety research for patients. Other initiatives prompted by these seminal reports are the Joint Commission National Patient Safety Goals (2002); National Quality Forum adverse events and "never events" list (2002); creation of the Office of National Coordinator for Health IT to computerize health care (2004); formation of the World Health Organization's Alliance for Patient Safety (2004); Institute for Healthcare Improvement (IHI) 100,000 Lives campaign (2005) and the 5 Million Lives Campaign (2008); Congressional authorization of Patient Safety Organizations created by the Patient Safety and Quality Improvement Act to promote blameless error reporting and shared learning (2005); "no pay for errors" initiative launched by Medicare (2008); and the $19 billion Congressional appropriation to support electronic health records (EHRs) and patient safety (Wachter 2010).

The AHRQ safety culture primer (n.d.) suggests that organizations should strive to achieve high reliability by being committed to improving healthcare quality and preventing medical errors, and to demonstrate an overall commitment to patient safety. That is, everyone and every level in an organization must embrace the **safety culture**. Key features of a safety culture identified by the AHRQ are as follows:

- Acknowledgment of the high-risk nature of an organization's activities and the determination to achieve consistently safe operations
- A blame-free environment where individuals are able to report errors or near misses without fear of reprimand or punishment
- Encouragement of collaboration across ranks and disciplines to seek solutions to patient safety problems
- Organizational commitment of resources to address safety concerns (AHRQ, n.d., para. 1)

An important part of the safety culture is cultivating a blame-free environment. Errors and near misses must always be reported so that they can be thoroughly analyzed. One can learn from mistakes and change organizational processes or culture to ensure patient safety. The Patient Safety and Quality Improvement Act of 2005 mandates the creation of a national database of medical errors and funded several organizations to analyze these data with the goal of shared learning to prevent medical errors. Organizations themselves can engage in **root-cause analysis** or **failure modes and effects analysis** to examine medical errors closely and to determine the system processes that need to be changed to prevent similar future errors (Harrison & Daly, 2009). A tool for implementing root-cause analysis developed by the National Center for Patient Safety is detailed at this website: http://www.patientsafety.gov/CogAids/RCA/index.html#page=page-1. Similarly, the IHI has a website dedicated to failure modes and effects analysis. "Failure Modes and Effects Analysis (FMEA) is a systematic, proactive method for evaluating a process to identify where and how it might fail, and to assess the relative impact of different failures in order to identify the parts of the process that are most in need of change" (IHI, n.d.1, para. 1). This powerful tool and shared experiences from other organizations can be viewed at http://www.ihi.org/ihi/workspace/tools/fmea/.

If one embraces a blame-free environment to encourage error reporting, then where does individual accountability fit? According to the ARHQ, one way to balance these competing cultural values (blameless versus accountability) is to establish a "just culture" where system or process issues that lead to unsafe behaviors and errors are addressed by changing practices or work-flows processes, and a clear message is communicated that reckless behaviors are not tolerated. The "just culture" approach accounts for three types of behaviors leading to patient safety compromises: (1) human error (unintentional mistakes); (2) risky behaviors (workarounds); and (3) reckless behavior (total disregard for established policies and procedures).

STRATEGIES FOR DEVELOPING A SAFETY CULTURE

Strategies for achieving a safety culture have been addressed frequently in the literature. The focus here is limited to those described by two key organizations, the AHRQ and the IHI. The AHRQ (n.d) provides access to data from two validated surveys, the Patient Safety Culture Survey and the Safety Attitudes Questionnaire. The AHRQ suggests that teamwork training, executive walk-arounds, and unit-based safety teams have improved safety culture perceptions, but have not demonstrated a significant reduction in error rates. The IHI (n.d.2) stresses that organizational leaders must drive the culture change by a visible commitment to safety and by enabling staff openly to share safety information. Some of the strategies suggested by the IHI include appointing a safety champion for every unit, creating an adverse event response team, and reenacting or simulating adverse events to understand better the organizational or procedural processes that failed.

A systems engineering approach to patient safety where technology manufacturers partner with organizations to identify risks to patient safety and promote safe technology integration is advocated by Ebben, Gieras, and Gosbee (2008). They note that **human-factors engineering** is "The discipline of applying what is known about human capabilities and limitations to the design of products, processes, systems, and work environments." Its application to system design improves "ease of use, system performance and reliability, and user satisfaction, while reducing operational errors, operator stress, training requirements, user fatigue, and product liability" (p. 327). For example, Ebben et al. describe the feel of an oxygen control knob that rotated smoothly between settings suggesting to the user that oxygen flows at all points on the knob, when in fact oxygen only flowed at specifically designated liter flow settings. Human-factors engineering testing would most likely reveal this design flaw and the setting knob could be improved to include discrete audio or tactile feedback (click into place) to the user to indicate a point on the dial where oxygen flows. They emphasize that testing human use factors provides more objective safety data than the subjective responses gained from user preference testing. "Understanding how the equipment shapes human performance is as important as evaluating reliability or other technical criteria" (Ebben et al., p. 329). Organizations that are purchasing medical technology devices should avail themselves of shared safety data on equipment maintained by several key organizations including Joint Commission, the Food and Drug Administration, and the Medical Product Safety Network (MedSun www.fda.gov/MedicalDevices/Safety/MedSunMedicalProductSafetyNetwork/default.htm).

Once the technology is integrated into the organization, biomedical engineers can become valuable partners in promoting patient safety through appropriate use of these technologies. For example, in one organization the biomedical engineers helped to revamp processes associated with the new technology alarm systems after they discovered several key issues: slow response times to legitimate alarms and multiple false alarms (promoting **alarm fatigue**) created by alarm parameters that were too sensitive. Strategies for addressing these issues included improving the nurse call system by adding "voice over internet protocol" telephones carried by all nurses that wirelessly receive alarms directly from technology equipment, thus reducing response times to alarms, feeding alarm data into a reporting database for further analysis, and encouraging nurses to round with physicians to provide input into alarm parameters that were too sensitive and were generating multiple false alarms (Williams, 2009). The Research Brief describes a study of Intelligent Agent (IA) technology to improve the specificity of physiologic alarms.

Clearly, there is more work to be done to create safety cultures in complex healthcare organizations and to reduce the incidence of errors. Many organizations are looking to informatics technology to help manage these complex safety issues by using smart technologies that provide knowledge access to users, provide automated safety checks, and improve communication processes.

Research Brief

The investigators used simple reactive intelligent agent (IA) technology to develop and test decision algorithms for improving the sensitivity and specificity of physiologic alarms. The IA technology was tested in a 14-bed cardiothoracic unit over 28 days, and was implemented in parallel to the usual physiologic patient monitor providing measures, such as systolic blood pressure, mean arterial pressure, central venous pressure, and cardiac index. Alarm data generated by both systems were compared and classified as to whether the alarm represented at true medical event requiring clinician intervention or a false-positive alarm. There were a total of 293,049 alarms generated by the usual physiologic monitoring system and 1,012 generated by the IA system after raw physiologic data were filtered using rule-based IA technology. The IA filtering system shows promise for improving the specificity of physiologic alarms and decreasing the number of false-positive alarms generated by artifacts, thus reducing the incidence of alert fatigue in clinicians.

Source: Blum, J., Kruger, G., Sanders, K., Gutierrez, J., & Rosenberg, A. (2009). Specificity improvement for network distributed physiologic alarms based on a simple deterministic reactive intelligent agent in the critical care environment. *Journal of Clinical Monitoring and Computing, 23*(1), 21–30. Retrieved from ProQuest Nursing & Allied Health Source. (Document ID: 1848695561).

INFORMATICS TECHNOLOGIES FOR PATIENT SAFETY

Healthcare technologies are frequently designed to improve patient safety, streamline work processes, and improve the quality and outcomes of healthcare delivery. Technology is not always the answer to patient safety, as the Joint Commission (2008) cautions, "the overall safety and effectiveness of technology in health care ultimately depends on its human users, and that any form of technology can have a negative impact on the quality and safety of care if it is designed or implemented improperly or is misinterpreted" (para. 2). Although technology may certainly help to prevent or reduce errors, one must always remember that technology is not a substitution for safety vigilance by the healthcare team in a safety culture.

Bates and Gawande (2003) urged the adoption of information technology (IT) processes to improve safety. They suggest that information technologies improve communication, reduce errors and adverse events, increase the rapidity of response to adverse events, make knowledge more accessible to clinicians, assist with decisions, and provide feedback on performance. They also describe the benefits of technology-based forcing functions that direct or restrict actions or orders implemented by computer technologies. For example, physicians are forced to write complete and accurate medication orders, are restricted from ordering an inappropriate dosing route for a medication, or are prompted to write corollary orders that should be included in the care regimen as part of the standard of care.

The Wired for Health Care Quality Act of 2005 began a series of funding streams to promote health IT, to promote sharing of best practices in health IT, and to help organizations implement health IT (Harrison & Daly, 2009). Many early adopters opted to focus technology and safety initiatives on medication ordering and administration processes. Medication errors are the most frequent and the most visible errors because the medication administration cycle has many poorly designed work processes with several opportunities for human error. Thus, **computerized physician order entry** (CPOE), automated dispensing machines, smart pump technologies for intravenous drug administration, and **bar code medication administration** (BCMA) frequently preceded the adoption of the EHR in many institutions because of the costs associated with implementing these technologies. In an ideal world, the EHR would be adopted concurrently as part of an interoperable health IT system. In the early EHR systems, clinicians were prompted by electronic alerts reminding them of important interventions that should be part of the standard of care, but these alerts tended to be generalized and not patient specific. For example, "Did you check the allergy profile?" or "Has the patient received a pneumonia immunization?" These early alert and care reminders are now evolving into more sophisticated **clinical decision support** (CDS) systems to promote accurate medical diagnoses and suggest appropriate medical and nursing interventions based on patient data. Other technologies designed to promote patient safety include wireless technologies for patient monitoring, clinician alerts, point-of-care applications, and radiofrequency identification (RFID) applications. Each of these is reviewed here, and the chapter concludes with a section discussing future technologies for patient safety.

TECHNOLOGIES TO SUPPORT THE MEDICATION ADMINISTRATION CYCLE

The steps in the medication administration cycle (assessment of need, ordering, dispensing, distribution, administration, and evaluation) have been relatively stable for many years. Each of the steps depends on vigilant humans to ensure patient safety resulting in the five rights of medication administration: (1) the right patient, (2) the right time and frequency of administration, (3) the right dose, (4) the right route, and (5) the right drug. Human error can be related to many aspects of the cycle. Distractions, unclear thinking, lack of knowledge, short staffing, and fatigue are a few of the factors that cause humans to deviate from accepted safety practices and commit medication errors. Technology integration into the medication administration cycle promises to reduce the potential for human errors in the cycle by performing electronic checks and providing alerts to draw attention to potential errors.

CPOE is an electronic prescribing system designed to support physicians and nurse practitioners in writing complete and appropriate medication and care orders for patients. When the CPOE is part of an EHR with a CDS system, the medication order is electronically checked against specific data in the patient record to prevent errors, such as ordering drugs that interact with a drug the patient is already taking, ordering a dose too large for the patient's weight, or ordering a drug contraindicated by the patient's allergy profile or renal function. Because it is impossible for and unreasonable to expect a clinician to remember each of the more than 600 drugs that require a dose adjustment in the case of renal dysfunction, safe dosing parameters are provided by the CPOE (Bates & Gawande, 2003). In a standalone CPOE system without a CDS system, the medication orders are simply checked by the computer against the drug database to ensure that the dose and route specified in the order are appropriate for the medication chosen. Specific benefits of CPOE include:

- Prompts that warn against the possibility of drug interaction, allergy or overdose
- Accurate, current information that helps physicians keep up with new drugs as they are introduced into the market
- Drug-specific information that eliminates confusion among drug names that sound alike
- Improved communication between physicians and pharmacists
- Reduced healthcare costs caused by improved efficiencies (The LeapFrog Group, 2008)

CPOE solves the safety issues associated with poor handwriting and unclear or incomplete medication orders. Orders can be entered in seconds and also entered from a remote site eliminating the use of verbal orders that are especially subject to interpretation errors. Orders are then transmitted electronically to the pharmacy reducing the potential for transcription errors common in the paper system, such as lost or misplaced orders, delayed dosing, or unreadable faxes. Thus, CPOE changes workflows for all clinical staff and physicians and it also changes health team communication patterns (Manor, 2010). As with any technology integration, there is a learning curve to gain proficiency, resistance to change, and users must learn to trust the system. Manor urges careful planning and training during implementation with plenty of staff support. She also reports on the need for a paper-based back-up system in the case of network or electrical outages or system maintenance.

The verification and dispensing functions of the pharmacy can also be assisted by technology. The pharmacist begins by verifying the allergy status of the patient and the medication reconciliation information to ensure that the new medication is compatible with other medication in the care regimen. This verifying function is computer based, and the medication order is electronically checked via the knowledge database. If the order is verified as safe and appropriate, the pharmacist proceeds to the dispensing process. Barcode medication labeling at a unit dose level was mandated by the Food and Drug Administration in 2004 with targeted compliance by 2006. A bar code is a series of alternating bars and spaces that represents a unique code that can be read by a special barcode reader. Bar code technology spans both the medication dispensing and administration steps in the medication administration cycle. In the pharmacy the barcode helps to ensure that the right drug and the right dose are dispensed by the pharmacy. Medications that are labeled with bar codes can also be dispensed by robots capable of reading the codes or by automated dispensing machines. Thus, barcode technology helps with the processes of procurement, inventory, storage, preparation, and dispensing (Cohen, 2002).

The processes of drug storage, dispensing, controlling, and tracking are easily carried out via an automated dispensing machine (alternatively named automated dispensing cabinets, unit-based cabinets, automated dispensing devices, or automated distribution cabinets). These devices have benefits for both the user and the organization, specifically in the areas of access security (especially with narcotic administration tracking), safety, supply chain, and charge functions (Institute for Safe Medication Practices, 2008).

Radiofrequency identifier (RFID) technology is rapidly gaining a foothold in healthcare technology and may soon be used in the medication administration cycle. Although more expensive than bar coding for packaging, the RFID tags are reprogrammable (Wicks, Visich, & Li, 2006) and issues associated with barcode printing imperfections and barcode scanner resolution can be mitigated (Snyder, Carter, Jenkins, & Frantz, 2010). As discussed later in this chapter, RFID technologies may also be an important component of a medication compliance system for patients.

BCMA systems help to ensure adherence to the five rights of medication administration. Whether the BCMA is part of the larger EHR or free-standing electronic medication administration system (eMAR), barcode technology provides a system of checks and balances to ensure medication safety. The nurse begins by scanning his or her name badge, thus logging in as the person responsible for medication administration. Next, the barcode on the patient's identification bracelet is scanned prompting the electronic system to pull up the medication orders. Next, the bar code on each of the medications to be administered is scanned. This technology checks to ensure that the five rights of medication administration are met. If there is a discrepancy between the order and the medication that was scanned or a contraindication for administration, an alert is generated by the system. For example, in an EHR system with CDS, the nurse may be prompted to check the most recent laboratory results for electrolytes before administering a potassium supplement. In a free-standing eMAR without CDS or EHR links, if the medication orders have recently been changed, the nurse is alerted to the change. When an alert is generated, the nurse must chart about the action taken. For example, an early dose might need to be given if the patient is leaving the unit for a diagnostic test.

Despite the promising advances in patient safety afforded by this technology, it is not fail-safe (Cochran, Jones, Brockman, Skinner, & Hicks, 2007). Medications that are labeled individually by the in-house pharmacist increase the potential for human error if the medication is given an incorrect barcode, such as a wrong dose or even the wrong medication. In addition, the barcode printers themselves may generate unreadable labels, leading to staff workarounds in the interest of saving time. Cochran et al. make the following recommendations to reduce BCMA errors:

- Purchase unit of use medications with manufacturer bar codes whenever possible.
- Double-check all hospital generated bar-code labels including compounded injectable medications before the product leaves the pharmacy.
- Carefully review all BCMA override reports. Address system workarounds through process change and staff education.
- Minimize false-positive warnings to reduce the likelihood that staff will ignore warnings for real errors.
- Ensure that an urgent need exists for all "stat" orders as pharmacy review and advantages of bar code administration are usually circumvented.
- Establish institutional policies and procedures that can be easily implemented when products fail to scan. Processes in pharmacy will likely be different than processes at the point of care (p. 300).

Smart pump technologies are designed for safe administration of high-hazard drugs and to reduce adverse drug events during intravenous medication administration. Smart pumps have software that is programmed to reflect the facility's infusion parameters, and a drug library that compares normal dosing rates with those programmed into the pump. Discrepancies generate an alarm alerting the clinician to a safety issue. A soft alarm can typically be overridden by a clinician at the bedside, but a hard alarm requires the clinician to reprogram the pump to fall within the facility's intravenous administration guidelines for the drug to be infused. All alarms generated by the smart pump are tracked along with the clinician's responses to them (Dulak, 2005). Smart pumps can be seamlessly integrated into BCMA systems and data can also be fed directly into the EHR. The IHI recommends the following steps to ensure safe implementation of smart pump technology:

- Prior to deploying these pumps, standardize concentrations within the hospital. Asking the nurse to choose among several concentrations increases the risk of selection error.
- Prior to deploying these pumps, standardize dosing units for a given drug (for example, agreeing to always dose nitroglycerin in terms of mcg/min or mcg/kg/min but not both). Asking the nurse to choose among several dosing units increases the risk of selection error.
- Prior to deploying these pumps, standardize drug nomenclature (for example, agreeing to always use the term KCl, but not Potassium chloride, K, Pot Chloride, or others). Asking the nurse to remember and choose among several possible drug names increases the risk of selection error.
- Perform a Failure Modes and Effects Analysis (FMEA) on the deployment of these devices.
- Ensure that the concentrations, dose units, and nomenclature used in the pump are consistent with that used on the Medication Administration Record (MAR), the pharmacy computer system, and the electronic medical record.
- Meet with all relevant clinicians to come to agreement on the proper upper and lower hard and soft dose limits.
- Monitor overrides of alerts to assess if the alerts have been properly configured or if additional quality intervention is required.
- Be sure the "smart" feature is utilized in all parts of the hospital. If the pump is set up volumetrically in the operating room but the "smart" feature is used in the ICU, an error may occur if the pump is not properly reprogrammed.
- Be sure there are upper and lower dose limits for bolus doses, when applicable.
- Engage the services of a human factors engineer to identify new opportunities for failure when the pumps are deployed.
- Identify a procedure for the staff to follow in the event a drug must be given which is either not in the library or when its concentration is not standard.
- Deploy the pump in all areas of the hospital. If a different pump is used on one floor and the patient is later transferred, this will create new opportuni-

ties for failure. Also, there may be incorrect assumptions about the technology available to a given floor or patient.

- Consider using "smart" technology for syringe pumps as well as large volume infusion devices (Institute for Healthcare Improvement, n.d. 3, para. 3).

CDS can enhance the medication administration cycle by promoting safety and improving patient outcomes. Clinical decision making is guided by targeted information delivery ensuring that the five rights of CDS are implemented: the right information provided to the right person in the right format through the right channel at the right time in workflow. For example, during medication selection, a CDS helps a clinician select an appropriate medication based on client data, such as clinical condition, weight, renal function, concurrent medications, and cost. A CDS ensures that the order is complete including checks for drug interactions, duplications, or allergy contraindications and ensures the right dose and right route are specified. During the verification and dispensing phase of the medication administration cycle, the CDS provides double checks for interactions, allergies, and appropriate dose orders. Consideration is also given to potential infusion pump programming issues, incompatibilities during infusion, and proper notation and dispensing when portions of a dose must be wasted. During the administration phase, the CDS assists with patient identification and current assessment parameters (i.e., blood pressure, glucose level) that may contraindicate the use of the medication at that point in time. Checks for interactions with foods or other medications, and timing and monitoring guidelines, are also provided to the clinician administering the medication. The CDS has patient education guidelines and printable handouts to assist clinicians in educating patients about their medications. The monitoring functions of the CDS provide a structured data reporting system to track side effects and adverse events across the population (HIMSS, 2009a).

There are several promising future technologies to assist patients with medication compliance after discharge. For example, eMedonline collects patient medication compliance data by scanning package barcodes or RFID medication tags and using personal digital assistant or smart phone technology to send compliance data to the server. Clinicians review the medication compliance data and provide education and feedback to patients to increase their compliance with proper medication administration (eMedonline, n.d.). The SIMpill Medication Adherence System uses Web-based technology to monitor patient compliance and provide reminders about taking medications or to refill prescriptions by sending text messages to the patient or caregivers (SIMPill 2008). Caps of pill bottles may contain RFID tags that monitor and collect data on when the bottle is opened, or contain flashing time reminders when a dose is due (Blankenhorn,

2010). Smart inhalers track asthma medication compliance using a micro-processor that records and stores medication compliance. They may also include visual and audio reminders to use the inhaler (Nexus 6, 2010). These are just a sampling of the newer technologies for medication adherence; more are expected in the future.

ADDITIONAL TECHNOLOGIES FOR PATIENT SAFETY

CDS systems have safety uses beyond the medication administration cycle. The robust data collection and data management functions help to ensure quality approaches to patient health challenges based on research evidence and clinical guidelines. A CDS may also ensure cost-effectiveness by alerting clinicians to duplicate testing orders, or suggesting the most cost-effective diagnostic test based on specific patient data (HIMSS, 2009b). Consider this description of the features of a CDS based on screen captures of a CDS system:

> The patient is a 75-year-old male with coronary artery disease (CAD), diabetes mellitus (DM), and elevated creatine kinase (CK). Assessment prompts and reminders on the screen for this patient include: no recent LDL test; BP is above goal; patient is due for pneumovax and influenza vaccines; patient is a current smoker, not thinking of quitting, last counseled with date; patient is overweight; patient is due for eye and ear checks. The patient management prompts include:
>
> - Lipid Management: No Recent LDL management is printed red with a series of checkboxes presenting choices to the clinician:
>   - Order lipid panel now; Order lipid panel with Direct LDL now; print instructions for fasting Lipid panel (link); print orders for outside lab request for lipid panel testing (link).
> - BP management: BP is above goal average over last 2 visits 130/80 goal is < 130/80
>   - Choices on checkboxes: Start another antihypertensive (help me choose) link
>   - Series of links listing current meds with opportunities to adjust each
> - Order Chem 7 now or order Chem 7 in (dropdown menu for timing of order)
> - Suggestions for referrals include
>   - Refer to nutritionist
>   - Refer to cardiac Rehab (help me choose link)
>   - Refer to BP Specialist (help me choose link)
> - Prompts for patient education handouts include:
>   - Print 'Control High Blood Pressure' link
>   - Print DASH diet instructions link
>   - Print exercise prescription (White, Shiffman, Middleton, & Cabán, 2008).

The prompts and instructions provided to the clinician are detailed and easy to navigate. Implementation of a CDS has the potential to optimize care by ensuring that all of the details of a patient's health issues are presented to the clinician for management, thus promoting individualized approaches to the total health of the patient based on best available evidence and clinical guidelines.

RFID technologies have both supply chain and patient care applications to patient safety. An RFID system contains a tag affixed to an object or to a person that functions as a radiofrequency transponder and provides a unique identification code, a reader that receives and decodes the information contained on the tag, and an antenna that transmits the information between the tag and the reader. When RFID tags are embedded in patient identification bracelets, they can help with patient tracking during procedures and testing, or function as part of the EHR communicating pertinent information to clinicians at the bedside. RFIDs may be part of the medication administration process, thus replacing bar-code technologies. They can be used to track medical supplies and equipment reducing staff time in locating such items. They may also be imbedded into surgical supplies to automate supply-counting procedures, thus reducing the likelihood that sponges or tools are erroneously left in the patient. RFIDs may also reduce the likelihood of wrong patient, wrong site surgical procedures (Revere, Black, & Zalila, 2010). RFIDs used in the medication supply chain protect patients by reducing the potential that a counterfeit medication is inadvertently introduced into the supply, and by providing for efficient medication recalls. Potential terrorist manipulation of the medication supply is also thwarted by RFID supply chain tracking technology. Blood and blood products can be efficiently tracked by RFID because specialized tags can detect temperature fluctuations and thus ensure that the blood or blood product was stored at the optimum temperature for safe administration (Wicks, Visich, & Li, 2006).

Smart rooms are being tested for wider use in healthcare facilities. As a caregiver enters the room, the RFID tag on their name badge announces to the patient on a monitor (typically mounted on the wall in the patient's line of sight) exactly who has entered the room and triggers "need to know" data by caregiver status to be displayed on the monitor in the room. For example, when a dietary aide enters the room, only dietary information is displayed, when a physician or nurse enters, all of the pertinent medical data from the EHR is available. Clinicians can review patient data in real time and chart at the bedside using touch screen technology, thus increasing productivity (Cronin, 2010). Some smart room technologies include workflow algorithms to alert clinicians as they enter the room about procedures that need to be implemented for the patient and can track individual clinician efficiency and effectiveness by aggregating data over time (Sharbaugh & Boroch, 2010).

New technologies to improve patient monitoring include **wearable** devices and wireless area networks, variously called "body area networks" or "patient area networks." The technologies provide the ability to wear a small unobtrusive monitor that collects and transmits physiologic data via a cell phone to a server for clinician review. Although most of these technologies are designed for monitoring chronic disease, they also have safety implications because they help to identify early warning physiologic signs of impeding serious health events (California Healthcare Foundation, 2007). A wireless chip on a disposable band-aid with a 5- to 7-day battery promises to be able to monitor the patient's heart rate and electrocardiogram, blood glucose, blood pH, and blood pressure, allowing for the collection of important clinical data outside the hospital (Miller, 2008). Wearable stress-sensing monitors detect electrical changes in the skin that may signal increased stress in autistic children who are unable to communicate an impending crisis. Caregivers are alerted to the potential crisis via wireless transmission and intervene to reduce the stress and prevent the crisis (Murph, 2010).

Robotics technologies are also being increasingly tested for safety and efficiency uses. Robotics have been used in minimally invasive surgery for some time; however, newer devices are including haptic (tactile) feedback to the surgeon, thus increasing the sense of reality during the procedure and reducing the potential for unsafe manipulation (June, 2010). A robot designed to assist with patient lifting promises increased safety for both patients and clinicians (Melanson, 2010). Finally, laser-guided robots are performing such routine functions as emptying and disposing of trash, cleaning rooms, delivering supplies and meals, and dispensing drugs (Savoy, 2010).

ROLE OF THE NURSE INFORMATICIST

The human side of patient safety is paramount. As technologies that can help to reduce errors and increase safety are integrated, health care professionals must also be improved. Therefore, not only must the technology be scrutinized and tested routinely, but the users must also be maintained and nurtured so that they are able to use the tools to the patient's benefit, avoiding harm and keeping the patient safe. Even the best CDS systems can contribute to mistakes by providing meaningless or harmful information. Nurse informaticists and the IT team in the facility must ensure that systems are properly configured and maintained. They should routinely monitor and check these systems while making sure that their human potential, the users, are capable of using the systems accurately to avoid errors. A technology and its user can never be left to their own devices.

Human inputting must focus on patient safety to raise the issues and sound out solutions. Nurse informaticists must be involved in all stages of the system development lifecycle with a focus on safety. Safety concerns and remedies need to be analyzed, synthesized, and integrated throughout the system development lifecycle to have a robust tool that provides meaningful information and enhances patient care while preventing errors and promoting patient safety. According to Effken and Carty (2002), "Creating a safe patient environment is a very complex issue that will require the combined knowledge and skill of clinical informaticists, informatics faculty, researchers, and system designers" (para. 16). The Research Brief describes the results of a survey on the impact of nurse informaticists on patient safety.

SUMMARY

Patient safety is an important and ubiquitous issue. This chapter explores the characteristics of a safety culture and technologies designed to promote patient safety. The need to evaluate errors carefully to determine why and how they occurred and how work-flow processes might be changed to prevent future errors of the same type is emphasized. Technology is changing rapidly and the culture of sharing related to technology implementation, error reporting, and troubleshooting prompts continuous process improvements. The key for organizations is to invest in their users and choose wisely so that the technologies they are adopting are interoperable and easily upgradable as technologies and safety practices evolve.

Organizations must make a commitment to a safety culture where everyone at every level is committed to patient safety at every moment. In an ideal world, everyone would first stop and think "Is this safe?" before every action, workarounds would not occur, and everyone would embrace rather than resist the technologies and work-flow processes designed to promote patient safety.

Research Brief

In 2009, HIMSS conducted an Informatics Nurse Impact Survey sponsored by McKesson (HIMSS, 2009c). This web-based survey yielded 432 acceptable responses over a 2-month period from December 2008 to February 2009.

One of the areas assessed was "value and impact of informatics nurse," on a scale of 1 to 7, with 7 being the highest rating:

> Respondents believe that informatics nurses involved in system analysis, design, selection, implementation and optimization of IT have the greatest impact on patient safety (6.21), workflow (6.17) and user/clinician acceptance (6.15). The area with the least impact was integration with other systems (6.03). These findings suggest the informatics nurse is a driver of quality of care and enhanced patient safety within their organization (p. 2).

This demonstrates the belief that nurse informaticists can greatly improve patient safety. The nurse executives who responded rated the positive impact of nurse informaticists on patient safety at 6.36 out of 7. In their conclusion, the researchers stated that:

> The role of informatics nurses is not limited to IT; this research also suggests that informatics nurses play an instrumental role with regard to patient safety, change management and usability of systems as evidenced by their impact on quality outcomes, workflow, and user acceptance. These additional areas highlight the value of informatics nurses—their expertise truly translates to the adoption of more effective, higher quality clinical applications in healthcare organizations (p. 11).

HIMSS. (2009c). *Informatics nurse impact survey sponsored by McKesson.* Retrieved from http://www.himss.org/content/files/HIMSS2009NursingInformaticsImpactSurveyFullResults.pdf

THOUGHT-PROVOKING Questions

www

1. What are the current patient safety characteristics of your organizational culture? Identify at least three aspects of your culture that need to be changed with regard to patient safety, and suggest strategies for change.

2. Describe a current technology that you use in patient care that would benefit from human factors engineering concepts. What are some ways this technology should be improved?

3. Identify a workaround that you have used and analyze why you chose this risk-taking behavior over behavior that conforms to a safety culture.

For a full suite of assignments and additional learning activities, use the access code located in the front of your book to visit this exclusive website: http://go.jblearning.com/mcgonigle. If you do not have an access code, you can obtain one at the site.

www

References

Agency for Healthcare Research and Quality (AHRQ.gov). (n.d.). *Patient safety primer: safety culture.* Retrieved from http://psnet.ahrq.gov/primer.aspx?primerID=5

Bates, D., & Gawande, A. (2003). Improving safety with information technology. *New England Journal of Medicine, 348,* 2526–2534.

Blankenhorn, D. (2010). *Can better tools overcome the medical compliance crazy?* Retrieved from http://www.zdnet.com/blog/healthcare/can-better-tools-overcome-the-medical-compliance-crazy/3925

Blum, J., Kruger, G., Sanders, K., Gutierrez, J., & Rosenberg, A. (2009). Specificity improvement for network distributed physiologic alarms based on a simple deterministic reactive intelligent agent in the critical care environment. *Journal of Clinical Monitoring and Computing, 23*(1), 21–30. Retrieved from ProQuest Nursing & Allied Health Source. (Document ID: 1848695561).

California Healthcare Foundation. (2007). *Healthcare unplugged: The evolving role of wireless technology.* Retrieved from http://www.chcf.org/~/media/Files/PDF/H/PDF%20HealthCareUnplugged TheRoleOfWireless.pdf

Cochran, C., Jones, K., Brockman, J., Skinner, A., & Hicks, R. (2007). Errors prevented by and associated with bar-code administration systems. *The Joint Commission Journal on Quality and Patient Safety, 33*(5), 293–301. Retrieved from http://www.scribd.com/doc/12844778/Errors-Prevented-by-and-Associated-With-BCMA

Cohen, M. (2002). Bar code labeling for drug products. Proceedings of the Food and Drug Administration's July 26, 2002, public meeting. Retrieved from http://www.ismp.org/pressroom/viewpoints/FdaBarCoding.asp

Cronin, M. (2010). *SmartRooms from IBM connect hospital staff to patient data.* Retrieved from http://medhealth.tmcnet.com/topics/medhealth/articles/95633-smartrooms-from-ibm-connect-hospital-staff-patient-data.htm

Dulak, S. (2005). Technology today: Smart IV pumps. Retrieved from http://www.modern medicine.com/modernmedicine/article/articleDetail.jsp?id=254828

Ebben, S., Gieras, I., & Gosbee, L. (2008). Harnessing hospital purchase power to design safe care delivery. *Biomedical Instrumentation & Technology, 42*(4), 326–331. Retrieved from ProQuest Nursing & Allied Health Source. (Document ID: 1548954831).

Effken, J., & Carty, B. (2002). The era of patient safety: Implications for nursing informatics curricula. *Journal of the American Medical Informatics Association (JAMIA), 9*(6 Suppl 1). Retrieved from http://www.ncbi.nlm.nih.gov/pmc/articles/PMC419434/

eMedonline. n.d. How eMedonline works. Retrieved from http://www.emedonline.com/about.asp?topic=howitworks

Harrison, J., & Daly, M. (2009). Leveraging health information technology to improve patient safety. *Public Administration and Management, 14*(1), 218–237. Retrieved from ABI/INFORM Global. (Document ID: 1685699891).

HIMSS. (2009a). Approaching CDS in medication management. Retrieved from http://healthit.ahrq.gov/images/mar09_cds_book_chapter/CDS_MedMgmnt_ch_1_sec_3_applying_CDS.htm

HIMSS. (2009b). *Clinical decision support (CDS) fact sheet.* Retrieved from http://www.himss.org/content/files/CDSFactSheet3-17-09.pdf

Institute of Medicine (2000). *To Err Is Human: Building a Safer Health System.* Kohn L, Corrigan J, Donaldson M, eds. Washington, DC: Committee on Quality of Health Care in America, National Academies Press. Retrieved from http://psnet.ahrq.gov/resource.aspx?resourceID=1579

Institute of Medicine (2001). *Crossing the Quality Chasm: A New Health System for the 21st Century.* Committee on Quality of Health Care in America, Institute of Medicine. Washington, DC: National Academies Press. Retrieved from http://psnet.ahrq.gov/resource.aspx?resourceID=1564

Institute for Healthcare Improvement (IHI.org). (n.d.1). *Failure modes and effects analysis tool.* Retrieved from http://www.ihi.org/ihi/workspace/tools/fmea/

Institute for Healthcare Improvement (IHI.org). (n.d.2.) *Develop a culture of safety.* Retrieved from http://www.ihi.org/IHI/Topics/PatientSafety/SafetyGeneral/Changes/Develop+a+Culture+of+Safety.htm

Institute for Healthcare Improvement (IHI.org). (n.d.3). *Reduce adverse drug events (ADES) involving intravenous medications: Implement smart infusion pumps.* Retrieved from http://www.ihi.org/IHI/Topics/PatientSafety/MedicationSystems/Changes/IndividualChanges/ImplementSmartInfusionPumps.htm

Institute for Safe Medication Practices. (April 19, 2007). *Smart pumps are not always smart on their own.* Retrieved from http://ismp.org/Newsletters/acutecare/articles/20070419.asp

Institute for Safe Medication Practices. (2008). *Guidance on the interdisciplinary safe use of automated dispensing cabinets.* Retrieved from http://www.ismp.org/tools/guidelines/ADC_Guidelines_Final.pdf

Joint Commission. (2008). *Sentinel event alert #42 safely implementing health information and converging technologies.* Retrieved from http://www.jcrinc.com/Sentinel-Event-Alert-42/

June, L. (2010). *Sofie surgical robot gives haptic feedback for a more humane touch.* Retrieved from http://www.engadget.com/2010/10/11/sofie-surgical-robot-gives-haptic-feedback-for-a-more/

Manor, P. (2010). CPOE: Strategies for success. *Nursing Management, 41*(5), 18. Retrieved from ABI/INFORM Global. (Document ID: 2044925551).

Melanson, D. (2010). *Yurina health care robot promises to help lift, terrify patients.* Retrieved from http://www.engadget.com/2010/08/13/yurina-health-care-robot-promises-to-help-lift-terrify-patients/

Miller, P. (2008). *Wireless chip on a band-aid to monitor patient's from home.* Retrieved from http://www.engadget.com/2007/02/28/philips-introduces-wireless-medical-tablet-powered-by-intels-mc/

Murph, D. (2010). *Affectiva's Q Sensor wristband monitors and logs stress levels, might bring back the snap bracelet.* Retrieved from http://www.engadget.com/2010/11/02/affectivas-q-sensor-wristband-monitors-and-logs-stress-levels/

Nexus 6. (2010). *What are smart inhalers?* Retrieved from http://www.smartinhaler.com/Researcher_SI.aspx

Revere, L., Black, K., & Zalila, F. (2010). RFIDs can improve the patient care supply chain. *Hospital Topics, 88*(1), 26–31. Retrieved from Health Module. (Document ID: 2119405721).

Savoy, V. (2010). *Robots to invade Scottish hospital, pose as 'workers'.* Retrieved from http://www.engadget.com/2010/06/21/robots-to-invade-scottish-hospital-pose-as-workers/

Sharbaugh, D., & Boroch, M. (2010). Hospital smart rooms are ready for rollout. Retrieved from http://www.buildings.com/tabid/3413/ArticleID/9675/Default.aspx

SIMpill. (2008). The SIMpill medication adherence solution. Retrieved from http://www.simpill.com/thesimplesolution.html

Snyder, M., Carter, A., Jenkins, K., & Frantz, C. (2010). Patient misidentifications caused by errors in standard barcode technology. *Clinical Chemistry, 56*(10), 1554–1561.

The LeapFrog Group. (2008). *Fact sheet: Computerized physician order entry.* Retrieved from http://www.leapfroggroup.org/media/file/FactSheet_CPOE.pdf

U.S. Department of Veteran's Affairs. (2009). *NCPS root cause analysis tools.* Retrieved from http://www.patientsafety.gov/CogAids/RCA/index.html#page=page-1

Wachter, R. (2010). Patient safety at ten: Unmistakable progress, troubling gaps. *Health Affairs, 29*(1), 165–173. Retrieved from ABI/INFORM Global. (Document ID: 194983018

White, J., Shiffman, R., Middleton, B., & Cabán, T. (2008). A National Web Conference on Using Clinical Decision Support to Make Informed Patient Care Decisions. Slide 63: Partners CDS Services: CAD/DM Smart, Form Slides 63-65. Presented at Agency for Healthcare Research and Quality September 19, 2008. Retrieved from http://healthit.ahrq.gov/images/sep08cdswebconference/textmostly/

Wicks, A., Visich, J., & Li, S. (2006). Radio frequency identification applications in healthcare. *Int J Healthcare Technology and Management, 7*(6), 522–540.

Williams, J. (2009). Biomeds' increased involvement improves processes, patient safety. *Biomedical Instrumentation & Technology, 43*(2), 121–3. Retrieved from ProQuest Nursing & Allied Health Source. (Document ID: 1692747971).

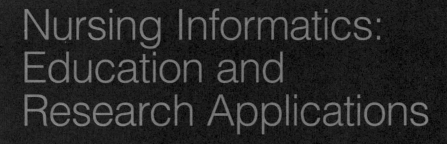

Nursing Informatics: Education and Research Applications

Nursing informatics (NI) provides more tools and capabilities than can at times be imagined. Just as NI has changed the way nursing is administered and practiced, it has also dramatically impacted research and educational practices.

Nursing research has evolved with technology. In the era of evidence-based practice, clinicians must continue to think critically about their actions. What is the science behind interventions? Things must no longer be done one way just because they have always been done that way. One should research the problem, use evidence-based resources, critically select electronic and nonelectronic references, consolidate the research findings and combine and compare the conclusions, present the findings, and propose a solution. One may be the first to ask why, and thus become a key player in making change happen. NI enhances and facilitates collaboration; improves access to online libraries; provides research tool transparency for collection, analysis, and dissemination of research knowledge; and facilitates the development of a common data language. NI provides organizational and informational support to advance translational research, helping to fill the gap between research findings and practice implementation. Repeat studies are needed to provide meaningful meta-analyses and systematic reviews of evidence to advance practice. Technology advancement in the area of incorporating evidence into clinical tools must continue. Removing the barriers to knowledge-seeking behavior and providing access to evidential resources promotes knowledge use and, in the end, improves patient outcomes.

Nursing education is evolving with the integration of NI tools to promote learning. The tools that are available must be used prudently by reflecting on and applying knowledge on teaching styles, learning styles, and other pedagogic concerns. As informatics capabilities continue to expand, a phenomenal amount of potential for virtual reality–embedded education looms on the horizon. Once the purview of gamers and geeks, virtual reality has exploded onto the academic scene. The use of virtual reality has the potential for cross-pollination between fields of inquiry across the curriculum, the university, and even learning systems. Many university departments will experiment with virtual reality in the hopes of staying current and appealing to their young and demanding "generation next" constituency. However, much of society loves the feel of books too much to dismiss them as archaic. There is room for both books and technology in education. Students, educators, and administrators will ultimately return to a modified form of face-to-face classroom teaching, even with the availability of newer and more adventuresome teaching technologies. Furthermore, after fast, high-burn technologies stop flooding the marketplace, and big business provides opportunities for proprietary online universities, modified traditions will take their place, creating new spaces for nontraditional students and members of the 'net generation, both anxious for technology use in the classroom for very different reasons.

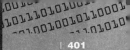

Foundation of Knowledge model.

FIGURE
V-1

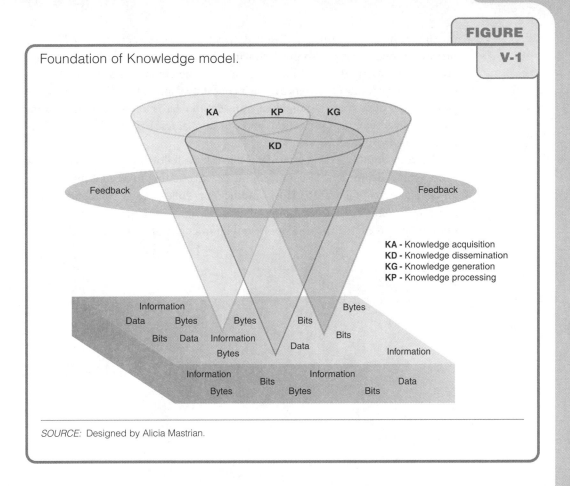

KA - Knowledge acquisition
KD - Knowledge dissemination
KG - Knowledge generation
KP - Knowledge processing

SOURCE: Designed by Alicia Mastrian.

The material in this book is placed within the context of the Foundation of Knowledge model (Figure V-1) to meet the needs of healthcare delivery systems, organizations, patients, and nurses. Nursing research is conducted to generate knowledge. In relation to the model, the nurse researcher is involved with every aspect from acquiring (collecting) and processing (analyzing) data and information; generating knowledge; and disseminating the results or findings (knowledge). Through this work, the researcher generates knowledge for the nursing profession. Knowledge generation is extremely important in the advancement of nursing science. Nursing education promotes scholarship and evidence-based teaching and learning. Through the sound integration of information management and technology tools, teaching and learning strategies promote the social and intellectual growth of the learner. As teachers and learners quest for knowledge, the pursuit of lifelong learning is instilled. Teachers and learners involved in the process of education are also involved with all levels of the model. Typically, they acquire and process data and information and generate and disseminate knowledge within the frame of reference of their educational institution. Their knowledge generation is on a limited, individual/course/school basis unless they become involved with developing publications and educational research that informs others in the nursing profession.

The reader of this section is challenged to ask the following questions: (1) How can I apply the knowledge I gain from my practice setting to benefit my patients and enhance my practice? (2) How can I help my colleagues and patients understand and use the current technology that is available? (3) How can I use my wisdom to help create the theories, tools, and knowledge of the future?

CHAPTER 23

Nursing Informatics and Nursing Education

Heather E. McKinney and Sylvia DeSantis

1. Describe nursing education in relation to the Foundation of Knowledge model.
2. Explore knowledge acquisition and sharing.
3. Assess technology tools and delivery modalities used in nursing education.
4. Compare and contrast knowledge assessment methods.

www

INTRODUCTION: NURSING EDUCATION AND THE FOUNDATION OF KNOWLEDGE MODEL

Nursing informatics facilitates the integration of information, data, and knowledge to support nurses, patients, and other providers in their various settings and decision-making roles (Carty & Ong, 2006). The **Foundation of Knowledge model** specifically prompts nurses to extend theoretical and metaphorical knowledge into practical, holistic determinations based on a variety of factors and contexts. Because competencies in informatics include but are not limited to **information literacy**, computer literacy, and the ability to use strategies and system applications to manage data, knowledge, and information (American Nurses Association, 2000), the ability of nursing students to use computer-mediated communication skills is essential to success in the nursing field and to improve patient safety.

The rise of telecommunications, computer-mediated communications, and virtual technologies has opened up opportunities for improving communication and extending care within the healthcare industry (Barnes & Rudge, 2005). Proponents of instructional

Key Terms **www**

Advocate
Asynchronous
Audiopods
Avatars
Blended hybrid
Blog
Case study
Collaboration
Compact disc read-only memory (CD-ROM)
Computer-assisted instruction (CAI)
Computer-based
Continuing education
Digital pen
Digital versatile disc or digital video disc (DVD)
Distance education
E-learning
Electronic mailing list
E-mail
Face to face
Foundation of Knowledge model
High fidelity
Hybrid
Hypertext
Information literacy
Instant message (IM)

Continues

applications of computer technology view it as a way to erase geographic boundaries for students, enhance the presentation of content, improve learning outcomes, and even tailor instruction to individual learning needs. When carefully matched with curricular objectives, technology becomes an efficient and affordable avenue through which nursing faculty may provide useful knowledge to their students, thus facilitating the learning process (Hebda, Czar, & Mascara, 2005). Far beyond the simple applications of word processing software or spreadsheets, technology applications have evolved greatly, taking advantage of modern capability in providing nursing and related healthcare students with simulations, complex **multimedia**, virtual reality–assisted clinical scenarios, and a host of information and literature-gathering Internet tools.

Case Study

WWW

For years, Victoria has been torn between the desire to practice nursing in the vibrant, metropolitan city, or in her peaceful, mountainous hometown in the country with her family. She wonders how the two experiences differ. How do the demands differ? How does the technology differ? To learn more about these differences, she explores a variety of education **scenarios**, including computer-based **virtual reality**, **simulations**, and real life scenarios in both urban and rural settings. How do you think the demands and technologies differ? How can virtual reality, simulations, and real life scenarios be designed to provide optimal education for nursing students? How might they be integrated into the nursing school curriculum to increase patient, practitioner, and hospital safety?

Knowledge Acquisition and Sharing

The shift from computer literacy to information literacy and management has drawn attention to interactivity and design as the most important components of interactive **Web-enhanced** and **Web-based** courses in providing effective learning environments. Thurmond (as cited in Carty & Ong, 2006, p. 523) discusses the four types of interactions related to Web-enhanced courses: (1) learner–learner, (2) learner–content, (3) learner–instructor, and (4) learner– interface interactions. In traditional learner–learner exchanges, students interact with one another to troubleshoot, work out challenges, and exchange solutions generated from different perspectives. Traditional and familiar, both learner–content and learner–instructor interactions expect students to work directly with course content or the faculty member and then participate in relevant course activities, such as tests and reviews. Learner–interface interaction includes the ways students access their coursework and their ultimate success or failure in finding, retrieving, and using what they need (Carty & Ong). When Web enhanced, these interactions include **online chats**, forum discussions, participation in **electronic mailing list** groups, **instant messaging,** blogging, and using **e-mail**, all of which ask the student to engage, digest, use, and disseminate information in new ways.

Hardware and Software Considerations

In the 21st century, nursing informatics has begun to rely heavily on technology usability, functionality, and accessibility. **Computer-assisted instruction** (CAI) has had an enormous impact on nursing informatics, with many computer-assisted instruction CAI programs offering individualized instruction in the form of customizable scenarios, frameworks, and programs for study. Additionally, computer-assisted instruction CAI contributes to better understanding of material by supporting all learning styles, types, and paces. Consequently, nursing skills have presented endless development potential for software development, making the effective use of software and hardware by educators and students a prime necessity (Riley, 1996).

Software is used to describe the instructions that direct a computer's hardware to work, whereas hardware describes physical computer components, such as a mouse, keyboard, and monitor. Software essentially translates commands into computer language, allowing the hardware to perform its functions. Without hardware and software, computer technologies are moot, and without software, hardware does not function (McHugh, 2006). Applications software refers to the various programs individuals use to communicate with others, do work, play games, or watch multimedia on a computer. The most common software package sold with computers is an office package that generally includes a word processing program, spreadsheet capability, a presentation graphics program (e.g., PowerPoint), and some kind of database management system. Software packages are available on **compact disc read-only memory (CD-ROM)**, **digital versatile disc** or **digital video disc (DVD),** or through the Internet, allowing the user to download the software directly from a vendor's website (McHugh, 2006).

When evaluating software or hardware for purchase, careful assessment of the products and services helps an educator, administrator, or student to make the best choices. Most important when evaluating software is to understand how congruently the software's functionality compares to learning goals and objectives. Although many programs are available for assisting a nurse practitioner who is evaluating software for particular learning purposes, the main criteria concern content (Is the information accurate? Is it relevant?); format (How is information visually presented? Is it in frames? Does it come with graphics?); documentation style (What's the tone? Is it scholarly and applicable?); and strategies

(Is the software useful for all students, including remedial students and accelerated students?) (Edwards & Drury, 2000).

Hardware decisions depend on the way a computer system will be used, in addition to cost, ease of use, and durability (Clochesy, 2004). Systems purchased for personal use may differ dramatically from those purchased for online learning laboratories or smart classrooms. Because the technology inherent to workstations, servers, and computers in general tends to change quite rapidly, discussing large system decisions with an information technology expert yields a better informed decision. Some factors to consider include where the system will be stationed (at home for personal use or in a learning laboratory for use by many students); how many desktops there will be (one or a few dozen); if it will be networked to a school's internal system; if printing will be available; and the level of security needed (Hebda et al., 2005).

Delivery Modalities

Nursing educators are discovering that current students are not responding in the same ways the educators did during their own tenure as students. Technology-laden students from the millennial age demand instant information delivered in an entertaining fashion, an expectation built on extensive exposure to e-mail, text messaging, online chatting, and the Internet (Ridley, 2007). Additionally, many nursing departments are facing an increase in student enrollment and a corresponding growth in faculty. Although new nursing faculty bring significant clinical experience to their academic positions, also apparent for some is an underlying tension and unfamiliarity with technologic advances, outcomes-based accreditation initiates, and teaching itself. Schools of nursing are scrambling to provide professional development for busy nursing faculty and introducing them to best practices in teaching (Shaffer, Lackey, & Bolling, 2006).

Learning is a multispatial function, and in the age of technology innovation, instructional delivery can inhabit many forms in both physical and virtual spaces. Spaces in academia are no longer defined by a class or its content, but instead by the learning the class is trying to promote. To this end, learning spaces should support multiple modes of learning and delivery, including reflection, discussion, and experience, and facilitate **face-to-face** and online interaction within and beyond classrooms. Truly innovative delivery, whether face-to-face classroom interaction, online engagement, or a **blended hybrid** of technology and traditional classroom teaching, supports learning activities rather than standing independently of them (Oblinger, 2005).

Face-to-Face Delivery

Ridley (2007) suggests that although it is the most widely used teaching method among nurse educators, traditional face-to-face lecture yields only a 5% information retention rate over a 24-hour period, compared with demonstration (30%), discussion groups (50%), practice activities (75%), and peer teaching (90%) (as cited in Sousa, 1995).

Additionally, the inability of physical space to keep pace with learning models also inhibits the benefits gained from face-to-face interaction between teacher and student. For example, collaborative learning grinds to a halt when class is held in a room with chairs bolted to the floor, facing a lectern (Oblinger, 2005); this kind of spatial arrangement prohibits a sense of classroom community by inhibiting easy peer interaction, reducing students' ability to see each other, and concentrating all attention on the professor.

Conversely, in a collaborative learning environment, the professor guides conversation and sets up discussion, acting less as classroom authority and more as facilitator, helping students maintain focus, gently guiding discussion, and ultimately empowering students to push knowledge boundaries in a safe and secure atmosphere of peer support. This inductive, epistemologic approach promotes active, critical thinking skills and assists students in learning not just facts, but how to learn. As future healthcare professionals determined to rely on quantification and rationale, nursing students benefit from face-to-face classroom interaction that hones student ability to manufacture new personal truths through interaction with people and ideas in ways that cannot always be measured and counted.

Ridley (2007) suggests that such interactive, cooperative learning strategies might include gaming, **role playing**, and **problem-based** learning. Because games are nonthreatening and fun, they promote critical thinking and teamwork by pushing students to work together in groups to find answers and achieve success. Role playing is similar in that it allows students to try on real-life scenarios by filling either prescripted or ad-libbed roles (doctor, nurse, patient, clinician, and so forth) without the fear or pressure of putting another's life at risk while trying to determine the best course of action or find a solution to a fictitious patient's health issue.

Problem-based learning, a well accepted form of interactive learning, takes assignments out of a contextual vacuum and applies real-life scenarios to problems or challenges. Students work in groups to solve the dilemma presented by real patient cases and build on prior knowledge, using higher level thinking skills and progressive inquiry to resolve the problem (Ridley, 2007).

Online Delivery

E-learning, online learning, and Web-based education have caused a significant shift in student–teacher relationships in nursing education and, according to Phillips (1999), "the Internet will offer a chance to make real profits from education, while offering students a choice about who will educate them and at what price" (para. 14). According to Oblinger (2005), not only are learning spaces no longer physical or formal, especially on campuses with wireless capabilities, but nursing students are also expecting to make use of wide ranges of cutting-edge technology during their academic tenure, exchanging the traditional sage on the stage for a technologically savvy guide on the side (Leasure, Davis, & Thievon, 2000) who gives up the role of gatekeeper and instead promotes and facilitates dialogue as central to teaching–learning (Aquino-Russell, Maillard Strüby, & Reviczky, 2007).

Student-centered and no longer limited to the domain of the classroom, laboratory, or even a patient's bedside, online learning allows educators to translate theory into practice, creating a virtual classroom space that promotes **collaboration**, engagement, discussion, and analysis.

Detractors of online learning initiatives suggest, however, that sharing an online space undermines the student–teacher relationship, makes building peer relationships difficult, and generally disrupts the normal classroom dynamic, thus creating an unfamiliar, uncomfortable atmosphere. Despite these concerns, studies show that not only do Web-based courses continue to gain in popularity, but they also enhance learning in ways that encourage students to share personal experiences and support. Researchers cite many factors that make online learning laudable, with accessibility and convenience being two of the most frequently cited issues (Aquino-Russell et al., 2007).

The **asynchronous** and time-independent elements of Web-based courses answer a huge need for flexible class times by today's growing population of nontraditional learners. Additionally, Web-based and place-independent learning allows participation by anyone, anywhere in the world, with access. Related to this issue is the democratizing effect of online learning, such that all students have the same opportunity to participate without judgment. Web-based classes provide an easily accessible permanent record, a convenience for both teachers and learners (Aquino-Russell et al., 2007).

Online learning has the capability to reenvision classroom interaction, and depending on the specific delivery mode, can even change basic pedagogic concepts. The best online delivery (whether through a chat, **blog**, or class) just like traditional classes in a physical space adheres to solid teaching parameters that ensure student investment and success. These include providing students with a clear set of learning activities and expected outcomes; relating content to real situations using **case studies** and simulation (problem-based learning); building in collaborative activities, such as team projects; building in an instructor's personality and presence; and setting up technology such that users build their confidence rather than experience failure and frustration (Winfield, Mealy, & Scheibel, 1998). Refer to Box 23-1 for more information.

BOX
23-1

A Day in the Life

Eric Doerfler

Some days, I feel like I cannot get away from technology. I teach three classes that I keep tabs on through a course management system. It is a great system, but when the network is down, it is hard to get anything done. I am a teaching assistant in another university, and that program also is all online. Every work day, I spend time in the electronic world of my students. Of my own courses I can say this: at least every 2 weeks I see their nonvirtual faces. I have a handheld computer for my schedule and my address book. I use software for my finances, and that synchronizes to the handheld computer. I type my patient notes into a word processor. When someone calls with a problem, I can boot up my laptop and get a reminder of what I did and why.

That is the upside. Although I sometimes feel too dependent on complex machines for what was once simpler, the access I have and the options I am offered have changed my daily life. Online discussion boards offer reticent students a less threatening environment in which to participate, so I see more class participation. Posting articles online reduces my department's copying costs and logistical aggravation. If I see a good article, I do not need to print it, send it down to the copy center, and wait. My calendars are backed up; if one computer does not work, another one does, and there is no way for me ever to lose my address book, check register, or other key documents!

It is more expensive, however, to live this way. Computers, peripherals, and ink cartridges all cost money. Life was cheaper when I bought a day planner each December and retired the last. Electronic health records almost drove my practice budget into deficit until I went back to typing them into the laptop and saving and printing them. As I make my way through each day, I do sometimes find myself wondering how and when this can all become less bothersome, disjointed, and complex, and more simple, interconnected, private, and reliable, without driving me and all of us into the poorhouse! Although I teach informatics, as I go along I find that less technology is more, and I have started to walk by all the latest gadgets, waiting for the inevitable evolution that will marry me to my machines without spoiling my humanity or my peace of mind.

Hybrid or Blended Delivery

Traditional courses are more frequently being offered as online, virtual classes (i.e., **distance education**), learning that occurs elsewhere than in the traditional classroom and consequently, requires special course design, planning, techniques, and communication. A **hybrid** of this delivery mode includes learning in which traditional classroom time is enhanced or broken up with online components, thereby creating a class in which blended learning occurs. Some forms of hybrid learning include Web-enhanced learning and learning that takes place in and makes use of smart classrooms (e.g., teaching in a wired room equipped with classroom learning technologies, such as the Blackboard Learning System).

Web-enhanced instruction, such as asking students to blog responses to a reading or class discussion, allows technically ambivalent institutions to participate in the technology revolution without huge budgetary expenditure and also addresses a preference by some faculty for a way to include innovation and technology in classes without giving up traditional classroom engagement. *Syllabus* magazine has reported that most distance learning courses used up to five media to reach students, including chats, telephone calls, forums, student Web pages, and group pages, in addition to print materials from laboratory manual study guides and textbooks, and samples of student work, quizzes, and tests (Hibbison, 2001). Faculty are reaching for multiple media and hybrid approaches to encourage student-centered learning, maximize teaching effectiveness, and take advantage of the best on-campus and online teaching and learning (Black & Watties-Daniels, 2006). Box 23-2 provides more information.

BOX 23-2

Open Source and Moodle, a Course Management System

Dee McGonigle and Kathleen Mastrian

Open source is being used in business and health care. Open source refers to standards and guidelines for writing software open source code. The power comes in the fact that it is often free to use. "Open source is a development method for software that harnesses the power of distributed peer review and transparency of process. The promise of open source is better quality, higher reliability, more flexibility, lower cost, and an end to predatory vendor lock-in" (Open Source Initiative, 2007, para. 1). Graham (2005) adds that "Ten years ago there seemed a real danger Microsoft would extend its monopoly to servers. It seems safe to say now that open source has prevented that. A recent survey found 52% of companies are replacing Windows servers with Linux servers" (para. 1). Open source is changing the way health care and education conduct their business. Educators are looking to open source software to help manage their online courses because they can have flexibility, reliability, and lower costs.

Continues

Modular Object-Oriented Dynamic Learning Environment (Moodle) is an open source course management system or learning management system. *About Moodle* (2008) describes Moodle as open source software for "producing Internet-based courses and web sites" (para. 1). *What is Moodle?* (n.d.) describes Moodle as a "learning management system that lets you provide documents, graded assignments, quizzes, discussion forums, etc. to your students with an easy to learn and use interface. Moodle is developed by a worldwide effort of over 75,000 students, faculty, and staff at over 6500 institutions around the world" (para. 1). Munoz and Van Duzer (2005) compared Blackboard and Moodle. They describe Moodle as "Open source (free!). Customizable by programming staff. Flexible for the instructor and developer. Supported by programmers world-wide" (para. 2).

Open source code and the promise of free or low-cost globally supported software continues to gain appeal. As more and more people turn to open source, the more robust it will become, because it is a community effort between users and programmers.

References

About Moodle. (2008). Retrieved from http://docs.moodle.org/en/About_Moodle

Graham, P. (2005). *What business can learn from open source.* Retrieved from http://www.paulgraham.com/opensource.html

Munoz, K., & Van Duzer, J. (2005). *Blackboard vs. Moodle: A comparison of satisfaction with online teaching and learning tools.* Retrieved from http://www.humboldt.edu/~jdv1/moodle/all.htm

Open Source Initiative. (2007). *Home.* Retrieved from http://www.opensource.org/

What is Moodle? (n.d.). Retrieved from http://www.humboldt.edu/~moodle/whatis.html

Smart classrooms, also known as digital and multimedia classrooms, integrate computer and audiovisual technologies by providing a ceiling-mounted projector with an access point at the front of the room, an instructor podium or workstation, sound, and network access. An enhanced smart classroom also provides networked student workstations instead of traditional desks, allowing students to follow along online and perform network or Web searches, chat, blog, or myriad other activities as dictated by the professor. For example, at the Penn State School of Nursing, users access announcements, course materials, faculty information, websites, and other tools through Blackboard, enabling the nursing faculty to extend learning beyond the physical classroom walls.

Surveys by WebCT, an online virtual learning environment system created in 1995 and now slowly being phased out in favor of other systems, confirm the growing realization among faculty that traditional campus courses can benefit from the interactive components of a website, forums, and chat, and that online courses also benefit from face-to-face contact. In another survey, faculty showed strong preference for Web-enhanced classroom instruction over either traditional classroom-only instruction or online-only distance education, observing that student achievement is maximized in courses that combine online and classroom elements (Hibbison, 2001).

Technology Tools

The **'net generation** or millennial generation (students who have grown up inside a wired world of instant access and online everything) are connected, digital, experiential, and social. Working in teams comes naturally to this peer group, and interacting in peer-to-peer situations is a familiar and common learning mode. These students desire information immediately, are skilled multitaskers, and are, according to Oblinger in a 2005 Educause learning initiative, "no longer the people our educational system was designed to teach" (Prensky, 2001). Certain social trends emerging from the morass of both traditional and innovative technology tools include the use of technologies attempting to meet the needs of these new learners; through the use of software, hardware, drivers, dedicated servers, plugins, and an Internet connection, students can chat, collaborate, play a game, or interact electronically with a peer in some way, all with little to no learning curve or effort. Because visual media is now the vernacular of a highly digital culture, students and faculty are also embracing technology tools that allow for the creation and interpretation of visual images (Oblinger, 2005). These tools might take the shape of interactive **tutorials**, a created city within a virtual reality landscape, or even a multimedia action maze that prompts users to choose different outcomes within a scenario. Regardless of the particular tool, technology can only perform as well as the pedagogy that drives it, thus creating a need for integration, support, and sustainability within nursing education programs willing to implement new instructional and assessment strategies (Bassendowski, 2005). Refer to Box 23-3 for more information.

Tutorials

Academic institutions face a multitude of challenges in trying to satisfy the information needs of users who are inundated daily by tons of information as part of their regular Web use. In addition to facing a technologic revolution, it seems that academia is facing a pedagogic revolution as well, trying to meet students' needs in innovative and engaging ways. One solution to providing students with information and the skills to find, evaluate, understand, and apply this information comes in the form of online tutorials (Bracke & Dickstein, 2002).

BOX

23-3

Digital Pen Technology Tool

Dee McGonigle, Kathleen Mastrian, and Nedra Farcus

Digital pens are actual writing implements that can also digitally capture handwriting or drawings. They are battery operated and generally come with a universal serial bus (USB) cradle that permits uploading captured materials to the desktop, laptop, or palmtop computer. Scribes can use them as a ballpoint pen and write on regular paper just as they would with a normal pen. To capture what one is writing or drawing digitally, it is necessary to write on digital paper. This paper is different from regular paper in that there are small dots that permit the digital pen to see what one is writing or drawing so it can be captured digitally. Some manufacturers are trying to create digital pens that use regular paper. If one wants to capture what one is working on, the pen must be instructed to save the work. There are memory limitations; the memory will generally hold around 40 pages of captured digital paper.

Digital pens have been around for a while, and some of the former models are probably still collecting dust in someone's office. A new resurgence in the digital pen, however, is reflective of the advances in technology. Fried (2008) states that,

> One thing all the new products have going for them is that they come at a time where Windows' support for digital ink has never been better. With Windows XP, only the stylus-based Tablet PC edition really supported pen input. With Windows Vista, though, the operating system supports more kinds of ink, including that from tablets like those from Wacom, as well as things like Iogear's Digital Scribe (para. 22).

Some of these new marvels use Bluetooth wireless technology to send captures directly to a computer. The file formats vary by manufacturer but are typically GIF or JPEG, making them easily shared and supported.

Think of the educational applications of being able to capture 40 pages of material and upload it to a computer for share and exchange. What about the impact on patient care? The city of Stockholm is slated to use digital pens in its healthcare delivery system. According to *City of Stockholm to Use Anoto's Digital Pen to Improve Elderly Care Services* (2007),

> The Anoto digital pens will primarily be used to facilitate documentation and information transfer, in order to improve the quality of elderly homecare in the city (para. 4).

> The technology has already been deployed successfully in Solna and Sundbyberg, two towns north of Stockholm, where homecare nurses use the digital pen to register their arrival and departure times on each visit and tick off the services delivered to each patient, on a digital form (para. 5).

The Logitech digital pen system can be used to document assessments. A digital camera in the pen captures a watermark pattern when the user writes on interactive

Continues

paper. The pen is then set in a USB cradle, and the data are uploaded into the computer where they are converted to text. The use of a digital pen system enables students to complete an assessment in the home with pen and paper and share the information with their professor or a research team for analysis within a short period of time.

The digital pen is being used for many applications in education and healthcare. Would this be something you would use?

References

City of Stockholm to use Anoto's digital pen to improve elderly care services. (2007, September). *Wireless News, 1.* Retrieved from ABI/INFORM Trade & Industry database (Document ID: 1343068491).

Fried, I. (2008). *Is the digital pen mightier?* Retrieved from http://www.usatoday.com/tech/products/cnet/2007-08-24-digital-pen_N.htm

Modern tutorials mimic lectures by guiding users through a series of objectives or tasks, usually allowing the user to do the work at his or her own pace (Edwards & Drury, 2000). Tutorials generally stand alone as autonomous multimedia that may use animation, text, graphics, sound, questions, and different kinds of interactivity to engage and intrigue the user. They tend to promote active learning by prompting the user to answer sets of questions, follow clickable **hypertext**, or complete quizzes. For example, users might be asked to fill in worksheets after reviewing anatomy concepts, take a quiz, post an answer to a question, or even click through a scenario by choosing the best course of action in a mock clinical situation.

Some tutorials, such as those used by medical students at the Morgan Stanley Children's Hospital of New York, are designed to be brief (10 minutes), interactive, very focused, and immediately relevant. In this case, medical students bustling through a busy clinical rotation who accessed the tutorials actually raised examination grades (Pusic, Pachev, & MacDonald, 2007).

Because most students benefit from being able to contextualize a lesson's framework and purpose, the most effective tutorials provide users with understandable navigation, such as a table of contents at its beginning, or additional navigational aids, such as icons, buttons, or text that indicate where and how they need to progress (Dewald, 1999). For example, Penn State University Libraries offers a nursing tutorial specifically designed to teach the tenets of evidence-based practice (http://www.libraries.psu.edu/instruction/ebpt-07/index.htm). Although any piece of the tutorial may be accessed at any time, it prompts the user to follow a linear path in applying the four basic steps of evidence-based practice to make the process easier and more understandable.

Effective tutorials surpass the simple presentation of information in a Web-based format; they instead address certain pedagogic and student-centered needs by identifying and taking into consideration specific factors, such as instructional content, the educator's purpose and teaching goal, the initiative's overall purpose, the potential need for special conceptual input, the learners' ultimate objectives in completing the tutorial, and the standards that determine what qualifies as successful completion of the tutorial (DeSantis, 2002).

Although most tutorials are created to stand alone, some may also benefit and supplement face-to-face instruction, such as the interactive information skills tutorial developed at the Institute for Health and Social Care Research in Salford, United Kingdom. This tutorial divides a traditional lecture series into chunks, incorporating questions that would normally arise during the session into the text, and providing hyperlinks. This allows users to browse to different parts of the tutorial, open a database in a new window to perform a practice search, and access other features (Grant & Brettle, 2006). Tutorials in all their iterations urge students to hone and develop effective critical thinking skills.

Simulations

Used within healthcare circles for more than 15 years, the use of simulations in nursing training has experienced a recent upsurge in popularity, in part caused by the new availability of high-quality simulation equipment and a reduction in price for this technology. Ranked by fidelity, or the level of realism the equipment resembles, simulation may take various forms, from **computer-based** simulation, in which software is used to simulate a subject or situation (e.g., an interactive tutorial featuring a nurse–patient situation), to full-scale simulation, in which all the elements of a healthcare situation are recreated using real physiology, people, and interaction to resemble an environment as closely as possible to immerse students in the experience (Seropian, Brown, Gavilanes, & Driggers, 2004).

Task and skill training ranks as the most popular form of simulation, during which students hone repetitive skills through interaction with a wide range of equipment, including such products as low-fidelity plastic intravenous arms and **high-fidelity** virtual reality trainers. The expectation is that students will learn to respond to a situation through a repeated practice-and-learn model of knowledge acquisition; however, because even basic nursing skills, such as administering an injection, require technical skill and interpersonal skill, task and skill training enjoys only limited usefulness within the Foundation of Knowledge model without additional clinical exposure or high-fidelity simulation. Even reasonable anatomic fidelity cannot simulate accurately the intensity and vagaries inherent in clinical situations, thus making it difficult for the student accurately to assess and integrate one's clinical judgment, knowledge, and acquisition of skills (Seropian et al., 2004).

The most useful teaching simulations combine high-fidelity equipment with **Real-time** demonstrations of simulated medical emergencies, such as those enacted by the patient simulator laboratory at the Patient Safety Institute, a training subcenter of the North Shore–Long Island Jewish Health System. Home to programmable human simulator mannequins (including an infant) that can exhibit a variety of symptoms resembling various patient scenarios, the patient simulator laboratory tests and trains nurses and staff responding to simulated medical emergencies using real-time demonstrations and gives immediate feedback on their video-recorded activities. Intended to help improve both clinical and decision-making skills, the mannequins mimic human responses, such as breathing, coughing, and speaking, and are anatomically accessible in their ability to be intubated, catherized, and auscultated (Spillane, 2006). The richest and most educationally useful simulation training for students results as a combination of best practices, current pedagogy, appropriate choice of simulation, clinical experience, and theory. See Chapter 24 for a comprehensive discussion of simulation.

Virtual Reality

In traditional virtual reality, the user receives multiple sensory inputs, either mediated or generated by a computer, through visual stimulation (glasses, goggles, and screens); audio input (earphones, microphones, and synthesizers); and touch (smells, gloves, and bodysuits). A form of simulation training and once considered a science fiction technology of the future, virtual reality healthcare training has been widely used by medical students and surgeons in training, allowing individuals to practice an operation before working on the patient (Turley, 2000). The most current spotlight in virtual reality systems focuses on **Second Life**, an online virtual world created by San Francisco-based Linden Lab in 2003 with multiple teaching applications.

Virtual worlds are online environments in which the residents are **avatars** who, in turn, represent individuals participating online. Virtual world participants have an opportunity to design nearly every aspect of their environment, from their avatars' clothing, gender, and appearance (EDUCAUSE, 2006), to more complex elements that openly lend themselves to teaching approaches supported by the Foundation of Knowledge model, such as how the avatars communicate, move, interact, and create. Because virtual worlds are so versatile in their setup, and preselected environments are highly customizable, healthcare instructors have the opportunity to create learner-led scenarios, rather than outcome-based models of knowledge development (EDUCAUSE), thus creating opportunities for "mediated immersion" (Dede, 2005), a "neomillennial learning style" (Skiba, 2007b, p. 156) that encourages the ability to negotiate multiple media and simulation-based virtual settings and communal learning, providing an important and valuable balance among experiential learning and guided mentoring (Dede).

No longer limited to the purview of computer geeks, virtual worlds like Second Life have not only gained the attention of large organizations, such as the American Cancer Society and the Centers for Disease Control and Prevention, but also educational institutions, such as Penn State University, Dartmouth College, and Harvard University (Skiba, 2007b). Because virtual worlds foster unintentional learning through gamer-like technology in which students discover and create knowledge to accomplish something, rather than experiencing traditional outcome-based learning, their experiences result in greater comprehension and deeper knowledge. In a virtual clinical scenario, for example, a simulated, immersive environment presents invaluable learning opportunities for the student assuming the role of healthcare provider. Faculty can monitor the interaction and interrupt as necessary to provide advice or suggestions, while students negotiate the real and virtual world components of the scenario and their avatar patients, thus becoming aware of how, why, and when to apply specific skills within a clinical setting (EDUCAUSE, 2006).

Because so much of the data nurses rely on is complex, and so many patient cues lack concrete language or responses, virtual worlds' animated, immersive, three-dimensional environment allows students to practice skills, try new ideas, and learn from their mistakes while receiving feedback from educators within a globally networked classroom environment. Some students may struggle to participate in virtual communities for various reasons. Increasing comfort with multidisciplinary learning among students and educators improves patient safety and encourages the refinement of best practices for effective integration of these tools into mainstream education (EDUCAUSE, 2006).

Internet Tools: Webcasts, Searching, Instant Messaging, Chats and Online Discussions, Electronic Mailing Lists, and Portals

The general consensus in nursing education suggests that any technology that allows users to interact and engage both materials and each other is useful. More specifically, the Foundation of Knowledge model qualifies this observation with the caveat that technology must display user-friendly capabilities to provide benefits to its users, thus allowing students not just to find information and each other online, but also to engage, challenge, and institute their discoveries. Providing nursing students easy, free Internet tools for reaching the first step of this equation (gaining access to materials and peers) has been addressed by a proliferation of communication technologies available to any user with an Internet connection. Beyond the gadgetry, with the development of new strategies, practices, applications, and resources in technology comes the need for instructional strategies that not only appeal to this newer generation of students but also enhance learning. These strategies, coupled with easily accessible and functional tools, encourage nursing students to see beyond the right answer, and instead seek out information that encourages them in developing approaches to issues and resolutions for problems (Bassendowski, 2005).

Webcasts

Webcasts, typically live presentations delivered by way of the Web, offer great potential for students and faculty to engage both information and each other globally, tapping students' multiple intelligences for them to access what they need. Because of the growing ease in producing streaming video and subsequently delivering it via larger bandwidth, Webcasts have grown in popularity and are especially favored by programs that feature distance education components. Although some institutions are creating their own Webcast delivery system, most users rely on a few standard providers who, in turn, present the Webcast online. Although often delivered live, allowing audience members to participate, many instructors use Webcasts as an access point for prerecorded archives of lectures and presentations by experts their students would not otherwise have the opportunity to see or hear. Studies show that students enthusiastically embrace Webcast technology, accessing archived presentations more repeatedly than traditionally filmed sessions of guest lecturers; this dynamic level of engagement aids students in better grasping the subject manner. Like much dynamic technology, Webcasts provide an innovative component that keeps students engaged but tend to work best when learners are provided with learning outcomes before viewing (Bell, 2003).

Searching

One of the most common and proliferate search tools in technology today is the **wiki.** Wikis are websites or hypertext document collections that allow users to edit and add content in an open-ended forum. The appeal of (and objection to) wikis resides in their ability to let anyone with an interest and an Internet connection participate in a once-exclusive community of knowledge creators and seekers. As an environment that encourages practice and learning, wikis support learning communities where students collaborate online (Skiba, 2007a). Higher education has evolved from a place of straightforward knowledge transmission to a place where one strives to become a member of an expert community, and wikis promise to create opportunity for individuals to participate in this community in heretofore untapped ways. Most objectionable about wikis is their lack of organizing principle (many are organized alphabetically) and the ability for anyone to edit entries, the latter of which creates new intellectual property right challenges. Wikipedia, for example, the best known wiki project on the Web, is an online encyclopedia of sorts whose open access policy regarding its content keeps educators and professionals wary of inaccurate information (Skiba, 2007a). For additional search information, see "Search Engines" in Chapter 26.

Instant Messaging

Instant messaging, one of many collaborative Web chat tools available to any user with a computer and Internet access, continues to establish itself as a working, useful tool for informatics learning, providing instant access to and communication between people, information, and technology. Although some instant message (IM) services even provide voice and video, all instant messaging clients (of which the three leading are Yahoo! Messenger [Y!M], AOL Instant Messenger [AIM], and MSN Messenger) provide real-time text, allowing users to interact in the form of an on-screen conversation through a technology that is free, already quite popular with users, Web-based, does not require additional hardware or software, and has a very low learning curve for those few to whom it is unfamiliar. Beyond having a real-time conversation, instant messaging (IMing) an individual also allows the user to share links, pictures, and files. This kind of easy accessibility allows students, when logged on, to collaborate; seek real-time help from professors or librarians; and engage others working on questions, studying for clinical examinations, or reviewing information or notes (Chase, 2007).

Chats and Online Discussions (Blogs)

Real-time chats occur all over the Internet, at each hour of every day. The best-known chat tools are instant messenger clients, but chatting also refers to real-time discussion venues in which users meet in virtual chat rooms to engage in conversations by posting messages; this provides a comfortable, recognizable way of communicating for 'net generation students used to surfing the Web and interacting online. In a chat, students can meet, discuss, and engage each other over any given topic. Chats take various forms, the most complex of which involve highly evolved virtual communities in which users step into various rooms where they interact with any other individuals in the room at the same time. Initially the exclusive purview of gamers or hardcore programmers creating private online communities, chat rooms now exist for a wide variety of topics and interests.

Web logs, also known as "blogs," have emerged as low-investment and easy-to-use writing tools that, through their very setup and appearance, enhance health professionals' communication, writing, reading, information-gathering, and collaboration skills (Maag, 2005). Blogs are a kind of online journal, created by individuals who then invite comments from visitors to that Web space. Compared to technically complex online projects, such as tutorials and various multimedia, blogs are immediate, free to set up and access with an Internet connection, and even easily negotiable by the technically ambivalent. Because by nature blogs present a built-in discussion area to the user, they are especially useful for study groups interested in reflecting on material and evaluating ideas in a collective, collaborative way (Shaffer et al., 2006).

Electronic Mailing Lists

One low-investment information-gathering tool for use by nursing professionals includes membership in an electronic mailing list. These electronic discussion groups use e-mail to communicate and promote communication and collaboration with others interested in a particular field of study (Hebda et al., 2005). Electronic mailing lists require very little to participate, usually just a free subscription and e-mail capability. Electronic mailing lists are available on any subject but most share common features, such as the need to subscribe and then log in to participate. The moderators of an electronic mailing list have specific instructions on how to post messages and how to set subscription controls. Posting information means that when one replies to a topic thread, one generally has sent information to every member of the list. Like other technologies, the capabilities of electronic mailing lists continue to change and expand, providing ongoing viability for use in nursing education.

Portals

Similar to electronic mailing lists in the way they deliver specific information to one's e-mail, a **portal** allows the personalization of a specific website. Portals organize information from Web pages into simple menus so that the user may choose what they want to view and how they want to view it (Hebda et al., 2005). For example, WebMD is one of the most popular and best-known portals, allowing users to create accounts, bookmark their favorite information, and sign up for e-mail notifications. Portals, like most Web technologies, require an Internet connection and a free subscription that allows one to log in.

Podcasts: Audiopods and Videopods

Podcasts are audio recordings linked to the Web that are then downloaded to an MP3 player (Gordon, 2007) or computer where the listener accesses the recording or video. An outgrowth of the Apple **iPod** market frenzy, podcasts are developed and delivered by way of the Internet and require minimal investment, which includes a microphone, an Internet connection, and (often free) editing software.

Although most listeners use an MP3 player (of which iPod is but one brand name) to access podcasts, a desktop computer works just as well (Oblinger, 2005).

Beyond possibilities for global accessibility to whatever information one may record, podcasts also allow for automatic updates in the form of a **really simple syndication (RSS)** (also known as "**resource description framework (RDF)** site summary") feed that lets subscribers receive automatic notification whenever a podcast is updated (Gordon, 2007). Refer to Box 23-4 for more information.

BOX
23-4

Podcasts

Jackie Ritzko

A basic Web search using the search term *nursing podcast* produced 1,220 hits on one search engine. But what does this mean in the context of nursing informatics? The implication is that there are many resources on the Internet that somehow involve podcasts with a nursing focus. How these sites might be of use to a professional in the nursing field is the focus of this box. Before any discussion of the educational uses of a technology tool can take place, there needs to be an understanding of the hardware, software, training, and support that is required to use the tool.

Podcast is a term coined from the words *iPod* and *broadcast.* The word *iPod* is the name given to a family of portable MP3 players from Apple Computer. MP3 is a common file format for electronic audio files. Audio files, or in particular MP3 files, can contain verbal speech, music, or a combination of both. MP3 files can be played or listened to using an MP3 player. MP3 players can be portable devices, such as the iPod, or an MP3 player can simply be software that is installed and used on a computer. One can now see that a podcast is simply an MP3 file that can be played on an MP3 player. Broadcast, in its simplest usage, refers to the ability to send out. In terms of podcast, broadcasting is the ability to share MP3 files in such a way that the files are delivered to the user whenever new versions are available through a subscription. This ability to share resources and access the most up-to-date resources is a great advantage especially for the educational community.

We will now discuss podcasts in terms of function ranging from the more basic to the more advanced: finding podcasts, listening to podcasts, creating podcasts, and sharing podcasts. Finding podcasts at a minimal level requires only an Internet connection and a Web browser. A basic Web search for the term *nursing podcast* found many sites. Performing a basic Web search, however, may provide a user with only limited search capabilities. An **MP3 aggregator** is a program that can facilitate the process of finding, subscribing to, and downloading podcasts. A commonly

Continues

known aggregator is Apple Computer's iTunes, which is a free program available as a download from apple.com. Although iTunes is common, it is not the only program of this type. Using such a program as iTunes gives one the ability to search for podcasts based on many criteria including category, author, or title. The iTunes program provides access to audio downloads that may be either songs or podcasts. In both cases, users find downloads that are free and those that require payment.

Because podcasts are MP3 audio files, an MP3 player is needed to listen to a podcast. As noted, this can be done on a computer with an MP3 player or on a portable MP3. There are two ways in which podcasts can be downloaded. They can be manually downloaded, or a user can subscribe to a podcast. In the case of a subscription, once a new track is added to the podcast, iTunes automatically delivers it to a computer. Continuing to use iTunes as an example, once a podcast is found, it can be downloaded from iTunes to a computer. Once on the computer, it can be listened to or transferred to a portable device.

One may also choose to produce or record podcasts. As with most technology solutions, there are typically hardware and software requirements. The hardware for recording a podcast can vary. In a stationary setup, a microphone can be connected to a desktop or laptop computer. Standalone audio recorders can also record podcasts, and some MP3 players have built-in recorders. Free recording software is available for most computer platforms.

There may be times when a podcast is created for the sole use of the creator. More often, however, a podcast is created with the intention of being shared and listened to by others. Podcasts can be stored on Web servers for distribution and can also be shared via tools, such as iTunes. A common area within iTunes where educational institutions are able to host podcasts is iTunesU.

Podcasts have many uses in education in general and more specifically in nursing education. Simple searches on the Web produce many hits for nursing podcasts. Informal learning can take place when a nursing student listens to podcasts. Listening to or creating podcasts may be a formal class assignment, providing new ways to interact with course material.

Short discussions of what is new in the field may appear as podcasts on the Internet, in particular in news and research sites. Learners may rely on the portability of MP3 players to take learning on the road. Commuters and walkers and joggers are often seen listening to MP3 players. Because creating podcasts is relatively easy and inexpensive, they can be produced by students as review files for common terms or they can be used for students to self-assess their ability to discuss topics. The uses of podcasts from an educational perspective are limitless.

Bringing the discussion of podcasts back to the Foundation of Knowledge model, for each task or process in the model, one can see how podcasts fit. Podcasts can be used to acquire new knowledge from sources on the Web. Listening to podcasts provides learners with another tool for learning in addition to readings and lectures, thus reaching a wider audience with varying learning styles. Because podcast creation is simple and inexpensive, podcasts are an ideal way to generate and disseminate knowledge.

Audiopods

Audiopod is a term used to describe a traditional or audio-based podcast. Participating in podcasting can exercise not just basic technology skills, but also writing, editing, and speaking skills. Writing scripts for a podcast can be an excellent exercise in critical thinking and information delivery, whereas the technology itself allows global access to information by faculty, teachers, and students anywhere at any time (Gordon, 2007). Both faculty and students can create audiopods with little difficulty, and most often use podcasts to share additional class materials, updates, and even entire lectures (Oblinger, 2005).

Videopods

Similar to audiopods in set-up and accessibility, a **videopod** is a podcast that provides video in addition to audio functionability. Faculty might use videopodcasts to demonstrate concepts, interview experts in the field, and even assess student progress (Gordon, 2007). Libraries and other institutions have even begun using the videopod as a learning alternative to the ubiquitous and often mocked information video, finding that highly mobile students are more readily embracing this technology (Oblinger, 2005).

Multimedia

As technologically savvy students continue to demand accessible, interactive learning tools to keep them engaged, an increasing number of instructors are experimenting with and incorporating multimedia into their courses. Generally, multimedia refers to a computer-based technology that incorporates traditional forms of communication to create a seamless and interactive learning environment, such as interactive tutorials, streaming video, and problem-solving programs. Nursing education has long relied on traditional multimedia, such as slide presentations, overhead projections, and training videos for **continuing education** (CE) of staff, classroom learning, and patient education (Edwards & Drury, 2000), but new advances in multimedia now allow faculty to add such innovations as simulations and virtual reality to their healthcare training, providing a way for students to learn procedural skills, such as insertion of needles and physical assessment, without any risks to an actual patient.

Research suggests that the seeing, hearing, doing, and interacting afforded by multimedia facilitates learning retention, with multimedia at least as effective as traditional instruction, but with the benefit of greater learner satisfaction. Authoring software, programs that allow users of varied technical skill to design and create Web pages and movies, has greatly facilitated the use of multimedia by faculty (Hebda et al., 2005), although the most effective multimedia relies on the careful and pedagogically appropriate combination of textual material, graphics, video, animation, and sound (Edwards & Drury, 2000), a distinctly separate skill set from teaching and instructing.

Beyond providing a flexible method of delivery for instructional information, multimedia promises to motivate students by requiring them to analyze evidence in ways that require higher-order thinking and problem-solving skills. Similarly, faculty can begin to think about their classes in new ways and accommodate different student learning styles (Oblinger, 2005). Refer to Box 23-5 for more information.

BOX 23-5

Personal Digital Assistant

Dee McGonigle and Kathleen Mastrian

The **personal digital assistant (PDA)** is a handheld or palmtop computer. PDAs have gained appeal because of their small size; they are usually designed to fit in a pocket, making them easily portable with impressive performance capabilities that allow one to store, access, and organize information, such as calendar entries, documents, spreadsheets, databases, notes, and to-do lists. The capabilities and access are limited by the processing speed and memory, and the faster and more robust are the memory capabilities, the more the unit costs. As one considers purchasing a PDA, it is important that the prospective buyer reflects on his or her current and future needs. One wants to be able to expand capabilities as needed without having to replace the PDA. Therefore, before selecting one, it is important to review all of the PDAs currently available. Interactive comparisons of various PDAs are available (CNET, 2008a), as are reviews of various models (CNET, 2008b). Softpedia (2007a) provides the latest news on handhelds and is typically updated daily, with an opportunity to download a user manual and view PDA reviews (Softpedia 2007c).

Most of today's PDAs use either the Linux, PocketPC (Windows), or PalmOS (Palm) operating systems. Because they can be used in networked environments including wireless configurations, they can theoretically keep the clinician in constant access to patient information, colleagues, and other necessary resources.

The applications available provide a wide range of functionality from simple to highly complex software tools. From a PDA nurses can use dosage calculators, drug and specialty databases, educational applications, or clinical forecasting tools; take dictation; or practice telenursing. Because the PDA is compact and one uses a stylus or scroll bars to manage information from inputting, accessing, and output, there are many add-ons available to enhance functionality and ease of use.

Continues

HOW TO USE A PDA

The PDA can have the following equipment: a display or touch screen, infrared (IR) port, USB connector, secure digital memory slot, clock icon, menu icon, sync icon, find icon, Web browser button, navigator button or pad, calendar icon, home icon, contacts icon, scroll button or bar, headphone jack, internal Bluetooth, internal Wi-Fi, speaker, multiconnector, reset button, stylus, microphone, or cell phone capabilities. The configuration of the PDA affects its performance and use. The navigation buttons and scroll functions allow the user to see, access, and open applications, files, and documents. Depending on the PDA selected, how one inputs data and commands varies. There are handwriting and voice recognition capabilities available but generally a mixture of a plastic stylus, touch screen, and handwriting recognition software is used. The handwriting software that recognizes the characters one writes and transfers them to letters and numbers is Graffiti on Palms and Block Recognizer for Pocket PCs. The Transcriber software used on the Pocket PC recognizes legible normal handwriting, printing, or a combination of writing and printing. Thus, users do not have to remember the character codes for the letters and numbers. Users can also type input using the soft keyboard, a small keyboard on the screen, or such add-ons as a small or full-size peripheral keyboard using a Bluetooth or USB connection.

Most current PDAs come with an expansion slot enabling the owner to increase storage space or memory. Secure digital is a common type of card that provides additional memory relatively inexpensively. For those considering purchase of a PDA, an expansion slot is a must-have item in today's environment.

PDAs usually come with office applications, sync software, Bluetooth, cables, and an IR port. The office applications could include word processing, spreadsheets, database, or presentation software. The sync (synchronize) software functions to sync or match and update information on both a computer and PDA. Bluetooth is a form of wireless connectivity that is commonly used in cell phones. Although it usually does not provide Internet access, it does facilitate file transfer between a PDA and a computer. One can purchase an adaptor if one has a PDA without Bluetooth. Cables are an inexpensive way to connect to a computer, essentially plugging the PDA into a computer. The downside of using cables is that the user must be near the computer to connect. The IR beams of light are used as a unidirectional means to transfer select data or entire programs wirelessly to other PDAs. The data and information are not exchanged or traded but rather transferred in only one direction. To obtain something in hard copy, one can beam a document to an IR-enabled printer. Most commonly, people beam their business cards. For example, if one attended a career fair or conference and visited exhibitor booths, one could beam their business card into a vendor's PDA. To beam across platforms, additional software is required.

As PDAs continue to evolve, so do their capabilities and connectivity. The Internet connectivity (Web browser and e-mail) provides the clinician with communication capabilities and constant access to real-time online data and information. Because the PDA is portable, connectivity must be ready whenever and wherever it is needed.

Continues

One way to establish connectivity is through the use of Wi-Fi compatibility, which provides for use at hot spots throughout the country, such as cafes, coffee shops, hotels, restaurants, and universities. It can also use the existing wireless network in an agency or office. This feature can be added to a PDA by purchasing a Wi-Fi adaptor.

Some cell phones, called **smartphones**, have limited PDA capabilities, whereas some PDAs are telephone enabled. Smartphones have limited PC functionality; they have an operating system and facilitate the use of e-mail and other applications. Based on one's practice setting, the addition of the phone features could be an important consideration.

APPLICATIONS

There are tremendous advantages to using a PDA in nursing practice. They can be used to track patients, as point-of-care devices, or as calculators. The PDA could take dictation at the bedside or on the go as the user travels between patients or appointments. As reference tools, they can provide ready access to clinical or drug databases; electronic textbooks and reference materials; online journals in real time, such as *MEDLINE* and the *Online Journal of Nursing Informatics*; and educational tools, such as study guides and care planning documents as those found in Dykes Library (2008) and PDA Cortex (n.d.). Users can transfer information within a network even when they are in the field. Using the network, they can send a note to a case manager, update a physician on the status of patients they visited in their homes, or even send prescriptions to the pharmacy. The PDA allows users to maintain their schedules or calendars and receive reminder alarms. One can even use a PDA for professional development, such as continuing education offerings or furthering academic education online. Whether one is an avid PDA user, is beginning to use a PDA, or is just contemplating purchasing one, it is best to get involved and participate in the list that discusses PDA use in nursing at http://www.rnpalm.com/nursing_pdas_listserv.htm.

The PDA also can enhance health care for patients. Nurses can monitor patients and send surveys and questionnaires; patients can submit responses to their healthcare provider or to the healthcare institution. The PDA can enhance patient access to clinicians, especially for patients who are mobile; the PDA can go where they go and they can keep in touch via e-mail, telephone, fax, instant messaging, or text messaging. They can maintain their appointment and medication schedule and receive patient education materials and access clinician-recommended websites and electronic mailing lists.

The educational arena has embraced this technology. Nursing instructors are communicating and sharing information with their learners and clinical settings using PDA technologies. Using wireless connectivity in class, instructors can receive instant feedback as to the understanding of their learners. PDAs can even assist with discussions and provide study aids, interactive exercises, and quizzes. For a nursing student, the reference materials and podcasts available for coursework can be stored on

Continues

a PDA for easy access. Students can upload and download clinical documents and information with an instructor and clinical setting staff. In the clinical setting, the easy access to robust reference tools and materials, such as dosage calculators, helps to reduce errors. The educational applications continue to expand as more software and capabilities become available.

This is certainly not an exhaustive list of PDA applications or equipment, and the truth of this information era is that the current will be the past by the time this book is in print. PDAs continue to evolve and become smaller and more robust (About.com, n.d.; Seko, 2005; Softpedia, 2007a; Softpedia, 2007c). As the future unfolds, so too will applications of PDAs in nursing.

References

About.com (n.d.). Palmtops/PDAs: Fossil wrist PDA FX2008 with Palm OS review. Retrieved from http://palmtops.about.com/od/palmhardware/fr/FossilWristPDA.htm

CNET. (2008a). PDA—CNET reviews. PDAs matching "PDA." Retrieved from http://reviews.cnet.com/4244-5_7-0.html?query=PDA&tag=srch&target

CNET. (2008b). CNET Reviews: What to look for in handhelds. Retrieved from http://reviews.cnet.com/4520-3127_7-5021319-1.html?tag=wtlf%5C%22%3Ehttp://computers.cnet.com/hardware/0-1087-8-20549052-1.html?tag=wtlf

Dykes Library. (2008). Popular freeware for PDAs. Retrieved from http://library.kumc.edu/resources/PDAFreebies.htm

PDA Cortex. (n.d.). The Journal of Mobile Informatics and PDA resources for healthcare professionals. Retrieved from http://www.rnpalm.com/

Seko, S. (2005). IR watch Ver 0.3: The version only for WristPDA. Retrieved from http://www.pamupamu.com/soft/irmoniw/irw.htm

Softpedia. (2007a). Handhelds area and latest handheld devices (RSS). Retrieved from http://handheld.softpedia.com/#devices

Softpedia. (2007b). Headline news: Handhelds news and latest handhelds news. Retrieved from http://news.softpedia.com/cat/Telecoms/Handhelds/

Softpedia. (2007c). Handhelds area and PDA manual 1.0 download (for the PocketPC). Retrieved from http://handheld.softpedia.com/get/Documents-E-Books/Pda-Manual-36435.shtml

Promoting Active and Collaborative Learning

Because of the shift within the teaching–learning context from the individual seeking answers to the group trying to construct new knowledge from available information, the most effective learning solutions require new digital communication skills, new pedagogies, and new practices (Costa, 2007). A collaborative, student-centered approach uses the best tenets of inductive teaching by imposing more responsibility on students for their own learning than the traditional lecture-based deductive approach. These constructivist methods are built on the widely accepted principle that students are constantly constructing their own realities rather than simply absorbing versions presented by their teachers. Collaborative methods often involve students' discussion of questions and in-class problem solving, with much of the work (in and out of class) done by students in groups rather than individually (Felder & Prince, 2007).

Johnson and Johnson (1990) have identified five significant elements for successful collaborative learning:

1. Face-to-face interaction between students, allowing them to build on each other's strengths
2. Mutual learning goals that, in turn, prompt students to exhibit positive interdependence rather than individualized competition
3. Equal participation in the work process and personal accountability for the work one contributes
4. Regular debriefing sessions as a group after meetings or presentations during which time feedback is shared and observations analyzed
5. Use of cooperative group process skills learned in the classroom

Although collaborative learning relies heavily on student investment and participation, institutions must ultimately create the best physical and electronic settings where collaboration is encouraged. This can be achieved with a sound educational and technologic infrastructure, reliability on proved working models, adaptable physical spaces, and even pedagogic support in the form of preceptors or mentors.

Especially useful for nursing students is the collaborative fieldwork model in which two or more students share a clinical setting and the same fieldwork educator. In this model, learning happens in a reciprocal fashion, with students constructing knowledge from watching each other and exchanging ideas. The most effective fieldwork experiences are highly structured with clear outlines of responsibilities, duties, and expectations, ensuring that the experience matches learner expectations. All activities performed by students, such as conducting evaluations, are done jointly, so that peers provide each other with objective feedback, leading to eventual increased self-confidence (Costa, 2007). In this way, suggests Costa, individuals with different viewpoints and experiences create a space where new knowledge emerges and existing knowledge can be restructured (as cited in Cockrell, Caplow, & Donaldson, 2000).

Libraries have also begun to recognize their role in students' success with and predisposition to collaborative learning with redesigned spaces that reflect students' need to huddle in small groups, sit closely together without barriers, chat about their work, and view digital information without physical hindrances, such as carrels or work stalls. A leader in this movement has been Indiana State

University, whose new information commons features completely overhauled furniture, software, monitors, processing power, and wireless access to the university's network. Students can now collect as a group at kidney-shaped tables; better see the information loaded on the flat-screen monitors; make use of brainstorming, design, and planning software; and discuss their work in a chat-friendly zone. Some faculty members have even scheduled classes at the learning stations, and students, including those in nursing, have responded enthusiastically to the evolved space (Gabbard, Kaiser, & Kaunelis, 2007).

In addition to adaptable physical spaces that encourage discussion and group work, students also require a supportive infrastructure that provides essential elements necessary to successful research and scholarship. These include professional development support in the form of workshops that help students acquire or refresh skill sets; presentation opportunities; and hardware, software, and resource support. One such example includes participation by nursing students at the University of Texas medical branch school of nursing in the scholarly talk about research series (STARS) in which students and faculty give presentations of their work before presenting at professional conferences (Froman, Hall, Shah, Bernstein, & Galloway, 2003), thus eliciting collegial feedback, collaborative troubleshooting, and shared research ideas.

Consider that simply adopting a collaborative, inductive method of learning will not necessarily lead to better learning and more satisfied students. As with any form of instruction, collaborative teaching methods need skilled and careful implementation. Because students are often resistant to instruction that makes them more responsible for their own learning, those who attempt an inductive learning method should adhere to best practices, such as providing adequate scaffolding-extensive support and guidance when students are first introduced to the method and gradual withdrawal of support as students gain more experience and confidence in its use (Felder & Prince, 2007).

Nursing preceptors and mentors, for example, can provide this kind of scaffolded support as clinically active role models (Armitage & Burnard, 1991) and problem-solving **advocates** and collaborators (Gagen & Bowie, 2005). Primarily concerned with the teaching and learning aspects of the relationship, preceptors help students learn by acting as clinical practitioner role models from whom the students can copy appropriate skills and behaviors. Kramer (1974) introduced the concept of nurse preceptor to address the disparity of the theory and practice gap, the difference between what is taught in class and what actually happens in nursing practice. Preceptors enhance clinical competence through direct role modeling, especially valuable in a field where competence and clinical ability are paramount (Armitage & Burnard). Mentors, similar to preceptors, provide equally valuable assistance to nursing students in the form of a facilitator. Mentors are most often used in nursing and education to support new professionals trying to fulfill the rigors of a new position while negotiating the stress inherent to a new environment (Gagen & Bowie). Mentors tend to address student needs through open conversation, student advocacy, feedback on student progress, facilitation, teaching, and general support (Neary, 2000).

Generally, these and other forms of institutional support promote students' adoption of a meaning-oriented approach to learning, as opposed to a surface or memorization-intensive approach. Collaborative, inductive learning promotes intellectual development that challenges the dualistic thinking that characterizes many entering college students, which holds that all knowledge is certain, professors have it, and the task of students is to absorb and repeat it (Felder & Prince, 2007, p. 55). Further, this kind of learning helps students acquire the self-directed learning and critical thinking skills that characterize the best scientists and engineers (Felder & Prince). The active, engaging elements of collaborative learning increase self-confidence, promote autonomy in students, and foster a commitment to lifelong learning (Costa, 2007), all necessities for the success of a new millennial information-literate student.

KNOWLEDGE ASSESSMENT METHODS

An integral and critical component of educational programming is the evaluation of different learning methods. An evaluation process relies on actions taken to measure outcomes, such as the attainment of learning. Process or formative evaluation takes place over the lifespan of a program and is ongoing, whereas summative evaluation is enacted at the end of a program or learning activity.

Both administrators and nursing educators across various programs are responsible for evaluating their programs; beyond gathering feedback from participants and learners an important but ultimately one-dimensional evaluative tool and effective program evaluation should be considered in relation to successes, failures, and how program revision might reinstate a program's effectiveness (Menix, 2007). Dickerson (2005) suggests that evaluation constitutes a substantial part of the work of the nurse educator as defined in the Scope and Standards of Practice for Nursing Professional Development (Dickerson, as cited in American Nurses Association, 2000).

Papers and Projects

When one is looking for feedback and assessment of a particular learning activity, data are best collected during and at the completion of the activity. During the activity, different factors assist in determining how well a teaching strategy is working; these factors include participant engagement (Are students listening? Is there notetaking? Does anyone have questions or comments?), ease of use of equipment and resources, and time required to complete an activity. Much in the way nursing practitioners modify care plans in the midst of an unsuccessful treatment, so should educators change course when it seems the learning experience is not progressing as planned (Dickerson, 2005).

Evaluation by participants at the end of a project is also valuable because learners can provide information related to the attainment of objectives and the teaching effectiveness of both the faculty and the learning materials while the experience is still fresh and memorable. Learner input, although sometimes considered biased and unreliable (e.g., student evaluations refuted by many faculty as useless), actually represent useful feedback to the success of a project or assignment (Dickerson, 2005). Faculty at the University of Colorado at Boulder address this issue by choosing samples of student work for evaluation by faculty or external reviewers to see how well students are meeting program skills and goals. Because these papers and projects are graded by an instructor as part of the course, this form of embedded assignment ensures that the students are still expending effort without having to do extra assessment-specific assignments (University of Colorado at Boulder, Office of Planning, Budget and Analysis, 2001).

When a paper assignment or project does fail, the outcome provides a valuable learning opportunity for all educators to look closely at the pedagogy, structure, goals, outcomes, and expectations of success of the proposed activity and determine what needs revising or reevaluating for what the educator would term "successful" completion. Although many educators and researchers evaluate programs for effectiveness and to maintain certain standards (Dickerson, 2005), most innovative is the educator who evaluates and observes superficial failures as learning opportunities to improve pedagogy and delivery.

Discussions

Although traditional in-class discussion seems almost outdated in light of the stunning advances in technology that allow learners to participate in every kind of activity from computer-guided online quizzes to interactive simulations, the educator as facilitator still holds value and importance in a traditional or even blended classroom. In one study, students exposed to competency-based, written self-learning modules and students exposed to competency-based, didactic lecture modules performed equally. A sample was selected from a group of registered nurses (RNs) who attended a mandatory yearly review of standards from the Occupational Safety and Health Administration (OSHA) and the The Joint Commission (accrediting organization for healthcare organizations). The 67 subjects were given pretests, were exposed to the same content material through two different kinds of presentations, and were then posttested. Results indicated no significant differences among scores of either group. This suggests that advantages of one teaching method versus another ultimately lie in the educator (Schlomer, Anderson, & Shaw, 1997). Self-direction, independence, and a willingness to collaborate all mark the millennial learner, but without guidance, pedagogic grounding, and even a basic contextualized introduction to concepts and materials, even self-motivated, highly information-literate learners flounder without assistance.

Testing

With legal and financial implications of employee and student performance a major concern for all providers and healthcare organizations, multiple requirements for competence in nursing practices within the healthcare system have been established by national agencies and associations, such as those suggested by the American Nurses Association. Of specific concern to educators and administrators is the gap exhibited by test takers who, although scoring exceptionally well on examinations, are unable to perform a clinical procedure or recognize a warning sign in a patient experiencing difficulty. Use of traditional testing as an evaluative tool has been in existence for decades, although research shows that criterion-based performance better measures skill levels while also identifying deficiencies (Redman, Lenburg, & Walker, 1999).

As a result, some schools, such as the University of Colorado's school of nursing, have redesigned their curricula and the competency-based curricular outcomes for their educational programs. These substantial programmatic changes have resulted in a unique approach to nursing at both the undergraduate and graduate levels, with a new focus on such competency-based outcomes as incompetent effective reflective practice (Redman et al., 1999, p. 3) and generation of nursing knowledge and leadership and social change for improved health of individuals, communities, populations, and global environments (Redman et al., p. 3).

Additionally, faculty at the University of Colorado at Boulder use embedded testing to assess outcomes, with goals built into examinations or other assignments. Student performance regarding these items is part of an outcomes assessment, and it is graded accordingly by an instructor as part of the course (University of Colorado at Boulder, Office of Planning, Budget and Analysis, 2001). Such changes promise to deliver substantial changes in the way nursing is taught, perceived, and executed.

Case Scenarios

Professional organizations are increasingly recommending performance-based assessments of students in professional degree programs, and enacting case scenarios provides an opportunity for students to practice procedural responses and improve patient safety. Case scenarios, a form of problem-based learning, are now even available through simulation software or virtual reality programming. This kind of testing, in which students must respond within context to a perceived situation rather than a theoretical or fact-based question, allows educators to gauge procedural knowledge; it allows them to gauge how a student executes a skill or applies concepts and principles to specific situations (Garavalia, 2002). For example, in a clinical context, a student could explain how to change a dressing, insert an intravenous line, or intubate an individual, but the knowledge is declarative rather than procedural and, thus, for some evaluators, not as valuable. Conditional knowledge is often also reflected in procedural knowledge, demonstrating a student's ability to know when and why action is or is not taken, and how.

The best assessment strategies are identified through consideration of the cognitive level of the objective, the nature of the task, and the best context for the assessment. Performance assessments can be used throughout a curriculum, not just as a final component of a practical or clinical experience. Most important is ensuring that the assessment tool and task matches the instruction and the stated learning objective (Garavalia, 2002).

Other: Portfolios

Viewed in the 1980s as realistic evaluative tools of student accomplishment and learning, **portfolios** in nursing education are rising in popularity as useful tools for documenting students' exposure to educational experiences. A nursing portfolio allows a student to document a variety of sometimes unquantifiable skills, such as creativity, communication, and critical thinking. Further, portfolios can reflect achievement of goals, self-evaluation, and professional development, also providing a way for returning students to log and document past work or life experiences in a creative but structured way without taking a standardized test. The usefulness of a portfolio for an undergraduate in a nursing program depends on a structured system of organization: an identification page with resume, a table of contents, separate and clearly marked sections, and so forth. In this way, portfolios can monitor program outcomes, positively influence employment and graduate school admission, and provide a clear snapshot of a student's strengths and abilities (Alexander, Baldwin, & McDaniel, 2002). See Chapter 11 for a comprehensive discussion of portfolios and professional collaboration tools.

KNOWLEDGE DISSEMINATION AND SHARING

Sharing stories and experience from a clinical point of view accomplishes much more than simply promoting camaraderie or empathy (although this kind of engagement is infinitely valuable in its own way); sharing experiences of clinical learning can help convey lifesaving information to other clinicians in a way that is more memorable and palatable and less imposing than warnings delivered outside a social context. Clinical and caring knowledge, often rooted in everyday exchanges, become socially embedded such that those with experience in particular clinical settings share common knowledge and understanding. The social embeddedness of caring and clinical knowledge is a result of shared and shaped collective understanding of practice and sometimes provides an alternative view.

The power of pooled knowledge in combination with knowledge produced in dialogue with others helps to limit tunnel vision and is a powerful strategy for maximizing the clinical knowledge of a group. Whether the nurse is networking, presenting, or seeking CE or recertification, an understanding of socially embedded knowledge coupled with the multiple perspectives of skilled practitioners allows for a rich and vibrant opportunity to apply nursing skill effectively (Benner, Tanner, & Chelsa, 1997).

Networking

Considered crucial to career development because of opportunities for collaboration and information exchange, networking encourages professional support by making successful professionals accessible to their colleagues. Further, developing interactive professional networks between academic and clinical nurses can benefit practice in diabetes, stroke, and mental health care, and in community nursing wherein practitioners are encouraged to collaborate (Gillibrand, Burton, & Watkins, 2002).

The value of networking to members of male-dominated professionals, such as law, business, and medicine, resides in opportunities to make contact with fellow professionals, and in turn, further careers. This observation is especially poignant for nursing, a predominantly female profession that, until recently, has rarely reaped the benefits of formal networking (Nicholl & Tracey, 2007).

Because nurses tend to gather their information from personal networks, such as colleagues or professional meetings, the increased availability of technology to assist in networking has greatly facilitated information exchange. Blogs, e-mail, websites, electronic mailing lists, and other communicative technologies have made collaboration and networking possibilities endless, allowing nurses to access and learn from colleagues' experiences. Using the Internet allows for the discovery of information heretofore unavailable through traditional information sources (Pravikoff & Levy, 2006), helping nursing professionals decide if, for example, pursuing research opportunities or collaboration on specific professional projects seems viable.

Formal networks, such as the International Nurse Practitioner/Advanced Practice Nursing Network (INP/APNN), unveiled in 2000, promote the exchange of knowledge, resources, and expertise in order to enhance the presence of nursing in primary health care. Created in response to the globalization of nurse practitioner and Advanced Practice Nursing Network APNN roles, the network enables the enhancement and advancement of practice both for countries just beginning to initiate advanced practice nursing APN roles and for those with experienced practitioners (Affara, Cross, & Schober, 2001).

Membership and participation in professional associations also provide ways to network and advance one's profession. Professional associations provide venues through which members may set standards for professional practice, establish codes of ethics, become involved in advocacy, engage in CE opportunities, access job banks, subscribe to professional journals, and act as a common voice for the profession. For example, the American Nursing Association of Occupational Health Nurses is instrumental in maintaining healthcare issues on the political agenda. Research shows that nurses hesitate to join professional organizations because of barriers associated with cost, distance to meetings, lack of activities in one's geographic area, and inability to attend meetings. Because networking creates fertile areas for the development of new ideas, partnership, jobs, and strategies, both national and state associations would benefit from creating greater opportunities for healthcare practitioners to earn CE credit and network with others in their field (Thackeray, Neiger, & Roe, 2005).

Presenting and Publishing

Much in the way the American Association of Colleges of Nursing (AACN) maintains standards for nursing education, professional journals also hold their contributors to similarly rigorous standards and provide a valuable venue in which nursing professionals might share ideology and innovations in the field. With the proliferation of online journals and nursing information available in multiple media, publishing remains an excellent way to participate in the dissemination of professional information. Both nursing magazines and journals reach considerable audiences; journal distinctions lie in their authorship and audience. Although journal articles are written by and for scholars, with refereed or peer-reviewed journals requiring a blind review by a group of reviewers to eliminate bias, magazine articles may be written by a professional in the field, an editor, freelancer, or other author. Publishing provides excellent opportunities to extend knowledge and share research.

Similar to publishing, making presentations at contemporary professional conferences allows nursing educators and students to gain experience and share scholarship with colleagues. Presentations must meet certain standards for an audience to find them credible and effective. Because an audience retains 50% of what they see and hear in a presentation versus 20% if they only hear it, experts suggest the use of audiovisual aids in making professional presentations most effective (Bergren, 2000). A noteworthy presentation could involve multiple levels of complexity, from a simple PowerPoint to an animated tutorial. Because technology and well-designed visuals do not make up for lack of preparedness or research, presenters should be aware of their target audience and details of the research being presented. Regardless of media or presentation style, audiovisual presentations should be designed consistently and simply, using colors and fonts that are easy to read and understand and audience-appropriate language.

Conferences often host poster presentations to share research findings, innovations, and exemplar programs in a low-investment but visually captivating way. Because posters are primarily visual, with little or no verbal supplementation, most important for consideration are room elements, such as size, space limitations, and lighting. The best nursing practitioner posters feature consistent visual components, such as appropriately sized, readable font and simple colors, and are based on a research concept or clinical objective (Berg, 2005). A high-tech alternative to a paper poster is an electronic poster continuously running PowerPoint presentation either projected for larger audiences or left to run from a laptop or desktop for smaller audiences (Bergren, 2000). Both publishing and presenting provide opportunities for the nursing practitioner to disseminate new knowledge and stay abreast of information in the field.

Continuing Education and Recertification

Nationally, nursing employers and institutions have, because of budgetary constraints, begun to eliminate CE programs traditionally reliant on classes, conferences, and workshops; consequently, reliance on outside agencies and technology has increased to meet this need. The traditional approach to obtaining CE credits has included home study offered by professional journals and organizations in which the client reads articles, answers related questions, and sends in the test form and fee. Although fairly straightforward, this technique provides little in the way of peer interaction (Hebda et al., 2005).

With the ubiquitous technology influx and the accessibility it affords, obtaining CE credits through e-learning is considered a beneficial delivery method for mandatory educational programs and other programs that provide employees with opportunities to maintain or improve skills. Benefits of e-learning for CE training include the ability to access information at any time (thus creating a flexible schedule) and experience instant feedback and individualized instruction by seeking out specific, additional information as needed.

E-learning can also benefit administrative support of CE credits by providing instantly accessible computerized records and other tracking features, such as records of success and completion, associated costs of program development, and staff productivity. Allowing nursing professionals to complete mandatory training on demand represents a huge benefit of e-learning, with the best programs allowing for customization to accommodate program revisions and regulation changes (Hebda et al., 2005).

In some cases, acquiring CE credits may also help one achieve recertification. Available through myriad professional organizations, recertification ensures that nurses are staying current in their fields and some specialties; for example, the field of pediatric nursing requires annual recertification to maintain professional status. During recertification, the Pediatric Nursing and Certification Board offers each certified pediatric nurse (CPN) options for ensuring she or he is maintaining national standards within the specialty of pediatric nursing (Pediatric Nursing Certification Board, 2007).

As an added benefit, some hospitals provide higher salaries to nurses who maintain certification. Additionally, 90% of nurse managers indicate they would prefer to hire a certified nurse over a noncertified nurse. The trend in magnet hospitals to encourage, reward, and promote certified nurses is spreading to other facilities and healthcare settings, with retirement centers and home health agencies now beginning to seek certified nurses for perceived extra benefit to their customers and a marketing advantage in hiring nurses with guaranteed levels of competence (Peterson, 2007).

One such program that facilitates educational programs for medical professionals around the nation and helps nurses reach recertification goals is the innovative Wake Area Health Education Center RN refresher program designed to return RNs to practice. Nurses participate in a series of medical and surgical didactic models, participate in clinical practicums, and work one-on-one with an RN preceptor who provides instruction and evaluation of skills over the course of 160 hours. Most notable about this program is the initiation of handheld devices for use by the refresher students who, as a result, more actively used the medical library and experienced great self-confidence with both knowing how to use technology and in their return to nursing practice. As of 2006, more than 50 healthcare organizations were partnering with Wake Area Health Education Center in providing the clinical practicum portion of the RN refresher program, and more than 1,100 RNs enrolled since its inception in 1990 (Colevins, Bond, & Clark, 2006). For information on CE, visit the American Nurses Association CE page at http://nursingworld.org/ce/cehome.cfm.

FUTURE

The future holds a phenomenal amount of potential for virtual reality–embedded education. Once the purview of gamers and geeks, virtual reality has exploded onto the academic scene with potential for cross-pollination between fields of inquiry across the curriculum, university, and even learning systems. All kinds of university departments will experiment with virtual reality in the hopes of staying current and pleasing to their young and demanding constituency; however, much in the way society loves the feel of a book too much to make it archaic, so too will students, educators, and administrators ultimately return to a compromised form of face-to-face classroom teaching, even in the face of newer and more adventuresome teaching technologies. Further, once fast, high-burn technologies stop flooding the marketplace and making education an even bigger business for proprietary online universities, modified traditions will take their place, creating new spaces for nontraditional students and the Internet generation, both anxious for technology use in the classroom for very different reasons.

SUMMARY

In an ideal world, nurses will work against the assumption that technology runs itself, and take proactive roles in helping to design the education necessary best to prepare them for real-world scenarios. Consider that flash is not substance, and drama is not depth; technology only performs as well as the pedagogy that undergirds and sustains it. Plan for and use technology with care so that its best features consequently enrich yours as an educator or learner.

THOUGHT-PROVOKING Questions

1. What are some of the forces behind the push toward a more wired learning experience in nursing education?

2. What technology do you find most beneficial to use in your practice or education setting? Why do you find this tool useful? From your perspective, how could this tool be enhanced?

For a full suite of assignments and additional learning activities, use the access code located in the front of your book to visit this exclusive website: http://go.jblearning.com/mcgonigle. If you do not have an access code, you can obtain one at the site.

References

Affara, F., Cross, S., & Schober, M. (2001). Discovering resources—Making global connections, international networking. *Journal of the American Academy of Nurse Practitioners, 13*(10), 445–448.

Alexander, J. G., Baldwin, M. S., & McDaniel, G. S. (2002). The nursing portfolio: A reflection of a professional. *The Journal of Continuing Education in Nursing, 33*(2), 55–59.

American Nurses Association. (2000). *Scope and standards of practice for nursing professional development*. Washington, DC: Author.

Aquino-Russell, C., Maillard Strüby, F. V., & Reviczky, K. (2007). Living attentive presence and changing perspectives with a Web-based nursing theory course. *Nursing Science Quarterly, 20*(2), 128–134.

Armitage, P., & Burnard, P. (1991). Mentors or preceptors? Narrowing the theory-practice gap. *Nurse Education Today, 11*, 225–229.

Barnes, L., & Rudge, T. (2005). Virtual reality or real virtuality: The space of flows and nursing practice. *Nursing Inquiry, 12*(4), 306–315.

Bassendowski, S. L. (2005). NursingQuest: Supporting an analysis of nursing issues. *Journal of Nursing Education, 46*(2), 92–95.

Bell, S. (2003). Cyber-guest lecturers: Using Webcasts as a teaching tool. *TechTrends, 47*(4), 10–14.

Benner, P., Tanner, C., & Chelsa, C. (1997). The social fabric of nursing knowledge. *The American Journal of Nursing, 97*(7), 16BBB–16DDD.

Berg, J. A. (2005). Creating a professional poster presentation: Focus on nurse practitioners. *Journal of the American Academy of Nurse Practitioners, 17*(7), 245–249.

Bergren, M. D. (2000). Power up your presentation with PowerPoint. *Journal of School Nursing, 16*(4), 44–47.

Black, C. D., & Watties-Daniels, A. D. (2006). Cutting edge technology to enhance nursing classroom instruction at Coppin State University. *ABNF Journal, 17*(3), 103–106.

Bracke, P. J., & Dickstein, R. (2002). Web tutorials and scalable instruction: Testing the waters. *Reference Services Review, 30*(4), 330–338.

Carty, B., & Ong, I. (2006). The nursing curriculum in the information age. In V. Saba & K. McCormick (Eds.), *Essentials of nursing informatics* (4th ed., pp. 517–532). New York, NY: McGraw-Hill.

Chase, D. (2007). Transformative sharing with instant messaging, Wikis, interactive maps, and Flickr. *Computers in Libraries, 27*(1), 7–56.

Clochesy, J. M. (2004). Hardware and software options. In J. Fitzpatrick & S. Montgomery (Eds.), *Internet for nursing research* (pp. 120–128). New York, NY: Springer Publishing Company.

Cockrell, K., Caplow, J., & Donaldson, J. (2000). A context for learning: Collaborative groups in the problem-based learning environment. *Review of Higher Education, 23*(3), 347–363.

Colevins, H., Bond, D., & Clark, K. (2006). Nurse refresher students get a hand from handhelds. *Computers in Libraries, 6–7*, 46–48.

Costa, D. M. (2007). The collaborative fieldwork model. *OT Practice, 12*(1), 25–26.

Dede, C. (2005). Planning for neomillennial learning styles. *EDUCAUSE Quarterly, 28*(1) [Online]. Retrieved from http://www.educause.edu/apps/eq/eqm05/eqm0511.asp?bhcp=1

DeSantis, S. (2002). *Re-envisioning the pedagogical bridge: The new instructional designer.* Presented at the Pennsylvania Association for Educational Communications and Technology, Hershey, PA.

Dewald, N. H. (1999). Transporting good library instruction practices into the Web environment: An analysis of online tutorials. *Journal of Academic Librarianship, 25*(1), 26–32.

Dickerson, P. S. (2005). Evaluation: Part I. evaluating learning activities. *The Journal of Continuing Education in Nursing, 36*, 191–192.

EDUCAUSE Learning Initiative. (2006, June). *7 things you should know about ... virtual worlds.* Retrieved from http://connect.educause.edu/Library/ELI/7ThingsYouShouldKnowAbout/39392?time=1209214921

Edwards, M. J. A., & Drury, R. M. (2000). Using computers in basic nursing education, continuing education, and patient education. In M. J. Ball, K. J. Hannah, S. K. Newbold, & J. V. Douglas (Eds.), *Nursing informatics: Where caring and technology meet* (pp. 49–68). New York, NY: Springer.

Felder, R., & Prince, M. (2007). The case for inductive teaching. *Prism, 17*(2), 55.

Froman, R. D., Hall, A. W., Shah, A., Bernstein, J. M., & Galloway, R. Y. (2003). A methodology for supporting research and scholarship. *Nursing Outlook, 51*(2), 84–89.

Gabbard, R. B., Kaiser, A., & Kaunelis, D. (2007). Redesigning a library space for collaborative learning. *Computers in Libraries, 27*(5), 6–12.

Gagen, L., & Bowie, S. (2005). Effective mentoring: A case for training mentors for novice teachers. *Journal of Physical Education, Recreation & Dance, 76*(7), 40–45.

Garavalia, L. S. (2002). Selecting appropriate assessment methods: Asking the right questions. *American Journal of Pharmaceutical Education, 66*, 108–112.

Gillibrand, W. P., Burton, C., & Watkins, G. G. (2002). Clinical networks for nursing research. *International Nursing Review, 49*(3), 188–193.

Gordon, A. M. (2007). Sound off! The possibilities of podcasting. *Book Links,* 16–18.

Grant, M. J., & Brettle, A. J. (2006). Developing and evaluating an interactive information skills tutorial. *Health Information and Libraries Journal, 23*(2), 79–88.

Hebda, T., Czar, P., & Mascara, C. (2005). *Handbook of informatics for nurses & health care professionals* (3rd ed.). Upper Saddle River, NJ: Prentice Hall.

Hibbison, E. (2001). *Hybrid courses.* Retrieved from http://vccslitonline.cc.va.us/mrcte/many_media.htm

Johnson, D. W., & Johnson, R. T. (1990). *Learning together and alone: Cooperative, competitive and individualistic learning.* Boston, MA: Allyn & Bacon.

Kramer, M. (1974). *Reality shock.* St. Louis, MO: Mosby.

Leasure, A., Davis, L., & Thievon, S. (2000). Comparison of student outcomes and preferences in a traditional vs. World Wide Web-based baccalaureate nursing research course. *Journal of Nursing Education, 39*, 149–154.

Maag, M. (2005). The potential use of "blogs" in nursing education. *CIN: Computers, Informatics, Nursing, 23*(1), 16–26.

McHugh, M. L. (2006). Computer hardware. In V. Saba & K. McCormick (Eds.), *Essentials of nursing informatics* (4th ed., pp. 517–532). New York, NY: McGraw-Hill.

Menix, K. D. (2007). Evaluation of learning and program effectiveness. *Continuing Education in Nursing, 38*(5), 201–208.

Neary, M. (2000). Supporting students' learning and professional development through the process of continuous assessment and mentorship. *Nurse Education Today, 20*, 463–474.

Nicholl, H., & Tracey, C. (2007). Networking for nurses. *Nursing Management, 13*(9), 26–29.

Oblinger, D. G. (2005). Learners, learning, & technology: The EDUCAUSE learning initiative. *EDUCAUSE Review,* 66–75.

Pediatric Nursing Certification Board. (2007). *About recertification.* Retrieved from www.pncb.org/ptistore/control/certs/cpn/index

Peterson, T. (2007, November 19). *Here's the skinny: What you need to do to become and stay certified.* Retrieved from www.medscape.com/viewarticle/562945

Phillips, V. (1999). *Internet changing economics of higher education.* Retrieved from http://www.cnn.com/TECH/computing/9905/05/neted.idg/index.html

Pravikoff, D. S., & Levy, J. R. (2006). Computerized information resources. In V. Saba & K. McCormick (Eds.), *Essentials of nursing informatics* (4th ed., pp. 517–532). New York, NY: McGraw-Hill.

Prensky, M. (2001). *Digital natives, digital immigrants.* On The Horizon. 9(5). Retrieved from www.marcprensky.com/writing/

Pusic, M. V., Pachev, G. S., & MacDonald, W. A. (2007). Embedding medical student computer tutorials into a busy emergency room department. *Academic Emergency Medicine, 14*(2), 138–148.

Redman, R., Lenburg, C. B., & Walker, P. H. (1999). *Competency assessment: Methods for development and implementation in nursing education.* Online Journal of Nursing. Retrieved from http://nursingworld.org/MainMenuCategories/ANAMarketplace/ANAPeriodicals/OJIN/TableofContents/Volume41999/No3Sep1999/InitialandContinuingCompetenceinEducationandPracticeCompetencyAssessmentMethodsforDeve.aspx

Ridley, R. T. (2007). Interactive teaching: A concept analysis. *Journal of Nursing Education, 46*(5), 206–209.

Riley, J. B. (1996). Educational applications. In V. K. Saba & K. A. McCormick (Eds.), *Essentials of computers for nurses* (2nd ed., pp. 527–573). New York, NY: McGraw-Hill.

Schlomer, R. S., Anderson, M. A., & Shaw, R. (1997). Teaching strategies and knowledge retention. *Journal of Nursing Staff Development, 13*(5), 249–253.

Seropian, M. A., Brown, K., Gavilanes, J. S., & Driggers, B. (2004). Simulation: Not just a manikin. *Journal of Nursing Education, 43*(4), 164–170.

Shaffer, S. C., Lackey, S. P., & Bolling, G. W. (2006). Blogging as venue for nurse faculty development. *Nursing Education Perspectives, 27*(3), 126–128.

Skiba, D. J. (2007a). Do your students Wiki? *Nursing Education Perspectives, 26*(2), 120–121.

Skiba, D. J. (2007b). Nursing education 2.0: Second Life. *Nursing Education Perspectives, 28*(3), 156–157.

Sousa, D. A. (1995). *How the brain learns.* Reston, VA: National Association of Secondary School Principals.

Spillane, J. (2006). Virtual reality takes on patient safety. *Nursing Spectrum (New York/New Jersey Metro Edition), 18A*(7), 13.

Thackeray, R., Neiger, B. L., & Roe, K. M. (2005). Certified health education specialists' participation in professional associations: Implications for marketing and membership. *American Journal of Health Education, 36*(6), 337–344.

Turley, J. P. (2000). Nursing's future: Ubiquitous computing, virtual reality, and augmented reality. In M. J. Ball, K. J. Hannah, S. K. Newbold, & J. V. Douglas (Eds.), *Nursing informatics: Where caring and technology meet* (pp. 49–68). New York, NY: Springer.

University of Colorado at Boulder, Office of Planning, Budget and Analysis. (2001). *Assessment methods used by academic departments and programs.* Retrieved from http://www.colorado.edu/pba/outcomes/ovview/mwithin.htm

Winfield, W., Mealy, M., & Scheibel, P. (1998). *In Distance Learning '98.* Proceedings of the annual conference on distance teaching and learning. August 5-7, 1998, Madison, WI.

CHAPTER 24

Simulation in Nursing Informatics Education

Nickolaus Miehl

Objectives

1. Describe the role of simulation in nursing informatics education.
2. Differentiate between the types of simulated electronic health records available for use.
3. Identify the limitations of using a live clinical information system for educational purposes.

www

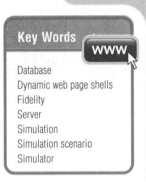

Key Words

www

Database
Dynamic web page shells
Fidelity
Server
Simulation
Simulation scenario
Simulator

INTRODUCTION

The patient call bell is ringing; you enter the room to find the patient verbalizing complaints of chest tightness. In a moment, the patient becomes unresponsive and a code is called. The team quickly responds initiating resuscitation measures per advanced cardiac life support (ACLS) protocol. You review the electronic health records (EHRs) with the attending physician while simultaneously discussing your assessment before the code. After a short while, the resuscitation efforts are successful and the patient is stable for transfer to the intensive care unit. You complete your documentation in the patient's EHR, the simulation scenario ends, and the debriefing begins. The instructor provides feedback on not only actions taken within the simulation scenario, but also on the use of the EHR as an important resource for patient information and documentation.

Perhaps it is the first day of a new course and rather than a lecture-based class with an accompanying textbook, the instructor uses an active learning approach with case studies delivered through an EHR interface to facilitate the learning and application of clinical concepts. In this example, rather than being part of an entire simulation scenario, the EHR itself is the learning tool providing learners with a hands-on learning opportunity centered on accessing and using the information contained within the patient record.

NURSING INFORMATICS COMPETENCIES IN NURSING EDUCATION

In the late 1990s it was identified that healthcare professionals needed to posses both skill and knowledge of informatics (American Association of Colleges of Nursing, 1997; Gassert, 1998; Pew, 1998). Additionally, information technology has been identified as a key measure in improving patient safety and quality of care (American Academy of Nursing, 2003; Institute of Medicine, 2000). In response to this increasing demand for practitioners to become skilled in this area coupled with the absence of research-based informatics competencies a Delphi study was used to identify informatics competencies for nurses at four different levels of practice (Staggers, Gassert, & Curran, 2002). In essence, this study created informatics competencies for entry-level nurses through informatics specialists and innovators with a focus on computer skills, informatics knowledge, and informatics skills.

Although informatics competencies for nurses have been identified, the degree to which schools of nursing have woven them into the curriculum varies greatly (Carty & Ong, 2006). In a study by Fetter (2009), a survey of graduating senior nursing students ranked the following competencies having no experience or minimal skill with: (1) using applications to document, (2) creating a careplan, (3) valuing informatics knowledge for practice, (4) valuing informatics knowledge for skill development, and (5) using applications for data entry.

The question becomes, what best practices exist so that students become prepared in informatics? In a position statement by the National League for Nurses (2008), results from a survey of nursing educators and administrators indicated that 50–60% of respondents said that informatics was integrated throughout the curriculum and that experience with nursing informatics was provided during clinical rotations. Findings also suggested that little clinically related informatics content or learning experiences are provided in the nursing programs. Personal digital assistants care planning software and clinical information systems were least likely to be incorporated into the courses. With emerging technologies in nursing and healthcare education, the use of simulation to allow students actively to use informatics in an authentic and realistic learning context is one potential approach.

A CASE FOR SIMULATION

In general terms, a **simulator** can perhaps best be described as a tool designed to emulate some aspect of the clinical practice environment and may be focused on a single task, or designed to mimic a complete patient care situation (Gaba & DeAnda, 1998). In its essence, it is any device used to create a realistic learning experience for the learner but it removes the risk associated with learning during hands-on patient care. It offers the unique ability to create a realistic learning environment that is safe, structured, and supportive for the learner (Bligh & Bleakley, 2006).

Simulators encompass a broad range of devices, such as partial task trainers, such as an IV insertion arm; screen-based simulations, including simulated EHRs; simulated environments replicating a realistic patient care area; and complex computer drive human patient simulation manikins. Although each of these simulation modalities can be used alone, they can be powerful learning tools when used together to create a realistic patient care scenario. The goal of **simulation**, according to Gaba (2004) is a seamless immersion into the simulated practice environment during which learners are drawn into the reality of the environment or task at hand. Hertel and Millis (2002) note that this is a cooperative process whereby learners come together in an authentic setting and begin to learn from one another.

Considering the realistic nature of simulation and its hands-on active approach to learning, it seems that the use of simulation modalities can be a powerful tool in moving student nurses, and any practitioner, toward achieving the informatics competencies. Recall the examples given at the beginning of this chapter. In the first example the EHR is part of a larger **simulation scenario** that mimics a real-life clinical case. In the second example, the EHR itself functions as a simulator and becomes a true-to-life learning tool. In either case, simulation is used to incorporate nursing informatics into the context of patient care, thereby giving students an authentic learning experience that can be applied in clinical practice.

INCORPORATING EHRs INTO THE LEARNING ENVIRONMENT

There are two main approaches to the incorporation of an EHR into the learning environment, whether used within a simulated clinical environment as part of a patient care scenario or as a stand-alone learning tool. The EHR can be created specifically for simulation purposes, ranging from a well-developed Microsoft Access database through commercially available products designed specifically for simulation purposes. A second option is the use of a real EHR system, either within a hospital-based simulation center or through a partnership with a healthcare facility or an EHR vendor.

There are certain advantages and disadvantages to each solution. Brown (2005) notes that whereas "live" documentation systems provide learners with a realistic experience and can be incorporated into the learning environment, they also present certain drawbacks: (1) they are designed for the patient care environment, not the learning environment, and therefore lack an efficient feedback mechanism for learners; (2) they are designed to work in real time, not simulated time, creating issues with data recall especially when a record may be used repeatedly over a period of months or years; and (3) if a system is overly complex, it may unintentionally focus the learning on the specific system, rather than the process of data retrieval and documentation. Refer to the Research Brief on the challenges of teaching clinical documentation skills in an EHR.

Research Brief

Faculty perceptions of the challenges of teaching undergraduate students proper clinical documentation in both paper-based and electronic systems are described in this qualitative research study by Mahon, Nickitas, and Nokes (2010). Participants (N = 25) were interviewed using both open- and closed-ended questions, and results were analyzed using a constant comparative method. The most common method of teaching documentation skills was some variation of demonstration-return-demonstration method. Faculty were concerned about the amount of time taken honing documentation skills in the actual clinical area, indicating a median of 2 hours of an 8-hour clinical day, and shared that there was seemingly little documentation taught in the classroom or laboratory. Faculty relied heavily on experts in the clinical setting and used their documentation as models for students to emulate. In the case of the electronic health record documentation, on-site nursing experts proficient in the use of the system were especially useful as role models. However, faculty was concerned that using the electronic system and the endless drop-down menus might actually interfere with the development of nursing expertise and critical thinking. One critical issue that was shared by faculty with regard to electronic documentation is that the clinical facility only provided the instructor with an access code so that all of the students in the clinical group used the one code to document, and there was limited access to computers on the clinical unit. The faculty was very concerned about the legal and ethical issues for appropriate documentation and for the provision of care, such as on-time medication administration in a group of 8–10 students with one access code. The authors suggest the need to integrate information competencies throughout the curricula and to provide opportunities for faculty development in informatics. They suggest that "faculty competencies in the area of informatics must be identified and standardized" and that faculty must learn to "model self-efficacy: the patience, support and persistence that characterize individual development within a professional discipline" (p. 620).

Mahon, P. Y., Nickitas, D. M., & Nokes, K. M. (2010). Faculty perceptions of student documentation skills during the transition from paper-based to electronic health records systems. *Journal of Nursing Education, 49*(11), 615. Retrieved from http://search proquest.com/docview/762454353?accountid= 13158

One system designed specifically for simulation is the internet-based medical chart (IMC), as described by Brown (2005). This system requires four components: (1) a **database**, (2) **dynamic web page shells**, (3) a **server**, and (4) computers with access to the Internet. With this system, a Microsoft Access database is created to hold administrative information about the simulation scenario and other pertinent overview information only accessible by the instructor, and simulated patient data, simulated patient documentation, student documentation entries, and learner feedback from instructors. Each time a learner logs into the IMC system via the Internet, the server custom creates the requested page using the existing database information, user-specific information, and the web page shells to create a realistic EHR for use by the student. Although this type of system offers a great deal of flexibility, because it is custom created by the end user and is certainly a cost-effective solution, it does require that the simulation instructor has a strong background in computer science and information technology to create and maintain the database and supporting materials.

One example of a commercially available solution is Elsevier's *Simulation Learning System* (2010). This system includes all of the elements needed for preparing, programming, running, and debriefing a simulation scenario, including a fully functional EHR. The EHR is linked to the simulation scenario and contains all of the pertinent patient information for learners to access before or during the simulation scenario. This system also incorporates the ability for learners to document just as they would in an actual clinical setting with the capability of submitting the documentation to the instructor for evaluation and feedback. A major strength of this type of system is that it is a prepackaged web-based solution that does not need to be created from the start.

Additionally, it includes all of the necessary tools for the instructor or simulation center staff to build the simulation scenario including (but not limited to) programming guides, staging and scripting information for the scenario, and debriefing guides. One potential disadvantage with any commercially available solution is the cost to purchase, which varies depending on the product and vendor.

Although the main disadvantages of a live system were discussed at the beginning of this section, it still remains that the use of a real EHR system provides learners with a truly authentic experience. One innovative solution was developed out of an academic-business partnership between the Cerner Corporation and the University of Kansas School of Nursing. The Simulated E-hEalth Delivery System incorporated the use Cerner Corporation's clinical information system and PowerChart application (Connors, Weaver, Warren, & Miller, 2002). This system was specifically adapted for educational purposes to address the learner's informatics needs. Similar to the IMC discussed previously, instructors developed the patient data stored within the Cerner Corporation's clinical information system database, creating virtual patients within the system. Students could navigate through the system and view pertinent patient data and document assessment information and create a plan of care within the PowerChart application. Additionally, the instructor could access student documentation for evaluation and feedback. Refer to the Research Brief for a discussion of a study on the use of the Simulated E-hEalth Delivery System.

This system, now known as Cerner's Academic Education Solution, has been introduced at both the University of Missouri-Kansas City and the University of Utah where a consortium

Research Brief

This qualitative research study by Kennedy, Pallikkathayil, and Warren (2009) describes the experiences and development of nursing process skills in nursing students (N = 5) using the Simulated E-hEalth Delivery System (SEEDS) learning innovation. In the SEEDS learning innovation, students were given written case studies and asked to enter the patient data in a simulated electronic health record and generate a care plan for the patient and family. The authors concluded that, "The technology provided an interactive venue for developing nursing process skills by linking assessment data from case studies with foundational concepts in nursing" (p. 99). "The exercise was authentic, dynamic, and learner centered" (p. 99). As a result of the themes discovered in this qualitative study, the authors propose two hypotheses for future research to explore learning outcomes resulting from the use of a simulated e-health system:

- During postclinical conferences, technologically competent students who use a modified electronic health record for documentation of patient data and care planning for the next day of practice will demonstrate more interactive discussion among students and teacher, experience greater learner satisfaction, and demonstrate better nursing process skills than will students who participate in the traditional postclinical group discussion about patient care.

- Following didactic instruction about nursing care of a patient with a specific disease, technologically competent students who use a modified electronic health record with embedded decision support to enter patient assessment data from a case study about the disease and then develop a care plan will communicate greater learner satisfaction, demonstrate better nursing process skills, and attain higher test scores on the specific topic than will students who organize the assessment data and develop a care plan with paper and pencil (p. 100).

Kennedy, D., Pallikkathayil, L., & Warren, J. J. (2009). Using a modified electronic health record to develop nursing process skills. *Journal of Nursing Education, 48*(2), 96. Retrieved from http://search.proquest.com/docview/203936907?accountid= 13158 has been created between the schools to collaborate on development and implementation strategies for using this system (Gassert & Sward, 2007). The Academic Education Solution is a fully functional clinical information system adapted for educational purposes to support and facilitate the development of informatics competencies in a realistic fashion.

CHALLENGES AND OPPORTUNITIES

The adoption and use of simulation technologies presents unique advantages and disadvantages. Using simulated medical records, as a stand-alone learning tool or in conjunction with a complete simulation scenario, provides the learner with an opportunity for a realistic, hands-on learning experience. Major considerations when looking to adopt a simulated EHR include (1) cost, (2) ease of use for the instructor and learner, (3) technical support from the vendor, (4) time to build or develop the patient database, (5) additional simulation materials included with the package, (6) flexibility of the system to be customized and used as a stand-alone tool or in the setting of a full-scale simulation scenario, and (7) overall **fidelity** or realism.

In 2006, a coalition comprised of experts from the fields of health care, informatics, business and industry, and nursing put forth the Technology Informatics Guiding Education Reform (TIGER) Initiative (TIGER, 2007). The aim of this group is to advance the integration of informatics core competencies into nursing education to provide better and safer care to patients. Seven key steps were established to meet the 10-year vision of the TIGER initiative. Of particular interest is the call to take an active role in the design and integration of informatics tools that are "intuitive, affordable, usable, responsive and evidence-based"(p. 5). This truly promotes new and innovative strategies for informatics education and significant opportunities for collaboration between industry, academia, and clinical practice.

WHAT DOES THE FUTURE HOLD?

Simulation will clearly play an important role in the development of informatics competencies for student nurses and practitioners. One theme of simulation-based learning is practicing just as a nurse would in the actual clinical setting. With regard to facilitating the growth of informatics competencies, it is no different. If there is an expectation for the use of clinical information systems and EHRs in the clinical setting, then the opportunity also exists for the incorporation into the classroom and simulated clinical setting.

Aside from using the simulated EHR in the setting of a clinical simulation scenario, there are also opportunities to incorporate the simulated EHR into the classroom in new and innovative ways. As mentioned in the beginning of the chapter in the second scenario, the EHR can be used as an active learning tool within the classroom. Rather than absorbing information from a book, the EHR can become a powerful way for learners to make important connections about caring for patients with a specific disease process or to learn concepts of pathophysiology or pharmacology.

THOUGHT-PROVOKING Questions

www

1. Consider your experience and learning with regard to EHRs. If you were to design a learning program centered on the use of EHRs, what would it look like? Consider the viewpoint of a student, a clinician, and a healthcare administrator.

2. Think about the clinical courses you have taken as a student. What opportunities and challenges exist to using an EHR as a major learning tool in conjunction with, or perhaps even replacing the required textbook?

3. If you were to design a simulation scenario incorporating the use of an EHR, which informatics competencies would you focus on and why?

For a full suite of assignments and additional learning activities, use the access code located in the front of your book to visit this exclusive website: http://go.jblearning.com/mcgonigle. If you do not have an access code, you can obtain one at the site.

www

References

American Academy of Nursing. (2003). Proceedings of the American Academy of Nursing conference on using innovative technology to decrease nursing demand and enhance patient care delivery. *Nursing Outlook, 51*, 1–41.

American Association of Colleges of Nursing. (1997). *A vision of baccalaureate and graduate nursing education: The next decade.* Washington, DC: Author.

Bligh, J., & Bleakley, A. (2006). Distributing menus to hungry learners: Can learning by simulation become simulation of learning? *Medical Teacher, 28*(7), 606–613.

Brown, M. C. (2005). Internet-based medical chart for documentation and evaluation of simulated patient care activities. *American Journal of Pharmaceutical Education, 69*(1–5), 204.

Carty, R., & Ong, I. (2006). The nursing curriculum in the information age. In V.K. Saba & K.A. McCormick (Eds.), *Essentials of nursing informatics* (4th ed., pp. 517–531). New York, NY: McGraw-Hill.

Connors, H. R., Weaver, C., Warren, J., & Miller, K. L. (2002). An academic-business partnership for advancing clinical informatics. *Nursing Education Perspectives, 23*(5), 228–233.

Fetter, M. (2009). Graduating nurses' self-evaluation of information technology competencies. *Journal of Nursing Education, 48*(2), 86.

Gaba, D. (2004). The future vision of simulation in health care. *Quality and Safety in Healthcare, 13,* 2–10.

Gaba, D., & DeAnda, A. A. (1998). A comprehensive anesthesia simulation environment: Recreating the operating room for research and training. *Anesthesiology, 69,* 387–393.

Gassert, C. A. (1998). The challenge of meeting patients' needs with a national nursing informatics agenda. *Journal of the American Medical Association, 3,* 263–268.

Gassert, C. A., & Sward, K. A. (2007). Phase I implementation of an academic medical record for integrating information management competencies into a nursing curriculum. *Studies in Health Technology and Informatics, 129*(Pt 2), 1392–1395.

Hertel, J. P., & Millis, B. J. (2002). *Using simulations to promote learning in higher education: An introduction.* Sterling, VA: Stylus.

Institute of Medicine. (2000). *To err is human: Building a safer system.* Washington, DC: National Academic Press.

National League for Nursing. (2008). *Preparing the next generation of nurses to practice in a technology-rich environment: An informatics agenda.* (Position Statement) New York, NY: Author.

Pew. (1998). *Recreating health professional practice for a new centaury: The fourth report of the pew health professions commission.* San Francisco, CA: Pew Health Professions Commission.

Simulation learning system. (2010). Retrieved from http://www.elsevieradvantage.com/simulations/sls/home.html

Staggers, N., Gassert, C. A., & Curran, C. (2002). A Delphi study to determine informatics competencies for nurses at four levels of practice. *Nursing Research, 51*(6), 383–390.

Technology Informatics Guiding Education Reform (TIGER). (2007). *The TIGER initiative: Evidence and informatics transforming nursing 3-year action steps toward a 10-year vision.* Retrieved from www.tigersummit.com

CHAPTER 25

Games, Simulations, and Virtual Worlds for Educators

Brett Bixler

1. Distinguish between learning environments as games, simulations, or virtual worlds.
2. Identify the different genres of games, simulations, and virtual worlds.
3. Compare and contrast games, simulations, and virtual worlds as informatics tools for nursing education.
4. Describe strategies choosing between a game, simulation, or virtual world as the best choice for instructional delivery in a given educational situation.

WWW

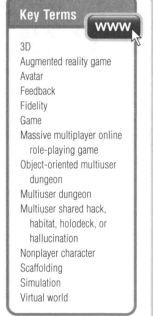

Key Terms   WWW

3D
Augmented reality game
Avatar
Feedback
Fidelity
Game
Massive multiplayer online role-playing game
Object-oriented multiuser dungeon
Multiuser dungeon
Multiuser shared hack, habitat, holodeck, or hallucination
Nonplayer character
Scaffolding
Simulation
Virtual world

INTRODUCTION

The use of educational games, simulations, and virtual worlds for education continues to grow, with a great deal of research effort and funds directed toward the discoveries of their best uses. Educational games, simulations, and virtual worlds all share some characteristics, and it is difficult to find a "pure" experience in any of the genres. Simulations may have game-like qualities, and virtual worlds may be used to present a simulation. This chapter introduces the reader to all three genres.

CASE SCENARIO

Joe sits down at the computer and logs into StratWorld, a virtual world that enables one to create their own team, then compete against other teams created by other StratWorld players. The developers of StratWorld create interesting challenges, part intellectual and part brute force, which teams strive to solve before other, competing teams solve them first.

After Joe logs on, he is presented with a three-dimensional (**3D**) view of a forest. Directly in front of him is a 3D figure that looks very much like Joe, except for broader shoulders, a more rugged face, and better skin complexion. This is Joe's **avatar**, his representation of self in StratWorld. Joe can change his avatar's appearance as he wishes, but he likes to stick to something close to the real thing. One of his opposing teams in StratWorld all prefer to appear as masses of glowing tubes. Joe thinks they are strange.

Today, he is recruiting for his virtual team, so he ducks into his inventory (a place to store stuff his avatar can wear and use) and dons his manager's jacket. "Joe's Team" is proudly displayed on the back. Joe is proud of the jacket; he created the lettering himself in a graphics program and uploaded it to StratWorld, then added it to a plain jacket and gave a copy to all new members of his team in StratWorld. As in many virtual worlds, clothes do make the man, woman, or thing.

Using the arrow keys and the mouse to manipulate his avatar, Joe begins to make his avatar walk down the forest trail. He is looking to recruit an Ogre for his team to beef up their physical offensive capabilities and replace the recent loss of Charlie the Unicorn. Ogres are big and strong, perfect for the task. Joe is a little nervous. He has never been to this part of StratWorld before, and explorations in new areas can be fraught with peril. After a brief sojourn, Joe comes upon an Ogre sitting in a daisy-strewn clearing, picking his teeth with a small sapling ripped from the ground. "Ogre!" Joe shouts. "I need someone to smash through things for my team. Interested?"

"What in it for me?" the Ogre asks, thumping his chest with the remains of the sorry sapling, splintering it in oblivion. "Darn! That was good toothpick!" The chirps of birds, the drone of insects in the foliage, all normal background noise here, suddenly stop. Joe picks up on this environmental clue, and just as in the real world when this happens, knows he is in danger.

Joe ponders the question. He knows he is talking to a **nonplayer character**, one that seems to have a brain behind the 3D façade, but in reality has very clever programming attached to it so it can seem to carry on an intelligent conversation. Some companies call this artificial intelligence, but both the creators of these environments and the scholars that study them hotly debate the proper use of that term. He also knows that the world is constructed so that he has to balance his profits from game wins with overhead costs, such as player salaries and equipment maintenance. He needs to make an offer to the Ogre. An offer too little will insult the Ogre, and a possible fight between it and Joe is the probable result. Joe's avatar could die, an inconvenience that will cost him time and loss of reputation with other StratWorlders. A generous offer will probably be accepted, but might bankrupt Joe over time. Joe needs to balance his needs and costs, and also think outside the box. It is a complex problem-solving situation!

"Ok, Ogre, here's the deal. Pay is $900 a month, and . . ." Joe attempts to continue, but the Ogre quickly rises in an aggressive manner. "Wait! Let me continue! I know that's a little less than normal, but I'll throw in a nice, new sapling each week for tooth maintenance! How about it?"

The Ogre sits back down and eyes Joe warily. "Just need to pick tooth's, not maintain ants. Contract for . . ." (the Ogre pauses to quickly count his fingers) "10 months?"

"Sure, sure, but if you are injured, you go to half pay until you can play again," Joe answers.

"I still get toothpick each week, even if hurt?"

"Absolutely. I mean, yes."

The Ogre leans forward on its haunches. "Sound good! You go. I follow."

"One more thing, Ogre. What do I call you?" Joes asks.

"Daisy! You managers sure stupid!"

Joe takes Daisy back to Joe's office by teleporting there, a way to move from one place to another with a simple click of a button. Joe pulls up a map of StratWorld, locates the land he owns, and clicks on it for instantaneous transport. Joes sends Daisy the Ogre down to practice smashing down walls in his training field, and then pauses for a moment to admire his recreation of his grandfather's old roll-top desk. He recreated it from an old photograph just for his office in StratWorld. Looking out the window, he sees Daisy running out on the training field. He sits down at his desk to go over his team's statistics. With the addition of Daisy to the team, he needs to recalculate all his strategies. He needs to determine how he can acquire a sapling each week for Daisy; where will he get one, and how much will it cost? Then he needs to send out an acceptance to a recent invitation from the game developers to participate in next week's challenge. A win will be sweet, but it will be a busy week of preparation! Before Joe hunkers down to work, he sends an instant message to Kathy, an admirable opponent in StratWorld he has competed against several times. Typing furiously and with a certain glee, he writes, "Hi Kathy, guess what? I'm gonna DUST your team in the next challenge!" Kathy's reply is swift: "Bring it on, Joe, bring it on!"

CASE SCENARIO DISCUSSION

This is a brief description of what occurs in many online virtual environments today. People create a presence in the environment, then manipulate events for a desired outcome. They explore, build things, interact with others, and try to achieve goals. The story is fictional; there is no StratWorld, but games do exist where people build teams and compete against one another. So, is StratWorld a simulation, a virtual world, or a game? What do you think? Think about simulations you have experienced or heard of, games you have played, and anything you have read about virtual worlds. Try looking up some definitions online. Write down your thoughts, and come up with some justifications that back your decision.

EDUCATIONAL GAMES

People voluntarily play **games** because they are fun, and embody many motivational aspects (Mastrian, McGonigle, Mahan, & Bixler, 2011). Great games provide an optimally challenging state between boredom and frustration (Csikszentmihalyi, 1990). Games exist within a set of rules (Kelley, 1988; Salen and Zimmerman, 2003), and players receive **feedback** from their interactions in the game and rule space.

An educational game, one designed for learning, is a subset of both play and fun, and is sometimes referred to as a "serious game" (Zyda 2005). It is a melding of educational content, learning principles, and computer games (Prensky, 2001). Educational games should emphasize the value of the experience (Nemerow, 1996). Mungai, Jones, and Wong (2002) state that the flow of an educational game may be under the designer's control more than a noneducational game, and feedback is used to stress competency, not just achievement. The trick in designing an educational game is to maintain the same "fun" state found in noneducational games (Koster, 2004).

There are many different types of games. Each type has a different potential for educational use (Mastrian, et al., 2011). To learn to respond quickly and hone reflexes, action games may be used. Adventure games may be used to discover the unknown, such as diagnosing a patient illness. Construction and building games could be used for building complex mental constructs that can only be understood through knowledge of their constituent parts and how they interrelate. Strategy games are great for nursing education teaching moments where careful, up-front planning is critical, and on-the-fly adjustments to one's plan may be needed to ensure its success.

In role-playing games, the player takes on the role of one or more characters and improves them as they progress through a storyline. Today, **massive multiplayer online role-playing games** are very popular, using the Internet to provide a shared, simultaneous experience for dozens or even hundreds of players. Role-playing games are an excellent way for nursing educators to guide students through any situation where a sequenced step-by-step introduction to the parts of the job or skill is required.

Fairly new are casual games, or mini games. These games are designed to be played in a short time span, or for a few minutes a day over several days, weeks, or even months. Many online browser-based games fit this category. Casual games may be useful for continuous reinforcement of basic concepts, for emulating a slowly changing environment, and for modifying the player's attitudes on a given topic over a period of time. These games to date are largely untapped as educational tools.

EDUCATIONAL SIMULATIONS

A **simulation** recreates a real-life set of conditions or events with as much **fidelity** as possible (Alessi, 1988). Aldrich (2010) contends that simulations develop cognition (Learning to Know skills); ethics and roles (Learning to Be skills); and application (Learning to Do skills). Unlike games, simulations are not necessarily designed to be fun.

Simulations may be experiential and task based, where the learner takes on a first-person role and executes a self-chosen series of decisions, manipulating the variables in the simulation toward a desired outcome (Gredler, 1996; Weatherford, n.d.).

Simulations may also be symbolic scenarios, where the learner directly manipulates variables, sees the results of changes, and then makes decisions on how to continue in the simulation. Spreadsheets are often used for this type of simulation. Symbolic simulations are good for discovering principles, misconceptions, and relationships, and for fostering understanding, prediction, and solution development (Mastrian, et al., 2011).

Simulations may use a process known as "**scaffolding**" (Guzdial, 1997; Jonassen, 1999) to assist in acquiring the accepted level of proficiency. An example of scaffolding is when corrective feedback is initially used, correcting user mistakes and ensuring success, and then the feedback fades away when it is no longer needed.

Medical simulations use realistic 3D computer models of humans to investigate new medical possibilities and to test assumptions (Learning to Know skills). Simulations of drawing blood and complex medical operations are used to teach "Learning to Do" skills. Refer to Chapter 24 for an in-depth discussion of simulations and nursing informatics skills to develop and run simulation scenarios.

VIRTUAL WORLDS

Wikipedia defines a **virtual world** as follows:

> A virtual world is a genre of online community that often takes the form of a computer-based simulated environment, through which users can interact with one another and use and create objects. Virtual worlds are intended for its users to inhabit and interact, and the term today has become largely synonymous with interactive 3D virtual environments, where the users take the form of avatars visible to others graphically. These avatars are usually depicted as textual, two-dimensional, or three-dimensional graphical representations, although other forms are possible (auditory and touch sensations for example). Some, but not all, virtual worlds allow for multiple users (2010, para. 1).

A 3D virtual world often mimics a real-world environment, although it also may include impossible abilities, such as flying unaided (Mastrian, et al., 2011). Users of virtual worlds are often quick to stress that virtual worlds in and of themselves are not games, although this confusion is easy to understand because virtual worlds share many of the same interface characteristics as 3D action and role-playing games.

The best use of virtual worlds for educational purposes may be when there is a need for an immersive experience coupled with a need for social interaction. For example, in the virtual world of Second Life, the Penn State University Harrisburg Campus has developed a virtual hacienda for students learning Spanish (Clark, 2009). Students interact with the environment and the objects in the hacienda while speaking to each other in Spanish, thus participating in authentic learning activities.

Virtual worlds need not be 3D. Predecessors to the 3D environment include **multiuser dungeons**, **object-oriented multiuser dungeons**, and **multiuser shared hallucinations**. All of these environments are text-based, where one receives environmental information as passages of text, and manipulates objects and talks to others by typing text commands. Multiuser dungeons, multiuser dungeons object-oriented, and multiuser shared hallucinations are still in use today.

CHOOSING BETWEEN EDUCATIONAL GAMES, SIMULATIONS, AND VIRTUAL WORLDS

Educational games, simulations, and virtual worlds all have a great deal of overlap. Games may be placed in virtual worlds, and simulations may have game-like elements. Yet, these three tools have distinctive characteristics, and by examining several key characteristics (goal orientation, competition, the fun factor, and exploratory learning and social interaction affordances) it becomes easier to choose the correct tool for teaching purposes.

Games are goal oriented and may be competitive in nature. Games should be fun and perhaps a bit "fantastical" and light-hearted. A particular game may or may not include exploratory learning and social interaction. Although simulations are also goal oriented, the competition is generally subdued. Simulations are generally more realistic and are not necessarily fun to use. A particular simulation may or may not include exploratory learning and social interaction. Virtual worlds in and of themselves do not have goals or competition; it is up to the player to construct them and add them to the world. Virtual worlds are not by default fun, although they may include the "fantastical." Virtual worlds generally lend themselves to exploratory learning and social interaction.

THE FUTURE OF GAMES, VIRTUAL WORLDS, AND SIMULATIONS

The use of games, virtual worlds, and simulations in Western society continues to increase. The combination of best practices supported by sound research, the ever-growing power of technology, and learners who grew up using these environments will lead to increases in their use (New Media Consortium, 2007).

In addition, games are becoming cheaper to produce and consume. Game development engines, long in the hands of only major game development companies, are now available at a cost that many can afford. Some games come with built-in development tools, an attempt by the game producers to use free labor to extend their product (Dyer-Witheford & de Peuter, 2009). The growth of "indie," or independent game companies is leading to a plethora of cheap yet high-quality games.

The same holds true for virtual worlds. New virtual worlds spring up all the time. Many offer free, if limited, accounts, and educators are exploring these spaces with increasing regularity, building fantastic learning environments.

Companies are tapping mobile devices as another avenue to push out their games. These devices are already used for a variety of communication and social functions. Why not build on that with casual games that rely on social interactions? Expect to see much more happening in this space in the near future.

Another related area of growth is **augmented reality games**. Augmented reality occurs when one uses a device, such as a smart phone, to overlay on the real world additional information (Klopfer & Squire, 2008). One might use the camera in the phone to view the stars at night and see on the phone's screen both the stars and the constellation labels and linking lines between the stars in a constellation. Augmented reality games use this concept in game-like ways, bringing people together physically and virtually to solve a series of challenges. In education, augmented reality games may be used to provide a fun way to collect and analyze data, to collaborate with other students, to access information resources, and to provide a new way to look at the world.

Serious games may also have a place in helping practicing nurses maintain or hone skills. Baker (2009) suggests that gaming has a place in continuing education.

> The science of nursing practices encourages us to ask questions, promote dialog, share lessons learned willingly and openly, and make the outcomes of our patients constructive and positive. The rigor or quality evaluation and research of the teaching and learning techniques offered by serious games can shed insight into future changes not conceived of at this moment. For example, if there were a serious game that could effectively assist nurses in maintaining the skill set required to care for a patient who is experiencing hypothermia, would that be worth the investment? If there were a game that

could reduce medication errors in the OR by 50% to 75% compared to what has been demonstrated in the past, would that have value? If it were found that after use of a serious game, a facility experienced zero errors in right site, right procedure, and right patient events during a 10-year period, would this be of value? (p. 173).

Other new games that can be used to educate health professionals were discussed by Skiba (2008). She describes Fold.IT, a game that challenges players to fold proteins as part of a research experience for Life and Death in the Age of Malaria, a game that simulates advice nurses would give to world travelers on health maintenance strategies, and 3DiMD, designed to facilitate skills training in teamwork for military environments. Two important websites to watch for emerging games are the Serious Games Initiative (www.seriousgames.org) and Games for Health (www.gamesforhealth.org).

Best uses of all these technologies and approaches still remain a bit murky. Fortunately, a great deal of research is underway whose findings will guide future educators toward the best uses of educational games, simulations, and virtual worlds. In an ideal world, educators would have a plethora of available, well-designed, and educator-certified games to choose from that mesh with the educational objectives of their classes, courses, and curricula.

THOUGHT-PROVOKING Questions

WWW

1. Games are supposed to be fun and voluntary. How can educators "force" a game on a student and expect it to remain fun and engaging?

2. It can take several hours of game play to learn the mechanics of some games, even longer for the more complex games. If subject matter learning can occur only after this initial game mechanic learning occurs, how can educators justify the amount of time a learner must spend within the game just to get to the point where learning begins?

3. How do educators acquire the training needed not just to "get by" in these new environments, but rather flourish, thrive, and mold the environments to their purposes?

For a full suite of assignments and additional learning activities, use the access code located in the front of your book to visit this exclusive website: http://go.jblearning.com/mcgonigle. If you do not have an access code, you can obtain one at the site.

WWW

References

Aldrich, C. (2010, August). *Virtual worlds, simulations and games for online educators.* Manga Online Seminar presented at Penn State University, University Park, PA.

Alessi, S. M. (1988). Fidelity in the design of instructional simulations, *Journal of Computer-Based Instruction, 15*(2), 40–47.

Baker, J. (2009). *Serious games and perioperative nursing.* Association of Operating Room Nurses. *AORN Journal, 90*(2), 173–175. Retrieved from Health Module. (Document ID: 1853293981).

Clark, G. (2009). These horses can fly! and other lessons from Second Life: The view from the virtual hacienda. In R. Oxford & J. Oxford (Eds.), *Second language teaching and learning in the net generation* (pp. 153–172). Honolulu, HI: National Foreign Language Resource Center.

Csikszentmihalyi, M. (1990). *Flow: The psychology of optimal experience.* New York, NY: Harper Collins.

Dyer-Witheford, N., & de Peuter, G. (2009). *Games of empire: Global capitalism and video games.* Minneapolis, MN: University of Minnesota Press.

Gredler, M. E. (1996). Educational games and simulations: A technology in search of a (research) paradigm. In D. H. Jonassen (Ed.), *Handbook of research for educational communications and technology.* New York, NY: Simon & Schuster Macmillan.

Guzdial, M. (1997). *Components of software-realized scaffolding.* Retrieved from http://www.cc.gatech.edu/gvu/edtech/SRS.html.

Jonassen, D. H. (1999). Designing constructivist learning environments. In C. M. Reigeluth (Ed.), *Instructional design theories and models: A new paradigm of instructional theory* (Vol. 2, pp. 215–239). Mahwah, NJ: Lawrence Erlbaum Associates.

Kelley, D. (1988). *The art of reasoning.* New York, NY: W. W. Norton.

Klopfer, E., & Squire K. (2008). Environmental detectives: The development of an augmented reality platform for environmental simulations. *Education Technology Research and Development, 56,* 203–228.

Koster, R. (2004). *A theory of fun for game design.* Scottsdale, AZ: Paraglyph Press.

Mastrian, K. G., McGonigle, D., Mahan, W. L., & Bixler, B. (2011). *Integrating technology in nursing education: Tools for the knowledge era.* Sudbury, MA: Jones and Barlett Learning.

Mungai, D., Jones, D., & Wong, L., (2002, August*). Games to teach by.* Paper presented at the 18th Annual Conference on Distance Teaching and Learning. Madison, WI.

Nemerow, L. G. (1996). Do classroom games improve motivation and learning? *Teaching and Change, 3*(4), 356–361.

New Media Consortium (2007). *Massively multiplayer educational gaming.* The Horizon Report 2007 Edition. Retrieved from http://www.nmc.org/horizonproject/2007/massively-multiplayer-educational-gaming.

Prensky, M. (2001). *Digital game-based learning* (1st ed.). New York, NY: McGraw Hill.

Salen, K., & Zimmerman, E. (2003). *Rules of play: Game design fundamentals.* Cambridge, MA: MIT Press.

Skiba, D. (2008). *Games for health.* Nursing Education Perspectives, 29(4), 230–232. Retrieved from ProQuest Nursing & Allied Health Source. (Document ID: 1538660701).

Weatherford, J. (n.d.). *Instructional simulations: An overview.* Retrieved from http://coe.sdsu.edu/eet/Articles/instrucsimu/start.htm.

Wikipedia. (2010). *Virtual world.* Retrieved from http://en.wikipedia.org/wiki/Virtual_World.

Zyda, M. (2005). From visual simulation to virtual reality to games. *Computer, 39*(9), 25–32.

CHAPTER 26

Nursing Research: Data Collection, Processing, and Analysis

Heather E. McKinney and Sylvia DeSantis

Objectives

1. Describe nursing research in relation to the Foundation of Knowledge model.
2. Explore the acquisition of previous knowledge through Internet and library holdings.
3. Assess informatics tools for collecting data and storage of information.
4. Compare tools for processing and analyzing quantitative and qualitative data.

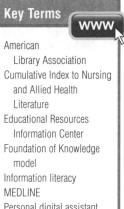

Key Terms

WWW

American
  Library Association
Cumulative Index to Nursing
  and Allied Health
  Literature
Educational Resources
  Information Center
Foundation of Knowledge
  model
Information literacy
MEDLINE
Personal digital assistant
PsycInfo

INTRODUCTION: NURSING RESEARCH AND THE FOUNDATION OF KNOWLEDGE MODEL

The **Foundation of Knowledge model** suggests that the most important aspect in information discovery, retrieval, and delivery is the ability to acquire, process, generate, and disseminate knowledge in ways that help those managing the knowledge reevaluate and rethink the way they understand and use what they know and have learned. These goals closely reflect the **Information Literacy** Competency Standards for Higher Education, presented by the **American Library Association** (ALA) in 2003 in response to changing perceptions of how information is created, evaluated, and used.

According to the ALA (2000), an information literate individual is able to do the following:

- Determine the extent of information needed
- Access the needed information effectively and efficiently
- Evaluate information and its sources critically
- Incorporate selected information into ones' knowledge base
- Use information effectively to accomplish a specific purpose

• Understand the economic, legal, and social issues surrounding the use of information and access and use information ethically and legally

In addition, new challenges arise for individuals seeking to understand and evaluate information because information is available through multiple media (graphical, aural, and textual). The sheer quantity of information does not by itself create a more informed citizenry without complementary abilities to use this information effectively. Most significantly, information literacy forms the basis for lifelong learning, forming a commonality to all learning environments, disciplines, and levels of education (Association of College and Research Libraries, 2000).

Case Study

During rounds Charles encounters a rare condition he has never personally seen, and only vaguely remembers hearing about in nursing school. He takes a few moments to prepare himself by searching the Internet. That evening, he researches even further to treat, administer, and assess the patient safely. He searches clinical databases online and his own school textbooks. Most of the information seems consistent, yet some factors vary. Charles wants to provide the highest quality in patient safety. He wonders which resources are best. Which are the most trusted? Which are the most accurate?

KNOWLEDGE GENERATION THROUGH NURSING RESEARCH

Information literacy is an intellectual framework for finding, understanding, evaluating, and using information activities. It is accomplished in part through fluency with information technology and sound investigative methods, but most importantly through critical reasoning and discernment. The Association of College and Research Libraries (2000) has suggested that information literacy initiates, sustains, and extends lifelong learning through abilities which may use technologies but are ultimately independent of them (p. 5).

Because nursing informatics combines all aspects of clinical practice, research, administration, and education (Ball, Hannah, & Douglas, 2000), the ability to recognize the need for a specific kind of information and locate, evaluate, and effectively use it (ALA, 1989) within the nursing informatics paradigm will catapult nurses ahead of other healthcare professionals in applying and engaging various facets of technology. However, because so few nurses have formal training in technology but still represent a disproportionate number of users, the ways in which nursing research integrates healthcare technology within nursing informatics creates an unseen challenge (McHaney, 2007). This potentially enormous impact on the future of health care and technology will determine the success of information-literate nurses: those who have learned how to learn and who understand the intricacies of how knowledge is organized, retrieved, and used in such a way that others can learn from them (ALA, 1989). Whether a nurse fills the role of administrator, manager, educator, or staff, integrating technology has become a necessity for every nurse in today's technologic marketplace (McHaney, 2007).

ACQUIRING PREVIOUS KNOWLEDGE THROUGH INTERNET AND LIBRARY HOLDINGS

In an environment of rapid technologic change coupled with an overwhelming proliferation of information sources, nurses face an enormous number of options when choosing how and from where to acquire information for their academic studies, clinical situations, and research. Because information is available through so many venues, libraries, special interest organizations, media, community resources, and the Internet in increasingly unfiltered formats, healthcare practitioners must inevitably question the authenticity, validity, and reliability of information (Association of College and Research Libraries, 2000).

Often, the retrieval of reliable research and information may seem to be a daunting task in light of the seemingly ubiquitous amount of information on the Web. Focusing on specific information venues not only aids this search but also assists in negotiating the endless maze of resources, allowing a nursing practitioner to find the best and most accurate information efficiently.

Professional Online Databases

Professional databases contribute to the Web, a source of online information generally invisible to all Internet users except those with professional or academic affiliations, such as faculty, staff, and students. Databases range from specific to general and act as collection points by aggregating information, such as abstracts and articles from many different journals; two such databases include the **Cumulative Index to Nursing and Allied Health Literature** (CINAHL) and **MEDLINE**. CINAHL, for example, specifically includes information from all aspects of allied health, nursing, alternative medicine, and community medicine. The MEDLINE database contains more than 10 million records, maintained and produced by the National Library of Medicine. Other databases, such as **PsycInfo** from the American Psychological Association and the **Educational Resources Information Center** (ERIC) database, may also benefit nursing. Many databases also offer full-text capabilities, meaning that entire articles are available online. The articles and abstracts contained within these databases have already passed the rigors of publication in professional journals and are thus considered viable and authentic peer-reviewed sources.

Libraries with subscriptions to databases often employ library professionals able to help patrons through the vast amounts of available electronic information;

using the expert research capabilities of a health science librarian at one's local university is the best way to learn how to conduct database searches that yield the most efficient and useful results. Also useful are websites that provide tutorials on best searching practices specifically for medically oriented databases, such as the Nursing Informatics Competency Project (http://library.med.nyu.edu/library/instruction/tutorials/nursing/index.html), which assists nursing students and professionals in using CINAHL's search engine efficiently.

Search Engines

Search engines allow users to surf the Web and find information on nearly anything, although many researchers steer clear of search engines because of the vast amounts of unsubstantiated information. Because no legitimacy needs to be provided for any information that appears on the Web, an author can make claims, substantiated or not, and still use the Web as a publishing venue. Despite the pitfalls associated with search engines in general, they still yield a bounty of useful information when used with discretion.

Different search engines produce different results for the same research. For example, one popular search engine ranks its results by number of hits a page or site has received. Consider that whereas the uppermost research results are relevant, the order in which results appear does not indicate quality or viability of the source.

Different Web address (domain) suffixes (com, .edu, .org, .gov, and so forth) indicate who is responsible for creating the website. Although an .edu site is hosted by an educational institution and for that reason may seem legitimate, consider that it could belong to a student stating personal opinion, gossip, or guesswork. In contrast, .gov sites are maintained by the government and nearly always have professional contact information. Web hosts develop new domain suffixes constantly, so although looking at the suffix can be useful, it should not be the only deciding factor when choosing to trust information.

One should not blindly trust information found on a Web page. When possible, check the date of the most recent update (how old is the page?); contact information (is there an available bibliography or sources?); links to external sources (do they seem relevant?); and previous attained knowledge from other reputable sources (is the information too unbelievable?).

Fees and information retrieval charges should be approached with skepticism. Private companies do offer information aggregate services for a fee. In these cases, users pay a flat monthly fee for access to collections of articles in a particular field. What users (especially those affiliated with an academic institution) may not realize is that they likely have free access to the same if not more complete information through their institution's library system.

Some legitimate databases and traditional newspapers who maintain a Web presence do provide access for a small fee, but just as many others simply ask users to register to see articles for free. Many nursing students and professionals affiliated with a university may find that their university library has already purchased access for the student body.

Electronic Library Catalogs

Nearly all higher education institutions have their library catalogs online. Although this is an obvious convenience for many students, some nursing professionals unused to working completely online may be intimidated by an e-catalog. Library professionals at the tiniest university and the busiest community college are available to demonstrate how to navigate a basic search of their library's catalog. Asking for assistance in learning how to access the vast assortment of journals, books, databases, and other resources available at one's college library is an excellent idea. Those in nursing programs at larger universities will likely find free classes that specifically teach users how to navigate and use the online catalog. If smaller colleges and universities do not offer these services, one should take advantage of the library's online tutorials, help pages, frequently asked questions pages, and online reference service (if available). Local public libraries often have subscriptions to popular databases and offer free classes on searching techniques to patrons, providing another free access point to the best information for one's research needs. Making full use of available library resources serves to strengthen information literacy skills, enabling learners to master content and extend their investigations, become more self-directed, and assume greater control over their own learning (Association of College and Research Libraries, 2000).

INFORMATICS TOOLS FOR COLLECTING DATA AND STORAGE OF INFORMATION

Nurses are already intimately familiar with data collection as daily agents of patient care documentation, patient monitoring, and interview data (Chang, 2001). In this way, formal nursing data sets are actually made up of gathered information, such as healthcare definitions, classification, and nursing information. Before data can be analyzed or critically reviewed to determine outcomes or assessment, it must be collected and aggregated. According to the Cleveland Clinic (2010):

> collaborative nursing-led research is enhanced by the ability to support these projects with patient data that is more easily extracted electronically (para. 12). Supporting these efforts and initiatives is a dedicated team of clinical and system analysts who provide support for the development and management of information databases, systems and processes to bring efficiency to nursing-driven quality and research endeavors through informatics (para. 13).

Nurses may generate and record data from their own observations or with the assistance of various devices. Free text (informational data, such as drug dosages administered, resources used, problems diagnosed) is recorded manually. Free text is then interpreted and organized by some standardizing principle, either manually or by computer. In this way, data (often qualitative data that cannot be traditionally measured) can be organized and processed. Data actually becomes information when these separate components are interpreted, organized, combined, and structured within a specific context to convey particular meanings (Hovenga & Sermeus, 2002).

Software designed to collect, sort, organize, store, retrieve, select, and aggregate data are database management systems. Nursing and health data may be separated into four basic types: (1) resource data (e.g., financial information); (2) patient and client demographics; (3) activity data (clinical data); and (4) health service provider data. These primary data are recorded manually or collected electronically, with manual collection providing a greater opportunity for error. Data that have been electronically recorded follow a programmed set of instructions built into the software, thus cutting down substantially on collection error. Of paramount importance in the collection process are the data collection form and computer interface used for inputting the data; these affect completeness, consistency, and accuracy (Hovenga & Sermeus, 2002).

Quantitative data collection tools or instruments include questionnaires, interviews, surveys, quizzes, assessments, e-mail interviews, and Web-based surveys. Questionnaires, one of the most popular forms of data collection, can be administered in hard copy, on paper, or programmed into a website where individuals may answer the questions electronically (Chang, 2001). Other electronic data collection tools include **personal digital assistants** and on-site laptops. A benefit of using electronic data collection is the ability to transmit data to another computer directly for compilation and analysis, thereby cutting down on error (Hebda, Czar, & Mascara, 2005).

An excellent example of innovative electronic data collection is the system used by participants in the Nightingale Tracker System pilot study, in which nursing students traveling to rural clinical sites submitted information into handheld devices while miles away from their preceptor-supervisors. Results suggest that, despite some technical challenges associated with the hardware, using the handheld technology enhanced students' learning (especially in the area of physical assessment), increased their confidence in practicing in community-based settings, and provided efficient data input capabilities (Ndiwane, 2005).

Harder to measure, nonnumerical qualitative data can be collected electronically in the form of a narrative or diary-like entry. Much in the way free text is analyzed and sorted, this narrative dialogue is assessed and then sorted according to the data collection's organizing principle (Chang, 2001).

TOOLS FOR PROCESSING DATA AND DATA ANALYSIS

Data analysis is the process by which data collected during the course of a study is processed to identify trends and patterns of relationships. Descriptive statistics allows the researcher to organize information meaningfully, thus facilitating insight by describing what the data show (Hebda et al., 2005). There exist a range of tools to facilitate analysis including specialized databases, word processing-spreadsheet-database applications, and statistical packages (Hovenga & Sermeus, 2002).

Quantitative Data Analysis

Quantitative data focuses on numbers and frequencies rather than experiences and meaning. Although the kind of data generated by quantitative collection is fairly straightforward and easy to analyze (responses to questionnaires, experiments, and psychometric tests) quantitative data analysis has come under criticism. Psychologists prefer to use a combination of quantitative and qualitative data, backing up research participants' explanations with statistically reliable information obtained by numerical measurement (Quantitative and Qualitative Data, n.d.).

In quantitative studies, variables represented by data are collected in numerical form. These values are then entered into specific fields that have predetermined meanings or are coded. Various quantitative data analyses can be applied to nursing research, such as intervention research, quality improvement studies, and outcomes research. One of the most common statistical packages on the market available for this kind of analysis is the Statistical Package for Social Sciences. Depending on the research goal, the researcher may use different types of analysis. Different statistical goals may require hypothesis testing, model building, descriptive and exploratory analyses, and others. For example, hypothesis testing is based on assumptions regarding the relative truth of the hypothesis, so a data analysis would compare actual outcomes with purported hypotheses (Chang, 2001).

Qualitative Data Analysis

Extremely varied in nature, qualitative data can include nearly any information that can be captured and is not numerical (Trochim, 2006a). Qualitative data are more concerned with describing meaning than in drawing statistical inferences; what is lost in reliability (faulty transcription, forgotten details, and so forth) is gained in validity (Quantitative and Qualitative Data, n.d.). Although qualitative data rely on judgments, they can still be manipulated numerically, much in the same way quantitative data can be open to judgment (Trochim, 2006b).

Some major types of quantitative data include in-depth interviews, direct observation, and written documents. Interviews include individual and focus group interviews and may be recorded in some way. Interviews differ from direct observation in their interactive nature. Direct observation differs from case to case and often means the researcher does not make contact with the respondent. Written documents might include a variety of written materials including memos, newspaper clippings, conversation transcripts, and books (Trochim, 2006a).

Computers can aid greatly in the storage, tabulation, and retrieval of qualitative data by acting as the equivalent of an electronic filing cabinet (Hebda et al., 2005). Data analysis can also be aided by simple data management programs, such as Excel Access, or NVivo, in which a user can categorize data and link categories with key words (Chang, 2001). Data can be converted into information and knowledge by either inductive or deductive reasoning. Most qualitative methods use an inductive approach in which one generates hypotheses (versus a deductive approach in which hypotheses are tested). Data analysis includes statistical analysis in which samples and populations are compared to discern whether the sample is biased or reflective of a true situation. Another aspect of analysis includes seeking relationships between a variable and events (Hovenga & Sermeus, 2002).

Future

The future of nursing informatics is growing as fast as technology itself. The more nurses participate in the development process of healthcare technology, the more efficient and effective nursing informatics may become. Nurses are urged to take an active role in the profession by providing real-world feedback during the design process and after implementation. Practical insights provide valuable data for technology evaluation and advancement in the field of nursing informatics.

SUMMARY

This chapter discusses the value of information literacy and its relationship to knowledge and lifelong learning. The reader is now acquainted with informatics tools useful to acquiring and assessing previous knowledge, and tools useful for collecting and storing and analyzing information. In an ideal world, information literacy and informatics tools will be used as a critical skill set for increasing healthcare efficiency, effectiveness, and safety in the 21st century.

THOUGHT-PROVOKING Question

How will the advent of information literacy affect nursing informatics in the 21st century?

For a full suite of assignments and additional learning activities, use the access code located in the front of your book to visit this exclusive website: http://go.jblearning.com/mcgonigle. If you do not have an access code, you can obtain one at the site.

References

American Library Association. (1989). *Presidential committee on information literacy: Final report.* Retrieved from http://www.ala.org/ala/acrl/acrlpubs/whitepapers/presidential.cfm

American Library Association. (2000). *Information literacy competency standards for higher education.* Chicago, IL: Author.

Association of College and Research Libraries. (2000). *Information literacy competency standards for higher education.* Retrieved from http://www.ala.org/ala/acrl/acrlstandards/standards.pdf

Ball, M. J., Hannah, K. J., & Douglas, J. V. (2000). Nursing and informatics. In M. J. Ball, K. J. Hannah, S. K. Newbold, & J. V. Douglas (Eds.), *Nursing informatics: Where caring and technology meet* (pp. 6–14). New York, NY: Springer.

Chang, B. L. (2001). Computer use in nursing education. In V. Saba & K. McCormick (Eds.), *Essentials of computers for nurses: Informatics for the new millennium* (3rd ed., pp. 445–456). New York, NY: McGraw-Hill.

Cleveland Clinic. (2010). *Nursing informatics.* Retrieved from http://my.clevelandclinic.org/nursing/informatics.aspx

Hebda, T., Czar, P., & Mascara, C. (2005). *Handbook of informatics for nurses & health care professionals* (3rd ed.). Upper Saddle River, NJ: Prentice Hall.

Hovenga, E. J. S., & Sermeus, W. (2002). Data analysis methods. In J. Mantas & A. Hasman (Eds.), *Textbook in health informatics: A nursing perspective* (pp. 113–125). Amsterdam: IOS Press.

McHaney, D. F. (2007, June–August). Embracing the integration of technology and care. *The Alabama Nurse, 34*(2), 1.

Ndiwane, A. (2005). Teaching with the Nightingale Tracker technology in community-based nursing education: A pilot study. *Journal of Nursing Education, 44*(1), 40–42.

Quantitative and qualitative data. (n.d.). Retrieved from http://www.holah.karoo.net/quantitative qualitative.htm

Trochim, W. M. K. (2006a). *Qualitative data.* Retrieved from www.socialresearchmethods.net/kb/qualdata.php

Trochim, W. M. K. (2006b). *Types of data.* Retrieved from www.socialresearchmethods.net/kb/datatype.php

CHAPTER 27

Translational Research: Generating Evidence for Practice

Jennifer Bredemeyer and Ida Androwich

1. Clarify the differences between evidence-based practice and translational research.
2. Describe models for introducing research findings into practice.
3. Identify barriers to research utilization in practice.

Key Words   WWW

Agency for
   Healthcare Research and
   Quality (AHRQ)
Context of care
Evidence
Evidence-based practice
   (EBP)
Iowa model
Meta-analysis
National Guideline
   Clearinghouse (NGC)
Open Access Initiative
Qualitative study
Quantitative study
Research utilization
Research validity
Translational research

INTRODUCTION

Mr. James is an 87-year-old man with osteoarthritis in his knees. He is frail, very thin, and requires assistance getting out of bed. Mary, a new registered nurse, is making her rounds with her team members and nurse's aide. Realizing Mr. James is at risk for skin breakdown and falls, she reviews the agency policy manual regarding pressure ulcer prevention and fall prevention. What other resources could Mary consult if she wanted more information on preventing these issues? If Mary wanted to know what current research suggests about preventing each of these conditions, how would she obtain this information?

This chapter introduces the concept of **translational research** and its role in **evidence-based practice** (EBP) with specific emphasis on nursing informatics. Before pursuing the content in this chapter, the reader should already have an understanding of nursing research, the Foundation of Knowledge model, and knowledge generation through nursing research. Key words and definitions used in this chapter are described briefly next. Classic sources (5 years or older) are used to enhance the reference base.

> If I limit what I speak about to what I know from experience to be true rather than what I think I am expected to say or what I am pressured to say, then I will have a contribution to make. (Camus, 1943).

CLARIFICATION OF TERMS

Evidence-based practice (EBP), translational research, and **research utilization** are all terms that have been used to describe the application of evidential knowledge to clinical practice. The following paragraphs explore the definitions of each topic. Although the terms are related, they have slightly different meanings and applications.

EBP, developed originally for its application to medicine, is defined by Sackett et al. (1996) as "The conscientious, explicit and judicious use of current best evidence in making decisions about the care of individual patients" (p. 71). The "best evidence" in this context refers to more than just research. Goode and Piedalue (1999) state that evidenced-based practice should be combined with other knowledge sources and "involves the synthesis of knowledge from research, retrospective or concurrent chart review, quality improvement and risk data, international, national, and local standards, infection control data, pathophysiology, cost effectiveness analysis, benchmarking data, patient preferences, and clinical expertise" (p. 15). EBP starts with a clinical question to resolve a clinical problem. For example, published research studies are used in healthcare quality as the evidence behind the development of practice algorithms designed to decrease practice variability, increase patient safety, improve patient outcomes, and eliminate unnecessary cost. Use of EBP promotes the use of clinical judgment and knowledge with procedures and protocols to what is scientifically proven rather than on what is customary or opinion.

Research utilization is the application of findings from one or more research studies in a practical application unrelated to the original study (Polit & Beck, 2008, p. 29) resulting in the generation of new knowledge. Stetler (2001, p. 274) defines research utilization as the "process of transforming research knowledge into practice." Research utilization can be self limiting if research is inconsistent or there is not enough research available to gain consensus regarding the answer to the clinical question (Kirchhoff, 2004).

Translational science (research) describes the methods used in translation of medical, biomedical, informatics, and nursing research into bedside clinical interventions. Woolf (2008) describes translational research in two ways: T1: the transfer of clinical research to its first testing on humans; or T2: the transfer of clinical research to an everyday clinical practice setting. Difficulties in translating research to the T2 setting exist when research applications do not fit well within the clinical context or practical considerations constrain the application in a clinical setting. Translational research is complicated by the follow-up analysis, practice, and policy changes that occur when adopting research into practice and consequently available evidence-based healthcare practices are often not fully incorporated into daily care (Titler, 2004, 2010). Organizational culture affects changes to a clinical application and establishes the groundwork and the support for change-making activities (2004). The study of how to promote the adoption of evidence in the healthcare context is called "translation science" (Titler, 2010).

HISTORY OF EBP

Research results are crucial to furthering EBP. The concept of using randomized controlled trials and systematic reviews as the gold standard against which one should evaluate the validity and effectiveness of a clinical intervention was introduced in 1972 by Archie Cochrane, a scientist and a physician (Cochrane, 1972). Cochrane's experiences as a prisoner of war and medical officer while interning during World War II led to his belief that not all medical interventions were needed and some caused more harm than good. Cochrane viewed the randomized clinical trial as a means of validating clinical interventions to limit the interventions to those that were scientifically based, effective, and necessary (Dickersin & Manheimer, 1998).

Cochrane's colleague, Iain Chalmers, began compiling a comprehensive clinical trials registry of 3,500 clinical trial results in the field of perinatal medicine. In 1988, after being published in print 3 years prior, the registry became available electronically. Chalmer's methods for compiling the trials databases became a model for future registry assembly. Eventually, the National Health Service in England, recognizing the value of and need for systemic reviews for all of health care, developed the Cochrane Center. The Cochrane Collaboration was initiated in 1993 and expanded internationally to maintain systematic reviews in all areas of health care (Dickersin & Manheimer, 1998).

EVIDENCE

The randomized controlled trial (RCT) is considered the most reliable source of evidence. Yet, RCTs are not always possible or available, and consequently, nurses must use critical analysis to base their clinical decision making on the best available evidence (Baumann, 2010.) The updated Stetler model of research utilization (Stetler, 2001) identifies internal and external forms of evidence. External evidence originates from research and national experts and internal forms of evidence originate from nontraditional sources, such as clinical experience and quality improvement data.

Evidence includes standards of practice, codes of ethics, philosophies of nursing, autobiographic stories, esthetic criticism, works of art, **qualitative studies,** and patient and clinical knowledge (Melnyk, Fineout-Overholt, Stone, & Ackerman, 2000). French (2002) summarizes evidence as "truth, knowledge (including tacit, expert opinion and experiential), primary research findings, meta-analyses and systematic reviews" (p. 254). Nurses may additionally draw on evidence from the **context of care**, such as audit and performance data, the culture of the organization, social and professional networks, discussion with stakeholders, and local or national policy (Rycroft-Malone et al., 2004, p. 86).

There has been concern from nurse theorists that nurses are being influenced too much by the medical model in accepting the randomized controlled trial as the only true source of evidence, thereby "reverting to the medical perspective" rather than incorporating "theory-guided evidence and diverse ways of knowing" (Fawcett, Watson, Walker, & Fitzpatrick, 2001, p. 115). The context change from medicine to nursing requires nurses to apply other knowledge and nursing theory. The use of research results alone as a basis for clinical decision making ignores other types of evidence inherent in nursing practice (Scott-Findlay & Pollock, 2004).

To use evidence in practice, the weight of the research, also called **research validity**, must be determined. Evidence hierarchies have been defined to grade and assign value to the information source. An example of an evidential hierarchy by Stetler and Brunell et al. (1998) prioritizes evidence into six categories:

1. **Meta-analysis**
2. Individual experimental studies
3. Quasiexperimental studies
4. Nonexperimental studies
5. Program evaluations, such as quality improvement projects
6. Opinions of experts

The hierarchy identifies meta-analysis as the best quality evidence because it uses multiple individual research studies to come to consensus. It is interesting to note that opinions of experts are the least significant and yet nurses most often seek the opinion of a more experienced colleague or peer when seeking information regarding patient care (Pravikoff, Tanner, & Pierce, 2005).

Qualitative research allows one to understand the way in which the intervention is experienced by the researcher and the participant and the value of the interventions to both parties (O'Neill, Jinks, & Ong, 2007). Qualitative research is not always considered in EBP, because methods for synthesizing the evidence do not currently exist. The Cochrane Qualitative Research Methods Group (CQRMG) is developing search, appraisal, and synthesis methodologies for qualitative research (Joanna Briggs Institute, n.d.).

BRIDGING THE GAP BETWEEN RESEARCH AND PRACTICE

The time between research dissemination and clinical translation may be significant, and the delay may adversely affect patient outcomes. Bridging the gap between research and practice requires an understanding of the key concepts and barriers, access to research findings, access to clinical mentors for research understanding, a reinforcing culture, and a desire on the part of the clinician to implement best practices (Melnyk, 2005; Melnyk, Fineout-Overholt, Stetler, & Allen, 2005). In the **Iowa model** of EBP, research and other evidential sources are adopted directly in the practice setting with the goal of developing a standard of care (Titler, 2007). Additionally, the groundwork required to create a conceptual framework supportive of an EBP includes workplace culture change and support of the change through leadership (Stetler, Brunell et al., 1998). Beliefs and attitudes, involvement in research activities, information seeking, professional characteristics, education, and other socioeconomic factors are potential determinants of research utilization (Estabrooks, Floyd, Scott-Findlay, O'Leary, & Gushta, 2003); however, meta-analysis points out that too much original research and not enough repetition of previous studies fails to advance the knowledge base. Developing countries are constrained economically from accessing research sources. Such organizations as the Cochrane Collaboration provide free reviews to fill this void. Still, knowledge dissemination strategies and education are required (The Cochrane Collaboration, 2004).

BARRIERS AND FACILITATORS

Barriers to the application of EBP include lack of time, lack of access to libraries within a facility, lack of technology confidence, lack of knowledge on how to search for information, lack of value assigned to using research in practice (Pravikoff et al., 2005), inadequate EBP knowledge and skills, lack of mentors in EBP, inadequate support and resources from administration, and insufficient time, (Melnyk, Fineout-Overholt, Stillwell, & Williamson, 2009). McKnight (2006) notes that nurses on the unit felt constrained by time and ethically obligated to provide patient care rather than spend time looking up evidence-based references. Nurses may also see the job of interpreting research as too complex or may see the organizational culture as a barrier to implementation (McCaughan, Thompson, Cullum, Sheldon, & Thompson, 2002).

Yet, Melnynk et al. (2009) note that there are a number of facilitators to the use of EBP. These include knowledge and skills in EBP; having a conviction that there is a value to using evidence in practices; practicing in a supportive culture with tools available to sustain evidence-based (EB) care, including access to computers and databases and EB content at the point of care; as well as the presence of EBP mentors.

THE ROLE OF INFORMATICS

Computers are used in all areas of research: (1) literature search databases, such as CINAHL; (2) online literature reference lists, such as RefWorks; (3) data capture, collection, and coding; (4) data analysis; (5) data modeling; (6) meta-analysis; (7) qualitative analysis; and (8) dissemination of results (e.g., via e-mail or Internet website) (Saba & McCormick, 2006). The context for nursing informatics has expanded to support dramatic changes in the way science is accomplished. Information need and the collaborative component of interdisciplinary research rely heavily on technology and informatics. Technologies, such as social networking (Web 2.0), improve collaboration. The use of technology and informatics in facilitating interdisciplinary and translational research is a key architectural component of the National Institutes of

Health reengineering of the clinical research enterprise as part of its road map initiative for medical research (National Institutes of Health, 2009).

An informatics infrastructure is critical to EBP. Bakken, Stone, and Larson (2008) discuss expanding the context of informatics to genomic health care, shifting research paradigms, and social Web technologies. The global collaborative nature of nursing research for 2010-2018 requires an expansion of the nursing research agenda to user information needs, data management, information support for nurses and patients, practice-based knowledge generation, and design evaluation methodologies. Giuse et al. (2005) describe the evolving role of the clinical informationist as a partner on the healthcare team for the purpose of providing timely clinical evidence into the clinical workflow. Although not specific to nursing informatics, the National Institutes of Health provides awards under its Clinical and Translational Science Award (CTSA) program to accelerate the transfer of research to the clinical setting (National Institutes of Health, 2009). The Quality and Safety Education in Nursing initiative (Cronenwett et al., 2009) cites key competencies (knowledge and skills) in both EBP and informatics.

As an example of the integration of informatics and the medical record, Matter (2006) describes the positive effects of a successful integration of referential links with EBP clinical content in the clinical pathway on patient outcomes. The pilot started in 2005 at Pinnacle Health in Pennsylvania involved two vendors, and combined the use of the electronic medical record with evidence-based electronic reference links to create a point of care tool that allowed clinicians to combine nursing care plans supported by the corresponding evidential link. Gains in the development of institutional guidelines, clinical collaboration, and 76% compliance with pain assessment 2 hours after administration were realized.

With the goal of promoting the use of research findings and tool use based on these findings, the **Agency for Healthcare Research and Quality** (AHRQ) became an active participant in pushing evidence forward into practice. The AHRQ is a government-sponsored organization with the mission of reducing patient risk from harm, decreasing healthcare cost, and improving patient outcomes through the promotion of research and technology applications focused on EBP. In 1999, AHRQ implemented its Translating Research into Practice Initiative (TRIP) to generate knowledge about evidence-based care (Agency for Healthcare Research and Quality, 2001). In the second Translating Research into Practice Initiative (TRIP-II), the focus was on improving the health care of the underserved and using information technology to affect translational research and health policy. AHRQ, in partnership with the American Medical Association and the American Association of Health Plans, developed the **National Guideline Clearinghouse** (NGC). NGC is a comprehensive database of evidentially based clinical practice guidelines and related documents that are regularly published through the NGC electronic mailing list and are available on the NGC website (National Guideline

Clearinghouse, 2010). The NGC website allows users to browse the website for the clinical guidelines, view abstracts and full-text links, download full-text clinical guidelines to PDA devices, obtain technical reports, and compare guidelines.

In addition, there are a growing number of printed and electronic resources available to assist in creating guidelines and offering information about EBP. A sampling of existing websites is shown in Table 27-1.

TABLE 27-1
The Role of Informatics: Online Evidence-Based Resources

Website	Description
Academic Center for Evidence-Based Practice (ACE) website: http://www.acestar.uthscsa.edu	The School of Nursing at the University of Texas Health Science Center at San Antonio sponsors the Academic Center for Evidence-Based Practice. The Center's ultimate goal is to bring research to practice to improve patient care, outcomes, and safety. The center is also home to the ACE Star model of Knowledge Transformation.
The Agency for Healthcare Research and Quality www.ahrq.gov	The agency for Healthcare Research and Quality contains a wealth of information regarding healthcare quality. There is no charge for access to the site or its resources.
BMJ Publishing http://www.bmjpg.com	The BMJ publishing group provides clinical databases by prescription. The BMJ Clinical Evidence site allows the download of some clinical papers and some interesting risk tools without charge.
The Center for Evidence-Based Practices (CEBP). http://www.evidencebasedpractices.org	The Center for Evidence Based Practices of the Orelena Hawks Puckett Institute focuses on research to practice initiatives related to early intervention, early childhood education, parent and family support, and family-centered practices.
Centre for Evidence Based Medicine. http://www.cebm.net	The Center for Evidence Based Medicine, located in Oxford in the UK, is devoted to developing and promoting evidence based resources for healthcare professionals. In addition to free articles the site also provides free teaching resources and presentation.
Cinahl http://cinahl.com	CINAHL information systems offers a multitude of online services, which include website link sources, CINAHL'S online nursing and allied health database, document delivery, and search services.
The Cochrane Collaboration http://www.cochrane.org	The Cochrane Collaboration provides reviews for free, but full-text articles are by subscription.
Entrez PubMed http://www.ncbi.nim.nih.gov/sites/entrez	Entrez PubMed is a service provided by The National Library of Medicine (NLM). The NLM was developed by the National Center for Biotechnology Information (NCBI), which provides access to life science journals and MEDLINE citations. Some of the journal links are free and some require a subscription.
PubMed Central http://www.pubmedcentral.nih.gov	PubMed Central (PMC) is a free digital archive of science-related articles managed by the NCBI. BioMed Central (an open-source online archive) may be accessed here.

Continues

TABLE 27-1
The Role of Informatics: Online Evidence-Based Resources—*continued*

Website	Description
The Joanna Briggs Institute http://www.joannabriggs.edu.au/about/home.php	The Joanna Briggs Institute was established in 1996 as a resource for best care practices. Joanna Briggs was first matron of the Adelaide Hospital in Australia and is recognized for her financial and organizational support. The Joanna Briggs Institute is a leader in developing evidence-based practices.
Information & Resources for Nurses Worldwide http://www.nurses.info/specialty_evidenced_based_orgs.htm	This website provides searchable links to evidence based practice organizations by specialty.
The Iowa Model of Evidence-Based Practice. http://www.uihealthcare.com/depts/nursing/rqom/evidencebasedpractice/iowamodel.html	This website provides a brief overview of the Iowa Model for Evidence Based Practice.
The Johns Hopkins Bloomberg School of Public Health http://www.jhsph.edu/epc	The Johns Hopkins Evidence Based Practice Center was established in 1997 and is one of 14 such centers producing comprehensive, systematic reviews for the AHRQ.
Trip Database. http://www.tripdatabase.com	Clinical search tool to allow clinicians to identify the best evidence for clinical practice.
University of Iowa College of Nursing http://www.nursing.uiowa.edu/consumers_patients/evidence_based.htm	The John A. Hartford Foundation Center of Geriatric Nursing Excellence at the University of Iowa has evidence based practice resources available at this site for a nominal fee.
World Views on Evidence-Based Nursing http://blackwellpublishing.com/wvn	Through Blackwell Publishing, this magazine, sponsored by Sigma Theta Tau, is dedicated exclusively to evidence-based nursing articles. The magazine is also offered online by subscription.

DEVELOPING EBP GUIDELINES

There have been several models developed to guide organizations into translating research into practice. Brief descriptions of the models are listed in Table 27-2. As an example, Titler (2007) identifies the steps in the Iowa model for translating research into practice as (1) identifying the problem, issue, or topic in nursing practice; (2) research and critique of related evidence; (3) adaptation of the evidence to practice; (4) implementation of the EBP; and (5) evaluation of patient outcomes and care practices. Careful analysis and discussion of the research or other forms of evidence in this scenario may reveal that given the context, implementation may not be practical. Following implementation, results must be monitored to determine if the application works for the context. Thoughtful discussion of the findings helps the clinical team determine if further research is

TABLE 27-2
Comparison of Model Approaches to Evidence-Based Practice

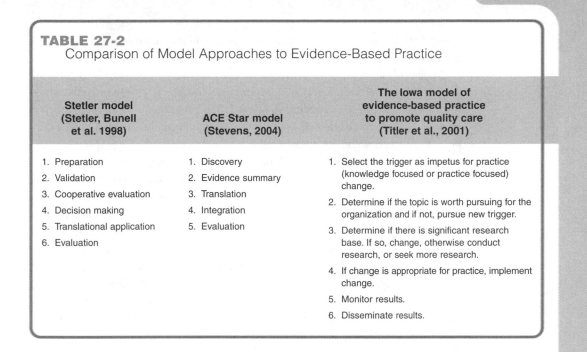

Stetler model (Stetler, Bunell et al. 1998)	ACE Star model (Stevens, 2004)	The Iowa model of evidence-based practice to promote quality care (Titler et al., 2001)
1. Preparation	1. Discovery	1. Select the trigger as impetus for practice (knowledge focused or practice focused) change.
2. Validation	2. Evidence summary	2. Determine if the topic is worth pursuing for the organization and if not, pursue new trigger.
3. Cooperative evaluation	3. Translation	3. Determine if there is significant research base. If so, change, otherwise conduct research, or seek more research.
4. Decision making	4. Integration	4. If change is appropriate for practice, implement change.
5. Translational application	5. Evaluation	5. Monitor results.
6. Evaluation		6. Disseminate results.

warranted or if further change is needed. As a practical application, evidence-based standards for care are developed by hospitals to meet the American Nurses Association/American Nurses Credentialing Center standards for achieving Magnet hospital recognition.

Information technology is important in synthesizing the research regardless of the model. Bakken (2001) recommends (1) standardized nomenclature required for the electronic health record (standardized terminologies and structures); (2) digital sources of evidence; (3) standards that facilitate healthcare data exchange among heterogeneous systems; (4) informatics processes that support the acquisition and application of evidence to a specific clinical situation; and (5) informatics competencies (p. 1999). Bakken's recommendations encourage an infrastructure that creates a database of experiential clinical evidence.

META-ANALYSIS AND GENERATION OF KNOWLEDGE

Systematic reviews combine results from multiple primary investigations to obtain consensus on a specific area of research. Studies are discarded from the review if they are not considered sound, thereby creating a reliable end result. The strength of the systematic review is its ability to corroborate findings and reach consensus. Systematic reviews show the need for more research by revealing the areas where quantitative results may be lacking or minimal. Bias may occur if selected studies are inadequate, if all sources of evidence are not investigated, or if publications selected are not adequately diverse (Lipp, 2005).

Meta-analysis, a form of systematic review, uses statistical methods to combine the results of several studies (Cook, Mulrow, & Haynes, 1997). **Quantitative studies** are typically used. According to Glass (1976), meta-analysis is the statistical analysis of a large collection of analysis results from individual studies for the purpose of integrating the findings (p. 3).

Kraft (2006) describes the documentation search strategy for meta-analysis as beginning with the identification of the studies through a search of bibliographic databases, identification of meta-analysis articles that match search criteria, elimination of articles that do not match search criteria, review of the reference lists in the meta-analysis for other articles that may relate to the topic, and review of each article for the quality and content. Additional sources should include unpublished works, such as conferences and dissertation abstracts, with the goal of obtaining as many relevant articles as possible. Gregson, Meal, and Avis (2002) identify the steps of a meta-analysis as (1) defining the problem followed by protocol generation, (2) establishing study eligibility criteria followed by literature search, (3) identifying the heterogeneity of results of studies, (4) standardizing the data and statistically combining the results, and (5) conducting sensitivity testing to determine if the combined results are the same. The often-cited criticism of meta-analysis is that emphasis is on quantitative, not qualitative, studies. Additionally, the analysis is only as good as the studies used (Gregson et al.). Collection and dissemination of these meta-analysis and systematic reviews are available in paper and on the Internet, although many such databases require a subscription.

The term "open access" refers to a worldwide movement to make a library of knowledge available to anyone with Internet access. The **Open Access Initiative** came about in response to the tremendous cost of research library access. Libraries pay large fees for journal subscriptions and the richness of library references are limited to what the budget allows. The cost of keeping current with research has caused library subscriptions to decline (Yiotis, 2005). Open access adds to the controversy with some journals charging authors for publications, which in itself may provide a financial barrier to publication of this form.

According to Suber (2004), open access refers to digital literature that is available to anyone with Internet access free of charge. There are two vehicles for open access: archives and journals. Open access journals are generally peer reviewed and freely available. The publishers of open access journals do not charge the reader but obtain funds for publishing elsewhere. Open access journals may charge the author or depend on other forms of funding, such as donations, grants, and advertising, to publish.

SUMMARY

These are amazing times. Technology has taken us faster and further than we ever thought possible. Healthcare jobs have become more technical and more complicated. In some ways technology has increased the margin for error. Some will continue to rely on little scraps of paper and systematic methods to keep themselves and their patients safe. One who becomes so tied to these things closes their mind to new innovations. The evolving quality culture and patient safety are dragging healthcare workers forward. For the benefit of the patients, health care must move forward.

Collaboration, improved access to online libraries, research tool transparency, a common data language, organizational and informational support, and continued research are a short list of needed items to advance translational research. Repeat studies are needed to provide meaningful meta-analysis and systematic reviews. Technology advancement in the area of incorporating evidence into clinical tools must continue. Removing the barriers to knowledge-seeking behavior and providing access to evidential resources will promote knowledge and in the end improve patient outcomes.

In the era of EBP, one must continue to think critically about their actions. What is the science behind our interventions? Healthcare workers must no longer do things one way just because they have always been done that way. Research the problem; use evidence-based resources; critically select electronic and nonelectronic references; consolidate the research findings and combine and compare the conclusions; present the findings; and propose a solution. One may be the first to ask why, and may be a key player in making change happen.

THE FUTURE

Titler (2007) indicates that future priorities should include development of theoretical formulations to guide research and systematic reviews so that they may be grouped by organizational context (e.g., primary care, outpatient). Focus on other forms of research, such as qualitative research, should also be incorporated into systematic reviews.

Given the vast amounts of data, Bakken et al. (2008) identifies areas of focus for nursing informatics in knowledge representation, data management, analysis, and predictive modeling in genomic health care and the need for policies and procedures to protect acquisition, dissemination, privacy, data security and confidentiality, and education in these areas. Informatics support nursing practice, education of healthcare consumers, and patient and knowledge generation. The technology is available now to incorporate evidence into reference links in clinical care plans. Incorporation of personalized clinical desktops to allow each clinician to have appropriate references (similar to Internet ad bot technology) provided to them may be possible. Time, research, and technology will tell.

THOUGHT-PROVOKING Questions

1. Twelve-hour shifts are problematic for patient and nurse safety, and yet hospitals continue to keep the 12-hour shift schedule. In 2004, the Institute of Medicine (Board on Health Care Services & Institute of Medicine, 2004) published a report that referred to studies as early as 1988 that discussed the negative effects of rotating shifts on intervention accuracy. Workers with 12-hour shifts realized more fatigue than workers on 8-hour shifts. In another study done in Turkey by Ilhan, Durukan, Aras, Turkcuoglu, and Aygun (2006), factors relating to increased risk for injury were age of 24 or less, less than 4 years of nursing experience, working in the surgical intensive care units, and working for more than 8 hours. As a clinician reading these studies, what would your next step be?

2. The use of heparin versus saline to maintain the patency of peripheral intravenous catheters has been addressed in research for many years. The American Society of Health System Pharmacists (ASHSP) published a position paper in January 2006 (American Society of Health System Pharmacists, 2006) advocating its support of the use of 0.9% saline in the maintenance of peripheral catheters in nonpregnant adults. It seems surprising that their position paper references articles that advocate the use of saline over heparin dating from 1991. What do you believe are some of the barriers that would have caused this delay in implementation?

For a full suite of assignments and additional learning activities, use the access code located in the front of your book to visit this exclusive website: http://go.jblearning.com/mcgonigle. If you do not have an access code, you can obtain one at the site.

References

Academic Center for Evidence-Based Practice. Retrieved from http://www.acestar.uthscsa.edu

Agency for Healthcare Research and Quality. (2001). *AHRQ profile: Quality research for quality health care.* Retrieved from http://www.ahrq.gov/about/profile.htm

American Society of Health System Pharmacists. (2006). ASHSP therapeutic position statement on the institutional use of 0.9% sodium chloride injection to maintain patency of peripheral indwelling intermittent infusion devices. *American Journal of Health System Pharmacy, 63,* 1273–1275.

Bakken, S. (2001). An informatics infrastructure is essential for evidence-based practice. *Journal of American Medical Informatics Association, 8,* 199–201.

Bakken, S., Stone, P.W., & Larson, E.L. (2008). A nursing informatics research agenda for 2008-18; Contextual influences and key components. *Nursing Outlook, 56,* 206–214.

Baumann, S. (2010). The limitations of evidence-based practice. *Nursing Science Quarterly, 23*(3) 226–230.

Board on Health Care Services & Institute of Medicine. (2004). *Keeping patients safe.* Washington, DC: The National Academies Press.

Camus, A. (1943). *The stranger.* London, United Kingdom: Penguin.

Cochrane, A.L. (1972) *Effectiveness and efficiency: Random reflections on health services.* London: Nuffield Provincial Hospitals Trust.

Cook, D. J., Mulrow, C. D., & Haynes, R. B. (1997). Systematic reviews: Synthesis of best evidence for clinical decisions. *Annals of Internal Medicine, 126*(5), 376–380.

Cronenwett, L., Sherwood, G., Pohl, J., Barnsteiner, J., Moore, S., Sullivan, D., Ward, D., & Warren, J. (2009). Quality and safety education for advanced nursing practice. *Nursing Outlook, 57*(6), 338–348.

Dickersin, K., & Manheimer, E. (1998). The Cochrane Collaboration: Evaluation of health care services using systematic reviews of the results and randomized control trials. *Clinical Obstetrics and Gynecology, 41*(2), 315–331.

Estabrooks, C. A., Floyd, J. A., Scott-Findlay, S., O'Leary, K. A., & Gushta, M. (2003). Individual determinants of research utilization: A systematic review. *Journal of Advanced Nursing, 42,* 73–81.

Fawcett, J., Watson, J., Walker, P. H., & Fitzpatrick, J. J. (2001). On nursing theories and evidence. *Journal of Nursing Scholarship, 33*(2), 115–119.

French, P. (2002). What is the evidence on evidence-based nursing? An epistemological concern. *Journal of Advanced Nursing, 37*(3), 250–257.

Giuse, N. B., Koonce, T. Y., Jerome, R. N., Gahall, M., Sathe, N. A., & Williams, A. (2005). Evolution of a mature clinical informationist model. *Journal of the American Medical Informatics Association, 12*(3), 249–255.

Glass, G. V. (1976). Primary, secondary and meta-analysis of research. *Educational Research, 5*(10), 3–8.

Goode, C. J., & Piedalue, F. (1999). Evidence-based clinical practice. *Journal of Nursing Administration, 29*(6), 15–21.

Gregson, P. R., Meal, A. G., & Avis, M. (2002). Meta-analysis: The glass eye of evidence-based practice? *Nursing Inquiry, 9*(1), 24–30.

Ilhan, M. N., Durukan, E., Aras, E., Turkcuoglu, S., & Aygun, R. (2006). Long working hours increase the risk of sharp and needlestick injury in nurses: A need for new policy implication. *Journal of Advanced Nursing, 56*(5), 563–568.

Joanna Briggs Institute. (n.d.). *Joanna Briggs Institute.* Retrieved from http://www.joannabriggs.edu .au/cqrmg/about.html

Kirchhoff, K. T. (2004). State of the science of translational research: From demonstration projects to intervention testing. *Worldviews on Evidence-Based Nursing 1*(S1), S6–S12.

Kraft, M. R. (2006). Meta-analysis: A research tool. *SCI Nursing Journal, 23*(2). Retrieved from http:// www.unitedspinal.org/publications/nursing/2006/08/27/research-corner/

Lipp, A. (2005). The systematic review as an evidence-based tool for the operating room. *Associate of Operating Room Nurses Journal, 81*(6), 1279–1287.

Matter, S. (2006). Empower nurses with evidence-based knowledge. *Nurse Management, 37*(12), 34–37.

McCaughan, D., Thompson, C., Cullum, N., Sheldon, T. A., & Thompson, D. R. (2002). Acute care nurses' perceptions of barriers to using research information in clinical decision-making. *Journal of Advanced Nursing, 39*(1), 46–60.

McKnight, M. (2006). The information seeking of on-duty critical care nurses: Evidence from participant observation and in-context interviews. *Journal of the Medical Library Association, 94*(2), 145–151.

Melnyk, B. M. (2005). Advancing evidence-based practice in clinical and academic settings. *Worldviews on Evidence-Based Nursing, 3,* 161–165.

Melnyk, B. M., Fineout-Overholt, E., Stetler, C., & Allen, J. (2005). Outcomes and implementation strategies from the first U.S. evidence-based practice leadership summit. *Worldviews on Evidence-Based Nursing, 2*(3), 113–121.

Melnyk, B. M., Fineout-Overholt, E., Stillwell, S., Williamson, K. (2009). Igniting a spirit of inquiry: An essential foundation for evidence-based practice. *American Journal of Nursing, 109*(11), 49–52.

Melnyk, B. M., Fineout-Overholt, E., Stone, P., & Ackerman, M. (2000). Evidence-based practice: The past, the present, and recommendations for the millennium. *Pediatric Nursing, 26*(1), 77–80.

National Guideline Clearinghouse. (2010). *National guideline clearinghouse.* Retrieved from http://www.guideline.gov/

National Institutes of Health. (2009). *Re-engineering the clinical research enterprise.* Retrieved from http://commonfund.nih.gov/clinicalresearch/overview-translational.asp

O'Neill, T., Jinks, C., & Ong, B. N. (2007). Decision-making regarding total knee replacement surgery: A qualitative meta-synthesis. *BMC Health Services Research, 7*(52). Retrieved from http://www.pubmedcentral.nih.gov/articlerender.fcgi?artid=1854891

Polit, D. F., & Beck, T. C. (2008). *Nursing research: Generating and assessing evidence for nursing practice* (8th ed.). Philadelphia, PA: Lippincott Williams & Wilkins.

Pravikoff, D. S., Tanner, A. B., & Pierce, S. T. (2005). Readiness of U.S. nurses for evidence-based practice. *American Journal of Nursing, 105*(9), 40–51.

Rycroft-Malone, J., Seers, K., Titchen, A., Harvey, G., Kitson, A., & McCormack, B. (2004). What counts as evidence in evidence-based practice? *Journal of Advanced Nursing, 47*(1), 81–90.

Saba, V. K., & McCormick, K. A. (2006). *Essentials of nursing informatics* (4th ed.). New York, NY: McGraw-Hill.

Sackett, D. I., Rosenberg, W.M., Gray, J.A., Haynes, R.B., Richardon, W.S. (1996). Evidence based medicine: What it is and what it isn't. *British Medical Journal 312,* 71–72.

Scott-Findlay, S., & Pollock, C. (2004). Evidence, research, knowledge: A call for conceptual clarity. *Worldwideviews on Evidence-Based Nursing, 1*(2), 92–97.

Stetler, C. B. (2001). Updating the Stetler model of research utilization to facilitate evidence-based practice. *Nursing Outlook, 49*(6), 272–279.

Stetler, C. B., Brunell, M., Giuliano, K. K., Morse, D., Prince, L., & Newell-Stokes, V. (1998). Evidence-based practice and the role of nursing leadership. *Journal of Nursing Administration, 28*(7/8), 45–53.

Stetler, C. B., Morsi, D., Rucki, S., Broughton, S., Corrigan, B., Fitzgerald, J., et al. (1998). Utilization-focused integrative reviews of nursing service. *Applied Nursing Research, 11*(4), 195–206.

Stevens, K. R. (2004). *ACE star model of EBP: Knowledge transformation.* Retrieved from http://www.acestar.uthscsa.edu/Learn_model.htm

Suber, P. (2004). *A very brief introduction to open access.* Retrieved from http://www.earlham.edu/~peters/fos/brief.htm

The Cochrane Collaboration. (2004). *Bridging the gaps across the income divide: A review of the Collaboration's efforts to date and recommendations for the future.* Retrieved from http://www2.cochrane.org/colloquia/abstracts/ottawa/O-006.htm

Titler, M. (2007). Translating research into practice: Models for changing clinician behavior. *American Journal of Nursing, 107*(6), 26–33.

Titler, M. G. (2004). Methods in translation science. *Worldviews on evidence-based nursing, 1,* 38–48.

Titler, M. G. (2010). Translation science and context. *Research Theory and Nursing Practice: An International Journal, 24*(1), 35–55.

Titler, M. G., Kleiber, C., Steelman, V., Rakel, B., Budreu, G., Everett, L., et al. (2001). The Iowa model of evidence-based practice to promote quality care. *Critical Care Nursing Clinics of North America, 13*(4), 497–509.

Woolf, S. H. (2008). The meaning of translational research and why it matters. *Journal of the American Medical Association, 299*(2), 211–213.

Yiotis, K. (2005). The Open Access Initiative: A new paradigm for scholarly communications. *Information Technology & Libraries, 24*(4), 157–162.

Imagining the Future of Nursing Informatics

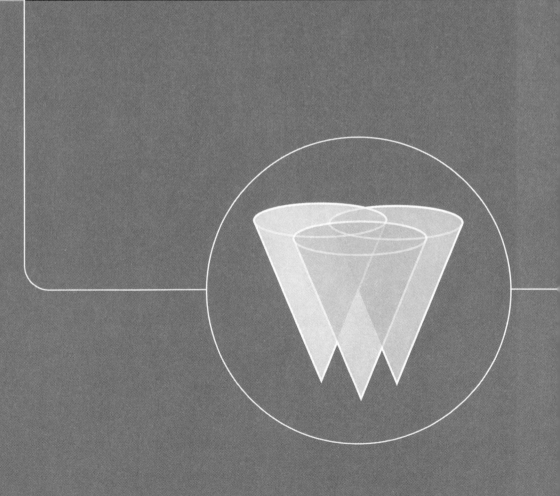

Nursing informatics is the synthesis of nursing science, information science, computer science, and cognitive science to manage and enhance healthcare data, information, knowledge, and wisdom for the dual betterment of patient care and the nursing profession. After reading the first five sections of this book, one should have a good idea of the current state of the science of nursing informatics. This final section helps the reader think about the future. The reader should envision his or her current practice setting and the nursing informatics applications he or she uses. What will come next? What should come next?

The material within this book is placed within the context of the Foundation of Knowledge model (Figure VI-1) to meet the needs of healthcare delivery sys-

FIGURE VI-1 Foundation of Knowledge model.

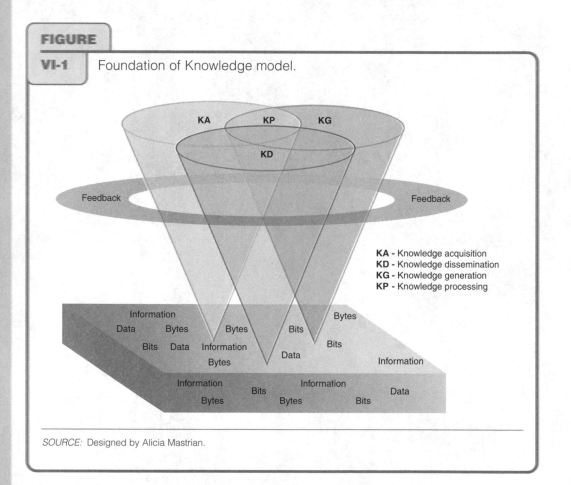

KA - Knowledge acquisition
KD - Knowledge dissemination
KG - Knowledge generation
KP - Knowledge processing

SOURCE: Designed by Alicia Mastrian.

tems, organizations, patients, and nurses. The first chapter, "Nursing Science and the Foundation of Knowledge Model," provides a thorough overview of the Foundation of Knowledge model, thus providing a framework that embraces knowledge so that readers can develop the wisdom necessary to apply what they have learned. Wisdom is the application of knowledge to an appropriate situation. In the practice of nursing science, one expects action or actions directed by wisdom. Wisdom uses knowledge and experience to heighten common sense and insight, allowing one to exercise sound judgment in practical matters. Wisdom is developed through knowledge, experience, insight, and reflection. Wisdom is sometimes thought of as the highest form of common sense resulting from accumulated knowledge or erudition (deep thorough learning) or enlightenment (education that results in understanding and the dissemination of knowledge). Wisdom is the ability to apply valuable and viable knowledge, experience, understanding, and insight while being prudent and sensible. Knowledge and wisdom are not synonymous because knowledge abounds with others' thoughts and information, whereas wisdom is focused on one's own mind and the synthesis of one's own experience, insight, understanding, and knowledge.

Reflect on the model while reading through this final section. The reader is challenged to ask, "How can I use my wisdom to help create the theories, tools, and knowledge of the future?"

CHAPTER 28

Bioinformatics, Biomedical Informatics, and Computational Biology

Dee McGonigle and Kathleen Mastrian

Objectives

1. Describe bioinformatics, biomedical informatics, and computational biology.
2. Appreciate the intertwining of bioinformatics and health care in biomedical informatics.
3. Imagine the future of health care based on genomics.

www

Key Terms

www

Allele
Bioinformatics
Biomedical informatics
Computational biology
Data set
Genome
Genomics
Haplotype
Human Genome Project
Informaticist

INTRODUCTION

The National Center for Biotechnology Information (NCBI) (2004a) states that "Biology in the 21st century is being transformed from a purely lab-based science to an information science as well" (para. 5). What must be remembered when delving into the new informatics frontier is that biologic systems are information systems. Consider that DNA essentially is a storehouse of information. Unlocking that information and learning how that information is transcribed to RNA and ultimately expressed as proteins promises interesting and cutting-edge developments in understanding diseases and managing them at the molecular level. This chapter introduces the reader to the exciting world of bioinformatics and provides a beginning understanding of the frontiers unleashed by the collection, mapping, storage, and sharing of genetic data.

BIOINFORMATICS, BIOMEDICAL INFORMATICS AND COMPUTATIONAL BIOLOGY DEFINED

Three terms are frequently used: (1) **bioinformatics**, (2) **biomedical informatics**, and (3) **computational biology**. As terms continue to be bandied about, it is important to comprehend what they mean to understand better these evolving fields. University of Texas at El Paso (2010) believes that "Bioinformatics is an interdisciplinary science with a focus on data management and interpretation for complex biological phenomena that are analyzed and visualized using mathematical modeling and numerical methodologies with predictive algorithms" (para. 1). University of Minnesota (2010) states

Bioinformatics is defined here as an interdisciplinary research area that applies computer and information science to solve biological problems. However, this is not the only definition. The field is being defined (and redefined) at present, and there are probably as many definitions as there are bioinformaticians (bioinformaticists?) (para. 1).

They identify the myriad of definitions for the "moving target named bioinformatics" (University of Minnesota, 2010, para. 2) that are reflected in those developed from 2000 to 2009. According to NCBI (2004a), "Bioinformatics is the field of science in which biology, computer science, and information technology merge to form a single discipline. The ultimate goal of the field is to enable the discovery of new biological insights" (para. 5). Network Science (2009) believes that

An absolute definition of bioinformatics has not been agreed upon. The first level, however, can be defined as the design and application of methods for the collection, organization, indexing, storage, and analysis of biological sequences (both nucleic acids [DNA and RNA] and proteins). The next stage of bioinformatics is the derivation of knowledge concerning the pathways, functions, and interactions of these genes (functional genomics) and proteins (proteomics) (para. 14).

Mulligen et al. (2008) wrote that

BioInformatics (BI) is a less mature scientific discipline which aims to research and develop algorithms, computational and statistical techniques which solve biological problems. Significantly, BI has experienced an exponential growth as a result of its importance to the understanding and interpretation of data generated by 'omics' technologies (para. 6).

The complete sequencing of the human genome has led to systems biology referred to as "omics" and has elevated scientists' ability from studying one gene or protein to being able to study fundamental biologic processes (Box 28-1).

National Human Genome Research Institute (NHGRI) (n.d.) tutorial on bioinformatics defines it as "the branch of biology that is concerned with the acquisition, storage, display, and analysis of the information found in nucleic acid and protein sequence data. Computers and bioinformatics software are the tools of the trade" (para. 4). Based on these definitions, one can get a flavor for what bioinformatics entails. It is clear that the definition for bioinformatics varies and there is not one definition that everyone agrees on at the present time.

Biomedicine applies bioinformatics to promote health. The Ohio State University Medical Center (2010) states that "Biomedical informatics is the study and process of efficiently gathering, storing, managing, retrieving, analyzing, communicating, sharing, and applying biomedical information to improve the

BOX

28-1

Omics

Kelly (2008) describes that "'ome' and 'omics' are suffixes that are derived from genome" (para. 1). National Public Radio (2010) credits botanist Hans Winkler with merging "the Greek words 'genesis' and 'soma' to describe a body of genes" (para. 1) in 1920. The term "genome" was born and genomics arose as the study of the genome.

Kelly (2008) continues to explain:

> Scientists like to append to these to any large-scale system (or really, just about anything complex), such as the collection of proteins in a cell or tissue (the proteome), the collection of metabolites (the metabolome), and the collection of RNA that's been transcribed from genes (the transcriptome). High-throughput analysis is essential considering data at the "omic" level, that is to say considering all DNA sequences, gene expression levels, or proteins at once (or, to be slightly more precise, a significant subset of them) (para. 1).

detection, prevention, and treatment of disease" (para. 2). Vanderbilt University (2010) believes that

> Biomedical Informatics is the interdisciplinary science of acquiring, structuring, analyzing and providing access to biomedical data, information and knowledge. As an academic discipline, biomedical informatics is grounded in the principles of computer science, information science, cognitive science, social science, and engineering, as well as the clinical and basic biological sciences (para. 1).

Gennari (2002) stated that, "Biomedical Informatics is the science underlying the acquisition, maintenance, retrieval, and application of biomedical knowledge and information to improve patient care, medical education, and health sciences research" (para. 1). He believes that "a primary feature of Biomedical and Health Informatics is its interdisciplinary nature: It connects computer science, medicine, biology and health care, and provides a synergy that goes beyond anything that researchers in any single domain can provide" (para. 3). According to Bioinformaticsweb.tk (2005), "Biomedical Informatics is an emerging discipline that has been defined as the study, invention, and implementation of structures and algorithms to improve communication, understanding and management of medical information" (para. 16). They go on to muddy the water with their description of bioinformatics.

Bioinformatics derives knowledge from computer analysis of biological data. These can consist of the information stored in the genetic code, but also experimental results from various sources, patient statistics, and scientific literature. Research in bioinformatics includes method development for storage, retrieval, and analysis of the data. Bioinformatics is a rapidly developing branch of biology and is highly interdisciplinary, using techniques and concepts from informatics, statistics, mathematics, chemistry, biochemistry, physics, and linguistics. It has many practical applications in different areas of biology and medicine (para. 1).

Biomedical informatics is a growing field, with significant applications and implications throughout the biomedical and clinical worlds. The authors believe that biomedical informatics is the application of bioinformatics to health care.

Computational biology is the action complement of bioinformatics and, therefore, biomedicine. NCBI (2004a) states that

Ultimately, however, all of this information must be combined to form a comprehensive picture of normal cellular activities so that researchers may study how these activities are altered in different disease states. Therefore, the field of bioinformatics has evolved such that the most pressing task now involves the analysis and interpretation of various types of data, including nucleotide and amino acid sequences, protein domains, and protein structures. The actual process of analyzing and interpreting data is referred to as computational biology. Important sub-disciplines within bioinformatics and computational biology include:

- the development and implementation of tools that enable efficient access to, and use and management of, various types of information
- the development of new algorithms (mathematical formulas) and statistics with which to assess relationships among members of large data sets, such as methods to locate a gene within a sequence, predict protein structure and/or function, and cluster protein sequences into families of related sequences (para. 6).

In 2000, the National Institutes of Health's (NIH) Biomedical Information Science and Technology Initiative Consortium defined bioinformatics and computational biology. They stated that "no definition could completely eliminate overlap with other activities or preclude variations in interpretation by different individuals and organizations" (NIH, 2000, para. 3). This consortium defined bioinformatics as "Research, development, or application of computational tools and approaches for expanding the use of biological, medical, behavioral or health data, including those to acquire, store, organize, archive, analyze, or visualize such data" (NIH, para. 4). The computational biology definition they derived was "The development and application of data-analytical and theoretical methods, mathematical modeling and computational simulation techniques to the study of biological, behavioral, and social systems (NIH, para. 5).

Bioinformatics tools help biomedical **informaticists** and healthcare personnel tackle the analysis of large **data sets**. The authors believe that biomedical informatics uses bioinformatics, whereas computational biology is their action complement. Therefore, using bioinformatics and computational biology to analyze and interpret intricate biologic events, biomedical informaticists promote health and improve patient care. Biomedical informatics and bioinformatics may seem similar but if one thinks of biomedical informatics as focusing on health care and patients, it helps distinguish between the two. Biomedical informaticists use bioinformatics methods to integrate large biologic and medical data sets to facilitate understanding of the human body and its biologic functioning; these efforts are geared toward improving health by defeating disease.

WHY ARE BIOINFORMATICS AND BIOMEDICAL INFORMATICS SO IMPORTANT?

The future of health care is based on **genomics**. Bioinformatics and computational biology have provided the tools to make it possible to analyze and interpret complex biologic processes. Through these developments, several projects have advanced understanding of the human **genome, haplotypes**, and the genomic changes related to disease.

In 2006, the Cancer Genome Atlas Project began (NHGRI, 2010). This "$100 million pilot will map the genomic changes in brain, lung and ovarian cancers to assess the feasibility of a full-scale effort to systematically explore the entire spectrum of genomic changes involved in every major type of human cancer" (para. 1). The goal of this project is to develop a "resource that will be used to develop new strategies for preventing, diagnosing and treating the disease" (para. 1).

The goal of the International HapMap Project (2006) is to

> develop a haplotype map of the human genome, the HapMap, which will describe the common patterns of human DNA sequence variation. The HapMap is expected to be a key resource for researchers to use to find genes affecting health, disease, and responses to drugs and environmental factors. The information produced by the Project will be made freely available (para. 1).

This international partnership of scientists has taken blood samples from clusters of related people, such as parents and children, from different international regions and from these samples they have been able to catalog some of the common variations in their DNA and investigate inherited **alleles**. As the name implies, haplotype map refers to a set of closely linked alleles on a chromosome that tend to be inherited together. The International HapMap Project states

> Most common diseases, such as diabetes, cancer, stroke, heart disease, depression, and asthma, are affected by many genes and environmental factors.

Although any two unrelated people are the same at about 99.9% of their DNA sequences, the remaining 0.1% is important because it contains the genetic variants that influence how people differ in their risk of disease or their response to drugs. Discovering the DNA sequence variants that contribute to common disease risk offers one of the best opportunities for understanding the complex causes of disease in humans (para. 3).

A major contribution has been the **Human Genome Project** (HGP), which began in 1990 and was completed in 2003 (Human Genome Program, 2010). The US Department of Energy and the NIH coordinated this program, which was designed to

- Identify all the approximately 20,000–25,000 genes in human DNA,
- Determine the sequences of the 3 billion chemical base pairs that make up human DNA,
- Store this information in databases,
- Improve tools for data analysis,
- Transfer related technologies to the private sector, and
- Address the ethical, legal, and social issues (ELSI) that may arise from the project (para. 2).

According to NHGRI (n.d.),

it was understood that to meet the project's goals, the speed of DNA sequencing would have to increase and the cost would have to come down. Over the life of the project virtually every aspect of DNA sequencing was improved. It took the project approximately four years to sequence its first one billion bases but just four months to sequence the second billion bases (para. 1).

During the month of January, 2003, 1.5 billion bases were sequenced. As the speed of DNA sequencing increased, the cost decreased from 10 dollars per base in 1990 to 10 cents per base at the conclusion of the project in April, 2003 (para. 2).

One of the most important aspects of bioinformatics is identifying genes within a long DNA sequence. Until the development of bioinformatics, the only way to locate genes along the chromosome was to study their function in the organism (in vivo) or isolate the DNA and study it in a test tube (in vitro). Bioinformatics allows scientists to make educated guesses about where genes are located simply by analyzing sequence data using a computer (in silico) (para. 8).

The other major piece brought out through the HGP was the realization that ethical, legal, and social issues (ESLI) arise from studying human genomes. They set aside a percentage of their annual budgets to research ESLI (HGP, 2008). Refer to Box 28-2 for questions raised regarding ESLI.

BOX

28-2

ESLI Questions Raised by the HGP

Who should have access to personal genetic information, and how will it be used?

Who owns and controls genetic information?

How does personal genetic information affect an individual and society's perceptions of that individual?

How does genomic information affect members of minority communities?

Do healthcare personnel properly counsel parents about the risks and limitations of genetic technology?

How reliable and useful is fetal genetic testing?

What are the larger societal issues raised by new reproductive technologies?

How will genetic tests be evaluated and regulated for accuracy, reliability, and utility? (Currently, there is little regulation at the federal level.)

How do we prepare healthcare professionals for the new genetics?

How do we prepare the public to make informed choices?

How do we as a society balance current scientific limitations and social risk with long-term benefits?

Should testing be performed when no treatment is available?

Should parents have the right to have their minor children tested for adult-onset diseases?

Are genetic tests reliable and interpretable by the medical community?

Do people's genes make them behave in a particular way?

Can people always control their behavior?

What is considered acceptable diversity?

Where is the line between medical treatment and enhancement?

Are genetically modified foods and other products safe to humans and the environment?

How will these technologies affect developing nations' dependence on the West?

Who owns genes and other pieces of DNA?

Will patenting DNA sequences limit their accessibility and development into useful products?

SOURCE: Human Genome Program. (2008). *Human Genome Project information: Ethical, legal, and social issues.* Retrieved from http://www.ornl.gov/sci/techresources/Human_Genome/elsi/elsi.shtml

Even though the HGP has ended, researchers are continuing to make improvements in DNA sequencing. They are advancing the bioinformatics and computational biology tools that are used in biomedical informatics. However, as Butte (2008) laments, "There is an absolute paucity of people trained to make use of these resources, to build the infrastructure, to ask these novel questions, and to even answer these questions" (p. 173).

These three projects are pivotal in genomics. The HGP focused on the DNA sequence from a single individual, the HapMap project focused on variation in the genome and on human populations, and the Cancer Genome Atlas Project is concerned with how cancer affects the genomes. As a result of these seminal projects, and a unique culture of data sharing unknown to date among biologic researchers, molecular data and measurement tools are now publicly available. Two examples of publicly available databases are the Gene Expression Omnibus maintained by the National Center for Biotechnology Information at the National Library of Medicine and ArrayExpress maintained by the European Bioinformatics Institute (Butte, 2008). As new researchers with both biology and computational expertise emerge, bioinformatics and computational biology projects will contribute new insights into disease mechanisms and therapeutic interventions.

WHAT DOES THE FUTURE HOLD?

It will take many more years of researching and applying bioinformatics and computational biology before the information in the human genome is understood in detail. Because these applications have the ability to allow one to analyze and interpret complex biologic processes, researchers are on the path to understanding the etiology of disease and of treatment interventions at the molecular level. Consider a typical day on any clinical unit. The advanced practice nurse who wants to prescribe a drug for a patient begins by reviewing the patient's genetic test results. The advanced practice nurse knows that this information must be assessed before prescribing so that the drug will treat the patient's illness successfully without harmful side effects. The patient will receive only the medication that he or she needs, and one that is designed to interfere with or enhance the specific molecular processes that are the signature for the patient's particular health challenge. The advances that bioinformatics and biomedical informatics promise will dramatically impact healthcare delivery as it is known. As explained by Rajappa, Sharma, and Saxena (2004),

> Understanding molecular mechanisms lead to better classification of disease and better management. A drop of blood from hypertensive patient gives gene expression profile by cDNA microarray analysis. It may reveal [Single Nucleotide Polymorphisms] SNPs related to hypertension and others which predispose a patient to diabetes mellitus or myocardial infarction and the clinician can determine which drugs are beneficial and which are harmful. This scenario has a whale of difference from the current 'trial and error' method of matching a patient with antihypertensives (p. 128).

Nurses can be involved in bioinformatics in many ways, including as nurse researchers helping to map molecular processes, and as educators and advocates helping patients and families to understand these complex biologic processes. For more information about the emerging roles of nurses in this exciting new field, visit the website of the International Society of Nurses in Genetics (http://www.isong.org/index.php).

SUMMARY

The focus of this book is on nursing informatics, but one can clearly see the connection between biomedical informatics and nursing informatics. The discipline of bioinformatics and its use in biomedical informatics epitomizes the junction of computer science, information science, computational biology, and health care. These new applications deal with the resources, devices, strategies, and methods needed to optimize the acquisition, processing, storage, retrieval, generation, and use of information in health and biomedicine. Biomedicine and its applications of bioinformatics support and manage all healthcare behaviors. It impacts how clinicians deliver health care to the infirmed, prevent disease, promote health, conduct research, and provide formal education for entry-level practitioners and continuing education for those who are currently practicing. This era of biomedical informatics, bioinformatics capabilities coupled with health care, includes informatics and computational biology algorithms and tools and clinical guidelines. It can be applied to the areas of nursing, pharmacy, laboratory, dentistry, medicine, and public health. Those living the profession of nursing know that the practice of nursing is intertwined with the management and processing of information including the new knowledge being generated by biomedical informatics.

On the biomedical side of informatics, one must be cognizant of the fact that medical data typically are extracted from personal, confidential, and legally protected medical records. The protection of human subjects must be paramount and all ESLI issues must be addressed.

Biomedical informatics provides knowledge about the effects of DNA disparities among individuals. Being able to study human genomes and biologic processing at the molecular level will revolutionize how care is diagnosed and provided. It is helping to prevent disease. If one can better understand an organism's biologic processes and genetic coding, one can better prevent or treat its attack on patients. Clinical care as it is known will change; it will become genomics based.

THOUGHT-PROVOKING
Question

WWW

After reading this chapter, one knows that the study of genomics is helping clinicians to understand better the interaction between genes and the environment. This new information and knowledge will continue to help clinicians find ways to improve health and prevent disease. How do you envision patient care will change based on genomics in 10 years, 20 years, or 50 years in the future?

For a full suite of assignments and additional learning activities, use the access code located in the front of your book to visit this exclusive website: http://go.jblearning.com/mcgonigle. If you do not have an access code, you can obtain one at the site.

WWW

References

Bioinformaticsweb.tk. (2005). *Bioinformatics resource portal: Bioinformatics definition*. Retrieved from http://bioinformaticsweb.net/definition.html

Butte, A. (2008). *Translational bioinformatics: Coming of age. Journal of the American Medical Informatics Association, 15*(6), 709–714. Retrieved from CINAHL database.

Gennari, J. (2002). *Biomedical informatics defined*. Retrieved from http://faculty.washington.edu/gennari/MedicalInformaticsDef.html

Human Genome Program. (2008). *Human Genome Project information: Ethical, legal, and social issues*. Retrieved from http://www.ornl.gov/sci/techresources/Human_Genome/elsi/elsi.shtml

Human Genome Program. (2010). *Human Genome Project information*. Retrieved from http://www.ornl.gov/sci/techresources/Human_Genome/home.shtml

International HapMap Project. (2006). *About the International HapMap Project*. Retrieved from http://hapmap.ncbi.nlm.nih.gov/abouthapmap.html

International Society of Nurses in Genetics (ISONG). (2010). *Welcome to ISONG*. Retrieved from http://www.isong.org/index.php

Kelly, R. (2008). *What are "omics" technologies?* Retrieved from http://www.reagank.com/2007/03/what_are_omics_technologies.php

Mulligen, E., Cases, M., Hettne, K., Molero, E., Weeber, M., Robertson, K., . . . Maojo, V. (2008). *Training multidisciplinary biomedical informatics students: Three years of experience. J Am Med Inform Assoc, 15*(2): 246–254. PMCID: PMC2274784. doi: 10.1197/jamia.M2488. Retrieved from http://www.ncbi.nlm.nih.gov/pmc/articles/PMC2274784/?tool=pubmed

National Center for Biotechnology Information. (2004a). *Bioinformatics*. Retrieved from http://www.ncbi.nlm.nih.gov/About/primer/bioinformatics.html

National Center for Biotechnology Information. (2004b). *Tools for data mining*. Retrieved from http://www.ncbi.nlm.nih.gov/About/tools/restable_data.html

National Human Genome Research Institute. (2010). *2006: The Cancer Genome Atlas (TCGA) Project started.* Retrieved from http://www.genome.gov/25520505

National Human Genome Research Institute. (n.d.) *NHGRI: Understanding the Human Genome Project CD-ROM: Mining the genome using bioinformatics (tutorial).* Retrieved as a tutorial download from http://www.genome.gov/19519278#al-5

National Institute of Health (NIH). (2000). *NIH working definition of bioinformatics and computational biology.* Retrieved from http://www.bisti.nih.gov/docs/CompuBioDef.pdf

National Public Radio. (2010). *Where the word genome came from.* Retrieved from http://www.npr.org/templates/story/story.php?storyId=128410577

Network Science – NetSci. (2009). *Terms and definitions in bioinformatics.* Retrieved from http://www.netsci.org/Science/Bioinform/terms.html

Ohio State University Medical Center. (2010). *College of Medicine, School of Biomedical Science: Biomedical informatics.* Retrieved from http://biomed.osu.edu/bmi/index.cfm

Rajappa, M., Sharma, A., & Saxena, A. (2004). *Bioinformatics and its implications in clinical medicine: A review. International Medical Journal, 11*(2), 125–129. Retrieved from CINAHL database.

Stanford University (n.d.). *The Stanford Center for Biomedical Informatics Research (BMIR).* Retrieved from http://bmir.stanford.edu/#one

University of Minnesota. (2010). *What is bioinformatics?* Retrieved from http://www.binf.umn.edu/about/whatsbinf.php

University of Texas at El Paso. (2010). *College of Science: Bioinformatics.* Retrieved from http://www.bioinformatics.utep.edu/

Vanderbilt University. (2010). *Department of biomedical informatics.* Retrieved from http://dbmi.mc.vanderbilt.edu/

CHAPTER 29

Emerging Technologies and the Generation of Knowledge

Peter J. Murray and W. Scott Erdley

Objectives

1. Outline the history of technology development and informatics applications.
2. Describe some of today's state-of-the-art technologies.
3. Predict the evolution of technology and its impact on knowledge generation in nursing.

WWW

The future is here. It's just not evenly distributed...
(William Gibson, novelist and visionary)

INTRODUCTION

Anyone foolhardy enough to try to predict the future holds himself or herself hostage to fortune as soon as the words are on the page—or in the case of many people's ways of writing today, as the data have been saved to the hard drive, flash drive, Google doc, iPad, cloud storage, or other medium. Many nursing colleagues have written about the future of nursing, and about the challenges and **changes** that will either affect nursing or that nursing might influence. The authors do not, therefore, claim to be doing anything radically new in this chapter; in the best tradition of "standing on the shoulders of giants" (especially in view of the increasing tendency of many to use tools, such as Google Scholar, for finding much of their literature), some of their works are used as a launch pad for explorations of the issues.

The authors have, for several years, been specifically working on projects and making conference presentations about some of the **emerging technologies** that are in both general, everyday use and in

Key Terms

WWW

Blogs
Change
Cloud storage
Electronic data interchange
Emerging technologies
Folksonomies
Futurologists
Genomics
Half-life of knowledge
HealthVault
Information mediator
Lab-on-a-chip device
Mobile e-health (mobile health, m-health)
Nanotechnology
Podcasts
Really simple syndication (RSS)
Relational databases
Social bookmarking
Social media
Social networking
Tags/tag clouds
Transistor
Transparent technology
Ubiquitous
Ubiquitous health (u-health)
Virtual peers
Virtual worlds

Continues

use and development within health care; and they have written and spoken at conferences about what the future might hold for nurses, nursing, and health care more generally. They were also fortunate, along with nursing colleagues from around the world, to be able to explore many of these issues during the NI2006 Post Congress conference (Murray, Park, Erdley, & Kim, 2007), from which they continue to draw and develop a number of the ideas and issues presented and discussed in this chapter.

This chapter presents an optimistic view of the future, one that some might say is unwarranted. It envisages a future with a high degree of continuing technologic development and general worldwide economic growth, and an absence of some of the possibilities that might bring much of the global infrastructure crashing down. The authors assume there will not be widespread global social breakdown; the predicted possible pandemics of avian and swine influenza, and other problems, will not happen; or catastrophic climate change will not produce as rapid effects as the worst prognostications suggest. However, the authors are aware many of these things could happen, to some degree or other.

Change is coming, and much of it is far enough advanced as to be virtually unavoidable. Demographic changes are occurring (changes to population age structures, increasing rates of dementia, crises in funding of health care and retirement) (Development Concepts and Doctrine Centre [DCDC], 2010) that will have a profound impact on all aspects of society, health, and care. Technology will not solve all future problems; some emerging technologies could create more problems than they solve. However, it is by having an awareness of likely and possible technologic developments that one can assess what impact they may have on the ways in which we work and live, and whether the many issues can be addressed.

Although not explicitly at each point addressing the four key areas of the Foundation of Knowledge model, the sections of this chapter do consider how emerging technologies may address the four areas of (1) knowledge acquisition, (2) knowledge processing, (3) knowledge generation, and (4) knowledge dissemination and feedback. We also do not focus explicitly on changes in health care and nursing technologies, but on the more general changes that might be adapted or adopted for use by nurses or within health care. The reader will also note that much of the "literature" cited is not from peer-reviewed academic journals, but rather from more popular or journalistic sources. Among major reasons for this are the rapidly evolving nature of the changes and discussions of the issues addressed, and the long lead-in time for scientific publication, which means that many of the issues have resulted in little scientific exploration.

One of the most important features for nursing informatics in the future, and one facing health care in general, is the vast amount of information available to everyone. Knowledge is growing exponentially (Siemens, 2005), and in many disciplines its useful life span can be measured in months, coupled with an ever-decreasing half-life (**half-life of knowledge** is the time span from when knowledge is gained to when it becomes obsolete). Many people believe there is now information overload; however, the present situation is nothing compared to the future amount of data and information that will have to be acquired, from new forms of patient monitoring, from advances in genomic medicine, and from the continuing explosion of knowledge generation and publishing. Additionally, all of the data and information need to be stored and manipulated if they are to be of use. Perhaps the key challenge for the future is to identify which emerging technologies will best provide the usable tools that nurses need to manage the knowledge explosion.

LOOKING BACK FROM THE FUTURE

Visions of societies of the future, both utopias and dystopias, have been produced by many people. Sometimes they have been science fiction writers, whereas **futurologists** (e.g., DCDC, 2010) have used scenario planning to examine possible alternatives for the future and then examine how they might be achieved or prevented and the implications for society. This technique was used in part in the NI2006 Post Congress workshop (Murray et al., 2007), but other useful scenarios that demonstrate possible emerging technologies also exist.

Easteal and Demosthenes (2005) postulate one such future containing some interesting and already very plausible possibilities. Some brief examples of the kinds of "what-if" thinking that may be helpful in exploring the implications of emerging technologies include the following:

- "Googlezon" (formed from a merger of Google and Amazon) used fact-stripping robots to create personalized news stories dynamically for delivery to health information portal subscribers (for patients, nurses, or family caregivers);
- Personalized "genoming" (the sequencing of an individual's genome) was a routine procedure;
- Biomedical research institutes had only executives and intellectual property lawyers as their permanent staff, with all the actual research outsourced and conducted under contract in India and China;
- "GoogleHealth" allowed individuals to store privately or publish their own health information, combining diverse information provided by patients, their own monitoring devices, and records supplied by hospitals, pathology and imaging services, and the general practitioner;
- GoogleHealth's search engines and social networking spaces allowed people to explore information held in "virtual populations" of individuals who were genetically and behaviorally like themselves, so they could see health trends in

these populations that had real and direct meaning to their lives, and adopt the best practices of their "**virtual peers**," so as to derive the same health benefits.

In 2005, when this scenario was written, these were speculative ideas. However, just 2 years later, Nobel laureate James Watson, codiscoverer of the DNA double helix and father of the Human Genome Project, become the first human to receive the data encompassing his entire personal genome sequence (Williams, 2007). Microsoft's **HealthVault**, along with Google Health, are now actual public online personal health record systems. Personalized information feeds using such tools as **really simple syndication** (RSS) now provide easy ways for people to receive the latest information from a range of multiple media sources that they can readily specify and customize. Search engine technology, combined with the forms of open information-sharing and tools underpinning **social networking** websites (e.g., Facebook and MySpace), could rapidly support the sharing of health behavior information. The future will be here more rapidly than many expect, and nurse informaticians need to be at least aware of, if not directly involved in determining, the many new emerging technologies and their possibilities for use within their domains of interest and practice.

HISTORICAL OVERVIEW

There are several ways to view the explosive growth of information technologies and applications (Saba & Erdley, 2006; Sackett & Erdley, 2002). Regardless of perspective, the growth tends to follow a long and often convoluted path from simple to complex in detail. An in-depth examination reveals the significance of these developments. Initial generations of computers, analog devices, focused on military uses, such as cryptography and weapons flight paths. Evolution proceeded from hardware to software for business administration and accounting tasks. The invention of **transistors** (solid-state semiconductors) resulted in the second generation of computers, digital devices much smaller and faster than analog computers. Silicon chips, smaller and more powerful than transistors, eventually replaced transistors, advancing the process of miniaturization. Future directions point toward a shift to advanced miniaturization (**nanotechnology**) for CPU and data storage capabilities and increased ubiquity of computational devices in general (Kurzweil, 2005).

One may also view computing history using eight time groupings, or demarcations, beginning with the pre-1800s. Sackett and Erdley (2002) presented a schema based on this model. The specific designations are pre- to mid-1800s, later 1800s, 1900–1950s, 1960s, 1970s, 1980s, 1990s, and early 21st century.

Pre-1800 computing primarily represents many forms of human communication (e.g., speech, oral history, hieroglyphics) (Sackett & Erdley, 2002). Examples of ancient tabulation devices include shells, rocks, and pieces of bone. Despite the individual impact of such devices as the abacus, growth and advancement of such devices was essentially influenced by the mobility of people and dispersion of ideas from the Old World to the New World (Sackett & Erdley).

The 1800s witnessed technologic developments, such as Babbage's difference engine in England (seen by many as the predecessor of the modern computer), and the invention of the telephone by Alexander Graham Bell. Bell's invention eventually provided the initial infrastructure on which computer connectivity began. From a software focus, a development of large significance was the first foray into standardized language (Dr. Peter M. Roget, author of Roget's Thesaurus of English Words and Phrases, based on synonyms, in 1852).

From the early 1900s through the 1950s, a number of hardware developments emerged with respect to computing (Z1, Colossus, Mark I, Electronic Numerical Integrator and Computer (ENIAC) and the Universal Automatic Computer (UNIVAC). In health care, one of the first computers to be used was the IBM 704, which also was one of the first computers to use magnetic core memory (invented by Wang) (Collen, 1995). The invention of transistors and subsequent integration into computational devices also helped shape the future of computing. Additional important developments include storing and running applications, a stored program concept by Neumann, and shift to a binary system from traditional base 10 (Collen).

The next decade (1960s) witnessed a substantial increase of activity and inventiveness providing important direction and substance to future computational needs. Transistor use in computers marked the end of first-generation computers and the beginning of the second generation. Kilby and Noyce's discovery of the ability of transistors to function as their own circuit boards greatly diminished the size and power requirements of computers, thus leading to minicomputers (Collen, 1995). Noyce and his colleagues also developed the first integrated silicon chip, which eventually led to the use of very-large-scale integration (VLSI) chips in the late 1960s (Collen). Noyce went on to found Intel in the late 1960s, which grew into one of the world's leading manufacturers of computational and other chips. These integrated circuits demarcated second-generation computers (Blum, 1986; Saba & McCormick, 1986).

Software applications grew substantially during this time. The Health Evaluation through Logical Processing (HELP) system was developed at the Latter Day Saints/LDS Hospital in Salt Lake City, Utah, in the late 1950s and early 1960s (Warner, Olmsted, & Rutherford, 1972). In 1962, Clark and Molnar of Massachusetts Institute of Technology (MIT) developed LINC (a laboratory-specific application) (Collen, 1995). The National Library of Medicine committed to computerization when it placed its journal collection, Medlars/Medline, onto a computer in 1963 (Collen). PLATO, from the late 1960s, was one of the first computer-based education programs. In health care, a number of landmark applications appeared including the Technicon Medical Information System (TMIS) initiated in 1965; the problem-oriented medical record (POMR) and problem-oriented medical information systems (PROMIS) in the 1960s; and the computer-stored ambulatory record (COSTAR) developed and implemented in the late 1960s using the Massachusetts General Hospital utility multiprogramming system (MUMPS) (Barnett et al., 1979).

In the 1970s, the focus of information technology in health care shifted away from hardware to software applications (Boutros, 1993; Brandejs, 1976; Collen, 1995; Elioutina & Tarasov, 1995; Hannah, Ball, & Edwards, 1999; Mandil, Moidu, Korpela, Byass, & Forster, 1993). The invention and subsequent use of the silicon chip in 1975 denoted a worldwide revolution in computer hardware and subsequent software developments. Shortly after this development, Paul Allen and Bill Gates founded Microsoft Corporation, which was destined to create an operating system of eventual global importance.

Internationally, from Canada and the United Kingdom, there are examples of computerized information systems in nursing practice. King's College Hospital in London pioneered computerized nursing care plans; Ninewells Hospital in Scotland implemented a real-time system for nursing documentation; and York Central Hospital in Richmond Hills, Ontario, implemented a computerized patient care system (Sackett & Erdley, 2002; Hayes & Barnett, 2008).

In the United States, hospital information systems (HISs) began adding care management and cost control functionality in the 1970s. Edgar F. Codd's work with **relational databases** provided the framework and underpinnings for growth in data collection, manipulation, and analysis (Haux, Knaup, & Schmucker, 1999). Examples of other United States HISs include Technicon at El Camino, California (a continuation of work from the mid-1960s) and PROMIS (Medical Center Hospital, Burlington, Vermont) (Collen, 1995). The Patient Care System (PCS) developed at Duke Medical Center, focused on nursing staffing. Refinement of PROMIS continued during this decade. MYCIN, a program designed to identify bacteria and recommend antibiotics (so named because of the typical suffix of antibiotics at the time), realized inexact reasoning in medicine (Shortliffe & Buchanan, 1975).

The decade of the 1980s witnessed continued growth of both the application and hardware arenas. The shift in computer focus from mainframe architecture to individual machines signaled a shift of power to the user. Hardware and software growth became collaborative in use and purpose. The U.S. Defense Agency Research Projects Agency (DARPA) network was developed to cope with communication in the event of an atomic war. The concept of "ethernet" by Bob Metcalf defined a form of communication over wires, which, along with developments in communication protocols, such as transmission control protocol/Internet protocol (TCP/IP), provided the framework for not only necessary communication but future collaborations (e.g., client–server architecture).

One of the more prominent software developments in the healthcare field in the early 1980s was Internist-1 (Miller, Pople, & Myers, 1982). This application applied symbolic reasoning to develop computer-assisted diagnoses through modeling physician behavior as a decision-support aid (van Ginneken, Koenderink & Dana, 1999). Other examples following in Internist-1's footprint include QMR, Internist-1's direct successor; DxPlain; Iliad; and Meditel. A hospital information systems project, based on the MUMPS, was initiated at Obafemi Awolowo University Teaching Hospital in Ile-Ife, Nigeria in 1988 (Daini, Makanjuola, & Ojo, 1993).

Technology applications "exploded" in the 1990s with the advent of increasingly sophisticated hardware, software, cheaper memory and speed, and the decreased cost of digital computer technology. From the development and use of the Internet to satellites to wireless innovations, from mainframes to minicomputers to microcomputers to work stations to global networks, the amount of knowledge generated and the necessity for management of increasingly complex information systems was evident everywhere and especially noticeable in health care.

International examples of information systems include CARE Telematics Project, led by the World Health Organization regional office for Europe (Zollner, 1995) and OPADE: Optimization of Drug Prescription Using Advanced Informatics (de Zegher et al., 1995), a joint venture between individuals from Belgium, France, Italy, Sweden, and the United Kingdom. TELENURSING was a European Commission-funded project

> . . . to promote standardized and formalized clinical nursing care data based on uniform definitions of data items with the purpose of developing countable and comparable nursing minimum data sets as a means of communicating nursing care information electronically between clinical setting, health care sectors nationally and European-wide and a means of producing Euro-Nursing Health statistics on people's need for nursing care (Mortensen & Nielsen, 1995, p. 115).

South America instituted several healthcare initiatives (Stammer, 2000) including swipe cards to validate patient identity and eligibility at public health centers.

As the healthcare market has become increasingly complex so has healthcare software. The number of software applications for health care numbers in the thousands with what seems to be a program for any and all purposes. In the last years of the 1990s healthcare informatics was swept up by both the Internet and the lure of the World Wide Web. The increased popularity of **electronic data interchange** (EDI) with its ability to reduce human errors, forever altered the financial aspect of health care. Carrying through to the early 21st century, this trend has continued with pledges to "computerize the nation's health records in five years, saving billions of dollars in healthcare costs and countless lives" (The White House, 2009). Regionalism and interoperability are now the buzzwords for healthcare informatics in the United States and increasingly abroad. Denmark has provided a health portal for its citizens and health providers, which is accessible for all and any healthcare concerns ranging from scheduling an appointment to reviewing laboratory results (The Danish eHealth Portal, 2008). Second-generation Web applications (**Web 2.0**) are increasing in popularity for both health care and the population in general in the United States and worldwide. Thus, knowledge and information continue to evolve from specific uses by individuals to growth, evolution, and application by the population. This shift will continue to impact the role of providers and health care in general.

This shift of information access, acquisition, and interpretation, for both provider and patient, may result in overload in terms of content and comprehension. Managing this overload will increasingly consume both providers and patients. How this issue will be managed is of great concern whether by an increased use of technology or a regression away from technology.

SOME TECHNOLOGIES OF TODAY

In many countries, not just the United States, much of the most recent focus of technology use in nursing and health care has been aimed at improving patient safety (e.g., reducing medication errors), as described by Oren, Shaffer, and Guglielmo (2003), among others. They point out, however, the limited research providing evidence of the impact of introducing these technologies on error reduction and the reduction of adverse events. The recent focus in the United States on developing "meaningful use" of electronic health records (e.g., Blumenthal, 2010) has reemphasized this focus. This perhaps reflects two interacting sets of issues: first, priorities for use of technologies often change in conjunction with changing political forces; and second, many technologies are changing so rapidly that, by the time they are evaluated in large-scale, controlled trial environments, they have been succeeded by a new generation of devices and applications. Patient safety issues are a strong driver to using technology today, and will probably continue to be so as long as politicians see benefit from such a focus; however, as other priorities, often political, emerge the focus will shift. One can already begin to see some of this changing focus with the emerging discussions on personal health records. In just one example of the plethora of materials on personal health records

(PHR) and personal health information management systems (PHIMS), the Post-Congress Workshop of the 10th International Nursing Informatics Congress (NI2009) explored a range of perspectives from multiple countries on the state of the art of development of PHIMS and some of the emerging issues that need to be addressed, including safety and confidentiality, patient engagement and empowerment, and standards and governance issues (Saranto, Brennan, & Casey, 2009).

However, many nurses often see technology as a hindrance or a barrier, rather than something that provides real benefit within their practice. Murray et al. (2007), for example, states "Much technology currently gets in the way of care, and there is a need for increasingly **transparent technology** [boldface added], which will need to function in the background; if you talk about the technology, it is not transparent" (p. 18). This may be for a wide variety of reasons but is often related to lack of consultation with end users in technology application to care processes. The true potential of technology to support nursing and health care will only come when it is both **ubiquitous** (everywhere) and transparent. The point has been made by Weaver et al. (2007), who says "small, inexpensive, unobtrusive" (p. 80) devices will facilitate future monitoring of patients and data collection. Kirovski, Oliver, Sinclair, and Tan (2007) suggest that the current generation of wearable physiologic sensors are obtrusive and so meet resistance from users. If they are to gain widespread acceptance, they need to provide for little or no change in the user's daily routine, with transparency being the key to widespread adoption.

Even the most cursory examination of the proceedings of any recent health or nursing informatics conference demonstrates the plethora of ways in which nurses are currently using a wide range of technologies to support and advance their practice. One can also begin to see adoption of the kinds of near-transparent and ubiquitous technologies just discussed. Taking examples from recent events by way of illustration, from the NI2006 International Congress on Nursing Informatics (Park, Murray, & Delaney, 2006), one can find examples from around the world of the following:

- Computerized decision support systems to prevent unnecessary visits to healthcare facilities in South Africa (Horner, Hanmer, & Mbananga, 2006)
- Wireless speech recognition and touchscreen triage support systems in emergency departments in Taiwan (Chang et al., 2006)
- Nurse-managed telehealth services in United Kingdom dermatology clinics (Lawton & Timmons, 2006)
- Use of open-source software for development of Web-based nursing informatics education in Germany (Schrader, 2006)

- Nurse-led development of a personal health record system in the United States (Lee, Delaney, & Moorhead, 2006)
- Demonstrated uses of wireless biomedical sensors for invasive monitoring in Norway (Oyri, Balasingham, & Hogetveit, 2006)

More recently, the NI2009 International Congress on Nursing Informatics (Saranto, Brennan, Park et al., 2009) also provided examples of technologies to support online knowledge management for e-health, use of virtual environments for education and clinical practice, and m-health applications.

Two reports focusing on nursing and technology also summarize some of the practical ways in which nurses are involved in using technologies. The report of the February 2007 Technology Informatics Guiding Education Reform (TIGER) Initiative summit (TIGER, 2007) defined a 3-year action plan toward achieving a 10-year vision to enable practicing nurses and nursing students to engage fully in the unfolding digital era of health care, thereby enabling nurses to use information technology (IT) seamlessly to provide safer, higher-quality patient care. Nine different collaborative teams were formed, to initiate Phase II, to address topics ranging from standards and interoperability to personal health records. Each committee submitted a report of its findings. TIGER is currently entering Phase III, which entails integrating recommendations elicited in Phase II into the nursing community at all levels of care and the development of online learning management systems to provide content delivery and interaction.

Among the examples of current use cited were Web-based patient health records, such as the U.S. Department of Veterans Affairs' MyHealtheVet (http://www.myhealth.va.gov), which patients can access from anywhere, and empowers them in making their own decisions about their health.

The 2004 report on technology's role in addressing the nursing crisis in Maryland (Technology Workgroup, Maryland Statewide Commission on the Crisis in Nursing, 2004), noting technology was not the solution to issues, acknowledges it could be a facilitator, demonstrated by pockets of innovation including:

- The use of wearable, hands-free communication badges (Vocera, 2007)
- Bar-coded medication administration schemes that have demonstrated reductions in error rates
- Use of intranets for providing current and consistent protocol and procedure information

However, in addition to the technologies available, there are changes occurring in the ways in which these technologies facilitate interaction, in particular through the emergence of a wide range of what are termed "Web 2.0" applications. Web 2.0 has many definitions and descriptions. O'Reilly (2005) first described it extensively, and many more recent descriptions still focus on interaction, the development of online communities, and support for collaboration and sharing as being the key elements. Among the technologies seen as contributing to Web 2.0 are **blogs** (**weblogs**), **wikis**, **podcasts**, "really simple syndication"(RSS) feeds, and other methods of providing many-to-many publication and communication. Social networking and social educational applications (Anderson, 2005), such as Facebook and Twitter, which facilitate interaction and collaboration, are also a central component of Web 2.0 (Murray & Maag, 2006).

Web 2.0 technologies allow for the possibility of increased participation among formal and informal online communities of users. As such, they are disruptive technologies that have the potential to transform the ways in which knowledge is generated and shared. There is not space within this chapter to explore at length the emerging tools and technologies generally labeled Web 2.0, nor to provide a detailed discussion of their potential implications. However, they are undoubtedly beginning to have profound impacts on the ways in which data, knowledge, and information (and perhaps even wisdom) are generated, and so it is worth summarizing some emerging ways in which they are being used within nursing and health care. However, detailed research studies on their use and effects are still relatively few, although there are emerging case study reports of their use in clinical practice and education (e.g., Anderson, Blumenthal, et al., 2010).

Maag (2006) described the use of podcasts of lecture materials with nursing students (the term podcast originated as an amalgam of broadcasting and Apple's proprietary iPod MP3 music player, although podcasts can be played on any computer or MP3 player). Although much argument still exists regarding whether podcasts will provide long-term benefits and changes to ways in which people learn, there is some evidence they can enhance the learning experience and engage learners. Maag (2005) is among those who have explored the potential use of blogs within nurse education, and she cites examples of small-scale evaluations within other educational contexts for teaching and research purposes. She concludes health professionals' writing, reading, and communication skills can be enhanced through the use of blogs, and blogs also facilitate collaborative and information-gathering skills. Other practical examples support the use of blogs within formal education (Godwin-Jones, 2003; Martindale & Wiley, 2004) for professional development, sharing information, interacting as part of a learning community, and building an open knowledge base. In addition, they have been used for encouraging informal knowledge sharing and professional development around health and nursing informatics conferences (Murray & Ward, 2004). Spallek, O'Donnell, Clayton, Anderson, and Krueger (2010) have explored the use of Web 2.0 tools, or as they are increasingly called, **social media** applications, in clinical practice, and through a series of vignettes have illustrated some current uses and identified research questions. The emergence of **social bookmarking**, **tags** and **tag clouds**, and **folksonomies** are providing opportunities for the exploration of new ways of linking, ordering, and searching information, based in large part on popularity of its use among a community. These tools have implications for the ways in which health and nursing informatics are classified.

SOME VIEWS OF WHAT WILL AFFECT THE FUTURE

Several nursing informaticians have concluded their books by looking to the future and imagining scenarios for the life and work of the 21st century nurse. McCormick (2001), writing a possible scenario for 2020, envisaged the nurse using voice recognition to interact with her computer (portable, of course) and with components of the hospital systems, telehealth applications for physiologic monitoring, use of genetic screening information in treatment decisions, and smart cards for storing a form of electronic health record. More than one third of the time from then until 2020 has passed, and many of these applications have become almost routine. The growth of networks (especially the Internet) means that we have already moved beyond some of the ideas in our development of ways of working.

Ball (2005) also advocates the use of technology, including wireless networks and personal digital assistants (PDAs), to reduce the time spent on documentation (and so potentially increase the time available for direct patient care). She perceives technology supporting new roles, such as an Internet guide to assist patients in accessing appropriate educational resources. McCormick et al. (2007), in discussing the American Medical Informatics Association (AMIA) Nursing Informatics Work Group's white paper on how the nursing informatics profession needs to set new directions, identified many areas that will impact the nature of nursing and health care in the future, although many of these were nontechnologic.

SOME OF THE ISSUES FROM NI2006

In mid-2006, following the NI2006 International Congress on Nursing Informatics in Seoul, Korea (Park et al., 2006), a group of nurse informaticians from around the world participated in an intensive workshop-based exploration of possible futures and the implications for nursing and nursing informatics. Some of the issues that they identified are worth exploring. It was acknowledged that nursing and nursing informatics would have to change. Among the new roles for nurses, arising out of current developments, was that of **information mediator**, but the implications of this were, again, the need for technology to support immediate access to up-to-date knowledge anywhere and anytime.

Many of the issues that were explored were not technologic or related to information technology. Discussions explored the many demographic changes that are known or can be predicted that are likely to occur, and that have been discussed by others exploring future trends (e.g., growing and ageing populations; changes in population structure, especially the numbers of productive working-age members able to contribute tax and other revenues to support healthcare systems; growing proportions of populations living in urban areas; and shifting global balances of power) (DCDC, 2010). Possible trends in healthcare provision and delivery as health policies and priorities change (e.g., moves toward less costly preventive or interventional measures, growing use of telehealth) and the impact these and other changes might have on the nature of nursing were also discussed.

Among the key issues that emerged from the discussions that are important for the international nursing informatics community to explore in coming years were

- The development of the concept, and a possible model, of u-nursing (ubiquitous nursing), which has implications for the practice of nursing and profound implications for all aspects of the education and continuing professional development of nurses (Oyri et al., 2007)
- The role of the nurse changing to become more of a knowledge professional, working in partnership with patients and their other caregivers
- The continuing growth of patient informatics, perhaps as a growth and evolution of the current concept of consumer health informatics, and with the increasing centrality of the patient as the controlling force in the entire enterprise
- The vast impact that genomics will have on all aspects of life, and in particular health care (Turley, Murray, Saranto, Ehnfors, & Seomun, 2007)

Such discussions of technologies as emerged were often focused on the interaction with these other changes. Among the issues discussed were nanotechnology; remote (e.g., wireless) monitoring of vital signs; wearable monitoring and treatment devices; ubiquitous access to computer networks; lifelong personal and electronic health records; and treatments, not only preventive and interventional, but also predictive of likely development of diseases, based in genetic medicine (Oyri et al., 2007).

Nanotechnology, and its specific applications within medicine and health care (nanomedicine), opens up many possibilities, including the development of minute biomedical devices the size of molecules that could provide drug delivery systems, precise targeting of therapies (e.g., delivery of drugs or radiation sources to individual cancer cells), or even nanorobots to undertake surgical procedures on cells. These types of technology are still in development stages. One project is the **lab-on-a-chip device** for undertaking comprehensive blood analyses (Schmidt, 2007). Staggers et al. (2008) note that because nanotechnology has potential applications in drug delivery devices and monitoring mechanisms, there are implications for the education of healthcare professionals about many issues, including the safe and ethical use of nanomaterials and their capabilities and limitations. Nurses and informaticians need to consider what, if any, would be the nursing or informatics role in such interventions. As Loescher & Merkle (2005) point out in relation to other emerging technologies, without knowledge of genomic technologies, reasons for their use, and the possible implications of genetic diagnosis and genomic-based treatments, nurses will be increasingly unable to provide the quality of care needed and demanded by patients. The same applies to all new and emerging technologies that may impact on or become integral parts of the delivery of health care, in whatever setting.

Although this chapter focuses on the technologies and can only summarize discussion of the issues, the technologies cannot be divorced from or considered in isolation from wider societal issues and the handling of increasingly large and complex volumes of data. Readers are directed to the Post Congress Conference proceedings for more detailed discussion (Murray et al., 2007).

Among the issues explicitly identified and implicitly emerging from the NI2006 discussions was that the amount of data available about all aspects of health care will increase tremendously. **Genomics**, proteomics, and the plethora of related "omics," many of which are often gathered in the general field of bioinformatics, will produce many challenges for the nature of health care, and for all forms of health informatics. As Martin-Sanchez et al. (2004) have suggested, there will be many technologic challenges, but also wider ethical and other issues to be addressed. They point out that, although new genetic and proteomic data provide the possibility of developing new therapies and of implementing new preventive measures, it is important to be able to deal with the large amounts of data generated. The new knowledge available and the new technologies will blur the distinctions between clinical and molecular information, while increased amounts of knowledge will lead to a greater need for genetic counseling as an even more important part of clinical, hands-on care. Martin-Sanchez et al. see a place for culture brokers (i.e., people who can translate between science and clinical care and between science and the self-caring citizen). As Turley et al. (2007) also points out:

> . . . from the genome information, we can determine the disease risks of a given patient, the drug allergies of that patient and to some extent the optimal drug treatments for individual patients. These all fall clearly within the purview of nursing concerns and the science of nursing, and have implications for truly personalized care (p. 56).

Other issues also emerge, such as the nature and amount of genomic data and information to be included in the electronic health record and how long it must be held, as well as a set of issues around the impact of the changes and emerging technologies on education for all health professionals. The necessity of collecting, storing, and manipulating huge amounts of genomic data will impact the technologies to be used. Grid technologies (unique configurations of distributed computing) are being explored as mechanisms for manipulating the data, but such issues as how the knowledge will be extracted from the data repositories and how it will be represented in usable form present challenges for the development of new technologies (Kuhn, Wurst, Bott, & Guise, 2006).

If, as many of the participants in the NI2006 Post Congress Conference suggest, one of the major roles of the nurse (and nurse informaticians) of the future will be that of a clinical knowledge worker (Weaver et al., 2007), then they will need to be familiar with the many new tools and technologies that will develop to enable them to retrieve, use, manipulate, present, and share the new knowledge with patients and other health professionals. The next section specifically explores some technologies and probable trends, but because new applications are being developed on a seemingly daily basis, the section does not dwell on any in detail, but explores some of the trends.

SOME EMERGING TECHNOLOGIES AND OTHER ISSUES THAT WILL IMPACT NURSING AND HEALTH CARE

For many years, the concept of e-health has existed, for which Oh, Rizo, Enkin, and Jadad (2005) have identified 51 unique published definitions. The definitions address not only health but also technology and commerce with a general tendency for health care to be viewed as a process rather than health as an outcome, and with technology seen both as a tool to enable a process/function/service and as a means to expand, to assist, or to enhance human activities rather than as a substitute for them. The European view of e-health, as developed by the Commission of the European Communities (2004), acknowledges the need for providing citizen-centered healthcare systems, respecting the diversity of Europe's multicultural, multilingual healthcare traditions. Examples of e-health developments include electronic health records, health portals, telemedicine and tele-health services, and wearable and portable monitoring systems.

A recent development is m-health (often termed **mobile e-health**, as opposed to simply mobile health), which according to some (e.g., WHO, 2007) includes health-related uses of mobile technologies including mobile telephones (and increasingly, Internet-enabled, wireless-connected smartphones), PDAs, tablet computers and sub-notebook microcomputers, remote diagnostic and monitoring devices, and global positioning systems (GPS) and geographic information system (GIS) mapping equipment.

M-health can be described in terms of the application to healthcare systems and processes of network technologies and mobile communications and devices (Istepanian, Laxminarayan, & Pattichis, 2006). The development and potential applications of m-health have been facilitated in recent years by the rapid rise in ownership and availability of mobile devices (cell phones; smartphones; PDAs; and more recently tablet-sized devices, such as the iPad) in many countries. There are now many examples, especially within developing countries in Africa and Asia, of m-health applications in such areas as AIDS/HIV monitoring and education (Murray, van Middelkoop, & Meyer, 2010; Mechael 2009). There is growing evidence of its impact on underserved populations and of transforming healthcare delivery in resource-poor environments (Akter & Ray, 2010).

More recently, recognizing the increasing pervasiveness of technology in all aspects of life, including health care, the concept of u-health has emerged. U-health (or **ubiquitous health** or health care) is based in the concept of ubiquitous computing, which is considered a third wave of computing wherein technologies become increasingly invisible, becoming incorporated into everyday use, and so fading into the background (Weiser, 1991). With true ubiquitous computing, which pervades all parts of the everyday environment, unobtrusively providing information and services, and with the very concept of the single device (computer) disappearing into the network (Bott, 2005), the real possibility of providing nurses and other healthcare professions with the information they need where and when they need it exists.

Oyri et al. (2007) suggest information and communications technologies will become ubiquitous within nursing, and that emerging technologies including nanotechnology, wireless sensors, and minimally invasive technologies will support not only health care but also wellness management. They suggest a model for u-nursing that "will focus on the provision of nursing for anyone or any organization, anytime, anywhere, through any networks and any devices" (p. 32).

Linked to these concepts has been the emergence of a considerable amount of research, especially funded by the European Commission, into body sensor networks, in particular wireless body area networks (WBAN) (Lymberis, 2010). These allow for data from a patient's or person's vital signs and movements to be collected by wearable or implantable sensors. The data, communicated via short-range wireless, can provide for real-time monitoring of health status (Liolios, Doukas, Fourlas, & Maglogiannis, 2010; O'Donovan et al., 2010; Santra, 2010).

Nanotechnology is a broad term developed and refined over the past few years. Originally focused on exceptionally small-scale technology, typically on the order of atoms, it has evolved to incorporate more than strictly engineering and structural meanings, such as its application to patient sensing as mentioned by Oyri et al. (2007). The potential for this technology is now becoming realized as clinicians are increasingly developing applications and investigating potential uses in medicine, such as disease detection or treatment (Kenwright & Pifer, 2010; Meetoo, 2009).

There is also discussion of whether society is shifting from a focus on information to one of knowledge. Generally considered to succeed the industrial age, the information age is one of information use resulting in wide-ranging social activity. This is manifest with the increasing popularity of applications, such as Facebook, MySpace, and Twitter. These and other such social media applications are increasingly becoming tools for health organizations and patients.

BEYOND WEB 2.0

General consensus sees the Web as evolving into something beyond its current status of 2.0. The current nomenclature, as initially named by O'Reilly, lends itself to a sequential progression to 3.0. Web 3.0 is considered to be the semantic Web. In essence Web 3.0 is a term used to define the many different ways for machines (computers) to understand words, and thus their meaning, on the Internet. These different ways are applications formally proposed by the World Wide Web Consortium. Web 3.0 is slowly gaining popularity but is not as common as Web 2.0.

Even the concept of Web 4.0, the iteration after 3.0, has been already discussed on the Web (e.g., Murray, 2009). The concept itself is even less defined than 3.0 with many definitions; however, it was formally presented at NI2009 with a subsequent blog posting. The concept has ranged from **wetware** (direct body-brain interfaces) to implantables, such as ocular viewing lens and more. It may seem without purpose to even conjecture about a concept like Web 4.0 but how can the future be known without trying to offer plausible aspects of it?

A TECHNOLOGY WISH LIST

There are doubtless many other technologies to cover, and some readers will say that should have been covered. Not addressed are the prospects for robotics in delivering aspects of care, even though there are well-documented examples of robotic surgery and even robots for delivering nursing care. Similarly, not explored are the possibilities of emerging **virtual worlds**, such as Second Life, and simulations. Also unaddressed are many of the technologies, such as wearable devices, that are being used to provide remote monitoring of physiologic parameters in care settings, including patients' own homes. These are certainly interesting and exciting developments, and one can only plead the excuse of lack of space in a printed text. Readers are urged to undertake their own explorations of these and other technologies.

A short wish list for some new technologies that the authors would like to see emerge in the next few years concludes this exploration. As with much of what was discussed previously, the seeds of these developments are already present, and they may be with us sooner than expected. Our technology wish list includes:

1. The kind of computer interface used in the film Minority Report: no mouse, no keyboard, just gesture-based interactions with virtual images projected into a vertical space at head height.
2. Ubiquity of computational devices to the extent that conversation and discussion of these devices will disappear from everyday social interactions; the technology will be transparent or invisible.
3. The ability to access information when and where it is wanted or needed, irrespective of modality, thereby maximizing mobility and other personal resources. This may lead to cell phones becoming the main avenue of access for more than text messages, speech, and video clips. Knowledge acquisition and use will then become ubiquitous and pervasive; new work roles will emerge to cope with this new and different technology.

WHAT THE FUTURE HOLDS: SUMMARY

The future will be different; however, it is likely that many of these changes are already in development or will be extrapolations of current developments and trends. There is always, however, the possibility of new developments, or unexpected consequences, of the development of emerging technologies.

This chapter has touched briefly on some of the emerging technologies that are likely to have an effect on nursing, nurse informatics, and health care in the near future, and that might impact and interact with the Foundation of Knowledge model. Some of the technologies have not been given as much coverage as hindsight will show that they ought to have received; this is, in part, because some of the emerging technologies are evolving so rapidly that it is difficult to predict what might emerge within the next few months, let alone the next few years, and the impacts they will have. Not much coverage has been given to the potential of Web 2.0, Web 3.0, and beyond as they are likely to deserve, again because the evolution is difficult to predict. New interfaces with technology (e.g., Apple's iPhone) have not been touched on, and little mention has been made of the emergence of virtual worlds.

The implications of social networking technologies that are major elements of Web 2.0 will have a significant impact on the amount of information and knowledge that is generated, and the ways in which it is used. It is known that new healthcare technologies will develop, most likely based in genomic and nanotechnologic sciences, and that they will lead to huge new volumes of data, with implications for what is captured and stored, for how long, and how it is used. It is also known that computing power and storage capabilities will lead to faster, smaller, more mobile, and more powerful devices with vastly greater capacities for storing data. Everyone will have the opportunity to be more connected, more readily, and more of the time, to many other people through the growth of wireless networks.

The major challenges will be to find the best tools and methods for managing, and to make the best use of the information that will be available not only 24/7, but 60/60/24/7 (i.e., every second of every day). For many, knowing what to keep up with, what is most relevant to practice, education, and research will be a challenge. Nurse informaticians have a good track record in finding ways to use information and will need to rise to that challenge.

The potential to generate more health data, for example from new forms of physiologic monitoring, or from the implications of the new "omics" sciences, will raise important new needs for storing that data, in both the short and long term, and for generating from it the information and knowledge needed to support clinical practice, research, and education. The key words to describe the changes in the ways in which nursing and healthcare knowledge are acquired, processed, generated, and disseminated are smaller, more integrated, more mobile, more wearable, more connected, and ubiquitous.

Devices for capturing and storing data will become smaller or more portable, and the amount of data that can be stored within a device will increase. Devices the size of today's cell phones are likely, as smartphone technology evolves, to have all the functionality and more of today's desktop computers. One can already see the integration of more functions into today's cell phones and newer, more portable tablet-sized devices, such as Apple's iPad, and this trend is likely to continue. Both of these trends make the information processing power available to nurses more mobile, enabling nurses to spend more time with patients and also develop new ways of interacting with patients and delivering care in a wide range of settings. Another emerging medium is **cloud storage,** which is a model of online storage where data is held on, and possibly distributed across, several virtual servers, rather than being hosted on dedicated servers. This has many implications that are only beginning to be explored, especially in terms of legal and ethical issues if, for example, health data is stored on servers that may be located outside of the jurisdiction of the country where the hospital or other health facility is physically located.

All of this increased computing power in mobile devices is of little use if mobile communications are restricted. Many health service facilities, for example, currently restrict staff access to certain external information resources, especially those that may involve social media. Access to information and use of information on the move will increase, as new forms of wireless communications are implemented, meaning that nurses are less restricted to particular physical spaces to interact with patients' records. One of the "hot topics" for discussion at the time of writing this chapter is whether the rise of "apps" running on smartphones and other mobile devices will mean the decline of web-based Internet use (apps is an abbreviation for application, meaning a piece of software that can run on the Internet, on a computer, or on another device) (Anderson & Wolff, 2010). Finally, although **wearable computing** may have more to offer in terms of capturing data from patients, there are many emerging tools that may mean the nurse will not be restricted to holding and handling physical devices, but may interact, through voice and other commands, with computing devices carried elsewhere on their persons. As nurses work in environments where they can be always connected to ubiquitous computing resources, they will no longer be able to say that they did not have access to the information they needed to undertake their roles. The challenge will be to find not only technologic ways of dealing with the available information, but also ways of using and prioritizing information, new ways of thinking, and new ways of interacting with information resources, so that they have the right information, at the right time, to do the right job, and are not overwhelmed with extraneous and irrelevant "noise." The technology is the easy part; the nontechnologic issues will be the greater, and perhaps more urgent, challenge.

This chapter explores some of the emerging technologies that are in both general use and in use and development within health care, and discusses what the future might hold for nurses, nursing, and health care more generally. Technology will not solve all our future problems; some emerging technologies could create more problems than they solve. However, it is by having an awareness of likely and possible technologic developments that nurses can assess what impact they might have on the ways in which we work and live. Although not explicitly at each point addressing the four key areas of the Foundation of Knowledge model, this chapter considers how some of the emerging technologies may address the four areas of (1) knowledge acquisition, (2) knowledge processing, (3) knowledge generation, and (4) knowledge dissemination or feedback. The focus is not explicitly on changes in health care and nursing technologies, but on the more general changes that might be adapted or adopted for use by nurses or within health care. In an ideal world, we would like to see the development of easy-to-use tools for nurses to manage the coming knowledge "explosion" as more information becomes available to support diagnosis, treatment, and care.

THOUGHT-PROVOKING Questions

www

1. This chapter raises several important issues related to nursing knowledge, not the least of which might be the uniqueness of nursing knowledge. Is this uniqueness requisite for future care by nurses or nursing informatics specialists?

2. Given that the future is relatively unpredictable, what might be said regarding what can be predicted and to what degree of certainty?

3. Will the new tools and technologies that nurses might use to manage the "knowledge explosion" be sufficient on their own, and how will they need to interact with human factors?

For a full suite of assignments and additional learning activities, use the access code located in the front of your book to visit this exclusive website: http://go.jblearning.com/mcgonigle. If you do not have an access code, you can obtain one at the site.

References

Akter, S., & Ray, P. (2010). mHealth - an Ultimate Platform to Serve the Unserved. In A. Geissbuhler & C. Kulikowski (Eds.), *Yearbook of Medical Informatics 2010* (pp. 94-100). Stuttgart: Schattauer.

Anderson, C., & Wolff, M. (2010). The Web is Dead. Long Live the Internet. *WIRED.* Retrieved from http://www.wired.com/magazine/2010/08/ff_webrip/all/1

Anderson, P., Blumenthal, J., Bruell, D., Rosenzweig, M., Conte, M., & Song, J. (2010). An Online and Social Media Training Curricula to Facilitate Bench-to-Bedside Information Transfer. In: Positioning the Profession: the Tenth International Congress on Medical Librarianship; Brisbane Australia, August 31–September 4, 2009. Retrieved from http://espace.library.uq.edu.au/eserv/UQ:179795/n4_2_Thurs_Blumenthal_205.pdf

Anderson, T. (2005). *Distance learning—Social software's killer AP?* Retrieved from http://auspace.athabascau.ca:8080/dspace/bitstream/2149/2328/1/distance_learning.pdf

Ball, M. J. (2005). Nursing informatics of tomorrow. *Healthcare Informatics, 2*(5): 74–75.

Barnett, G., Justice, N., Somand, M., Adams, J., Waxman, B., Beaman, P., et al. (1979). COSTAR—A computer-based medical information system for ambulatory care. In J. van Bemmel (Ed.), *Yearbook of medical informatics—The promise of medical informatics* (pp. 262–273). New York, NY: Schattauer.

Blum, B. (1986). *Clinical information systems.* New York, NY: Springer-Verlag.

Blumenthal, D. (2010). Launching HITECH. *New England Journal of Medicine, 362*:5.

Bott, O. J. (2005). Ubiquitous health care systems: A new paradigm for medical informatics? In R. Haux & C. Kulikowski (Eds.), *IMIA Yearbook of Medical Informatics 2005: Ubiquitous Health Care Systems* (pp. 213–218). Stuttgart: Schattauer.

Boutros, S. (1993). Egyptian experience with microcomputers in monitoring and evaluating of health care programmes. In S. Mandil, K. Moidu, M. Korpela, P. Byass, & D. Forster (Eds.), *Health informatics in Africa HELINA 93* (pp. 58–63). Amsterdam, Netherlands: Excerpta Medica.

Brandejs, J. (1976). *Health informatics Canadian experience.* New York, NY: American Elsevier Publishing Company.

Chang, P., Sheng, Y-H., Sang, Y-Y., Wang, D-W., Hsu, Y-S., & Hou, I-C. (2006). Developing and evaluating a wireless speech-and-touch-based interface for intelligent comprehensive triage support systems. In H-A. Park, P. J. Murray, & C. Delaney (Eds.), *Consumer-centered computer-supported care for healthy people. Proceedings of NI2006* (pp. 693–697). Amsterdam: IOS Press.

Collen, M. F. (1995). *A history of medical informatics in the United States: 1950–1990.* Indianapolis, IN: American Medical Informatics Association.

Commission of the European Communities. (2004). *E-Health–Making healthcare better for European citizens: An action plan for a European e-health area. COM (2004) 356 final.* Brussels, Belgium: Author.

Daini, O., Makanjuola, R., & Ojo, J. (1993). A hospital information system in a Nigerian university teaching hospital. In S. Mandil, K. Moidu, M. Korpela, P. Byass, & D. Forster (Eds.), *Health Informatics in Africa HELINA 93* (pp. 86–89). Amsterdam, Netherlands: Excerpta Medica.

The Danish eHealth Portal. (2008). Retrieved from https://www.sundhed.dk/Artikel.aspx?id=11006.105

Development, Concepts and Doctrine Centre (DCDC). (2010). *Strategic Trends Programme: Global Strategic Trends - Out to 2040* (4th ed.). Swindon, UK: DCDC, Ministry of Defence. Retrieved from http://www.mod.uk/NR/rdonlyres/38651ACB-D9A9-4494-98AA-1C86433BB673/0/gst4_update 9_Feb10.pdf

deZegher, I., Venot, A., Milstein, C., Sene, B., deRosis, F., DeCarolis, B., et al. (1995). OPADE: optimization of drug prescription using advanced informatics in health informatics in health. In M. F. Laires, M. J. Ladeira, & J. P. Christensen, (Eds.), *The new communications age health care telematics for the 21st century* (pp. 251–259). Amsterdam, Netherlands: IOS Press.

Easteal, S., & Demosthenes, P. (2005). *View from the future. Bio-ITWorld.com.* Retrieved from http://www.lifescientist.com.au/article/451/view_from_future/?fp=&fpid=&pf=1

Elioutina, S., & Tarasov, V. (1995). Current state and perspectives of healthcare informatics in Russia. *International Journal of Bio-Medical Computing, 39*, 163–167.

Godwin-Jones, R. (2003). *Emerging technologies. Blogs and wikis: environments for on-line collaboration. Language learning and technology.* Retrieved from http://llt.msu.edu/vol7num2/pdf/emerging.pdf

Hannah, K., Ball, M., & Edwards, M. (1999). *Introduction to nursing informatics* (2nd ed.). New York, NY: Springer-Verlag.

Haux, R., Knaup, P., & Schmucker, P. (1999). Commentary—Medical and health information systems; the boundaries are still fading. In A. McCray & J. van Bemmel (Eds.), *Yearbook of medical informatics 1999* (pp. 235–237). New York, NY: Schattauer.

Hayes, G. & Barnett, D. (Eds.). (2008). *UK health computing: Recollections and reflections.* Swindon, UK: The British Computer Society.

Horner, V., Hanmer L., & Mbananga, N. D. (2006). A consumer decision support system for common health ailments in South Africa. In H-A. Park, P. J. Murray, & C. Delaney (Eds.). *Consumer-centered computer-supported care for healthy people. Proceedings of NI2006* (p. 1027). Amsterdam: IOS Press.

Istepanian, R., Laxminarayan, S., & Pattichis, C. S. (Eds.). (2006). *M-Health: Emerging mobile health systems.* Berlin, Germany: Springer.

Kenwright, K., & Pifer, L. (2010). Focus: nanotechnology. Nanotechnology: nanomedicine. *Clinical Laboratory Science, 23*(2), 112–116. Retrieved from CINAHL Plus with Full Text database.

Kirovski, D., Oliver, N., Sinclair, M., & Tan, D. (2007). Health-OS: A position paper. Proceedings of the 1st ACM SIGMOBILE International Workshop. Retrieved from http://portal.acm.org/citation .cfm?id=1248077

Kuhn, K. A., Wurst, S. H. R., Bott, O. J., & Guise, D. A. (2006). *Expanding the scope of health information systems: Challenges and developments. IMIA Yearbook of medical informatics 2006.* Stuttgart, Germany: IMIA and Schattauer GmBH.

Kurzweil, R. (2005). *The singularity is near. When humans transcend biology.* London: Gerald Duckworth & Co. Ltd.

Lawton, S., & Timmons, S. (2006). The relationship between technology and changing professional roles in health care: A case study in teledermatology. In H-A. Park, P. J. Murray, & C. Delaney (Eds.), *Consumer-centered computer-supported care for healthy people. Proceedings of NI2006* (pp. 669–671). Amsterdam: IOS Press.

Lee, M., Delaney, C., & Moorhead, S. (2006). Building a personal health record from nursing perspective. In H-A. Park, P. J. Murray, & C. Delaney (Eds.), *Consumer-centered computer-supported care for healthy people. Proceedings of NI2006* (pp. 25–29). Amsterdam: IOS Press.

Liolios, C., Doukas, C., Fourlas, G., & Maglogiannis, I. (2010) An overview of body sensor networks in enabling pervasive healthcare and assistive environments. In PETRA '10, Proceedings of the 3rd International Conference on Pervasive Technologies Related to Assistive Environment. June 23-25, 2010. Samos, Greece. University of Texas at Arlington, TX.

Loescher, L. J., & Merkle, C. J. (2005). The interface of genomic technologies and nursing. *Journal of Nursing Scholarship, 37*(2), 111–119.

Lymberis, A. (2010). Advanced wearable sensors and systems enabling personal applications. *Lecture Notes in Electrical Engineering, 75*, 237–257.

Maag, M. (2005). The potential use of 'blogs' in nursing education. *CIN: Computers, Informatics, Nursing, 23*(1), 16–24.

Maag, M. (2006). Podcasting and MP3 players: Emerging education technologies. *CIN: Computers, Informatics, Nursing, 24*(1), 9–13.

Mandil, S., Moidu, K., Korpela, M., Byass, P., & Forster, D. (Eds.). (1993). *Health informatics in Africa HELINA93.* Amsterdam, Netherlands: Excerpta Medica.

Martin-Sanchez, F., Iakovidis, I., Norager, F., Maojo, V., de Groen, P., Vander Lei, J., et al. (2004). Synergy between medical informatics and bioinformatics: Facilitating genomic medicine for future health care. *Journal of Biomedical Informatics, 37*(1), 30–42.

Martindale, T., & Wiley, D. A. (2004). *An introduction to teaching with weblogs.* Retrieved from http://teachable.org/papers/2004_blogs_in_teaching.pdf

McCormick, K. A. (2001). Future directions. In V. K. Saab & K. A. McCormick (Eds.), *Essentials of computers for nurses: Informatics for the new millennium* (3rd ed., pp. 519–527). New York, NY: McGraw-Hill.

McCormick, K. A., Delaney, C. J., Brennan, P. F., Effie, J. A., Kendrick, K., Murphy, J., et al. (2007). Guideposts to the future—An agenda for nursing informatics. *Journal of the American Medical Informatics Association, 14*(1), 19–24.

Me-too, D. (2009). Practice development. Nanotechnology: the revolution of the big future with tiny medicine. *British Journal of Nursing (BJN), 18*(19), 1201–1206. Retrieved from CINAHL Plus with Full Text database.

Michael, P. (2009). *mHealth in the Millennium Villages Project. Earth Institute at Columbia University.* Retrieved from http://cghed.ei.columbia.edu/sitefiles/file/Mobile_Health_within_MVP%20 (1).pdf

Miller, R., People, H., & Myers, J. (1982). INTERNIST-1: An experimental computer-based diagnostic consultant for general internal medicine. *New England Journal of Medicine, 307*, 468–476.

Mortensen, R., & Nielsen, G. (1995). Tokenising. In M. F. Laires, M. J. Ladeira, & J. P. Christensen, (Eds.), *Health in the new communications age health care telematics for the 21st century* (pp. 115–126). Amsterdam, Netherlands: IOS Press.

Murray, P.J. (2009, June 29). *Looking Towards "Web 4.0" in Health and Nursing.* Blog post of http://www.hi-blogs.info

Murray, P. J., & Maag, M. (2006). *Towards health informatics 2.0: Blogs, podcasts and Web 2.0 applications in nursing and health informatics education and professional collaboration: A discussion paper.* Retrieved from http://www.differance-engine.net/hiblogs/media/publications/murraymaaghi20%20july06.pdf

Murray, P. J., Park, H-A., Erdley, W. S., & Kim, J. (Eds.). (2007). Nursing informatics 2020: Towards defining our own future. In *Proceedings of NI2006 Post Congress Conference.* Amsterdam: IOS Press.

Murray, P.J, van Middleton, I., & Meyer, S. (2010). Nursing informatics in South Africa: From a historical overview to the emergence of Hers, Telehealth and m-Health. In C.A. Weaver, C. W. Delaney, P. Weber & R.L. Carr (Eds.), *Nursing informatics for the 21st century: An international look at practice, education and EHR trends.* Chicago, IL: HIMSS.

Murray, P. J., & Ward, R. (2004). Engaging in healthcare informatics—Let's use the technology. *BJHC& IM, 21*(10), 14.

O'Donovan, T., O'Donoghue, J., Sreenan, C., et al. (2010). A context aware wireless body area network (BAN). In *Proceedings of the 3rd International Conference on Pervasive Computing Technologies for Healthcare 2009.*

Oh, H., Rizo, C., Enkin, M., & Jadad, A. (2005). What is ehealth (3): A systematic review of published definitions. *Journal of Medical Internet Research, 7*(1), e1. Retrieved from http://www.jmir.org/2005/1/e1

O'Reilly, T. (2005). *What is Web 2.0: Design patterns and business models for the next generation of software.* Retrieved from http://oreilly.com/web2/archive/what-is-web-20.html

Oren, E., Shaffer, E. R., & Guglielmo, B. J. (2003). Impact of emerging technologies on medication errors and adverse drug events. *American Journal of Health-System Pharmacy, 60*(14), 1447–1458.

Oyri, K., Balasingham, H., & Hogetveit, J. O. (2006). Implementation of wireless technology in advanced clinical practice. In H-A. Park, P. J. Murray, & C. Delaney (Eds.), *Consumer-centered computer-supported care for healthy people. Proceedings of NI2006* (pp. 730–733). Amsterdam: IOS Press.

Oyri, K., Newbold, S., Park, H-A., Honey, M., Coenen, A., Ensio, A. et al. (2007). Technology developments applied to healthcare/nursing. In P. J. Murray, H-A. Park, W. S. Erdley, & J. Kim (Eds.), *Nursing informatics 2020: Towards defining our own future. Proceedings of NI2006 Post Congress Conference* (pp. 21–37). Amsterdam: IOS Press.

Park, H-A., Murray, P., & Delaney, C. (2006). *Consumer-centered computer-supported care for healthy people. Proceedings of NI2006.* Amsterdam: IOS Press.

Saba, V. K., & Erdley, W. S. (2006). Historical perspectives of nursing and the computer. In V. K. Saba & K. A. McCormick (Eds.). *Essentials of nursing informatics* (4th ed., pp. 9–28). New York: McGraw-Hill.

Saba, V. K., & McCormick, K. A. (1986). *Essentials of computers for nurses.* Philadelphia, PA: J. B. Lippincott Company.

Sackett, K. M., & Erdley, W. S. (2002). The history of health care informatics. In S. P. Englebardt & R. Nelson (Eds.). *Health care informatics: An interdisciplinary approach* (pp. 453–457). St. Louis, MO: Mosby.

Salata, O. V. (2004). *Applications of nanoparticles in biology and medicine. Journal of Nanobiotechnology, 2.* Retrieved from http://www.jnanobiotechnology.com/content/2/1/3

Santra, T. (2010). Mobile health care system for patient monitoring. *Communications in Computer and Information Science, 101*, Part 3, 695–700.

Saranto, K., Brennan, P.F., & Casey, A. (Eds.). (2009). *Personal health information management—Tools and strategies for citizens' engagement.* Kuopio, Finland: University of Kuopio. Retrieved from http://www.uku.fi/vaitokset/2009/isbn978-951-27-1321-9.pdf

Saranto, K., Brennan, P.F., Park, H-A., Tallberg, M., & Ensio, A. (Eds.). (2009). *Connecting health and humans. Proceedings of NI2009 the 10th International Congress on Nursing Informatics.* Amsterdam: IOS Press.

Schmidt, K. F. (2007). *Nanofrontiers: Visions for the future of nanotechnology. Project on Emerging Nanotechnologies 6. Woodrow Wilson International Center for Scholars.* Retrieved from http://www.nano techproject.org/file_download/181

Schrader, U. (2006). Managing a lecture in nursing informatics in a blended learning format—A bottom-up approach to implement an open-source Web-based learning management system. In H-A. Park, P. J. Murray, & C. Delaney (Eds.), *Consumer-centered computer-supported care for healthy people. Proceedings of NI2006* (pp. 559–562). Amsterdam: IOS Press.

Shortliffe, E., & Buchanan, B. (1975). A model of inexact reasoning in medicine. *Math Biosci, 23*, 351–379.

Siemens, G. (2005). *Connectivism. A learning theory for the digital age.* Retrieved from http://www.constructict.com/blog/wp-content/themes/kiwi/featurepics/WBLEAlan/LinkedDocuments/ConnectivismLearninginttheDigitalAge.doc

Spallek, H., O'Donnell, J., Clayton, M., Anderson, P., & Krueger, A. (2010). Paradigm shift or annoying distraction: Emerging implications of Web 2.0 for clinical practice. *Applied Clinical Informatics, 1*:96–115. Retrieved from http://aci.schattauer.de/de/contents/archive/issue/1062/manuscript/12955/download.html

Staggers, N., McCasky, T., Brazelton, N., & Kennedy, R. (2008). Nanotechnology: the coming revolution and its implications for consumers, clinicians, and informatics. *Nursing Outlook 56*(5): 268–74.

Stammer, L. (2000). Brazil & its neighbours. *Healthcare Informatics, 17* (8): 26–8, 30, 32

Technology Workgroup, Maryland Statewide Commission on the Crisis in Nursing (2004). *Technology's role in addressing Maryland's nursing shortage: Innovations & examples.* Retrieved from http://maryland.nursetech.com/F/NT/MD/NursingInnovations2004.pdf

The White House (2009). *Weekly address: President Barack Obama discusses new White House Report on an American Recovery and Reinvestment Plan.* Retrieved from http://www.whitehouse.gov/the-press-office/weekly-address-president-barack-obama-discusses-new-white-house-report-american-rec

TIGER. (2007). *The TIGER Initiative: Evidence and informatics transforming nursing: 3-year action steps toward a 10-year vision.* Retrieved from https://www.tigersummit.com/uploads/TIGERInitiative_Report2007_bw.pdf

Turley, J. P., Murray, P. J., Saranto, K., Ehnfors, M., & Seomun, G-A. (2007). What if nurses get what they have always sought: Totally personalized care? Trends affecting nursing informatics. In P. J. Murray, H-A. Park, W. S. Erdley, & J. Kim (Eds.), *Nursing informatics 2020: Towards defining our own future. Proceedings of NI2006 Post Congress Conference* (pp. 55–72). Amsterdam: IOS Press.

van Ginneken, B, Koenderink, J. & Dana, K. (1999). Texture histograms as a function of irradiation and viewing direction, International Journal of Computer Vision, 31, pp. 169–184.

Vocera. (2007). *Vocera communications badge: Wearable instant voice communication.* Retrieved from http://www.vocera.com/downloads/voc_sys_datasheet_1206.pdf

Warner, H., Olmsted, C., & Rutherford, B. (1972). HELP—A program for medical decision-making. *Computers and Biomedical Research, 5*(1), 65–74.

Weaver, C., Kennedy, R., Erdley, W. S., Kim, J., Chang, P., Schrader, U. & Maag, M. (2007). Health care in 2020. In P. J. Murray, H-A. Park, W. S. Erdley, & J. Kim (Eds.), *Nursing informatics 2020: Towards defining our own future. Proceedings of NI2006 Post Congress Conference* (pp. 73–83). Amsterdam: IOS Press.

Weiser, M. (1991, *September*). The computer for the twenty-first century. *Scientific American, 265* (3): 94–104.

Wikipedia. *Semantic Web.* Retrieved from http://en.wikipedia.org/wiki/Semantic_Web

Williams, L. (2007). *Nobel laureate James Watson receives personal genome in ceremony at Baylor College of Medicine.* Retrieved from http://www.bcm.edu/news/packages/watson_genome.cfm

World Health Organization. (2007). *WHO brainstorming session on mhealth. Med-e-Tel Conference, Luxembourg, Luxembourg.* Retrieved from http://www.medetel.lu/download/2007/parallel_sessions/abstract/0418/WHO_m-HEALTH_Brainstorm_Notes.pdf

Zollner, H. (1995). The CARE telematics project. In M. F. Laires, M. J. Ladeira, & J. P. Christensen, (Eds.), *Health in the new communications age, health care telematics for the 21st century* (pp. 279–289). Amsterdam: IOS Press.

Nursing Informatics and the Foundation of Knowledge

Dee McGonigle and Kathleen Mastrian

1. Assess nursing as a knowledge-intensive profession.
2. Explore the contribution of nursing informatics to the foundation of knowledge.

WWW

Key Terms WWW

Comprehensive
  Health Enhancement
  Support System (CHESS)
Codify
Data
Data-centric
Information
Information technology (IT)
Knowledge
Knowledge acquisition
Knowledge-centric
Knowledge dissemination
Knowledge Domain Process
  (KDP)
Knowledge generation
Knowledge management
  system (KMS)
Knowledge repositories
Knowledge worker
Nursing informatics (NI)

INTRODUCTION

Throughout this book the reader has learned about the many facets of **nursing informatics** (NI) and the interfacing of nurse **knowledge workers** and technology. The Foundation of Knowledge model (Figure 30-1) has provided a framework for examining the dynamic interrelationships between **data**, **information**, and knowledge used to meet the needs of healthcare delivery systems, organizations, patients, and nurses. The importance of knowledge management in nursing is emphasized by taking this one last opportunity to ensure that the reader understands and appreciates the value of knowledge management in the nursing profession, and the role that technology has in **knowledge acquisition**, **knowledge generation**, **knowledge dissemination**, and knowledge processing.

FOUNDATION OF KNOWLEDGE REVISITED

A review of the Foundation of Knowledge model that provides a framework for the development of this text is useful. At its base, the model has bits, bytes (computer terms for chunks of information), data, and information in a random representation. Growing out of the base are separate cones of light that expand as they reflect upward and represent knowledge acquisition, knowledge generation, and knowledge dissemination. At the intersection of the cones and forming a new cone is knowledge processing. Encircling and cutting through the knowledge

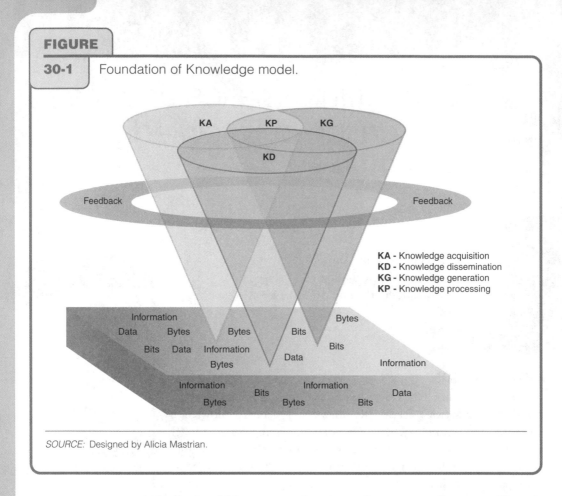

FIGURE 30-1 Foundation of Knowledge model.

KA - Knowledge acquisition
KD - Knowledge dissemination
KG - Knowledge generation
KP - Knowledge processing

SOURCE: Designed by Alicia Mastrian.

cones is feedback, which acts on and may transform any or all aspects of knowledge represented by the cones. Now, imagine the model as a dynamic figure with the cones of light and the feedback rotating and interacting rather than remaining static. Knowledge acquisition, knowledge generation, knowledge dissemination, knowledge processing, and feedback are constantly evolving for nurse scientists. The transparent effect of the cones is deliberate and is intended to suggest that as knowledge grows and expands its use becomes more transparent; that is, the user is not even consciously aware of what aspect of knowledge he or she is using at any given moment during her or his practice.

If you are an experienced nurse, think back to when you were a novice. Did you feel like all you had in your head were bits of data and information that did not form any type of cohesive whole? As the model depicts, the processing of knowledge as an individual in professional practice begins a bit later (imagine a time line applied vertically) with early experiences on the bottom and expertise growing as the processing of knowledge kicks in. Early on in nursing education conscious attention is focused mainly on knowledge acquisition, and the learner depends on their instructors and others to process, generate, and disseminate knowledge. As the learner becomes more comfortable with the science of nursing, they begin to take over some of the other knowledge functions. However, to keep up with the explosion of information in nursing and health care, one must continue to rely on the knowledge generation and dissemination of others. In this sense, nurses are committed to lifelong learning and the use of knowledge in the practice of nursing science.

As nurse knowledge workers, information is the primary resource, and when one deals with information it is done in overlapping phases. The nurse is acquiring, processing or assimilating, and retaining, and using this information to generate and disseminate knowledge. However, it is not a sequential phasing; instead, there is a constant gleaning of data and information from the environment, massaging it into knowledge bases so that it can be applied and shared (disseminated).

Knowledge is thought of as either explicit or tacit. Explicit knowledge is the knowledge that one can convey in letters, words, and numbers. This can be exchanged or shared in the form of data, manuals, product specifications, principles, policies, theories, and the like. Nurses can disseminate and share this knowledge publicly or on the record and scientifically or methodically. A nursing model or theory that is well developed and easily explained and understood is an example of explicit knowledge. Tacit knowledge, however, is individualized and highly personal or private, including one's values or emotions. This type of knowledge is difficult to convey, transmit, or share with others because it is one's own insights or slant on things, perceptions, intuitions, sense, hunches, or gut feelings. Tacit knowledge reflects skills and beliefs, and that is why it is difficult to explain or communicate it to others. Lake (2005) states:

> From close examination of and reflection on the literature it is possible to infer nursing prioritization of the patient need for care as it is initially taught to nursing students and is then developed in practice and influenced by practice setting. The process of nursing prioritization of the patient need for care involves discretionary judgment and ongoing assessment throughout and between unfolding patient situations. It is best understood from studies addressing clinical decision-making in nursing through the interpretive paradigm and in the plain language descriptions of nurse decision-making. The principles of such decision-making are discussed only in very general terms and the rationale remains the tacit knowledge of nursing (p. 152).

How nursing students and practicing nurses learn is directly affected by their practice experiences within their own personal frame of reference. The quality of clinical decision making is directly related to experience and knowledge. Knowledge is situational. Explicit and tacit knowledge is used to conduct assessments, diagnoses, intervention implementation, and evaluation of nursing actions for each individual patient. **Knowledge management system**s (KMSs) must blend these knowledge needs and provide knowledge bases and decision support systems to inform clinical decision making. Each person processes and assimilates knowledge in a unique way influenced by unique perspectives.

KNOWLEDGE USE IN PRACTICE

One way to capture and **codify** tacit knowledge is to engage in reflection and reflective practice. Schutz (2007) believes that reflection is a way of both learning about practice and a basis for changing practice. One must engage in reflective practice because

> reflective practice can enable a practitioner to find a means in which to put this personal or experiential knowledge into words and to find a way of considering why the situation turned out as it did and whether future practice might be different (Schutz, p. 27).

Some healthcare organizations are encouraging reflective practice to codify tacit knowledge and thus to build an organization's knowledge base. Sharing experiences in a Nursing Practice Council is one example of a means to encourage collaboration and knowledge sharing among professionals. Joining a list-serv or a community of practice is another example of collaboration to build knowledge. Watson (2007) describes knowledge audits, narratives, and storytelling as means of surfacing tacit knowledge and assessing the knowledge resources within an organization. He describes the use of **information technology** tools for knowledge management in an organization, such as intranets, extranets (shared intranets among several like organizations), knowledge directories, blogs, and wikis. Recent research suggests that organizations that embrace and encourage knowledge transfer among workers not only sustain and build professional competence and organizational engagement, but also enhance the quality of the work-life for professionals (Leiter, Day, Harvie, & Shaughnessy, 2007).

According to Gent (2007), there are three types of knowledge workers: (1) knowledge consumers, (2) knowledge brokers, and (3) knowledge generators. This breakdown of knowledge workers is not mutually exclusive but instead people transition between them as situations and experience, education, and knowledge change. Knowledge consumers are mainly users of knowledge who do not have the expertise to provide the knowledge they need for themselves. Novice nurses can be thought of as knowledge consumers who use the knowledge of experienced nurses or who search information systems for the knowledge necessary to apply to their practice. As responsible knowledge consumers, they must also question and challenge what is known to help them learn and understand. Their questioning and challenging facilitate critical thinking and the development of new knowledge. Knowledge brokers know where to find information and knowledge; they generate some knowledge but are mainly known for their ability to find what is needed. More experienced nurses and nursing students become knowledge brokers out of necessity, needing to know. Knowledge generators are the "primary sources of new knowledge" (para. 2). These are nursing researchers and nursing experts—the people who know. They are able to answer questions, craft theories, find solutions to nursing problems or concerns, and innovate practice.

The healthcare industry, the nursing profession, and patients all benefit as nurses develop nursing intelligence and intellectual capital by gaining insight into nursing science and its enactment, practice. NI applications of databases, knowledge management systems, and repositories where this knowledge can be analyzed and reused facilitates this process, enabling knowledge to be disseminated and reused.

To be able to enhance the acquisition, processing, generation, dissemination, and reuse of nursing knowledge, nurses must codify or be able to articulate knowledge structures so that they can be captured within the KMSs. According to Markus (2001):

> Synthesis of evidence from a wide variety of sources suggests four distinct types of knowledge reuse situations according to the knowledge reuser and the purpose of knowledge reuse. The types involve shared work producers, who produce knowledge they later reuse; shared work practitioners, who reuse each other's knowledge contributions; expertise-seeking novices; and secondary knowledge miners. Each type of knowledge reuser has different requirements for knowledge repositories (para. 1).

Markus refers to the **knowledge repositories** as "organizational memory systems" (2001, para. 1). These memory systems gained popularity for help desk personnel who could access and reuse knowledge of solutions to similar problems on which clients seek help. Health care is an arena that could use the KMSs or knowledge repositories. Hsia, Lin, Wu, and Tsai (2006) recognize that nurses are "knowledge intensive" (para. 4) professionals who are "required to take new nursing knowledge and experience that can be acquired through various net-enabled applications or the Internet. Nursing professionals are being asked to do more with less in such contexts, while their nursing care responsibilities have increased" (para. 4). The information technology capabilities are expanding to develop and support a "**knowledge-centric** [boldface added] view rather than simply a **data-centric** view [boldface added]" (Hsia et al., para. 4). Nurse knowledge workers must be able to access, use, and share these new informatics tools because "a well-designed IT-based knowledge management system (KMS) has become an ever more central force in improving the quality of care in competitive e-health environments" (Hsia et al., para. 4). Capturing the explicit and tacit forms of knowledge is paramount to truly harness nursing knowledge. As knowledge repositories evolve to enhance sharing and repurposing of knowledge, nurses will be able to easily access, process, evaluate, reuse, generate, and disseminate knowledge.

This book uses the Foundation of Knowledge model reflecting that knowledge is power, and for that reason, nurses focus on information as a key resource. The application of the model was described in each section of the book to help the reader understand and appreciate the foundation of knowledge in NI. All of the various nursing roles—practice, administration, education, research, informatics—involve the science of nursing. Nurses are knowledge workers, working with information and generating information and knowledge as a product. They are knowledge acquirers, providing convenient and efficient means of capturing and storing knowledge. They are knowledge users, individuals or groups who benefit from valuable, viable knowledge. Nurses are knowledge engineers, designing, developing, implementing and maintaining knowledge. They are knowledge managers, capturing and processing collective expertise and distributing it where it can create the largest benefit. They are knowledge developers or generators, changing and evolving knowledge based on the tasks at hand and information available.

Nursing science is dependent on knowledge generation, and NI should facilitate all aspects of nursing especially in the generation of knowledge and translational research where we attempt to bridge the gap between what we know (research) and what we do (practice). Swan, Lang, and McGinley (2004) describe NI and a common nursing language as an important vehicle to access stores of clinical information that can be used as the basis for research and to help answer the question, "What do nurses do?" "Embedding nursing language within informatics structures is essential to make the work of nurses visible and articulate evidence about the quality and value of nursing in the care of patients, groups, and populations" (para. 27). In this text, it has been established that NI is a vital tool for clinical decision making, especially when one is able to demonstrate how nurses structure and process information. An important direction for the future is to study the impact of NI on nursing science. For example, Goossen (2000) suggests the need for further study of nursing decision making and the need to model this process. He also suggests that one needs to focus on the evaluation of technology systems themselves and the human–technology interface.

As the HITECH Act is implemented, the use of electronic health records (EHRs) is an expectation in America and they must be designed to enhance patient outcomes through content enrichment and improved caregiver decision making. As bioinformatics and computational biology continue to evolve, their integration into the EHR is inevitable. Nursing informaticists must facilitate the inclusion of computational tools and algorithms to help handle the collection, organization, analysis, processing, presentation, and dissemination of biologic data to help address biologic questions and unravel biologic issues. It is imperative that current research strategies, such as those used to search for biomarkers, and new pharmacologic treatments be included in the EHR. In this bioinformatics era, one must be able to delineate biomarkers and have the necessary alerts, follow-ups, and reminders built into the system to make all caregivers aware of the bioinformatics information, such as the analysis of genes causing hypertension, cardiovascular, and diabetes diseases. Bioinformatics and computational biology will complement all of the current methods and aid in the analysis of populations and tracking selected diseases' progression. Consequently, nursing informaticists must be proactive in the development of policies and ethically based solutions to safeguard the genetic data in EHRs, the patient care implications of bioinformatics and computational biology in this bioinformatics era.

A paradigm shift is occurring from healthcare facility–owned machine-based computing to off-site, vendor-owned cloud computing. Web browser–based login accessible data, software, and hardware could link systems together and reduce costs. Hospitals with shrinking budgets and extreme IT needs are exploring the successes in other industries, such as Amazon's S3. As providers strive to implement potent EHRs, they are looking for the cloud-based models that offer the necessary functionality without having to assume the burden associated with all of the hardware, software, application, and storage issues. However, in the face of the HITECH Act and its associated penalties, the challenges must be overcome to realize the benefits. The advantages and disadvantages of cloud computing must be fully explored in light of the challenges faced by both the healthcare providers as they strive to maintain security while relinquishing control, and the vendors who are responsible for developing and maintaining this new cloud-based EHR environment.

NI can also be used to facilitate nursing administration and managerial studies of the work of nursing. Numerous opportunities for data mining in NI have been described. Goossen (2000) suggests two approaches to data mining. The first approach involves a general search looking for repeated instances or patterns without preconceived notions about what will be found. Findings from the eyes-wide-open look at the database may suggest patterns that warrant more structured data mining, consistent with Goossen's second approach. Some of the larger healthcare systems store all of the clinical information from all of the affiliated hospitals and clinics in a central data warehouse. General data scans and analyses looking for patterns may suggest a trend toward better outcomes for patients with congestive heart failure in one of the affiliate hospitals. This identification of such a trend clearly begs for further analyses. A nurse researcher or administrator could ask, "What are the factors contributing to these better outcomes and how can they be put into practice across the system?" Other research studies might focus on assessing the effectiveness of strategic planning and organizational goal setting or studying workflow and communication processes in an organization. Poissant, Pereira, Tamblyn, and Kawasumi (2005) present the results of a systematic literature review on the time efficiency impacts of EHRs in the clinical setting. There are numerous other examples of research aimed at advancing the state of the science of NI. Bakken (2006) provides one of the most comprehensive overviews of the effects of NI on patient safety. In her opening remarks, she writes, "The health information technologies deployed as part of the national framework must support nursing practice in a manner that enables prevention of medical errors and the promotion of patient safety and contributes to the development of practice-based nursing knowledge as well as best practices for patient safety" (para. 1). Shaw and colleagues (2006) summarize 15 years of research on the **Comprehensive Health Enhancement Support System (CHESS),** a computer-based system designed to help underserved breast cancer patients manage their disease. A study of comparing routine instruction with computer-assisted video instruction about home exercise and the effects on compliance with the regimen and patient satisfaction is yet another example of research opportunities related to NI (Lysack, Dama, Neufeld, & Andreassi, 2005). As a final example, Hering, Harvan, D'Angelo, and Jasinski (2005) studied the effects of a specially designed Web page related to surgical teaching on patient acquisition of information and overall satisfaction with the surgical experience. We invite you to read each of these studies in more detail.

Knowledge management and transfer in healthcare organizations are likely to be studied in greater depth as understanding of professional knowledge is increased and processes to capture and codify it are improved. The model is not perfect, and others have developed models of knowledge that are more complex. For example, Evans and Alleyne (2009) constructed the Knowledge Domain Process (KDP) model to represent knowledge construction and dissemination in an organization. Yet, they caution,

> the KDP model, like all models, is an abstraction aimed at making complex systems more easily understood. While the model presents knowledge processes in a structured and simplified form, the nature and structure of the processes themselves may be open to debate (p. 148).

In the future, there will be many more attempts to capture, represent, and explain knowledge processes in professional practice. It is hoped that the reader is convinced that for the nursing profession to evolve, knowledge must be dynamically generated, disseminated, and assimilated. This dynamic interplay means that as knowledge is generated, disseminated, and assimilated, new questions about the impact of NI that will help new knowledge to be generated and assimilated and so on will arise. The assimilation of new knowledge in a profession is a multifaceted approach of individual perception, challenges, and collective thought applied to the practice of nursing. Nurses challenge what is known, and want to acquire, process, generate, and disseminate knowledge.

SUMMARY

As a result of reading this book, you should have a deeper understanding of knowledge and informatics and the power they have to inform the science of nursing. It is hoped that you also gained valuable insights into the core principles of NI and the NI practice specialty. The future is exciting. The previous chapter in this section was an excellent insight into what will and can be. This chapter should motivate you to continue to learn more and perhaps delve into the science of NI in a nursing research role. Readers are invited to become active participants in molding the future of both nursing and informatics sciences.

THOUGHT-PROVOKING Questions WWW

Become informatics savvy and ask yourself the following questions:

1. How can I apply the knowledge I gain from my practice setting to benefit my patients and enhance my practice?
2. How can I help my colleagues and patients understand and use the current technology that is available?
3. How can I use my wisdom to help create the theories, tools, and knowledge of the future?

For a full suite of assignments and additional learning activities, use the access code located in the front of your book to visit this exclusive website: http://go.jblearning.com/mcgonigle. If you do not have an access code, you can obtain one at the site.

References

Bakken, S. (2006). Informatics for patient safety: A nursing research perspective. *Annual Review of Nursing Research, 24*, 219–254. Retrieved from ProQuest Nursing & Allied Health Source database. Document ID: 1106698271

Evans, M., & Alleyne, J. (2009). The concept of knowledge in KM: A knowledge domain process model applied to inter-professional care. *Knowledge and Process Management, 16*(4), 147. Retrieved from ABI/INFORM Global. Document ID: 1890423631

Gent, A. (2007). *Three types of knowledge workers.* Retrieved from http://incrediblydull.blogspot.com/2007/10/three-types-of-knowledge-workers.html

Goossen, W. (2000). Nursing informatics research. *Nurse Researcher, 8*(2), 42. Retrieved from ProQuest Nursing & Allied Health Source database. Document ID: 67258628

Hering, K., Harvan, J., D'Angelo, M., & Jasinski, D. (2005). The use of a computer Website prior to scheduled surgery (a pilot study): Impact on patient information, acquisition, anxiety level, and overall satisfaction with anesthesia care. *AANA Journal, 73*(1), 29–33. Retrieved from ProQuest Nursing & Allied Health Source database. Document ID: 795995771

Hsia, T., Lin, L., Wu, J., & Tsai, H. (2006). A framework for designing nursing knowledge management systems. *Interdisciplinary Journal of Information, Knowledge and Management.* Retrieved from http://www.ijikm.org/Volume1/IJIKMv1p013-022_Hsia02.pdf

Lake, S. (2005). *Nursing prioritization of the patient need for care: Tacit knowledge of clinical decision making in nursing.* Retrieved from http://researcharchive.vuw.ac.nz/bitstream/10063/22/6/thesis.pdf

Leiter, M., Day, A., Harvie, P. & Shaughnessy, K. (2007). Personal and organizational knowledge transfer: Implications for worklife engagement. *Human Relations, 60*(2), 259–283. Retrieved from ABI/INFORM Global. Document ID: 1260239891

Lysack, C., Dama, M., Neufeld, S., & Andreassi, E. (2005). Compliance and satisfaction with home exercise: A comparison of computer-assisted video instruction and routine rehabilitation practice. *Journal of Allied Health, 34*(2), 76–82. Retrieved from ProQuest Nursing & Allied Health Source database. Document ID: 855324561

Markus, M. (2001). Toward a theory of knowledge reuse: Types of knowledge reuse situations and factors in reuse success. *Journal of Management Information Systems, 18*(1), 57–94. Retrieved from http://jmis.bentley.edu/articles/v18_n1_p57/index.html

Poissant, L., Pereira, J., Tamblyn, R., & Kawasumi, Y. (2005). The impact of electronic health records on time efficiency of physicians and nurses: A systematic review. *Journal of the American Medical Informatics Association, 12*(5), 505–516. Retrieved from ProQuest Nursing & Allied Health Source database. Document ID: 908812431

Schutz, S. (2007). Reflection and reflective practice. *Community Practitioner, 80*(9), 26–9. Retrieved from ProQuest Nursing & Allied Health Source. Document ID: 1331520781

Shaw, B., Gustafson, D., Hawkins, R., McTavish, F., McDowell, H., Pingree, S. & Ballard, D. (2006). How underserved breast cancer patients use and benefit from ehealth programs: Implications for closing the digital divide. *American Behavioral Scientist, 49*(6), 823–834. Retrieved from ABI/INFORM Global database. Document ID: 974889131

Swan, B., Lang, N., & McGinley, A. (2004). Access to quality health care: Links between evidence, nursing language, and informatics. *Nursing Economics, 22*(6), 325–332. Retrieved from Health Module database. Document ID: 768191851

Watson, M. (2007). Knowledge management in health and social care. *Journal of Integrated Care, 15*(1), 27–33. Retrieved from ProQuest Nursing & Allied Health Source. Document ID: 1221495781

Abbreviations

3D	Three dimensional
ABC	Alternative billing codes
ADT	Admission, discharge, and transfer system
AHRQ	Agency for Healthcare Research and Quality
AI	Artificial intelligence
ALA	American Library Association
Alt	Alternate key on the computer keyboard
ALU	Arithmetic logic unit
ANA	American Nurses Association
ANGEL	A New Global Environment for Learning
ANSI	American National Standards Institute
API	Application programming interface
ARG	Augmented Reality Game
ARRA	American Recovery and Reinvestment Act
b	Bit
B	Byte
BCMA	Bar Code Medication Administration
BI	Bioinformatics
BIOS	Basic input/output system
bit/s or bps	Bits per second
BMP	Bitmap image
BRFSS	Behavioral risk factor surveillance system

CAI	Computer assisted instruction
CASE	Computer-aided software engineering
CBIS	Computer-based information system
CCC	Clinical care classification
CD	Compact disc
CDC	Centers for Disease Control and Prevention
CD-R	Compact disc recordable
CD-ROM	Compact disc-read only memory
CD-RW	Compact disc recordable and rewritable
CDS/CDSS	Clinical decision support/clinical decision support system
CHESS	Comprehensive Health Enhancement Support System
CHF	Congestive heart failure
CHI	Consolidated health informatics
CI	Cognitive informatics
CINAHL	Cumulative Index to Nursing & Allied Health Literature
CIO	Chief information officer
CIS	Clinical information systems
CMIS	Case management information system
CMP	Civil Monetary Penalties
CMS	Course management system; content management system; Centers for Medicare and Medicaid Services
CNPII	Committee for Nursing Practice Information Infrastructure
COPD	Chronic obstructive pulmonary disease
CPGs	Clinical practice guidelines
CPOE	Computerized physician order entry; computer-based provider order entry
CPU	Central processing unit
CRA	Community risk assessment
CRT	Cathode ray tube
CSS	Cascading style sheets
CTA	Cognitive task analysis
CTO	Chief technical officer; chief technology officer
Ctrl	Control key on the computer keyboard
CWA	Cognitive work analysis
DBMS	Database management system
DHR	Digital health record
DRAM	Dynamic random access memory
DSDM	Dynamic system development method

DSS	Decision support system
DVD	Digital versatile disc; digital video disc
DVD-R	Digital video disc-recordable
DVD-RW	Digital video disc-recordable and rewritable
DW	Data warehouse
EB	Exabyte
EBP	Evidence-based practice
EDI	Electronic data interchange
EEPROM	Electronically erasable programmable read-only memory
EHR	Electronic health record
ELSI	Ethical, legal and social issues
EMR	Electronic medical record
EPROM	Erasable programmable read-only memory
ERD	Entity relationship diagram
ERIC	Education Resources Information Center
ESC	Escape key
ESLI	Ethical, social, and legal implications
F key	Function key on the computer keyboard
FHIE	Federal Health Information Exchange
FMEA	Failure Modes and Effects Analysis
F/OSS or FOSS	Free/open source software
FPROM	Field programmable read only memory
FPU	Floating point unit
GB	Gigabyte
GHz	Gigahertz
GLBA	Gramm-Leach-Bliley Act
GUI	Graphical user interface
HCI	Human–computer interaction
HCT	Human–computer technology
HGP	Human Genome Project
HHA	Home health agency
HIE	Health information exchange
HIPAA	Health Insurance Portability and Accountability Act
HIS	Hospital information system

HIT	Health Information Technology
HITECH	Health Information Technology for Economic and Clinical Health Act
HL7	Health Level 7
HMIS	Health management information system
HMO	Health maintenance organization
HTI	Human–technology interaction
HTML	Hypertext markup language
ICNP	International classification of nursing practice
IDE	Integrated drive electronics
IEEE	Institute of Electrical and Electronics Engineers
IHIE	Indiana Health Information Exchange
IM	Instant message
IN	Informatics nurse
INS	Informatics nurse specialist
I/O	Input/output
IP	Internet protocol
IS	Information system
ISO	International Standards Organization or International Organization for Standardization
IT	Information technology
KB	Kilobyte
KMS	Knowledge management system
LAN	Local area network
LCD	Liquid crystal display
LOINC	Logical Observation Identifiers Names and Codes
LOS	Length of stay
LTC	Long-term care
MAN	Metropolitan area network
MB	Megabyte
MCIS	Managed care information system
MHDC	Massachusetts Health Data Consortium
MHz	Megahertz
MMIS	Medicaid management information systems
MMORPG or	Massive multiplayer online role-playing game simply MMO

Modem	Modulator-demodulator
Moodle	Modular Object-Oriented Dynamic Learning Environment
MOO	Object-Oriented MUD
MoSCoW	Must have, Should have, Could have, and Would have
MP3	MPEG-1 Audio Layer-3
MPEG	Moving Picture Experts Group
MPI	Master patient index
MRI	Magnetic resonance imaging
MUD	Multiuser dungeon
MUSH	Multiuser Shared Hack, Habitat, Holodeck, or Hallucination
NANDA-I	North American Nursing Diagnosis Association-International
NCPHI	National Center for Public Health Informatics
NGC	National Guideline Clearinghouse
NGI	Next-generation Internet
NHANES	National Health and Nutrition Examination Survey
NHII	National Health Information Infrastructure
NHIN	National Health Information Network
NHQR	National Healthcare Quality Report
NI	Nursing informatics
NIC	Nursing Intervention Classification; network interface cards
NIDSEC	Nursing Information and Data Set Evaluation Center
NIS	Nursing information system
NIST	National Institute of Standards and Technology
NLS	National language support
NMDS	Nursing minimum data set
NMMDS	Nursing management minimum data set
NOC	Nursing outcome classification
NPC	Nonplayer character
NPI	National provider identifier
OASIS	Outcomes and assessment information set
OCR	Office of Civil Rights
ONC	Office of the National Coordinator for Health Information Technology
OS	Operating system
OSI	Open systems interconnection
OWL	Web ontology language

PACS	Picture archiving and communication system
PADS	Planned accelerated discharge protocols
PB	Petabyte
PBL	Problem-based learning
PC	Personal computer
PCA	Patient-controlled analgesia
PCI	Peripheral component interconnection
PCIS	Patient care information system
PDA	Personal data assistant; personal digital assistant
PERS	Personal emergency response system
PHI	Protected health information; public health informatics
PHR	Personal health record
PNDS	Perioperative nursing data set
POSIX	Portable operating system interface for UNIX
PPS	Prospective payment system
PROM	Programmable read-only memory
PrtSc or Prnt Scrn	Print screen key
PS/2	Personal system/2
PT/INR	Prothrombin time/international normalized ratio
QA	Quality assurance
RAD	Rapid application development
RAM	Random access memory
RATS	Readiness assessment tests
RDBMS	Relational database management system
RDF	Resource description framework
RFI	Radiofrequency Identifier
RFID	Radio frequency identification
RHIO	Regional health information organization
RIS	Radiology information system
ROM	Read-only memory
RSS	Really simple syndication
RSVP	Rapid Syndromic Validation Project
RU	Research utilization
SCSI	Small computer system interface
SDLC	Systems development life cycle
SDO	Standards developing organization

SDRAM	Synchronous dynamic random access memory
SGML	Standard generalized markup language
SNOMED CT	Systematic Nomenclature of Medical Clinical Terms
SOX	Sarbanes-Oxley Act
SPRC	Suicide Prevention Resource Center
SQL	Structured English Query Language
TELOS	Technologic and systems, Economic, Legal, Operational, and Schedule feasibility
TB	Terabyte
TCP	Transmission control protocol
TPO	Treatment Payment Operations
URL	Uniform resource locator
USB	Universal serial bus
VNA	Visiting Nurse Association
VoIP	Voice-over-Internet protocol
VR	Virtual reality
W3C	World Wide Web Consortium
WAN	Wide area network
WWW	World Wide Web
XML	Extensible markup language
YB	Yottabyte
YRBSS	Youth Risk Behavior Surveillance System
ZB	Zettabye

Glossary

60/60/24/7 Every second of every day.

3D Three dimensional.

Acceptable use A corporate policy that defines the types of activities that are acceptable on the corporate computer network, identifies the activities that are not acceptable, and the consequences for violations.

Accessibility Ease of accessing the information and knowledge needed to deliver care or manage a health service; the extent to which a system is usable by as many users as possible.

Acquisition The act of acquiring, to locate and hold. We acquire data and information.

Acuity system System that calculates the nursing care requirements for individual patients based on severity of illness, specialized equipment and technology needed, and intensity of nursing interventions; determines the amount of daily nursing care needed for each patient in a nursing unit.

Administrative processes The processes used by administration, such as the electronic scheduling, billing, and claims management systems including electronic scheduling for inpatient and outpatient visits and procedures; electronic insurance eligibility validation; claim authorization and prior approval; identification of possible research study participants; and drug recall support.

Admission, discharge, and transfer (ADT) system System that provides the backbone structure for the other types of clinical and business systems (Hassett & Thede, 2003); it contains the groundwork for the other types of healthcare information systems since it includes the patient's name, medical record number, visit or account number and demographic information such as age, sex, home address, and contact information. They are the central source for collecting this type of patient information and communicating it to the other types of healthcare information systems including clinical and business systems.

Advocate To act in the patients' best interest; to act and/or speak on our patients' behalf; to make the healthcare delivery system responsive to our patients' needs.

Advocate/policy developer A nurse informatics specialist who is key to developing the infrastructure of health policy. Policy development on a local, national, and international level is an integral part of this role.

Agency for Healthcare Research and Quality (AHRQ) An agency within the Department of Health and Human Services (DHHS), that supports health services research initiatives.

Aggregate data Any types of data that can be referenced as a single entity, but that also consist of more than one piece of data. Collect, gather, and report data that is related and kept together in a way that addresses that relationship; for example the population of a state is an aggregate of the populations of its cities, counties, and regions.

Alarm Fatigue Multiple false alarms by smart technology causing workers to ignore or respond slowly to them.

Alerts Warnings or additional information provided to clinicians to help with decision making; the action of the clinician or system triggers the generation of an alert. An example of when an alert could be generated would be if the patient's serum potassium level is high and he is on potassium chloride, the system would alert the nurse on the screen (soft copy alert) with or without audio and/or by a printed (hard copy alert) warning; also known as triggers.

Alleles One member of a pair or series of genes that occupy a specific position on a specific chromosome.

Alternatives Choice between two or more options.

American Library Association (ALA) U.S.-based organization that promotes libraries and library education internationally.

American National Standards Institute (ANSI) An organization dedicated to promoting consensus on norms and guidelines related to the assessment of health agencies.

American Recovery and Reinvestment Act (ARRA) An economic stimulus package enacted in February 2009 that was intended to create jobs and promote investment and consumer spending during the recession. This act has also been referred to as the Stimulus or Recovery Act. There was a push for widespread adoption of health information technology and Title XIII of **ARRA** was given a subtitle: Health Information Technology for Economic and Clinical Health (**HITECH**) Act. Through this act, healthcare organizations can qualify for financial incentives based on the level of meaningful use achieved; the HITECH Act specifically incentivizes health organizations and providers to become "meaningful users."

A New Global Environment for Learning (ANGEL) A course management system designed to support classroom learning in academic settings.

Analysis Separating a whole into its elements or component parts. Examination of a concept or phenomena, its elements, and their relations.

Antiprinciplism Theory that emerged with the expansive technological changes and the tremendous rise in ethical dilemmas accompanying these changes. Opponents of principlism include those who claim that its principles do not represent a theoretical approach and those who claim that its principles are too far removed from the concrete particularities of everyday human existence; the principles are too conceptual, intangible, or abstract, or disregard or do not take into account a person's psychological factors, personality, life history, sexual orientation, religious, ethnic, and cultural background.

Antivirus software A computer program that is designed to recognize and neutralize computer viruses, malicious codes that replicate over and over and eventually take over the computer's memory and interfere with normal functioning.

Application Refers to the implementation software of a computer system. This software allows users to complete tasks such as word processing, developing presentations, and managing data.

Archetype Broad or general, idealized model of an object or concept from which similar instances are derived, copied, patterned, or emulated. Original model after which other similar things are patterned. First form from which varieties arise or imitations are made.

Arithmetic logic unit (ALU) Essential building block of the central processing unit (CPU) that digitally performs arithmetic and logical functions.

Artificial intelligence (AI) The field that deals with the conception, development, and implementation of informatics tools based on intelligent technologies. This field attempts to capture the complex processes of human thought and intelligence.

Asynchronous That which is not synchronous. Not in real time, or does not occur or exist at the same time, having the same period or time frame. Learning anywhere and anytime using Internet and World Wide Web software tools (course management systems, e-mail, electronic bulletin boards, Web pages, etc.) as the principal delivery mechanisms for instruction.

Attribute Quality or characteristic; field or element of an entity in a database.

Audiopod Utility to download podcasts.

Augmented Reality Game (ARG) The use of a device, such as a smart phone, to overlay on the real world bringing people together physically and virtually to solve a series of challenges.

Authentication Processes to serve to authenticate or prove who is accessing the system.

Autonomy Right of individual to choose for herself/himself.

Avatar Image on the Internet that represents the user in virtual communities or other interactions on the Internet; 3-dimensional or 2-dimensional image representing one user on the Internet.

Bar Code Medication Administration (BCMA) A system using bar code technology affixed to the medication, the patient ID bracelet, and the nurse ID badge to support the five rights of medication administration.

Behavioral Risk Factor Surveillance System (BRFSS) An assessment system initially designed to collect information on the movement of mentally impaired persons from state-operated facilities into community settings. The assessments have been expanded to include other populations and are designed to determine the effectiveness of programs in meeting healthcare needs of at-risk populations.

Beneficence Actions performed that contribute to the welfare of others.

Binary system System used by computers. A numeric system using two symbols: 0 and 1.

Bioethics The study and formulation of healthcare ethics. Bioethics takes on relevant ethical problems experienced by healthcare providers in the provision of care to individuals and groups.

Bioinformatics The application of computer science, information science, and cognitive science principles to biological systems, especially in the human genome field of study.

Bioinformatics (BI) An interdisciplinary science that applies computer and information sciences to solve biologic problems.

Biomedical Informatics Interdisciplinary science of acquiring, structuring, analyzing, and providing access to biomedical data, information, and knowledge to improve the detection, prevention, and treatment of disease.

Biometrics Study of processes or means to uniquely recognizing individual users (humans) based upon one or more intrinsic physical or behavioral attributes or characteristics. Authentication devices that recognize thumb prints, retinal patterns, or facial patterns are available. Depending on the level of security needed, organizations will commonly use a combination of these types of authentication.

BIOS Basic input/output systems, binary input/output systems, basic integrated operating system, or built-in operating system that resides or is embedded on a chip that recognizes and controls the computer's devices.

Bioterrorism The use of pathogens or other potentially harmful biologic agents to sicken or kill members of a targeted population. Informatics database applications are used to track strategic indicators, such as emergency room visits, disease case reports, frequency and type of lab testing ordered by physicians and/or nurse practitioners, missed work, and over-the-counter medication purchases, that may indicate an outbreak that can be attributed to bioterrorism.

Bit (b) Unit of measurement that holds one binary digit, 0 or 1. The smallest possible chunk of data memory used in computer processing, exhibited as either 1 or 0, making up the binary system of the computer.

Blended A term used to describe a program format in which students take courses both face to face and online. A program of study that combines face-to-face courses and online courses.

Blended/hybrid An approach to education that combines traditional face-to-face instruction with technology based instruction.

Blog Interactive, online weblog. Typically a combination of what is happening on the Web as well as what is happening in the blogger's or the creator's life. A blog is as unique as the blogger or person creating it. Thought of as a diary and guide.

Blogger Someone who creates and maintains a blog. A person who blogs.

Borrowed theory Theories borrowed or made use of from other disciplines; as nursing began to evolve, theories from other disciplines such as psychology, sociology, etc., were adopted to try to empirically describe, explain, or predict nursing phenomena. As nursing theories continue to be developed, nurses are now questioning whether or not these borrowed theories were sufficient or satisfactory in their relation to the nursing phenomena they were used to describe, explain, or predict.

Brain The central information processing unit of humans. An organ that controls the central nervous system, is responsible for cognition and the interpretation, processing, and reaction to sensory input.

Browser Software used to locate and display Web pages. Also known as a Web browser or Internet browser.

Building block Basic element or part of nursing informatics such as information science, computer science, cognitive science, and nursing science.

Bus Subsystem that transfers data between a computer's internal components or between computers.

Byte (B) Unit of memory equal to eight bits or eight informational storage units and represents one keystroke; e.g., any push of a key on a keyboard such as pressing the space bar, a lower case a or an upper case T, for example; a chunk of memory that consists of eight bits, and is considered to be the best way to indicate computer memory or storage capacity.

Cache memory Smaller and faster memory storage used by the central processing unit (CPU) to store copies of frequently used data in main memory.

Call centers Registered nurse-staffed facilities at which nurses typically act as case managers for callers or perform patient triage.

Care ethics An ethical approach to solving moral dilemmas encountered in health care that is based on relationships and a caring attitude toward others.

Care plan A set of guidelines that outline the course of treatment and the recommended interventions that will achieve optimal results.

Case management information system (CMIS) Computer programs and information management tools that interact to support and facilitate the practice of case managers.

Case study An account of a nursing informatics activity, event, or problem containing some of the background and complexities actually encountered by a nurse. The case is used to enhance one's learning about nursing informatics principles, practices, and trends. Each case describes a series of events that reflect the nursing informatics episode as it actually occurred.

Casuist approach Approach to ethical decision making that grew out of the concern for more concrete methods of examining ethical dilemmas. Casuistry is a case-based ethical reasoning method that analyzes the facts of a case in a sound, logical, and ordered or structured manner. The facts are compared to the decisions arising out of consensus in previous paradigmatic or model cases.

Centers for Disease Control and Prevention (CDC) An agency of the United States Department of Health and Human Services that works to protect public health and safety related to disease control and prevention.

Centers for Medicare and Medicaid Services (CMS) The largest health insurer in the United States, particularly for home healthcare services, and for the elderly, for healthcare services.

Central processing unit (CPU) Processors that execute computer programs, thought of as the brains, controlling the functioning of the computer; the computer component that actually executes, calculates, and processes the binary computer code instigated by the operating system and other applications on the computer. It serves as the command center that directs the actions of all other components of the computer, and manages both incoming and outgoing data.

Central stations Multifunctional telehealthcare platforms for receiving, retrieving, and/or displaying patients' vital signs and other information transmitted from telecommunications-ready medical devices.

Certification System that validates that a nurse possesses certain skills and knowledge or is competent to complete a task. Competence and skill level determined by or based on an external review, assessment, examination, or education.

Certified EHR Technology An EHR that meets specific governmental standards for the type of record involved, either an ambulatory EHR used by office-based healthcare practitioners or an inpatient EHR used by hospitals. The specific standards to be met are set forth in federal regulations.

Change A transition to something different.

Chat Real-time electronic communications; users type what they want to say, and it is displayed on the screens of all participants in the same chat. Internet relay chat (IRC) is the Internet protocol for chat.

Chief information officer (CIO) Person involved with the information technology infrastructure of an organization. This role is sometimes called chief knowledge officer.

Chief technology officer or chief technical officer (CTO) Person focused on organizationally based scientific and technical issues and responsible for technological research and development as part of the organization's products and services.

Chronic disease Range of long-term diseases, such as congestive heart failure, diabetes, and respiratory ailments.

Civil Monetary Penalties (CMP) The Social Security Act authorizes the Secretary of HHS to seek civil monetary penalties (CMPs) and assessments for many types of conduct.

Clinical analytics Process of analysis by which clinical data is used to help make decisions and develop predictive analytics.

Clinical database A collection of related patient records stored in a computer system using software that permits a person or program to query the data in order to extract needed patient information.

Clinical decision support (CDS) A computer-based program designed to assist clinicians in making clinical decisions by filtering or integrating vast amounts of information, and providing suggestions for clinical intervention. May also be called a clinical decision support system (CDSS).

Clinical documentation system Array or collection of applications and functionality; amalgamation of systems, medical equipment, and technologies working together that are committed or dedicated to collecting, storing, and manipulating healthcare data and information and providing secure access to interdisciplinary clinicians navigating the continuum of client care. Designed to collect patient data in real time to enhance care by providing data at the clinician's fingertips and enabling decision making where it needs to occur— at the bedside. Also known as clinical information system (CIS).

Clinical guidelines That which provides a guide to decisions and criteria for specific practice areas.

Clinical information system (CIS) Array or collection of applications and functionality; amalgamation of systems, medical equipment, and technologies working together that are committed or dedicated to collecting, storing, and manipulating healthcare data and information and providing secure access to interdisciplinary clinicians navigating the continuum of client care. Designed to collect patient data in real time to enhance care by providing data at the clinician's fingertips and enabling decision making where it needs to occur— at the bedside. Also known as clinical documentation system.

Clinical outcomes Patient's results and consequences from clinical interventions.

Clinical practice council Group that uses the information generated by the clinical information systems (CIS) to design clinical education programs. Also called nursing practice council.

Clinical practice guidelines (CPGs) Informal or formal rules or guiding principles that a healthcare provider uses when determining diagnostic tests and treatment strategies for individual patients. In the electronic health record they are included in a variety of ways such as prompts, pop-ups, and text messages.

Clinical transformation The complete alteration of the clinical environment; widespread change accompanies transformational activities and clinical transformation implies that the manner in which work is carried out and the outcomes achieved are completely different than the prior state, which is not always true in the case of simply implementing technology. Technology can be used to launch or in conjunction with a clinical transformation initiative; however, the implementation of technology alone is not justifiably transformational ability; therefore, this term should be used cautiously to describe redesign efforts.

Cloud computing Web browser-based login-accessible data, software, and hardware; could link systems together and reduce costs.

Cloud storage Data storage provided by networked online servers that are typically outside of the institution whose data is being housed.

Coded terminology Nursing terminologies that are given a specific and standardized designation so that they can be easily entered into computerized nursing documentation systems, searched for, and easily retrieved.

Codify To classify, reduce to code, or articulate.

Cognitive That which uses one's capacity to think. Process of cognition is important to generate knowledge. Conscious intellectual or mental activity such as thinking, reasoning, and remembering, it includes imagination or the ability to imagine and the ability to learn.

Cognitive activity Any process or task (activity) that involves the capacity to think, reason, imagine, and learn.

Cognitive informatics (CI) Field of study made up of the disciplines of neuroscience, linguistics, artificial intelligence and psychology. The multidisciplinary study of cognition and information sciences, which investigates human information processing mechanisms and processes and their engineering applications in computing.

Cognitive science The interdisciplinary field that studies the mind, intelligence, and behavior from an information processing perspective.

Cognitive task analysis (CTA) Examination of the nature of a task by breaking it down into its component parts and identifying the performers' thought processes.

Cognitive walkthrough A technique used to evaluate a computer interface or a software program by breaking down and explaining the steps that a user will take to accomplish a task.

Cognitive work analysis (CWA) A multifaceted analytic procedure developed specifically for the analysis of complex, high-technology work domains.

Collaboration The sharing of ideas and experiences for the purposes of mutual understanding and learning.

Column Field or attribute of an entity in a database.

Communication science Area of concentration or discipline that studies human communication.

Communication software Technology programs used to transmit messages via e-mail, telephonically, paging, broadcast such as MP3, Internet such as instant messaging, voice-over-Internet protocol (VoIP), or lists, etc.

Communication system Collection of individual communications networks and transmission systems. In health care, it includes call light systems, wireless phones, pagers, e-mail, instant messaging and any other devices or networks that clinicians use to communicate with patients, families, other professionals, and internal and external resources.

Communications hub A device that captures and assists in the transmission of information from peripheral equipment. A processor organizes the data, appropriately encrypts it to assure confidentiality, and transmits it to appropriate decision makers. Data can be transmitted via traditional phone lines, the Internet, or over wireless networks. Typically the hub will be a small box, to which peripheral equipment is connected.

Community risk assessment (CRA) A comprehensive examination of a community to identify factors that potentially affect the health of the members of that community. Often used in public health program planning.

Compact disc read-only memory (CD-ROM) Disc that can hold approximately 700 megabytes of data accessible by a computer.

Compact disc-recordable (CD-R) Compact disc that can be used once for recording.

Compact disc-rewritable (CD-RW) Compact disc that can be recorded onto many times.

Compatibility The ability to work with each other or other devices or systems; e.g., software that is compatible with a computer.

Compliance Conforming or performing in an acceptable manner; correctly following the rules.

Comprehensive health enhancement support system (CHESS) A computer-based system designed to help underserved breast cancer patients manage their disease.

Computational Biology The action complement of bioinformatics and therefore, biomedicine; it is the actual process of analyzing and interpreting data.

Computer A machine that stores and executes programs; a machine with peripheral hardware and software to carry out selected programming.

Computer-aided software engineering (CASE) Systematic application of computer software tools and techniques to assist engineering practice.

Computer assisted instruction (CAI) Any instruction that is aided by the use of a computer.

Computer-based That which uses the computer to interact; the computer is the base tool.

Computer-based information system (CBIS) Combinations of hardware, software and telecommunications networks that people build and use to collect, create, and distribute useful data, typically in organizational settings.

Computer science Branch of engineering (application of science) that studies the theoretical foundations of information and computation and their implementation and application in computer systems. The study of storage/memory, conversion and transformation, and transfer or transmission of information in machines—that is computers—through both algorithms and practical implementation problems. Algorithms are detailed unambiguous action sequences in the design, efficiency, and application, and practical implementation problems deal with the software and hardware.

Computerized physician order entry systems (CPOE) A system that automates the way that orders have traditionally been initiated for patients. Clinicians place orders within these systems instead of using traditional handwritten transcription onto paper. These systems provide major safeguards by ensuring that physician orders are legible and complete, thereby providing a level of patient safety that was historically missing with paper-based orders. These systems provide decision support and automated alert functionality that was previously unavailable with paper-based orders.

Conceptual framework Framework used in research to chart feasible courses of action or to present a desired approach to a study or analysis. Framework built from a set of concepts that are related to a proposed or existing system of methods, behaviors, functions, relationships, and objects. A relational model. A formal way of thinking or conceptualizing about a phenomenon, process, or system under study.

Conferencing software Electronic communications system or software that supports and facilitates two or more people meeting for discussion. One of the high-end systems offers telepresence (creates a life-like experience allowing people to feel as if they were present in person—it would be as though the nurse were physically there with the patient—so people can work, learn, and play in person over the Internet or have an effect at a remote location).

Confidentiality All personal information that must be safeguarded by ensuring that access is limited to only those who are authorized.

Connectionism A component of cognitive science that uses computer modeling through artificial neural networks to try to explain human intellectual abilities.

Connectivity Ability to hook up to the electronic resources necessary to meet the user's needs. The ability to use computer networks to link to people and resources. The unbiased transmission or transport of Internet protocol packets between two end points.

Consequences Outcomes or products resulting from our decision choices.

Consolidated health informatics (CHI) A collaborative effort to adopt health information interoperability standards, particularly health vocabulary and messaging standards, for implementation in federal government systems.

Consultant A person hired to provide expert advice, opinions, and recommendations based on his or her area of expertise.

Context of care The setting, services, patient, environment, and professional and social interactions surrounding the delivery of patient interventions.

Continuing education Coursework or training completed postbaccalaureate, often for the purpose of recertification.

Continuous learner One who gleans lessons or learns from success as well as failures, or who constantly searches for information to add to one's knowledge base.

Copyright A legal term used by many governments around the world that gives the inventor or designer of an original product sole or exclusive rights for a limited time; the same laws that cover physical books, artwork, and other creative material are still applicable in the digital world.

Core business system System that enhances administrative tasks within healthcare organizations. Unlike clinical information systems whose aim is to provide direct patient care, these systems support the management of health care within an organization. These systems provide the framework for reimbursement, support of best practices, quality control, and resource allocation. There are four common core business systems: (1) admission, discharge and transfer (ADT), (2) financial, (3) acuity, and (4) scheduling systems.

Core sciences The branches of study and knowledge that form the foundation of nursing informatics, including nursing, computer, and information sciences. Some, including the editors of this text, believe that cognitive science should also be included in the list of NI foundational sciences.

Courage The strength to face difficulty.

Course management system (CMS) Software system designed for both faculty and students that supports educational episodes including tools for grading, learner assessment, content presentation/interaction, and communication. These systems provide for the support of learning activities throughout course delivery; proprietary examples include ANGEL, Blackboard, WebCT, Learning Space, and eCollege.

Covered entity An entity that is a healthcare provider that conducts certain transactions in electronic form (called here a "covered healthcare provider"), a healthcare clearinghouse, or a health plan that electronically transmits any health information in connection with transactions (billing and payment for services or insurance coverage) for which HHS has adopted standards. An entity that is one or more of these types of entities is referred to as a "covered entity" in the Administrative Simplification regulations.

Creativity software Programs that support and facilitate innovation and creativity (intellectual process relating to the creation or generation of new ideas, concepts, or new relationships between currently existing ideas or concepts); allow users to focus or concentrate more on creating new things in our digital age and less on the mechanics or workings of how they are created or developed.

Culture broker Person who can translate between science and clinical care and between science and the self-caring citizen.

Cumulative Index to Nursing and Allied Health Literature (CINAHL) A comprehensive nursing and allied health literature database.

Data Raw fact that lacks meaning.

Data-centric Data is the central focus.

Data dictionary Software that contains a listing of the tables and their details including field names, validation settings, and data types.

Data file A collection of related records.

Data gatherer One involved in the direct procurement of raw facts (data). Raw fact (data) collector.

Data mart Collection of data focusing on a specific topic or organizational unit or department created to facilitate management personnel making strategic business decisions; could be as small as one database or larger such as a compilation of databases; generally smaller than a data warehouse.

Data mining A process of utilizing software to sort through data in order to discover patterns and ascertain or establish relationships. This process may help to discover or uncover previously unidentified relationships among the data in a database.

Data set Collection of interrelated data.

Data warehouse (DW) An extremely large database or repository that stores all of an organization's or institution's data and makes this data available for data mining. A combination of an institution's many different databases that provides management personnel flexible access to the data.

Database A collection of related records stored in a computer system using software that permits a person or program to query the data in order to extract needed information; may consist of one or more related data files or tables.

Database management system (DBMS) Software program/s and the hardware used to create and manage data.

Decision making Output of cognition. Outcome of our intellectual processing.

Decision support Recommendations for interventions based on computerized care protocols. The decision support recommendations may include such items as additional screenings, medication interactions, or drug and dosage monitoring.

Decision support/outcomes manager Person charged with reviewing the effects of interventions suggested by the computerized decision support system.

Decision support system (DSS) Computer applications designed to facilitate human decision-making processes. Usually DSSs are rule-based, using a specified knowledge base and a set of rules to analyze data and information and provide recommendations typically through the use of a knowledge base and rules to make recommendations to users.

Degradation Loss of quality; e.g., in telecommunications, it is the loss of quality in the electronic signal.

Desktop Computer's interface that resembles the top of one's desk, where one keeps things one wants to access quickly, such as paper clips, pens, paper, etc. On the computer's desktop, one can customize the look and feel to have easy access to the programs, folders, and files on the hard drive that one uses the most.

Digital divide The gap between those who have and those who do not have access to online information.

Digital health record (DHR) An electronic record of patient assessments that are collected over time, typically by a telemonitoring device. For example, daily assessments of weight and blood pressure can be captured electronically and graphically displayed to allow for the detection of subtle trends.

Digital pen Actual writing implement that can also digitally capture handwriting or drawings. It is battery operated and generally comes with a universal serial bus (USB) cradle that permits uploading captured materials to one's desktop, laptop, or palmtop computer. The user can use it as a ballpoint pen and write on regular paper just as he would with a normal pen, or he can capture it digitally after writing on digital paper.

Digital video disc-recordable (DVD-R) Disc on which a user can record once.

Digital video disc-recordable and rewritable (DVD-RW) Disc on which a user can record many times.

Digital video disc or digital versatile disc (DVD) Optical disc storage format that can generally hold or store more than six times the amount of data that a CD can.

Dissemination A thoughtful, intentional, goal-oriented communication of specific, useful information or knowledge.

Distance education Education provided from a remote location.

Document To capture and save information for later use.

Documentation Communication in the form of written or typed text, audio, video, graphics, photographs, pictures or any blending of these means used to describe some characteristics or elements of an object, system, or practice; for example, nursing documentation generates information about a patient (individual, family, group, community, populations) that describes the care and/or services that have been provided and allows for the communication necessary between nurses and other healthcare providers.

Domain name Series of alphanumeric characters that forms part of the Internet address or URL, such as psu.edu which denotes Penn State's address.

Drill-down Means of viewing data warehouse information by going down to lower levels of the database to focus on information that is pertinent to her/his needs at the moment.

Duty One's feeling of being bound or obligated to carry out specific tasks or roles based on one's rank or position.

Dynamic random access memory (DRAM) Type of RAM chip requiring less space to store the same amount on a similar SRAM (static RAM) chip; however, DRAM requires more power than SRAM since DRAM needs to keep its charge by constantly refreshing.

Dynamic system development method (DSDM) An agile software development strategy based on the rapid application development model that is iterative and used in the system development life cycle (SDLC) and project management.

Dynamic Web page shells Web pages that can be custom scripted to provide realistic case scenarios during a simulation experience.

E-brochure Electronic brochure. Patient education material that is typically tied to an agency Web site, and may include such information as descriptions of diseases and their management, medication information, or where to get assistance with a healthcare issue.

E-health Healthcare initiatives and practice supported by electronic or digital media. The most typical use is in patient and family education where information is communicated electronically.

E-learning Electronic learning or learning that is facilitated by electronic means such as computers and the Internet. E-learning, online, and Web-based education has caused a significant shift in student–teacher relationships in nursing education.

E-mail Electronic mail. To compose, send, receive, and store messages in electronic communication systems.

E-mail client Program that manages e-mail functions.

E-portfolio Personalized collections of evidence from coursework, experiences outside of the classroom, and reflective commentary related to this evidence that can be shared with others electronically; categorized electronic presentation of one's skills, education, and examples of work and/or career achievements.

Educational Resources Information Center (ERIC) A comprehensive educational resources database. An international database of educational literature.

Educator Sage, leader, and/or guide who assists in the process or practice of learning.

eHealth Initiative Initiative developed to address the growing need for managing health information and to promote technology as a means of improving health information exchange, health literacy, and healthcare delivery.

Electronic communication Any exchange of information that is transmitted electronically.

Electronic data interchange (EDI) Specific set of standards for exchanging information between/among computers (computer to computer).

Electronic health record (EHR) A computer-based data warehouse or repository of information regarding the health status of a client, replacing the former paper-based medical record; it is the systematic documentation of a client's health status and health care in a secured digital format, meaning that it can be processed, stored, transmitted, and accessed by authorized interdisciplinary professionals for the purpose of supporting efficient, high quality health care across the client's healthcare continuum. Also known as electronic medical record (EMR).

Electronic mailing list Automatic mailing list server such as LISTSERV that sends an e-mail that is addressed to the list to everyone who has subscribed to the list automatically. Similar to an electronic bulletin board or news forum.

Electronic medical record (EMR) See electronic health record (EHR).

Electronically erasable programmable read-only memory (EEPROM) A non-volatile storage chip used in computers and other devices to store small amounts of volatile data, e.g., calibration tables or device configuration.

Emerging technologies New technology that is likely to impact health care in a significant way such as nanotechnology or biotechnology.

Empiricism That knowledge which is derived from our experiences or senses.

Empowerment Promoting self-actualization. Achieve power or control one's own life.

Enterprise Integration Electronically linking healthcare providers, health plans, government, and other interested parties to facilitate electronic exchange and use of health information among all stakeholders.

End-users Target users or consumers of software and computer technology; software or computing applications should be designed for the end user, the one who will be using it in the end.

Entity See covered entity.

Entity relationship diagram (ERD) Diagram that specifies the relationship among the entities in the database. Sometimes the implied relationships are apparent based on the entities' definitions; however, all relationships should be specified as to how they relate to one another. There are typically three relationships, one to one, one to many, and many to many.

Entrepreneur One who assumes the risks of beginning an enterprise or business and accepts responsibility for organizing and managing the organization.

Enumerative approach Nursing terminology in which words or phrases are represented in a list or a simple hierarchy; gives an explicit and exhaustive listing of all the objects that fall under the concept or term in question.

Epidemiology The study of identifying things that come upon the people. Incidence, prevalence, and control of disease. Case finding.

Epistemology Study of the nature and origin of knowledge; what it means to know.

Erasable programmable read-only memory (EPROM) Type of computer memory chip that retains its data when its power supply is switched off, and can be erased with ultraviolet light.

Ergonomics In the United States, this term is used to describe the physical characteristics of equipment, for example, the optimal fit of a scissors to a human hand. In Europe, the term is synonymous with human factors. It is the interaction of humans with physical attributes of equipment or the interaction of humans and the arrangement of equipment in the work environment.

Ethical decision making The process of making informed choices about ethical dilemmas based on a set of standards differentiating right from wrong. The decision making reflects an understanding of the principles and standards of ethical decision making, as well as philosophical approaches to ethical decision making. Requires a systematic framework for addressing the complex and often controversial moral questions.

Ethical dilemma A difficult choice or issue that requires the application of standards or principles to solve. Issues that challenge us ethically.

Ethical, social, and legal implications (ESLI) Consideration and understanding of the ethical, social or legal connections or aspects of an issue that relates to a moral question of right and wrong.

Ethicist Expert in the arbitrary, ambiguous, and ungrounded judgments of other people. Ethicists know that they make the best decision they can based on the situation and stakeholders at hand.

Ethics A process of systematically examining varying viewpoints related to moral questions of right and wrong.

Eudaemonistic A system of ethical evaluation that involves consideration of what actions lead to being an excellent and happy person.

Events Occurrences that might be significant to other objects in a system or to external agents; for example, creating a laboratory request is an example of a healthcare event in a laboratory application. An event is defined and it could be a triggering event for the task or workflow; a task or workflow can have several triggering events.

Evidence Artifacts, productions, attestations, or other examples that demonstrate what an individual's knowledge, skills, or valued attributes are.

Evidence-based practice (EBP) Nursing practice that is informed by research generated evidence of best practices.

Exabyte (EB) One quintillion bytes of computer memory.

Execute To carry out software's or a program's instructions.

Expert system A type of decision support system that implements the knowledge of one or more human experts.

Extensibility System design feature that allows for future expansion without the need for changes to the basic infrastructure.

Extensible markup language (XML) Computer language that began as a simplified subset of standard generalized markup language (SGML). Its major purpose is to facilitate the exchange of structured data across different information systems, especially via the Internet. It is considered an extensible language since it permits its users to define their own elements allowing customization to enable purpose-specific development.

Face-to-face Most widely used teaching method among nurse educators where teacher and learners meet together in one location at the same time.

Failure Modes and Effects Analysis (FMEA) A systematic evaluation of a process to determine how and why it failed to produce the desired results.

Fair use Doctrine that permits the limited use of original works without copyright holder's permission; an example would be quoting or citing an author in a scholarly manuscript.

Federal Health Information Exchange (FHIE) A federal information technology (IT) healthcare initiative that enables the secure electronic one-way exchange of patient medical information from the Department of Defense's legacy health information system, the Composite Health Care System (CHCS), for all separated service members to Veterans Affairs' (VA) VistA Computerized Patient Record System (CPRS). The point of care in veterans affairs.

Feedback Input in the form of opinions about or reactions to something such as shared knowledge. In an information system, feedback refers to information from the system that is used to make modifications in the input, processing actions, or outputs.

Fidelity The extent to which a simulation mimics the processes of a real environment.

Field Column or attribute of an entity in a database.

Field study Study in which end users evaluate a prototype in the actual work setting prior to its general release. Also called field test, alpha test, or beta test.

Financial system System used to manage the expenses and revenue for providing health care. The finance, auditing, and accounting departments within an organization most commonly use financial systems. These systems determine the direction for maintenance and growth for a given facility. Financial systems often interface to share information with materials management, staffing, and billing systems to balance the financial impact of these resources within an organization. These systems report the fiscal outcomes in order to track them against the organizational goals of an institution. Financial systems are one of the major decision-making factors as healthcare institutions prepare their fiscal budgets. These systems often play a pivotal role in determining the strategic direction for an organization.

Firewall A common tool used by organizations to protect their corporate networks when they are attached to the Internet. A firewall can be either hardware or software or a combination of both. A firewall examines all incoming messages or traffic to the network. The firewall can be set up to only allow messages from known senders into the corporate network. Firewalls can also be set up to look at outgoing information from the corporate network.

FireWire Apple Computer's version of a high performance serial bus used to connect devices to a computer.

Firmware Hardware and software programs or data written onto ROM, PROM, and EPROM.

Flash drive Small, removable storage device.

Flash memory Special type of EEPROM that can be erased and reprogrammed in blocks instead of one byte at a time. Many modern PCs have their BIOS stored on a flash memory chip so that it can easily be updated if necessary.

Folksonomies Organization and classification of online content by users; derived from folk and taxonomy. Users tag information with key words to make it easier to index and search vast amounts of information.

Foundation of Knowledge model Model that proposes that humans are organic information systems constantly acquiring, processing, and generating information or knowledge in both their professional and personal lives. The organizing framework of this text.

Free/open source software(F/OSS or FOSS) Free to copy and reuse or repurpose the software by providing access to the source code; free and open use of software source code.

Futurologist Guru who is a forward thinker and looks to the future.

Game A structured activity undertaken for enjoyment.

Genome Hans Winkler is credited with merging "genesis" and "soma" (genome) to describe a body of genes.

Genomics The study of the genome.

Gigabyte (GB) Unit of measure used to express bytes of data storage and capability in computer systems; 1 gigabyte equals 1,000 megabytes.

Gigahertz (GHz) Unit of measure used to express speed and power of some components such as the microprocessor; 1 gigahertz or GHz is equal to 1,000 megahertz.

Good Favorable outcome in ethics.

Gramm-Leach-Bliley Act (GLBA) Federal legislation in the United States to control how financial institutions handle the private information they collect from individuals.

Graphical user interface (GUI) Software that provides a user-friendly desktop metaphor interface that is made up of the input and output devices as well as icons that represent files, programs, actions, and processes.

Graphics card A board that plugs into a personal computer to give it display capabilities.

Grey gap A term used to reflect the age disparities in computer connectivity; there are fewer persons over age 65 who use computer technology than those in younger age groups.

Gulf of evaluation The gap between knowing one's intention (goal) and knowing the effects of one's actions.

Gulf of execution The gap between knowing what one wants to have happen (the goal) and knowing what to do to bring it about (the means to achieve the goal).

Hacker Computer savvy individual most commonly thought of as a malicious person who hacks or breaks through security to steal or alter data and information, but it can also be computer aficionados who band together in clubs and organizations or who use their skills as a hobby.

Half-life of knowledge The time span from when knowledge is gained to when it becomes obsolete.

Haplotype Set of closely linked alleles on a chromosome that tends to be inherited together.

Hard disk Magnetic disk that stores electronic data.

Hard drive Permanent data storage area that holds the data, information, documents, and programs saved on the computer, even when the computer is shut off. The actual physical body of the computer and its components.

Hardware Physical or tangible parts of the computer. Computer parts that one can touch and that are involved in the performance or function of the computer, such as the keyboard and monitor.

Harm Physical or mental injury or damage. Unfavorable outcome in ethics.

Health disparities The health status differences between different groups of people, especially minorities and nonminorities; the gaps between the health status of minorities and nonminorities in the United States are ongoing even with the advances in technology and healthcare practices.

Health information exchange (HIE) Organization that prepares and organizes people and resources to manage healthcare information electronically across organizations within a community or region.

Health Information Portability and Accountability Act (HIPAA) Law signed by President Bill Clinton in 1996 addressing the need for standards to regulate and safeguard health information and making provisions for health insurance coverage for employed persons who change jobs.

Health Information Technology (HIT) Consists of the hardware, software, integrated technologies or related licenses, intellectual property, upgrades, or packaged solutions sold as services that are designed for or support the use by healthcare entities or patients for the electronic creation, maintenance, access, or exchange of health information.

Health Information Technology for Economic and Clinical Health (HITECH) Act Title XIII of ARRA that was enacted in February of 2009 was given a subtitle: Health Information Technology for Economic and Clinical Health (HITECH) Act. Under this act, healthcare organizations can qualify for financial incentives based on the level of meaningful use achieved; the HITECH Act specifically incentivizes health organizations and providers to become "meaningful users."

Health Level 7 (HL7) An accredited standards-developing organization that is committed to developing standard terminologies for information technology that support interoperability of healthcare information management systems.

Health literacy The acquisition of knowledge that promotes the ability to understand and to manage one's health.

Health management information system (HMIS) An information system that is specially intended to support and help with the planning, resource allocation and management of health programming to make healthcare more effective and efficient; information system that plans and manages health programs not the actual delivery of healthcare.

Healthcare information Information that is related to health and well being of a person, especially information related to therapeutic (care) interactions between people and healthcare providers.

Healthcare Provider A qualified person delivering appropriate health care professionally to an individual, group, family, community, or population in need of healthcare services; this term includes hospitals, skilled nursing facilities, nursing homes, long term care facilities, home health agencies, hemodialysis centers, clinics, community mental health centers, ambulatory surgery centers, group practices, pharmacies and pharmacists, laboratories, physicians, and therapists.

HealthVault Microsoft's online personal health record system.

Heuristic evaluation An evaluation in which a small number of evaluators (often experts in relevant fields such as human factors or cognitive engineering) evaluate the degree to which the interface design complies with recognized usability principles (the "heuristics").

High-fidelity A high level of realism generated by the equipment used in simulations.

High Hazard Drug A drug known to cause significant adverse side effects when administered inappropriately; a drug subject to frequent administration errors.

Home health agency (HHA) Organization that delivers part-time and intermittent skilled services including nursing and other therapeutic services in the patient's home.

Home health care Alternate site for healthcare services typically focusing on posthospital discharge patient needs.

Home telehealth care Home healthcare clinical and educational services provided via telecommunications-ready tools.

HONcode One of the two most common symbols that power users look for to identify trusted health sites.

Hospital information system (HIS) An information system intended to manage the clinical, financial and administrative needs of the hospital; refers to the paper-based as well as computer-based information processing that manages the functional aspects (administrative, financial and clinical) of a hospital.

Human Factors Engineering Recognizing the limitations of human performance and developing products to overcome these limitations.

Human Genome Project (HGP) A 13-year project designed to identify all of the 20,000–25,000 genes in human DNA; determine the sequences of 3 billion chemical base pairs in human DNA; create databases to store this information; and address the resultant ethical, legal, and social issues (ELSI).

Human–computer interaction (HCI) The study of how people use computers and software applications and the ways that computers influence people.

Human–computer interface The hardware and software through which the user interacts with the computer.

Human–technology interaction (HTI) How users interact with technology. The study of that interaction.

Human–technology interface The hardware and software through which the user interacts with any technology (e.g., computers, patient monitors, telephone, etc.).

Hybrid That which defines individual courses in which instruction is delivered using multiple formats such as online, face to face, print-based, or audio or videoconference such as PicTel.

Hypertext Clickable words that allow users to access another document at a remote location.

Indiana Health Information Exchange (IHIE) Collaborative effort among institutions in Indiana to provide high quality patient care and enhance safety and efficiency.

Industrial Age Late 18th and early 19th centuries when there were major changes in manufacturing, farming, and transportation; inventions and innovations led these changes.

Informaticist A person with specialized training or certification in informatics; one who is a specialist in using technology to manage health data and information.

Informatics A specialty that integrates the specialty's science, computer science, cognitive science, and information science to manage and communicate data, information, knowledge, and wisdom in a specialty's practice.

Informatics innovator Process of making enhancements or improvements and creative, novel, and inventive solutions in the informatics specialty.

Informatics nurse (IN) A nurse with specialized skills, knowledge, and competencies in informatics. An RN with an interest or experience working in an informatics field. A generalist in the field of informatics in nursing.

Informatics nurse specialist (INS) An RN with formal, graduate education in the field of informatics or a related field and is considered a specialist in the field of nursing informatics.

Informatics solution A generic term used to describe the product an informatics nurse specialist recommends after identifying and analyzing an issue. Informatics solutions may encompass technology and nontechnology products such as information systems, new applications, nursing vocabulary, or informatics curricula.

Information Data that are interpreted, organized, or structured. Data that is processed using knowledge or data made functional through the application of knowledge.

Information Age Period at the end of the 20th century, when information was easily accessible using computers, networks, and the Internet.

Information literacy Recognizing when information is needed and having the ability to locate, evaluate, and effectively use the needed information.

An intellectual framework for finding, understanding, evaluating, and using information.

Information mediator New nursing role arising out of the need for technology to support immediate access to up-to-date knowledge anywhere and anytime.

Information science The science of information, studying the application and usage of information and knowledge in organizations and the interfacings or interaction between people, organizations, and information systems. An extensive, interdisciplinary science that integrates features from cognitive science, communication science, computer science, library science, and social sciences.

Information system (IS) The manual and/or automated components of a system of users or people, recorded data, and actions used to process the data into information for a user, group of users, or an organization.

Information technology (IT) Use of hardware, software, services, and supporting infrastructure to manage and deliver information using voice, data, and video or the use of technologies from computing, electronics, and telecommunications to process and distribute information in digital and other forms. Anything related to computing technology, such as networking, hardware, software, the Internet, or the people who work with these technologies. Many hospitals have IT departments for managing the computers, networks, and other technical areas of the healthcare industry.

Information user The person who accesses and makes use of information made available to her/him.

Informatique French term that refers to the computer milieu.

Infrastructure Structural elements that provide the framework supporting a system. In the case of information technology, infrastructure refers to the architecture of the computer system, its operating system and various other systems that are fundamental to its operation.

Input Data and information entered into a computer system.

Input devices Hardware and software used to enter data and information into a computer.

Input/output system (I/O) (Pronounced "eye-oh.") The term I/O is used to describe any program, operation or device that transfers data to or from a computer and to or from a peripheral device.

Instant message (IM) Form of real-time communication between two or more people based on typed text conveyed via computers connected over a network.

Integrated drive electronics (IDE) Technology where the drive controller is located on the drive itself instead of being a separate controller connected to the motherboard.

Integration Assimilating or combining to make whole; in computer terminology, the process through which different technologies, software and hardware components, are synchronized and combined to make a functional and structural system.

Integrity Quality and accuracy. Employees need to have confidence that the information they are reading is in fact true. To accomplish this, organizations need clear policies to clarify how data is actually inputted, who has the authorization to change such data and to track how and when data are in fact changed.

Intelligence Mental ability to think logically, reason, prepare, ideate, assess alternative solutions to problems, problem solve by choosing a proposed solution, think abstractly, comprehend and grasp ideas, understand and use language, and learn.

Interactions Interfacing with users commonly using tasks or notifications.

Interactive technologies Technologies that promote or support user communication with other persons (e.g. email) or technologies that depend on a user response (e.g. games).

Interdisciplinary knowledge team A team composed of members of various disciplines in a healthcare organization who each contribute their unique knowledge to the team in problem-solving or management situations.

Interface Mechanism or a system used by separate things to interact. For example, if one wants to change a CD in a CD player, one could use a remote; one is not related to the CD player but can interact with it using the remote control. Therefore, the remote control becomes the interface that enables that person to tell the CD player which CD to play.

International Organization for Standardization (ISO) An international network supporting collaboration among the standards developing agencies of numerous countries for the development of consistent standards in a multitude of industries to support a global economy. ISO is best known in the technology industries for the ISO 9000 standards.

International Standards Organization or International Organization for Standardization (ISO) A non-governmental group that connects or bridges the public and private sectors to develop and publish international standards that assimilate the latest expert knowledge to provide practical tools for tracking economic, environmental and societal challenges.

Internet A worldwide system of computer networks whose connectivity promotes worldwide communications via computers.

Internet2 A nonprofit consortium which develops and deploys advanced network applications and technologies, for education and high-speed data transfer purposes. Led by 212 universities, it is also known as University Corporation for Advanced Internet Development.

Internet browser Software used to locate and display Web pages. Also known as Web browser or browser.

Interoperability Ability of various systems and organizations to work together to exchange information.

Intranet A computer network contained within an enterprise and which has restricted access. Has the look and feel of the Internet, often providing links to the Internet. The purpose varies, but can include employee and departmental directories, policies and procedures, internal and external resources, schedules, and updates on programs and business. The benefits are browsing capabilities and the ability to maintain contact information and phone numbers in a central location, with easy dissemination.

Intrusion detection devices Both hardware and software that allow an organization to monitor who is using the network and what files that user has accessed.

Intrusion detection system Method of security that uses both hardware and software detection devices as a system that can be set up to monitor a single computer or an entire network. Corporations must diligently monitor for unauthorized access of their networks.

Intuition A way of acquiring knowledge that cannot be obtained by inference, deduction, observation, reason, analysis, or experience.

Iowa model A model that facilitates the translation of research evidence into clinical practice. Also known as the Iowa model of evidence based practice.

iPod The name given to a family of portable MP3 players from Apple Computer.

Iteration To replicate and refine a method until it meets your goal or the desired result; each repetition is referred to as an iteration.

Jump drive Small, removable storage device.

Justice Fairness. Treatment of everyone in the same way.

Key field Within each database record, one of the fields is identified as the primary key or key field. This primary key contains a code, name, number, or other bit of information that acts as a unique identifier for that record. In a healthcare system, for example, a patient is assigned a patient number or ID that is unique for that patient.

Keyboard Set of keys resembling an actual typewriter that permits the user to input data into a computer.

Know-do gap Situation that exists because solutions to global health problems exist but are not implemented in a timely fashion because of the lack of access to important health information. The Internet connections in developing countries are widely scattered and may not be efficient/sufficient for viewing healthcare information.

Knowledge The awareness and understanding of a set of information and ways that information can be made useful to support a specific task or arrive at a decision; abounds with others' thoughts and information. Information that is synthesized so that relationships are identified and formalized. Understanding that comes through a process of interaction or experience with the world around us. Information that has judgment applied to it or meaning extracted from it. Processed information that helps to clarify or explain some portion of our environment or world that we can use as a basis for action or upon which we can act. Internal process of thinking or cognition. External process of testing, senses, observation, and interacting.

Knowledge acquisition The act of acquiring or getting knowledge.

Knowledge brokers People who know where to find information and knowledge. They generate some knowledge but are mainly known for their ability to find what is needed. More experienced nurses and nursing students become knowledge brokers out of necessity—needing to know.

Knowledge builder Person who examines, interprets, and compares clinical data and trends with an eye toward improving clinical practice based on the available evidence.

Knowledge-centric Knowledge is the central focus.

Knowledge consumers Users of knowledge who do not have the expertise to provide the knowledge they need for themselves.

Knowledge dissemination Distribution and sharing of knowledge.

Knowledge Domain Process (KDP) model Model that represents knowledge construction and dissemination in an organization.

Knowledge exchange The product of collaboration when sharing an understanding of information promotes learning to make better decisions in the future.

Knowledge generation Creating new knowledge by changing and evolving knowledge based on one's experience, education, and input from others.

Knowledge generators Nursing researchers and nursing experts—the people who know; they are able to answer questions, craft theories, find solutions to nursing problems or concerns, and innovate practice.

Knowledge management system (KMS) A repository of information that contains the latest collective expertise based on experience and research. The knowledge is typically stored in a computerized system that promotes easy access for use.

Knowledge processing The activity or process of gathering or collecting, perceiving, analyzing, synthesizing, saving or storing, manipulating, conveying, and transmitting knowledge.

Knowledge repositories Collections of information made available to an organization's workers to support and inform their work.

Knowledge user Individuals or groups who benefit from valuable, viable knowledge.

Knowledge workers Those who work with information and generate information and knowledge as a product.

Lab-on-a-chip device A nanotechnology device designed to perform blood analyses.

Laboratory information system Report on blood, body fluid, and tissue samples along with biological specimens that are collected at the bedside and received in a central laboratory. These systems provide clinicians with reference ranges for tests indicating high, low, or normal values in order to make care decisions. Often the laboratory system provides result information directing clinicians toward the next course of action within a treatment regimen.

Laptop Portable battery-powered computer also known as a notebook that the user can take with him or her.

Legacy system Old computer systems or programs that are not replaced because the institution does not want to expend the resources; they can cause problems especially in interfacing with newer systems.

Liberty The independence from controlling influences.

Library science An interdisciplinary science that integrates law, applied science, and the humanities, to study issues and topics related to libraries (collection, organization, preservation, archiving, and dissemination of information resources).

Local area network (LAN) Organizationally based network; joined together locally.

Logic A system of thinking that uses principles of inference and reasoned ideas to govern action.

Long-term care facility A healthcare institution designed to support the needs of those who need ongoing care, especially the aged.

Longevity Usability beyond the immediate clinical encounter. Long-term value.

Main memory Computer's internal memory.

Mainframe Extremely high-performance computer that is smaller than supercomputer, used for high-volume, processor-intensive computing. Computers used by some large businesses and/or for scientific processing purposes.

Malicious code Software that includes spyware, viruses, worms, and Trojan horses.

Malicious insider An insider or employee who sabotages or adds malicious codes or hacks into systems to cause damage or to steal data and information.

Mask Method that a proxy server uses to protect the identity of a corporation's employees while surfing the World Wide Web. The proxy server keeps track of which employees are using which masks and directs the traffic appropriately.

Managed care information system An information system that crosses organizational boundaries in order that data can be obtained at any and all of the patient areas; these information systems make it possible for nurses and physicians to make clinical decisions while being mindful of their financial ramifications.

Massachusetts Health Data Consortium (MHDC) A consortium of regional healthcare organizations that collects data, publishes comparative information, supports and promotes electronic standards, educates, and researches.

Massive multiplayer online role-playing game (MMORPG or simply MMO) A game using the Internet to provide a shared, simultaneous experience for dozens or even hundreds of players.

Master patient index A tool that identifies, compares, removes duplicate entries, combines, and cleans the patient record so it can be added to the master index; provides a comprehensive and single view of a patient via their record while establishing a master index of all patients.

Meaningful use The American Recovery and Reinvestment Act of 2009 specifies three main components of meaningful use: (1) the use of a certified EHR in a meaningful manner, such as e-prescribing; (2) the use of certified EHR technology for electronic exchange of health information to improve quality of health care; and (3) the use of certified EHR technology to submit clinical quality and other measures. The criteria for meaningful use will be staged in three steps over the course of the next 5 years. Stage 1 (2011 and 2012) sets the baseline for electronic data capture and information sharing. Stage 2 (expected to be implemented in 2013) and Stage 3 (expected to be implemented in 2015) will continue to expand on this baseline and be developed through future rule making.

Medical home/health information exchange An information technology platform that enables the seamless exchange of important patient information among many providers in a healthcare system. Typically the Primary Care Physician (Medical Home) initiates the collection of patient data, coordinates the care of the patient and helps to maintain the accuracy of such data. Other care providers access the information and add to it as they provide services to patients.

Medical informatics A specialty that integrates medical science, computer science, cognitive science, and information science to manage and communicate data, information, knowledge, and wisdom in medical practice.

Medicaid management information systems (MMIS) An integrated group of procedures and computer processing operations (subsystems) developed at the general design level to meet principal objectives of control and administrative costs; service to recipients, providers, and inquiries; operations of claims control and computer capabilities; and management reporting for planning and control.

Medication management devices Range of telecommunications-ready medication devices to remind or otherwise alert patients to medication compliance needs.

MEDLINE A database that contains more than 10 million records, maintained and produced by the National Library of Medicine.

Megabyte (MB) Unit of measure used to express the amount of data storage and capability in computer systems; 1 megabyte equals 1,000 kilobytes.

Megahertz (MHz) Unit of measure used to express the speed and power of some components such as the microprocessor.

Memory Data stored in digital format; generally refers to random access memory (RAM).

Meta-analysis A form of systematic review that uses statistical methods to combine the results of several research studies.

Metrics Measurements or a set of measurements to quantify performance; they provide understanding about the performance of a process or function. Typically, within clinical technology projects one identifies and collects specific metrics about the performance of the technology or metrics that capture the level of participation or adoption. Equally important is the need for process performance metrics. Process metrics are collected at the initial stage of a project or problem identification. Current state metrics are then benchmarked against internal indicators. When there are no internal indicators to benchmark against, a suitable course of action is to benchmark against an external source, such as a similar business practice within a different industry.

Microprocessor Chip that integrates the processor onto one circuit, incorporating the functions of the central processing unit (CPU) and continues to evolve processing capacity.

Milestones A predetermined planned occurrence that indicates the completion or achievement of a deliverable.

Mind The brain's conscious processing; encompasses thought processes, memory, imagination and creativity, emotions, perceptions, and inner drive or will.

Mobile e-health (mobile health, m-health) Health-related uses of mobile technologies including mobile phones (and increasingly, Internet-enabled, wireless-connected smartphones), personal digital assistants (PDAs), tablet computers and, sub-notebook microcomputers, remote diagnostic and monitoring devices, and Global Positioning System (GPS)/geographic information system (GIS) mapping equipment.

Model of terminology use A domain content model that is optimized for the management of particular entities within an informational and/or operational context.

Modem Hardware that allows a user to send and receive information over the phone or cable lines, for example, with a computer. It enables Internet connectivity via a telephone line or cable connection through network adaptors situated within the computer apparatus.

Monitor Computer display that allows the user to view text and graphic images.

Moral dilemma Situation for which there is no clear evidence that one of several alternatives is morally right or wrong.

Moral rights Ethical privileges.

Morals Social conventions about right and wrong human conduct that are socially constructed and tacitly agreed upon as good or right.

MoSCoW An approach where the team works with the stakeholders to develop a prioritized requirements list and a development plan; MoSCoW approach stands for Must have, Should have, Could have, and Would have.

Motherboard A key foundational computer component. All other components are connected to it in some way (either via local sockets, attached directly to it, or connected via cables). The essential structures of the motherboard include the major chipset, super I/O chip, BIOS, read-only memory (ROM), bus communications pathways, and a variety of sockets that allow components to plug into it.

Mouse A small device that one can roll along or scroll to control the movement of the pointer or cursor on a display and click to search for and/or execute features.

MP3 aggregator A program that can facilitate the process of finding, subscribing to, and downloading podcasts. A commonly known aggregator is Apple Computer's iTunes, which is a free program available as a download from apple.com. Using a program such as iTunes gives one the ability to search for podcasts based on many criteria including category, author, or title. iTunes provides access to audio downloads, which may be either songs or podcasts.

MPEG-1 Audio Layer-3 (MP3) Digital or electronic audio programming format.

Multimedia A computer-based technology that incorporates traditional forms of communication to create a seamless and interactive learning environment.

Multispatial Relating to the need for educators in the age of technology to account for both physical and virtual spaces and their relationship to the learning process.

Multiuser dungeon (MUD) A computer program, usually running over the Internet, that allows multiple users to participate in virtual-reality role-playing games.

Multiuser shared hack, habitat, holodeck, or hallucination (MUSH) Like MUDs and MOOS, but with the ability of the user to extend the "world" by adding new rooms, objects, and features.

Nanotechnology Microscopic technology on the order of one billionth of a meter.

National Center for Public Health Informatics (NCPHI) Center created in 2005 by the Centers for Disease Control and Prevention (CDC) to provide leadership in the field of public health informatics.

National Guideline Clearinghouse (NGC) A comprehensive database of clinical practice guidelines developed as a result of research. The NGC Web site allows users to browse for the clinical guidelines, view abstracts and full-text links, download full-text clinical guidelines to personal digital assistive (PDA) devices, obtain technical reports, and compare guidelines.

National Health Information Infrastructure (NHII) An initiative set forth to improve the effectiveness, efficiency, and overall quality of health and health care in the United States. A comprehensive knowledge-based network of interoperable systems of clinical, public health, and personal health information that would improve decision making by making health information available when and where it is needed. The set of technologies, standards, applications, systems, values, and laws that support all facets of individual health, health care, and public health. The NHII is voluntary and not a centralized database of medical records or a government regulation.

National Healthcare Quality Report (NHQR) A report that explores the quality of health care in the United States; it has been issued by the AHRQ every year since 2003.

Nationwide Health Information Network (NHIN) An agency of Health and Human Services charged with the development of a safe, secure, interoperable health information infrastructure.

National Health and Nutrition Examination Survey (NHANES) A survey sponsored by the Center for Disease Control and Prevention (CDC) combining both questionnaires and physical examination to collect data on the health and nutritional status of adults and children in the United States.

National Institute of Standards and Technology (NIST) A nonregulatory federal agency within the US Department of Commerce that was founded in 1901; its mission is to promote United States innovation and industrial competitiveness by advancing measurement science, standards, and technology in ways that enhance economic security and improve the quality of life. From automated teller machines and atomic clocks to mammograms and semiconductors, innumerable products and services rely in some way on technology, measurement, and standards provided by NIST.

National provider identifier (NPI) A standard 10-position unique identifier (code) mandated by HIPAA legislation and designed to replace previous provider identifiers.

Negligence A departure from the standard of due care, prudent reasonable care, toward others, including intentionally posing risks that are unreasonable as well as unintentionally, but carelessly, imposing risks.

Net generation Students used to surfing the Web and interacting online.

Network Connection of computers that can be local and/or organizationally based, joined together into a local area network (LAN), on a wider area scope (such as a city or district) using a metropolitan area network (MAN), or from an even greater distance (e.g., a whole country or continent or the Internet in general) using a wide area network (WAN) configuration.

Network accessibility The ability of the network to be accessed by the right user to obtain what they need when they need it.

Network availability Network information being accessible when needed.

Network security Refers to the specific precautions taken to ensure that the integrity of a network is safe from unauthorized entry and that the data and information stored on the network are only accessible by authorized users.

Neuroscience The study of the nervous system.

New England Health EDI Network (NEHEN) An example of an implementation model for building regional health information organizations that are functional, sustainable, and growing while reducing administrative costs.

Next-Generation Internet (NGI) A government project to develop new, faster technologies to enhance research and communication.

Nicomachean Vocabulary of technical terms used in a particular field, subject, science, or art. Terminology.

Nonmaleficence Doing no harm.

Nonplayer character (NPC) An individual in a simulation, virtual world, or game that is controlled by the program, not another person.

Nonsynchronous That which is not in real time or does not occur or exist at the same time, having the same period or time frame. Occurring anywhere and anytime using Internet and World Wide Web software tools (course management systems, e-mail, electronic bulletin boards, Web pages, etc.) as the principal delivery mechanisms.

Nursing informatics (NI) A specialty that integrates nursing science, computer science, and information science to manage and communicate data, information, knowledge, and wisdom in nursing practice.

Nursing informatics competencies A set of essential skills related to informatics deemed appropriate for various levels of nursing practice.

Nursing knowledge A body of facts accumulated over time from experience, education, and research that are used to make nursing decisions.

Nursing science The ethical application of knowledge acquired through education, research, and practice to provide services and interventions to patients in order to maintain, enhance, or restore their health; to advocate for health, and to acquire, process, generate, and disseminate nursing knowledge to advance the nursing profession.

Nursing terminology Body of the terms used in nursing. Terminology for nursing.

Nursing theory Concepts, propositions, and definitions that represent a methodical viewpoint and provide a framework for organizing and standardizing nursing actions.

Object-oriented MUD (MOO) Similar to a MUD, but with more advanced programming features.

Office of Civil Rights (OCR) Part of HHS and is responsible for enforcing HIPAA. It provides significant information and guidance to clinicians who must comply with the Privacy and Security Rules. It has been tracking complaints and investigating violations since 2003.

Office of the National Coordinator for Health Information Technology (ONC) This office is within the US Department of Health and Human Services (HHS) and was established through the HITECH Act. The ONC is headed by the National Coordinator, who is responsible for overseeing the development of a nationwide HIT infrastructure that supports the use and exchange of information.

Office suite Software that is generally distributed together with a consistent user interface that is designed for knowledge workers and clerical personnel. These software packages can interact with each other to enhance productivity and ease of use.

Online Something accomplished while connected to or using a computer.

Online chat Synchronous interaction with another person facilitated by an Internet connection technology.

Ontological approach Theory that considers ontology development (domain analysis) and its mapping to object models (specification of infrastructure). Based on enumerating all concepts used in a domain and in providing their formal definitions according to suitable formalisms (usually logic based).

Ontology Study of that which is compositional in nature and a partial representation of the entities within a domain and the relationships that hold between them. An explicit specification of a conceptualization.

Open Access Initiative A worldwide movement to make a library of knowledge available to anyone with Internet access.

Open source software (OSS) Computer software where the source code is made available for use and/or modification without charge. The developers share code in the hopes that the software will evolve as others modify and improve upon the base.

Open systems interconnection (OSI) A model of standardization for communications in a network developed to insure that various programs would work efficiently with one another.

Operating system (OS) The most important software on any computer. It is the very first program to load on computer start-up and is fundamental for the operation of all other software as well as the computer's hardware.

Order entry management A program that allows a clinician to enter medication and other care orders directly into a computer including laboratory, microbiology, pathology, radiology, nursing, medicine, supply orders, ancillary services, and consults.

Order entry system A system that automates the way that orders have traditionally been initiated for patients. Clinicians place orders within these systems instead of using traditional handwritten transcription onto paper. They provide major safeguards by ensuring that physician orders are legible and complete, thereby providing a level of patient safety that was historically missing with paper-based orders. These systems provide decision support and automated alert functionality that was previously unavailable with paper-based orders.

Outcome Changes, results, and/or impacts from inputting and processing.

Output Changes that exit a system and that can activate or modify processing.

Palmtop or palm computer Miniature or small computer that fits in the palm of the hand.

Parallel port Interface for connecting an external device that is capable of receiving more than one bit at a time.

Password A code established by the user to identify her/him when she/he enters the system. Most organizations today enforce a strong password policy. Strong password policies include using combinations of letters, numbers, and special characters such as plus (+) signs and ampersands (&). Policies typically include the enforcement of changing passwords every 30 or 60 days.

Patient care information system (PCIS) Patient-centered information systems focused on collecting data and disseminating information related to direct care. Several of these systems have become mainstream types of systems used in health care. The four systems most commonly found include (1) clinical documentation systems, (2) pharmacy information systems, (3) laboratory information systems, and (4) radiology information systems.

Patient care support system System of components that make up each of the specialty disciplines within health care and their associated patient care information systems. The four systems most commonly found include (1) clinical documentation systems, (2) pharmacy information systems, (3) laboratory information systems, and (4) radiology information systems.

Patient-centered Change from a focus on illness/healthcare professional to a focus on the patient/person with patients becoming active participants in their own healthcare initiatives. Patients as active participants receive services designed to meet their individual needs and preferences, under the guidance and counsel of their healthcare professionals. Data, observations, interventions, and outcomes focused on direct patient care.

Patient outcomes Measurable effects resulting from best practice treatment interventions that improve/stabilize the course of health over time.

Patient informed consent Document that a patient signs to agree to treatment. Document that a home healthcare patient signs to agree to receive telehealthcare services in addition to conventional home health care.

Patient support The total array of tools and software that can be used to provide information and assistance to help meet the healthcare needs of consumers.

Payor organization Those organizations that contract with healthcare agencies and service providers to attempt to manage healthcare costs.

Perception The process of acquiring knowledge about our environment or situation by obtaining, interpreting, selecting, and organizing sensory information from seeing, hearing, touching, tasting, and smelling. Sensory experience foundational to formulating knowledge.

Performance improvement Enhancing or improving performance. Quality indicators.

Performance improvement analyst Person who analyzes performance improvement initiatives. Person who is intimately involved in the design of the system used by nursing.

Peripheral biometric (medical) devices Range of telecommunications-ready measurement devices, such as blood pressure cuffs and blood glucose meters, that typically use the household telephone jack to transmit patient data to a central server location.

Peripheral component interconnection (PCI) Mechanism for attaching peripheral devices to a motherboard that can be via computer bus, expansion slots, or integrated circuits.

Peripheral devices Devices with a digital readout typically used in home telehealth and whose output is capable of being captured by computer. Generally this equipment is self-administered by the patient or family caregiver. Examples of the most commonly used peripheral devices include: a weight scale, blood pressure monitor, pulse oximeter, thermometer, glucometer, spirometer, prothrombin/international normalized ratio (PT/INR) meter, digital camera (to capture images of wounds), and a personal digital assistant-based or telephonic self-reporting device.

Personal computer (PC) Computer made for individual use or directly used by an end user.

Personal digital assistant (PDA) A handheld device, miniature or small computer or palmtop that uses a pen for inputting instead of a keyboard. Also called a handheld computer. Also known as personal digital assistive.

Personal emergency response systems (PERS) Signaling devices for patients to access emergency and other care needs.

Petabyte (PB) A unit of information or computer storage equal to one quadrillion bytes, or 1,000 terabytes.

Pharmacy information system Information system that facilitates the ordering, managing, and dispensing of medications for a facility. It also commonly incorporates allergies and height and weight information for effective medication management; streamline the order entry, dispensing, verification, and authorization process for medication administration while they often interface with clinical documentation and order entry systems so that clinicians can order and document the administration of medications and prescriptions to patients while having the benefits of decision support alerting and interaction checking.

Picture archiving and communication system (PACS) Systems that are designed to collect, store, and distribute medical images such as computed tomography (CT) scans, magnetic resonance imaging (MRI) and X-rays; replace traditional hard copy films with digital media that is easy to store, retrieve, and present to clinicians. These systems may also be stand-alone systems, separate from the main radiology system, or they can be integrated with radiology information systems (RIS) and computer information systems (CIS). The benefit of PACS systems is their ability to assist in diagnosing and storing vital patient care support data.

Plug and play What a user can do to add new devices to a computer easily without having to manually install and reconfigure the computer to accept the device.

Podcast A digital media file or collection of related files that are distributed over the Internet using syndication or subscription feeds for playback on portable media players such as MP3 players, laptops, and personal computers. Subscribe using RSS feeds. Online media delivery. Enhanced podcasts contain slides and pictures. Vodcasts contain videos.

Policy Basic principle that guides behavior and performance and is enforced: for example, in a corporation, corporate policy would be enforced by corporate administration or the United States government would enforce public policy.

Population health management A term adopted by healthcare management companies to express their goal of achieving optimum health outcomes at a reasonable cost. The management process involves data collection and trend analyses that are used to predict clinical outcomes.

Port Interface between a computer and other devices or other computers.

Portability Ability to be transported easily. For example, users can easily take handheld computers wherever they go.

Portable operating system interface for UNIX (POSIX) A uniform set of standards adopted by the Institute of Electrical and Electronics Engineers (IEEE) and the International Organization for Standardization (ISO) that define an interface between programs and operating systems. The standardization ensures that software can be easily ported to other POSIX-compliant operating systems.

Portals Tools for organizing information from Web pages into simple menus on one's desktop. Also, multifunctional telehealthcare platforms for receiving, retrieving, and/or displaying patients' vital signs and other information transmitted from telecommunications-ready medical devices.

Portfolio A collection of evidence used to demonstrate knowledge and skill achievement. A nursing portfolio provides the opportunity for a student to document a variety of sometimes unquantifiable skills, such as creativity, communication, and critical thinking.

Power supply A device that supplies electrical energy or power; the device that provides the electrical energy or power to the computer; a battery can be a source of energy or power.

Presentation Act of presenting or showing; typically uses presentation software in a slide show format. The most commonly used presentation software in the United States is Microsoft PowerPoint.

Primary key A field within a record also known as the key field. This field contains a code, name, number, or other bit of information that acts as a unique identifier for that record. In a healthcare system, for example, a patient is assigned a patient number or ID that is unique for that patient.

Principlism A foundation for ethical decision making. Principles were expansive enough to be shared by all rational individuals, regardless of their background and individual beliefs.

Privacy An important issue related to personal information, about the owner or about other individuals, that is included for sharing with others electronically and the mechanisms that restrict access to this personal information.

Problem-based Typically refers to a type of student-centered instructional strategy where students collaboratively solve problems and reflect on their experiences.

Problem solving Cognitive process of critically thinking through a problem or issue to determine a course of action.

Process analysis Breaking down the work process into a sequential series of steps that can be examined and assessed to improve effectiveness and efficiency; explains how work takes place, gets done, or how it can be done.

Process owners Those who directly engage in the workflow to be analyzed and redesigned and have the ultimate responsibility for the performance of the process. They are the individuals who can speak about the intricacy of process, including process variations from the normal. When constructing the team include individuals who are able to contribute information about the exact current state workflow and offer suggestions for future state improvement.

Processing Acting on something by taking it through established procedures in order to convert it from one form to another. Examples include: information is processed data, and we process a credit application to get a loan.

Product developer One who designs, creates, and builds a product; for example, a computer program, network, and/or system. One who employs productivity software to create a product.

Productivity software Programs or software that help us compose, create, or develop. An example is the Microsoft Office suite of productivity tools, which offers word processing, spreadsheet, database, presentation, and Web tools to help us complete our tasks both professionally and personally.

Professional development Acquisition of skills required for maintaining a specific career path or to general skills offered through continuing education, including the more general skills area of personal development. It can be seen as training to keep current with changing technology and practices in a profession or in the concept of lifelong learning.

Professional networking Connecting with other professionals in a field with a predetermined and focused purpose as well as an identified target audience in mind.

Programmable read-only memory (PROM) Form of digital memory where the setting of each bit is locked on a chip by a fuse or antifuse. Such PROMs are used to store programs permanently, and thus are useful in applications where the programming needs to be permanent. The device cannot be erased, therefore it must be replaced if changes are deemed necessary in the system.

Project manager Responsible for the success of a project by managing the planning and enactment of the project.

Protected health information (PHI) Any and all information about a person's health that is tied to any type of personal identification.

Prototype Original mock-up or first model; original form which is studied, tested and processed before duplication.

Proxy server Hardware security tool to help protect an organization against security breaches.

PsycINFO A comprehensive database in the field of education and psychology.

Psychology The field that studies the mind and behavior.

Public health The science of protecting the well-being of communities and the population through education, research, intervention, and prevention.

Public health informatics (PHI) An aspect of informatics focused on the promotion of health and disease prevention in populations and communities.

Public health interventions Actions taken to promote and secure the well-being of a population or a community.

Publishing The process of production and dissemination of information.

Qualified Electronic Health Record EHR containing health-related information on an individual that consists of his or her demographic and clinical health information including medical history and a list of health problems and supports entry of physician orders; a qualified EHR can capture and query information relevant to healthcare quality and be able to exchange electronic health information with and assimilate such information from other sources to provide support for clinical decision making.

Qualitative study A type of research design that focuses on the human experience of a phenomenon using words, concepts, language, and meanings rather than numbers to capture the essence of the subject under study. Subjective study.

Quality A level or grade of excellence; relative merit; a distinct or essential characteristic, attribute or property.

Quality assurance (QA) The systematic process of assessing and testing to verify that a product or service being developed or used is meeting its specified requirements; focuses on discovering and correcting defects before they become part of the final product.

Quantitative study Research that looks at the what, where, and when to provide understanding of phenomena based on quantifying data and using statistical measures; depending on the research, can ascertain cause and effect relationships. Objective study.

Query A form of questioning. A request for information; an example would be a database query.

QWERTY Name given to the typical computer keyboard layout, derived from the six letters in the first row below the numeric or number row.

Radio frequency identification (RFID) chip ID chip that stores the information for retrieval.

Radio Frequency Identifier (RFI) A reprogrammable chip that communicates with a reader to aid in identifying an object.

Radiology information system (RIS) Information system designed to schedule, report, and store information as it relates to diagnostic radiology procedures. One common feature found in most radiology systems is a picture archiving and communication system (PACS). The benefit of RIS and PACS systems is their ability to assist in diagnosing complex cases and storing vital patient care support data.

Random access memory (RAM) Volatile, temporary storage system that allows the processor to access program codes and data while working on a task. RAM is lost once the system is rebooted, shut off, or loses power.

Rapid application development (RAD) A method using prototyping and reiteration to develop products sooner and of superior quality.

Rapid Syndromic Validation Project (RSVP) System where local healthcare professionals report cases such as influenza. Data is analyzed centrally and the resulting information is shared with appropriate local authorities in an attempt to identify outbreaks early and prevent the spread of contagious diseases.

Rationalism An ethical position that contends that knowledge is derived from deductive reasoning and not from the senses.

RDF site summary Resource description framework site summary. See really simple syndication.

Read-only memory (ROM) Essential permanent or semipermanent, nonvolatile memory that stores saved data and is critical in the working of the computer's operating system and other activities. ROM is primarily stored in the motherboard but may also be available through the graphics card, other expansion cards, and peripherals.

Real environment data Refers to patient data collected in the home during telehealth monitoring. This data is typically more reflective of the true patient situation because it is collected in the "real" environment and not the "artificial" environment of a healthcare agency.

Real time Human time; occurs live with users or learners interacting at the same time.

Real-time telehealth Live interactions between two or more clinicians, usually performed with videoconferencing equipment.

Really simple syndication (RSS) A form of Web feed formats used to publish frequently updated content in podcasts, blog entries, or even news headlines. Subscribers receive update notices whenever new content is added or a site is updated. Also known as RDF site summary (RSS 1.0 and RSS 0.90) and rich site summary (RSS 0.91).

Reasoning Way of thinking, calculating, interpreting, or introspectively rethinking or critically thinking through an issue; reflective thought to reason or think through one's ideas and alternatives.

Record Row in a relational database representing one patient, for example. Also called a tuple. Group of related fields in a database. To record or capture audio and video using specific devices.

Reflective commentary Narrative comments that focus on why an individual thinks specific evidence is important, the ways in which he values what he has learned, or why he thinks it is important for his profession.

Regional health information exchange See Regional health information organization.

Regional health information organization (RHIO) A regional network of healthcare organizations and providers who exchange information related to the health of the population. The goal is to work together without duplication to provide cost effective health care and promote community well-being.

Relational Database A database that can store and retrieve data very rapidly. Relational refers to how the data is stored in the database and how it is organized.

Relational database management system (RDBMS) A system that manages data using the relational model. A relational database could link a patient's table to a treatment table, for example, by a common field such as the patient ID number field.

Reporting The act of using of documents or information system outputs to convey information to stakeholders.

Reporting and Population Health Management The data collection tools to support public and private reporting requirements including data represented in a standardized terminology and machine-readable format (IOM, 2003).

Reports Documents that contain data or information based on a query or investigation designed to yield customized content in relation to a situation and a user, group of users, or an organization; designed to inform, reports may include recommendations or suggestions based on programming and other embedded parameters.

Repository Central place where data are collected, stored, and maintained. Central location for multiple databases or files that can be distributed over a network or directly accessible to the user. Location for files and databases so that the data can be reused, analyzed, explored, or repurposed.

Research utilization (RU) The process of moving new understandings generated in research into practice.

Research validity A conclusion that can be drawn about the conduct of the research based on an analysis of the research design and methods (internal validity) and the applicability of the findings to the general population (external validity).

Resource description framework (RDF) A structure of consistent semantics adopted by the World Wide Web Consortium (W3C) to promote encoding, exchange and reuse of metadata.

Results management An approach to evaluating the outcomes of a process to determine if the process was useful or valuable.

Reusability The extent to which software or other work-related artifacts can be used in more than one computing program or software system.

Rights Privileges; include the right to privacy, confidentiality, etc.

Risk assessment Determination of risk or danger, such as assessing for risk factors related to heart disease.

Robotics The designing, development, and implementation of robots or machines to carry out tasks typically performed by people.

Role playing Situation that allows students to try on real-life scenarios by filling either prescribed or ad-libbed roles (doctor, nurse, patient, clinician, etc.) without the fear or pressure of putting another's life at risk while trying to determine the best course of action or find a solution to a fictitious patient's health issue.

Root Cause Analysis Similar to a failure modes events analysis to discover why a process is faulty or produces an undesired result.

Row A record in a database; also known as a tuple.

Safety culture An organizational commitment to patient safety and the prevention of medical errors.

Sarbanes-Oxley Act (SOX) Legislation that was put in place to protect shareholders as well as the public from deceptive accounting practices in organizations.

Scaffolding Adding initial support for a task and then gradually removing this support over time.

Scenario Mock description of a situation or series of events.

Scheduling system A system designed to track resources within a facility while managing the frequency and distribution of those resources. For example, resource-scheduling systems provide information about operating room utilization, or availability of intensive care unit beds and regular nursing unit beds.

Second Life A proprietary virtual reality tool that allows users to create virtual communities.

Secure information Information that is protected from error, unauthorized access, and other threats that can compromise its integrity and safety.

Security Protection from danger or loss. In informatics, one must protect against unauthorized access, malicious damage, and incidental and accidental damage and enforce secure behavior and maintain security of computing, data, applications, information, and networks.

Security breach Any security violation.

Self-control Self-discipline. Strength of will.

Sensor and activity monitoring systems Systems for tracking activities of daily living of seniors and other at-risk individuals in their places of residence. Additional applications are sensors' use in detecting anomalies or problems such as faucets and stoves left turned on.

Serial port An interface for connecting an external device that is capable of receiving only one bit at a time, such as a mouse, a modem, and some printers.

Server A computer or a group of computers that link computers together or provide services to a group of computers.

Shoulder surfing Watching over someone's back as she is working. This is still a major way that confidentiality is compromised.

Simulation An imitation of a real-life event or circumstance; in nursing education, the replication of a clinical scenario developed to provide an opportunity for practice in a mock situation.

Simulation Scenario A virtual case situation developed in a simulation laboratory to mimic a clinical practice situation.

Simulator A mechanical or electronic device that provides an environment in which a simulation can occur. Some of these may be quite large.

Situational awareness The ability to detect, integrate, and understand critical information that leads to an overall understanding of a problem or situation.

Six Sigma/Lean Business management tactic that seeks to improve the quality of process outputs by identifying and removing the causes of imperfections (errors) and reducing inconsistency and variability in processes; Lean and Six Sigma are a complementary combination of activities that focus on doing the right steps and actions (Lean) and doing it right the first time (Six Sigma).

Small computer system interface (SCSI) Set of standards for physically connecting and transferring data between computers and peripheral devices. The SCSI standards define commands, protocols, and electrical and optical interfaces. Standardization among commercial products help to ensure that devices will interface with many different systems.

Smart Pump Machine used to infuse medication with dose-checking technology and safeguards designed to help avert medication errors.

Smart Room Patient room that is equipped with technologies to increase patient safety and improve patient care.

Smartphone A cell phone that has limited personal digital assistant capabilities. Smartphones have limited personal computer functionality; they have an operating system and facilitate the use of e-mail and other applications.

Social bookmarking Saving bookmarks or Internet URLs to a public Web site instead of on the user's private computer. The purpose is to share and grow the list of Web sites related to a specific topic. As users add bookmarks they also typically add keyword tags that aid in search and organization processes.

Social engineering The manipulation of a relationship based on one's position in an organization. For example, someone attempting to access a network may pretend to be an employee from the corporate information technology office who then simply asks for an employee's digital ID and password. A second example of social engineering is a hacker impersonating a federal government agent. After talking an employee into revealing network information, the hacker basically has an open door to enter the corporate network.

Social media Web-based technologies that support interactions or communication among people who belong to a social group.

Social networking Subscribing to and utilizing Web-based applications for the purpose of sharing personal information with others.

Social sciences Collection of academic/scientific fields or disciplines concerned with the study of the human aspects of our world/environment.

Software Anything that can be stored electronically; it is divided into two types—system (software that includes the operating system and other software necessary for the computer to function) and application (software that allows users to complete specific tasks, e.g., word processors, spreadsheet software, presentation software, database managers, and media players).

Sound card A computer expansion card that facilitates the input and output of audio signals to/from a computer under control of computer programs. Also known as an audio card.

Spreadsheet Text and numbers located in cells on a grid and the software necessary to process formulas and other computations such as creating graphs and charts.

Spyware A program that may contain malicious code that may attack or attempt to "take over" a computer. Spyware may also be nonmalicious in intent and monitor the user's behavior in an attempt to gain information about the user for targeted advertising.

Staff development The process of providing opportunities for professional growth and skills development. Computer information systems are frequently used to assist with the ongoing education and development of nursing staff members since the medium can embed the prompts, information, and related questions in the nursing documentation system with a link to an appropriate clinical protocol.

Stakeholder An individual or group with the responsibility for completing a project, influencing the overall design, and is most impacted by success or failure of the system implementation.

Standard Benchmark. Criterion. Rule. Norm. Principle.

Standard generalized markup language (SGML) Metalanguage, markup language for documents. Extensible markup language (XML) began as a simplified subset of SGML.

Standardized nursing terminology A body of terms used in nursing that is in some ways approved by an appropriate authority or by general consent.

Standardized plan of care That which presents clinicians with treatment protocols to maximize their outcomes and support best practices.

Standards developing organization (SDO) Guidelines, standards, and rules to help healthcare entities collect, store, manipulate, dispose of, and exchange secure protected health information. Many SDOs are working to help develop standards. HIPAA guarantees the security and privacy of health information and curtails healthcare fraud and abuse while enforcing standards for health information.

Static medium Something that cannot be updated; for example, a print-based brochure may be outdated almost as soon as it is printed.

Store-and-forward telehealth transmission Application of telehealth care, in which images and other clinical data are captured and transmitted to specialist clinicians.

Structured English Query Language (SQL) Pronounced "sequel"; is a database querying language not a programming language. It is a standard language for accessing and manipulating databases. It simplifies the process of retrieving information from a database in a functional or usable form while facilitating the reorganization of data within the databases.

Suicide Prevention Community Assessment Tool Risk assessment method that addresses general community information, prevention networks, and the demographics of the target population as well as community assets and risk factors.

Summaries Condensed versions of the original designed to highlight the major points.

Supercomputer Fastest computer; designed to run special applications that require numerous calculations.

Surveillance The act of watching for trends in health-related data for early detection of health threats.

Surveillance data systems A networked computer system designed to use health-related data trends to predict the probability of an outbreak of a contagious or infectious disease, or to detect morbidity and mortality trends in a geographic area as a precursor to public health planning or response.

Synchronous Real time or occurring at the same time, having the same period or time frame. Learning anywhere and anytime in real time using any real time delivery modalities such as traditional face-to-face, Internet, and World Wide Web software tools (course management systems, chat, e-mail, electronic bulletin boards, audio-video communication tools, etc.).

Synchronous dynamic random access memory (SDRAM) Most common type of dynamic random access memory found in personal computers.

Syndromic surveillance A specialized system of data collection to detect trends in the incidence and severity of a specific disease or health-related syndrome and plan the public health response.

Synthesis Combining parts of existing material or ideas into a new entity or concept.

Systems development life cycle (SDLC) Stages involved in the life of a system, typically an information system; model used in the project management of a system's development effort from feasibility to its demise.

Table A collection of related records in a database.

Tags/tag clouds A collection of keywords (tags) that describe the contents of Web sites related to a topic of interest that are then organized by importance using differing colors and font sizes and styles (cloud). Many tag clouds are navigable; that is, the tags are hyperlinks to Web pages.

Task analysis Analytic technique that focuses on how a task must be accomplished, including detailed descriptions of task-related activities, task characteristics and complexity, and the environmental conditions required for a person to perform a given task.

Tasks Actions that are value-added and necessary. For example, some tasks come about because of workarounds or for other unsubstantiated reasons. Tasks that are considered non–value added and are not necessary for the purpose of compliance or regulatory reasons should be eliminated from the future state process.

Technologist Person skilled in the use of technology.

Technology Method by which people use knowledge and tools. Knowledge used to solve problems, control and adapt to our environment, and extend human potential. Generally people use technology to refer to machines or devices such as computers and the infrastructure that supports them. A simplistic example, examining cell phones and planes—they are technologies that are tangible—one can see and touch them but cannot see and touch the vast infrastructures supporting them such as the wireless communications between the device (cell phone) and the cell towers nor can one see and touch the electronic guidance used by the device (plane) to navigate the skies.

Telecommunications Broadcasting or transmitting signals over a distance from one person to another person or from one location to another location for the purpose of communication.

Telehealth Telecommunication technologies used to deliver health-related services or to connect patients and healthcare providers to maximize patients' health status. A relatively new term in our medical/nursing vocabulary, referring to a wide range of health services that are delivered by telecommunications-ready tools such as the telephone, videophone, and computer.

Telehealth care Health services delivered by telecommunications-ready tools, usually supervised by a nurse or other clinician.

Telehealth hardware Equipment that captures objective vital signs data. Some systems use interactive self-reporting devices to capture subjective information on how a patient feels as well. The values obtained from the patient are then collected and transmitted by a communication hub. Peripheral devices used in home telehealth can include any item with a digital readout. Generally this equipment is self-administered by the patient or family caregiver.

Telehealth software Computer programs designed to collect and interpret health data gathered remotely via a telehealth communications system.

Telemedicine Health services delivered by telecommunications-ready tools supervised or directed by a physician.

Telemonitoring Remote measurement of patients' vital signs and other necessary data.

Telenursing Health services delivered by telecommunications-ready tools supervised or directed by a nurse.

Telepathology Use of telecommunications technology to facilitate the transmission and transfer of pathology data for the purposes of diagnosis, education, and research. Transmission and exchange of image-rich pathology data between remote locations.

Telephony Telephone monitoring of patients at their residences by off-site telenurses.

Teleradiology Use of telecommunications technology to electronically transmit and exchange radiographic patient images with the consultative text or radiologist reports from one location to another.

TELOS strategy Is an approach that provides a clear picture of the feasibility of a project; TELOS stands for Technologic and systems, Economic, Legal, Operational, and Schedule feasibility.

Terabyte (TB) A measurement term for data storage capacity. The value of a terabyte is 1,024 gigabytes.

Term At its simplest level, a word or phrase used to describe something concrete, e.g., leg, or abstract, e.g., plan.

Terminology Vocabulary of technical terms used in a particular field, subject, science, or art; concerned with the collection, description, processing, and presentation of terms belonging to specialized areas of usage of one or more languages; nomenclature.

Thick or fat client A computer connected to a network designed primarily for data processing and not communications or storage.

Thin client A computer that conveys input and output from the user to the server and back, but does no processing.

Three dimensional (3-D) A geometric model of the physical universe in which we live; the three dimensions are typically length, width, and depth (or height), although any three directions can be chosen, given that they do not lie in the same plane.

Three dimensional (3-D) computer graphics Graphics that use three-dimensional representations of geometric data stored in the computer for the purposes of performing calculations and rendering images. These images may be stored for later viewing or displayed in real-time.

Throughput The amount of work a computer can do in a given time period; a measure of computer performance that can be used for system comparison.

Thumb drive Small removable storage device.

TIGER initiative Group called the Technology Informatics Guiding Education Reform—or TIGER—team. This is a team of nursing leaders who developed a vision for utilizing information technology to transform nursing practice.

Touch screen The display used as an input device for interacting with or relating to the display's materials or content. The user can touch or press on the designated display area to respond, execute, or request information or output.

Transistor Solid-state semiconductors that resulted in the second generation of computers. Digital devices much smaller and faster than analog computers.

Translational research Research that is conducted with a vision toward transforming clinical nursing practice (translating into practice).

Transparent Done without conscious thought.

Transparent technology Technology that is not visible or recognizable by the user, therefore allowing the user to focus on the function or output and not the challenges of the technology itself.

Transput Input and output activities collectively.

Treatment Payment Operations (TPO) Is the treatment of patients, the payment for services, or the operations of the entity; providers and other covered entities were not required to include in the accounting any disclosures that were made to facilitate the treatment of patients, the payment for services, or the operations of the entity. This is commonly known at the "TPO exception." This exception ended in January 2011 for providers that recently implemented new EHR systems. For those providers with EHR systems that were implemented before the HITECH Act, the TPO exception ends in January 2014. It is easy to understand why this exception is ending. Because all providers implement comprehensive EHR systems, it will be very easy to generate an electronic record with an accounting of anyone who accessed a patient's record.

Trend General movement—a line of development. Process of getting others to emulate one's actions.

Trending Process of collecting and analyzing patient data that is collected over time via telehealth technology. Trending analysis provides a more accurate picture of health status than the analysis of episodic data collected during an agency visit.

Triage Process of assessing patients who are ill or injured and determining the need for intervention based on the severity of the health issue. Some software programs used in telehealth monitoring systems provide this function by comparing actual data with a preset standard and then alerting clinicians that an intervention is necessary.

Trojan horse Malicious code capable of replicating within a computer that is hidden in data or a program that appears to be safe.

Trust-e One of the two most common symbols that power users look for to identify trusted health sites.

Truth Fact. Certainty. Sincere action, character, and fidelity.

Tuple A record in a database; also known as a row.

Tutorial Learning materials available to the learner, who must then be self-directed to study the specific topical area presented.

U-health Is based on the concept of ubiquitous computing, wherein technologies become increasingly invisible as they are incorporated into everyday use so much so that they are not even thought of while the person is performing; also known as ubiquitous health or ubiquitous health care.

U-nursing Based on the concept of ubiquitous computing, nurses will provide care to anyone, anytime, anywhere using emerging transparent (ubiquitous) technologies and devices that support nursing care and practice.

Ubiquitous Existing or being everywhere at the same time; widespread.

Ubiquitous health (u-health) The concept of health care that is so present in one's daily life that it seems invisible or in the background.

Ubiquity State of being everywhere at once (or seeming to be everywhere at once). Presence in many places especially simultaneously. With changing models of healthcare delivery, information and knowledge should be available anywhere.

Uncertainty Ambiguity. Insecurity. Vagueness.

Universal serial bus (USB) That which connects to a myriad of plug-in devices, such as portable Flash drives, digital cameras, MP3 players, graphics tablets, light pens, and so on using a plug and play connection without rebooting the computer.

Usability The ease with which people can use an interface to achieve a particular goal. Issues of human performance during computer interactions for specific tasks within a particular context.

User friendly Programs and peripherals that make it easy to interact or use computers. Design of a program to enhance the ease with which the user can utilize and maximize the productivity from computer programs.

User interface Mechanisms or systems used by users to interact with programs.

Values Relative worth of an object or action such as aesthetic beauty or ethical value.

Veracity Right to truth.

Video adapter card A board or card that is inserted or plugged into a computer to provide display capabilities.

Videopod Self-contained system with a video transmitter.

Virtual memory The use of hard disk space temporarily when the user is running many programs simultaneously. This temporary use frees up RAM to allow programs to run simultaneously and seamlessly.

Virtual peers Virtual populations of individuals who are genetically and behaviorally alike.

Virtual reality (VR) Technology that simulates reality in a virtual medium.

Virtual world World that exists in cyberspace where people can establish avatars, purchase land, and interact with others. Emerging virtual worlds such as Second Life are changing the meaning of social networking.

Virtue Certain ideals toward which we should strive that provide for the full development of our humanity. Attitudes or character traits that enable us to be and to act in ways that develop our highest potential; examples are honesty, courage, compassion, generosity, fidelity, integrity, fairness, self-control, and prudence. Like habits, they become a characteristic of a person. The virtuous person is the ethical person.

Virtue ethics Theory that suggests that individuals use power to bring about human benefit. One must consider the needs of others and the responsibility to meet those needs.

Virus Malicious code that attaches to an existing program and executes its harmful script when opened.

Visiting Nurse Association (VNA) A nonprofit home healthcare agency.

Voice recognition A type of software that allows the user to input data or to navigate the Web using voice commands. Voice interactivity should help to reduce the disparity associated with those who have limited keyboard or mousing skills.

Waterfall model An early systems development life cycle (SDLC) model that is linear in nature, meaning that when one phase ends you move onto the next phase and do not go back unlike its modern counterparts that stress iterative development.

Wearable computing Devices that one can don or put on as one would other articles of clothing or watches, jewelry, etc. Wearable devices are being used to provide remote monitoring of physiological parameters in care settings, including patients' own homes.

Wearable Technology A small unobtrusive monitor worn by a patient that collects and transmits physiologic data via a cell phone to a server for clinician review.

Web 2.0 Developing tools for social networking. The implications of the social networking technologies that are major elements of Web 2.0 will have significant impact on the amount of information and knowledge that is generated, and the ways in which it is used.

Web-based Originating from the World Wide Web.

Web enhanced That which uses the World Wide Web to enhance or promote functions or tasks such as effective learning and skill acquisition.

Web publishing The design and development of Web pages that include links to digital files that are all uploaded to Web servers so that these files are accessible to others via Web browsers.

Web quest A search of the World Wide Web for information.

Web servers Multifunctional telehealthcare platforms for receiving, retrieving, and/or displaying patients' vital signs and other information transmitted from telecommunications-ready medical devices.

Webcast Media distributed over the Internet as a broadcast; uses streaming media technology to facilitate downloading and participation. It could be distributed in real time, live, or recorded for asynchronous interaction.

Weblog A Web site that contains the contributions of single or multiple users about a particular topic or issue. Similar in nature to a threaded discussion board or a personal diary, weblogs or blogs can provide insight into the perceptions of the contributors about the topic.

Wetware Direct body-brain interfaces. A reference to the human mind or central nervous system when interfaced with a computer; derived from computer terminology such as software and hardware.

Wi-Fi Wireless technology brand owned by Wi-Fi Alliance, which is used to improve the interoperability of wireless networking devices.

Wiki Server software that allows users to create, edit, and link Web page content from any Web browser. Server software that supports hyperlinks. The simplest online database; used to develop collaborative Web sites.

Wisdom Knowledge applied in a practical way or translated into actions; uses knowledge and experience to heighten common sense and insight to exercise sound judgment in practical matters. Sometimes thought of as the highest form of common sense resulting from accumulated knowledge or erudition (deep, thorough learning) or enlightenment (education that results in understanding and the dissemination of knowledge). It is the ability to apply valuable and viable knowledge, experience, understanding, and insight while being prudent and sensible. It is focused on our own minds; the synthesis of our experience, insight, understanding, and knowledge. The appropriate use of knowledge to solve human problems. It is knowing when and how to apply knowledge.

Word processing Creating documents using a word processing software package such as Microsoft Word.

Work process See workflow.

Workaround A way invented by users to bypass the system to accomplish a task. Usually indicate a poor fit of the system or technology to the workflow or user. Devised ways to beat a system that does not function appropriately or is not suited to the task it was developed to assist with; for example, one might remove the armband from the patient and attach it to the bed if the bar code reader fails to interpret bar codes when the bracelet curves tightly around a small arm.

Workflow Is a progression of steps (tasks, events, and interactions) that comprise a work process; involve two or more persons; and create or add value to the organization's activities. In a sequential workflow, each step is dependent on the occurrence of the previous step; in a parallel workflow, two or more steps can occur concurrently. The term "workflow" is sometimes used interchangeably with process or process flows, particularly when used in the context of implementations; a sequence of connected steps in the work of a person or team of people, that is, the process or flow of work within an organization; a virtual illustration of the "real" work or steps (flow) that workers enact to complete their tasks (work). The purpose of examining and redesigning workflow is to streamline the work process by removing any unnecessary steps that do not add value or might even hinder the flow of work.

Workflow analysis Is not an optional part of clinical implementations but is a necessity for safe patient care fostered by technology. The ultimate goal of workflow analysis is not to "pave the cow path" but rather create a future state solution that maximizes the use of technology and eliminates non–value add activities. Although there are many tools to accomplish workflow redesign the best method is the one that compliments the organization and supports the work of clinicians. Redesigning how people do work evidentially creates change and therefore the nursing informaticist needs to apply change management principles for the new way of doing things to take hold. Workflow analysis has been described in this chapter within the context of the most widely accepted tools that are fundamentally linked to the concepts of Six Sigma and Lean.

World Wide Web (WWW) An international network of computers and servers that offers access to stored documents written in HTML code, and access to graphics, audio, and video files.

Worm A form of malicious code. A self-replicating computer program that uses a network to send multiple copies of itself to other computers, subsequently tying up bandwidth and incapacitating networks.

Yottabyte (YB) A unit of information or computer storage equal to one septillion bytes.

Youth Risk Behavior Surveillance System (YRBSS) An epidemiologic survey conducted by the CDC to identify and track the most common health risk behaviors that lead to illnesses and mortality among youth.

Zettabyte (ZB) A unit of information or computer storage equal to one sextillion bytes.

Index

Page numbers followed by *t* or *f* indicate information in tables or figures, respectively. Those followed by *b* indicate information in boxes.

quantitative studies, 480
telehealth, 345–346, 346*b*
translational, 310, 471, 481, 595
Wide-ranging Online Data for Epidemiologic
Research, 372
research utilization (RU), 472
definition of, 472, 588
Stetler model of, 473
research validity, 474, 589
researchers, 129, 136
resource data, 466
resource description framework (RDF) site
summary, 421, 589
results management, 289, 589
resumes, 190
reusability, 111, 589
RFI. *See* radiofrequency identifier
RFID. *See* radiofrequency identification
RHIO. *See* regional health information
organization
rich site summary (RSS 0.91), 588
rights, 71
definition of, 589
five rights of knowledge, 23–24
five rights of medication administration, 386
of knowledge, 23–24
moral rights, 82–83, 577
Office of Civil Rights (OCR), 173–174, 580
patient rights, 173, 179
RISs. *See* radiology information systems
risk assessment, 370
community health risk assessment, 370–371
community risk assessment (CRA), 371
definition of, 589
HIMSS 2010 Security Survey, 258
steps ascribed to, 370
threat and risk assessment, 370
risk assessment tools, 371
risk management strategies, 260
Robert Wood Johnson Foundation, 56
robotics, 394, 589
Roget, Peter M., 507
role playing, 407, 589
role-playing games, 454
ROM. *See* read-only memory
root-cause analysis, 383, 589
rows, 222*b*, 589
RP-7. *See* Remote Presence Robot
RSS. *See* really simple syndication
RSS 0.90, 588

RSS 0.91, 588
RSS 1.0, 588
RSVP. *See* Rapid Syndromic Validation Project
RU. *See* research utilization
rural healthcare, 330

S

Safe Harbor, 177*b*
safety
with medical devices, 384
patient safety, 395
problems, 234
recommended steps to ensure safe implementation of smart pumps, 390–391
Safety Attitudes Questionnaire, 384
safety culture, 382–383
definition of, 589
key features of, 383
promoting patient safety, 381–382
strategies for developing, 384–385
Sarbanes-Oxley (SOX) Act, 176*b*–177*b*, 589
scaffolding, 455, 589
scenarios
definition of, 589
real-life, 407
simulation scenarios, 590
symbolic, 455
scheduling systems, 218–219, 589
school-aged children
promoting health literacy in, 358–359
Web quests for older school-aged children,
358
School of Nursing (University of Colorado),
432
Screencast-o-matic, 52*b*
SCSI. *See* small computer system interface
SDLC. *See* systems development life cycle
SDOs. *See* standards-developing organizations
SDRAM. *See* synchronous dynamic random
access memory
Seaman's Church Institute of New York, 318
search engines, 464–465
searching, 418–419, 480
Second Life, 416, 456, 589
security. *See also* network security
definition of, 590
of e-portfolios, 193
of health information, 19, 23, 167, 168*b*–169*b*,
172–174, 180–181, 342
HIMSS 2010 Security Survey, 258–259